Veterinary Anatomy

VETERINARY ANATOMY

The Regional Gross Anatomy of Domestic Animals

Vitthal R. Bhamburkar
Ex. Dean
Nagpur Veterinary College
Maharashtra Animal and Fishery Sciences University
Seminary Hills, Nagpur - 440006
Maharashtra

Illustrations by
Sanjay B. Banubakode
Head
Department Veterinary Anatomy and Histology
Nagpur Veterinary College
Maharashtra Animal and Fishery Sciences University
Seminary Hills, Nagpur - 440006
Maharashtra

nipa

NEW INDIA PUBLISHING AGENCY
New Delhi – 110 034

NEW INDIA PUBLISHING AGENCY
101, Vikas Surya Plaza, CU Block, LSC Market
Pitam Pura, New Delhi 110 034, India
Phone: + 91 (11) 27 34 17 17 Fax: + 91 (11) 27 34 16 16
Email: info@nipabooks.com
Web: www.nipabooks.com

Feedback at feedbacks@nipabooks.com

ISBN: 978-93-86546-48-7

Composed, Designed and Printed in India

Preface

Since the beginning of veterinary education in India, Veterinary Gross Anatomy was taught in the form of Systemic Anatomy. Each of the various systems viz- Skeletal, Muscular, Blood vascular (circulatory), Nervous, Endocrine etc were taught separately in greater details. However, it was long felt necessary to switch over to regional pattern for study of anatomy. This will make easy to understand the anatomical features of all relevant parts of different systems together in the given location (region). Probably with these views the Veterinary Council of India has recently revised the course curriculum of anatomy and introduced the regional approach of teaching veterinary anatomy. The teaching fraternity of veterinary anatomy in India have widely appreciated and accepted this change in the veterinary anatomy curriculum. However there is a need to provide appropriate study and teaching material in the new format. Hope, this book entitled "Veterinary Anatomy- the Regional Gross Anatomy of Domestic Animals" shall fulfill these urgent needs and will reach to the expectations of the students and teachers. This book has been specifically designed to make the so called tough and dry subject of veterinary anatomy as more easy and interesting to learn and practice.

The text of this book with regional approach of teaching and studying veterinary gross anatomy has been divided in six divisions. The first division comprises the basics of veterinary anatomy described in the conventional form of systemic anatomy while the remaining five divisions comprise regionwise description of gross anatomy. Each of these regional divisions contains the description of all anatomical structures *viz*. bones, joints, muscles, viscera, blood vessels, lymphatics nerves, etc located in the respective region of the animal body viz. head, neck, thorax, abdomen, pelvis and the fore and hind limb. Bovine animal, the ox, has been considered as a model species for detail description of the anatomical features, while the major differences or remarkable features in other species like horse, dog, sheep and goat, pig and fowl have been described under a separate heading as Comparative Anatomy. In addition to this, a separate section on Applied Anatomy has been introduced at the end of each regional division. This will makes it easy to understand the applications of the anatomical features that form the basis of surgical, diagnostic, medical and obstetrical techniques in the solution of clinical disorders which is the main purpose of regional pattern of learning the anatomy. Because of these distinctive features, the book has become a little voluminous and therefore, had to be split into two parts. PART-1 comprises first three divisions viz-General Systemic Anatomy, Anatomy of Head and Neck and the Anatomy of **Thorax** while PART-2 comprises the next three divisions viz- the Anatomy of Abdomen and Pelvis, the Anatomy of Fore limb and the Anatomy of Hind Limb.

Adequate efforts have been made to be in line with the recently revised syllabus of veterinary anatomy prescribed by the Veterinary Council of India in accordance with the Veterinary Council of India -Minimum Standards of Veterinary Education- Degree Course (B.V.Sc. & A.H.) Regulation- 2016 with a few exceptions.

Vitthal R. Bhamburkar

Acknowledgement

Round about the year 2000-01, late Professor Emeritus Dr. U. B. Singh, the past President of Indian Association of Veterinary Anatomists (IAVA) and ex Professor and Head of Anatomy and Dean of the College of Veterinary Science APAU Hyderabad had entrusted me the work of writing some chapters for the revision of the book 'The Anatomy of Ox' (ICAR Publication). It was a project awarded to him by the ICAR. However, that project was abandoned because of his sudden death. Thereafter sometime in the year 2005-06, Dr. K. S. Roy who had just retired as Dean of the College of Veterinary Science, Ludhiana was awarded the same project by ICAR. He too had allotted me some chapters of that book for revision. But he could not complete that project because of health problems. Thus on two occasions in the past, the opportunity came to me to write but it was aborted in the middle. Although these two attempts turned up as aborted, it kindled the instinct in me for writing a book on Veterinary Anatomy at appropriate time and that time has come up now. Hence, I express my first and foremost gratitude to late Dr. U. B. Singh and my worthy friend Dr. K. S. Roy.

I gratefully acknowledge the authors, editors and publishers of the books, articles, which have been used as resource material and data base for this book. The names of these authors, editors, publishers and Research Scientists have been reflected under the Bibliography. The valuable information received from several websites on internet is also acknowledged gratefully.

In the initial stages of strategic planning, organizing and designing the construction of this book I received valuable suggestions and insightful feedback from my all-time trustworthy Dr. S. B. Banubakode, the present Head of the Anatomy Department of Nagpur Veterinary College. The success of producing this work would not have been possible without his precious help. I am profusely grateful to him for his graceful support.

After deciding the basic framework of the book, the next main task was to search and collect the source material. This facility was most efficiently and pleasantly provided by Mr. S. N. Gawande, the University Librarian of Maharashtra Animal and Fishery Sciences University, Nagpur. I am delighted to express my sincere thanks to this wonderful ever helping and cheerful personality.

For illustrations, I relied heavily on Dr. Banubakode. He worked very hard for preparing illustrations with the help of his other colleagues in the Anatomy Department Drs. N. C. Nandeshwar, Ms. Rupali Charjan and Umesh Mainde. His doctoral candidates studying under him for Ph.D. degree course, Drs. Amol Salankar and Ms. Jigyasa Rana did a marvelous job. I gratefully acknowledge their contribution in the creation of this book.

The Publisher M/S New India Publishing Agency (NIPA) deserves special thanks for having accepted my suggestions in the entire process of creating this wonderful work. In my conversations with him I found Mr. Sumit Jain, the publisher a gentleman.

Throughout the period of writing this book, I received wholehearted support and encouragement from my family, specially from my daughters Tejaswini and Vrushali, son-in-law Umesh and Amit, my wife Shailaja and a senior member of the family Adv. V. G. Bhamburkar. All of them deserve special thanks and appreciation from me. Amit in particular with his skills in computer applications, has greatly helped me in Editing of this book. It was done during my stay with him in California (U.S.). His contribution in creating this work is highly appreciated and acknowledged.

Vitthal R. Bhamburkar

Contents

Section-F: Sense Organs and Common Integument

PART-1.2: ANATOMY OF HEAD AND NECK

Section-A: Musculo-Skeletal Component

Section-B: Organs and Glands

Section-C: Blood Vessels and Lymphatics

Section-D: Nerves

Section-E: Applied Anatomy

PART-1.3: ANATOMY OF THORAX

Section-A: Musculo-Skeletal Component

Section-B: Thoracic Cavity and Viscera

Section-C: Blood Vessels and Lymphatics

Section-D: Nerves

Section-E: Applied Anatomy

PART-II

PART-2.1: ANATOMY OF ABDOMEN AND PELVIS

Section-A: Musculo-skeletal Component

Section B: Viscera

Section-C: Blood Vessels and Lymphatics

Section-D: Nerves

Section-E: Applied Anatomy

PART-2.2: ANATOMY OF FORE LIMB

Section-A: Musculo-Skeletal Component

Section-B: Blood Vessels and Lymphatics

Section-C: Nerves

Section-D: Applied Anatomy

PART-2.3: ANATOMY OF HIND LIMB

Section-A: Musculo-Skeletal Component

Section-B: Blood Vessels and Lymphatics

Section-C: Nerves

Section-D: Applied Anatomy

Introduction

Anatomy is a branch of biology concerned with the study of form and structure of organisms and their parts. When it is concerned with the structure of animals, it becomes Anatomy of Animals or **Veterinary Anatomy**. The comparative description of the form and structure of the body parts in different species of animals comprises the **Comparative Anatomy**. Originally the word anatomy has been derived from a Greek word meaning as ''cut open' or dissection. The dissection of animal body provides the means of describing the appearance and position, form, size, shape, colour, and texture of different parts of the body and their structures and the systematic description arising out of this, constitutes the **systematic or descriptive anatomy**. The **Gross Anatomy** is the examination and study of different body parts and structures with unaided eyesight while that with the aid of optical devises is called **Microscopic Anatomy (Histology)**. The progressive development of these various parts and structures of the body leading to acquire their full functional form constitutes the **Developmental Anatomy (Embryology)**. The gross anatomy can be studied with naked eye with the help of simple dissecting instruments such as scalpel and forceps. Now a day, for more specific and advance anatomical studies, newer techniques like Sonography, Angiography, Endoscopy, Magnetic Resonance Imaging etc are used in the study of gross anatomy. Similarly, for microscopic anatomy, although light microscopy is widely used, a vast number of advanced technologies are available and their use depends on the specific purpose of the study. These include Phase Contrast Microscope, Fluorescence microscope, Electron Microscope, X ray, MRI, CT Scan etc. There are two forms or ways of study of gross anatomy. The first one is named as **Systematic or Systemic Anatomy** and the other one is named as **Regional or Topographic Anatomy**.

Systemic Anatomy: In Systemic Anatomy, the animal body is considered as made up of different systems, each of which consists of a group of different parts, organs, or apparatus relevant to a particular physiological function of the body regardless of their position or location in the body (e.g. Respiratory system,

Digestive system) or relevant to their tissue make-up (Muscular System, Skeletal System).

Classification based on a group of organs relevant to their physiological function

Locomotor System – consists of organs of locomotion, i.e. - bones and cartilages (**Skeletal System**), joints or articulations (**Articular System)** and muscles (**Muscular System)**

Digestive System – consists of organs of prehension and digestion of food i.e. mouth and GI tract and their accessory glands.

Respiratory System – consists of organs of respiration i.e. nasal passage, trachea, bronchi and lungs.

Urinary System - consists of organs of excretion i.e. kidneys, ureters, urinary bladder and urethra.

Genital System – consists of organs of male and female genital organs i.e. internal and external genitalia of male and female animals along with their accessory glands.

Endocrine System: – consists of the ductless glands producing different hormones that control the physiological activities and regulate the normal functions of the body.

Cardio Vascular (Blood vascular) or Circulatory System – consists of organs of blood and lymph circulation including the heart, the vessels and the glands.

Nervous System – consists of the organs of central, peripheral and autonomic nervous system i.e. brain, spinal cord, cranial nerves, peripheral nerves and autonomic including the sympathetic and parasympathetic nerves.

Integumentory and sensory organ System – consists of the organs of integument i.e. Skin, hoofs, and horns and the organs of common senses i.e. eye, ear etc.

Classification based on tissue make-up of the organs or group of organs of the body

Osteology is the study of bones and cartilages (skeleton) that protect and support the soft parts and organs of the body.

Myology is the study of skeletal muscles and tendons that cover and play over the bones, body cavities and other places all over the body of the animal.

Arthrology or Syndesmology is the study of joints that helps in movements of the bones, and muscles effecting locomotion and other visible movements of different parts of the animal body.

Splanchnology is the study of visceral organs, their membranes and the accessory glands that include mostly the organs of digestive, respiratory, urinary and genital systems.

Endocrinology is the study of endocrine glands that helps in the functioning and functional coordination of various organ systems.

Angiology is the study of the organs and vessels of blood and lymph circulation.

Neurology is the study of neural organs and structures that helps in controlling and coordinating the activities and functions of all the organs and organ systems of the body.

Aesthesiology is the study of organs of different senses e.g. sense of vision (eye), sense of hearing (ear), sense of touch (skin) etc.

Regional Anatomy: The regional or topographic study of gross anatomy, however, deals with the anatomical description of various parts, organs or structures in a particular region, location, position or site of the animal body. It provides better perception of coordination and correlation of different organs and organ systems in the animal body. In the regional or topographic pattern of anatomy, the animal body is considered as consisting of six divisions namely, the head, neck, trunk, tail, and the fore limb and hind limb. However, for the convenience of description it is described in the following five divisions namely

(1) Anatomy of Head and Neck

(2) Anatomy of Thorax

(3) Anatomy of Abdomen and Pelvis

(4) Anatomy of Fore Limb

(5) Anatomy of Hind Limb.

In addition to those mentioned above as systematic or systemic anatomy and regional or topographic anatomy, there are some other terms often used for gross anatomy related to the application of the knowledge of gross anatomy for other specific purposes. These are as under.

Applied Anatomy is concerned with the application of anatomical facts in relation to physical examination of the animal body and surgical or any other clinical procedures used in the diagnosis and treatment of animals e.g. identifying the cardiac and pulmonary areas on the body surface for clinical examination of heart and lungs or identifying the site of supraorbital or infraorbital foramen used for supraorbital or infraorbital nerve block. Applied anatomy can also be termed as **Surface Anatomy** or **Clinical anatomy.**

Radiographic Anatomy is the term used when the anatomical knowledge of the internal organ or a part of animal body is applied for diagnosis or treatment of that particular internal organ or part through radiographic or radiological means. Some times radiology and radiography is used as a tool for studying anatomy.

Forensic Anatomy is the most recent term framed for the application of anatomical knowledge for investigative purposes in the field of Forensic Science or Forensic medicine.

Topographic Terms

The topographic terms used for gross description of various organs, parts or structures in this book are as far as possible close to those recommended by the International committee on Veterinary Anatomical Nomenclature (I.C.V.A.N.) and published in the Nomina Anatomica Veterinaria (N.A.V.) 1973.

In a quadruped animal standing on the ground, the surface directed towards the ground or towards the belly of the animal is termed as **ventral** and opposite to that i.e. the surface directed upward towards the backbone of the animal is termed as **dorsal**. The surface directed towards the front side i.e. head of the animal is termed as **cranial** or **anterior** surface and that directed towards the tail or rear side is termed as **caudal** or **posterior** surface. The surface that is facing towards the median plane of the animal body is termed as **medial** surface and the opposite i.e. facing outside laterally is termed as **lateral** surface. With respect to the structures, parts or organs in the head region the terms **rostral** for those facing towards the nose and the term **caudal** for those facing backward away from nose are used. For parts, organs or structures such as long bones and muscles in the limbs, the terms **proximal extremity** and **distal extremity** are used for the upper and lower ends respectively. For the planes or surfaces of the bones of forelimb below carpus, the terms **dorsal** and **palmer** are used while those in the hind limb, below the tarsus, are termed as **dorsal** and **plantar** respectively. The directional terms such as forward and backward are replaced by the terms craniad and caudad respectively. Those for outward and inward are replaced by the terms laterad and mediad. The terms upward and downward are replaced by the terms dorsad and ventrad respectively.

Topographic planes

For orientation of these anatomical terms, some auxiliary planes have been formed and are used in the description of anatomy of domestic animals. The plane passing vertically through the central axis and dividing the body longitudinally into two halves is termed as **median** or **middle plane**. The planes running parallel to the median plane away from the centre of the body is termed as **sagittal** plane. The plane cutting the long axis of the body perpendicular to the median plane is termed as **transverse plane** and the plane parallel to horizon at right angles to the vertical plane as **horizontal plane** of the animal body.

Part-I.I: GENERAL SYSTEMIC ANATOMY

SECTION- A
LOCOMOTOR SYSTEM

Animal locomotion is defined as a variety of movements effected by animal body resulting into progression of the animal from one place to other place. It also includes those movements effected by different parts of the body even when the animal is in static position either in a standing or sitting posture. In order to perform this function of locomotion, the animal body is provided with skeletal and muscular framework. Such a framework not only provides a strong support and stability to animal body for performing the movements but also protects the other soft organs or organ systems of the body. In addition, it provides the basis for the characteristic confirmation of individual species. To locomote, animal requires both, the propulsive and control mechanisms. The diverse propulsive mechanism involves the contractile structure- the skeletal muscles attached to a strong base of skeleton made of hard bones of different form, size and shapes joined or articulated to each other at various joints or articulations with the help of other elements like cartilages and ligaments. Thus, a joint force of propulsion is effected by **skeletal, articular** and **muscular** elements and their **systems** resulting into animal locomotion. However, the control mechanism to initiate and coordinate the actions of these three elements i.e. bones, muscles and joints is conducted by nervous system which shall be dealt with under a separate chapter on nervous system.

1

Skeletal System (Osteology)

In domestic animals, skeleton (Fig. 1-1) is a framework that is formed of bones, cartilages and ligaments binding together giving the specific shape, form and support to the body. In addition, the skeletal framework surrounds the major cavities of the body giving protection to other soft visceral organs of the body. There are three major parts of skeleton in the animal body (1) the axial skeleton (2) the appendicular skeleton and (3) the splanchnic skeleton.

The axial skeleton consists of the skull, vertebral column, ribs, and sternum.

The appendicular skeleton consists of the bones of fore limb and hind limb

The splanchnic skeleton includes some of the bones embedded in the substance of visceral organs in the body such as os cordis in ox and os penis in dog.

Bones

The bones forming the skeleton of the body are of different shape, size, form and the constituting tissue material. The number of different types of bones of any species may differ in various stages of the growth of the animal. So also the numbers of various bones differ from species to species.

Classification of bones

Long bones: The long bone is elongated, cylindrical in shape and form. The middle cylindrical part of long bone is termed as shaft or diaphysis. The two ends of the cylinder are enlarged. These are called extremities or epiphyses. The shaft is tubular and it encloses the cavity called as medullary cavity that is occupied by medulla or bone marrow. The long bones mostly occur in the limbs where they act as supporting pillars of the body e.g. humerus in fore limb and femur in hind limb.

Flat bones: Flat bone is flat and plate like expanding in two directions. It affords large area on its surfaces for attachment of muscles e.g. scapula, the shoulder bone and provide protection to the subjacent structures or organs which they

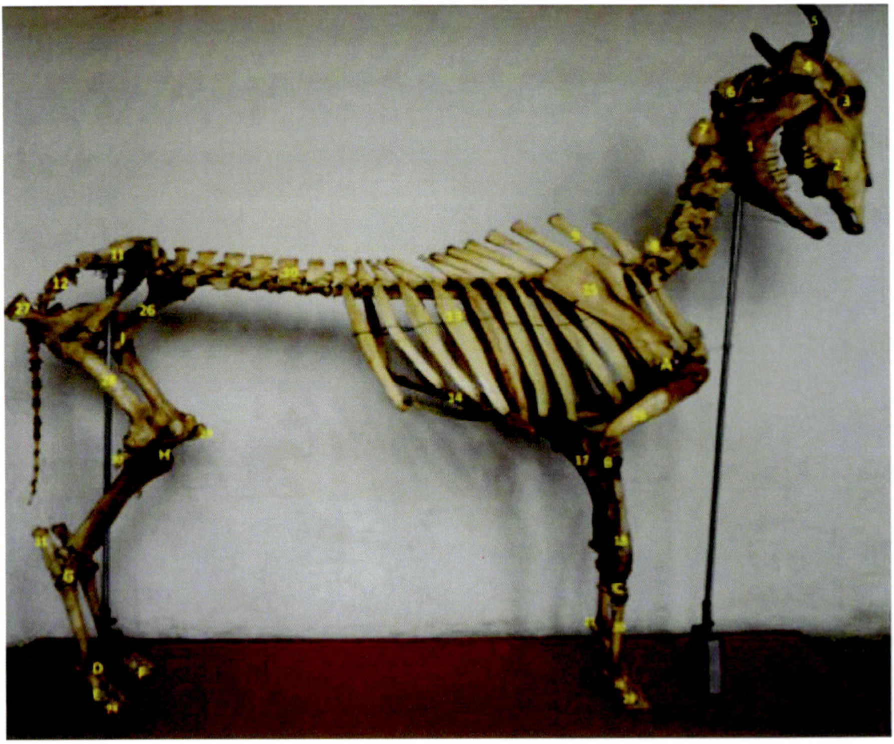

Fig.1-1: Skeleton of ox

1. Mandible
2. Maxilla
3. Orbit
4. Temporal Fossa
5. Cornual process
6. Atlas
7. Axis
8. Seventh Cervical vertebra
9. Second thoracic
10. llnd lumbar vertebra
11. Sacrum
12. Coccygeal vertebra vertebra
13. Rib
14. Costal cartilage
15. Scapula
16. Humerus
17. Ulna
18. Radius
19. Carpal
20. Metacarpal
21. Proximal sessamoid
22. First phalanx
23. Second Phalanx
24. Third phalanx
25. Distal sessamoid
26. Os coxae
27. Tuber coxae
28. Femur
29. Patella
30. Fibula
31. Fibular tarsal

A. Shoulder joint
B. Elbow joint
C. Carpal joint
D. Fetlock joint
E. Pastern joint
F. Coffine joint
G. Hock joint
H. Stifle joint
I. Hip joint

cover e.g. bones of skull. It is comprised of a pad like structure made of two layers of compact bone covering a layer of soft bone and a marrow in the middle.

Short bones: Short bone is usually small and presents similar dimensions in length, breadth and thickness. It helps in diffusing the concussion when lying between the two large bones, in diminishing friction caused due to running of tendons over the bones and in increasing the leverage to muscles and tendons attached to or running over other bones. e.g. Patella lying on distal extremity of femur and the sesamoid bones developed in the capsules of some joints. The internal constitution of these bones is similar to that of flat bones.

Irregular bones: Irregular bone is, as the name indicates, irregular in shape and is always median in position. Thus, these bones are unpaired. e. g. the vertebrae comprising the vertebral column and some cranial bones forming the base of the cranium. The internal constitution of these bones is similar to that of flat bones. These bones provide extra leverage to the strong muscles covering the bony skeleton of the body.

Structure of bone

Bone is formed of two types of osseous tissue. The outer shell of the bone is made up of dens white tissue called as **compact tissue** while the inner spongy mass of soft substance is called as **cancellated tissue**. Thin strands of cancellated tissue intercross each other forming a mesh with tiny marrow spaces containing red marrow. In the long bone, the compact tissue forming the shell of the bone is thickest in shaft and it thins out towards the extremities. The cancellated tissue is, however, sparingly low in amount in the shaft while it forms the bulk of the extremities of the long bones. In the flat bones, short bones and irregular bones, the bulk of the tissue mass inside the bone is occupied by the cancellated tissue sandwiched between two thin outer layers of the compact tissue. The thin fibrous covering adhering to the outer surface of the bone is called **periosteum** while a thin fibrous membrane lining the internal medullary cavity is called **endosteum**. The epiphyseal ends of long bones in the early growing stage of life of the animal are mostly cartilaginous or in some cases the process of ossification of epiphyseal end starts. In such a situation, the shaft i.e. diaphysis and the extremities i.e. epiphysis are separated by cartilaginous epiphyseal discs. In these long bones, the part of the shaft adjacent to the epiphyseal disc is called as **metaphysis**. The appearance of metaphysis examined by X ray is considered as the factor for deciding the age of animal and it varies from species to species.

Properties of bones

Physical properties: When exposed in living animal, the bone appears bluish pink in colour. A fresh dead bone is yellowish white and. when macerated or boiled, it becomes white. It is hard and resistant to pressure. It possesses elasticity and toughness.

Chemical properties: Bone consists of organic matter (tissue component) and inorganic matter (chemical component) in a proportion of approximately 1:2. The hardness and strength of the bone is because of the presence of inorganic mineral salts and the elasticity and pliability of the bone is due to the presence of organic matter. The composition of inorganic substances includes calcium phosphate (85 per cent), calcium carbonate (12 per cent) and calcium fluoride, magnesium phosphate and magnesium carbonate combined (3 per cent). The organic matter mainly consists of a protein called as bone collagen or ossein. This protein is in the form of membrane, cartilage, marrow vessels, nerves etc and the tissue fluids. The wet bone on boiling yields gelatin. Decalcification by immersing the bone in dilute hydrochloric acid dissolves the inorganic salts and make it pliable and soft without affecting its form and size. So also, removal of organic matter by heat does not change the general form of the bone but reduces its weight remarkably and makes it fragile.

Features of bones

The bones on their surfaces present various types of features for the purpose of attachment of muscles, providing the passages for running the muscles, tendons, ligaments, vessels, nerves etc over them. These features are in the form of projections and depressions. Various terms used for describing these features are as under.

A **process** is a general term for a prominence on the bone.

A **spine** is the term used for a process in the form of elongated and pointed projection.

A **ridge** is a term used for linear and thick elevation.

The **head** is a rounded articular enlargement at the end or extremity of the long bone. The head is normally joined with the shaft by the neck.

A **condyle** is somewhat cylindrical and ovoid articular eminence at the end of long bone. The **epicondyle** is a nonarticular eminence attached to the condyle.

A **tubercle** is a small rough projection.

The **tuberosity** is a prominent rough projection.

A **trochanter** is an excessively developed projection on the long bone.

A **trochlea** is a special type of articular surface developed in the form of pulley.

A **facet** is a small flat or slightly undulating articular surface on the body of the bone.

A **foramen** is a small perforation or a canal or conduit passing into the bone through which the vessels and nerves enter the bone.

The hiatus is a small depression on the surface of the bone for accommodating more than one foramen at the same location.

A **fossa** is a comparatively larger size of depression on the surface of the bone used for attachments of the tendons of muscles and ligaments.

A **fovea,** a **groove** and a **sulcus** are smaller size of usually linear depressions on the bone surface for attachment of muscle tendon and ligament.

A **glenoid cavity** is a shallow articular depression for the lodgment of head of the long bone.

A **cotyloid cavity** is a term used for a cavity which is sufficiently deep in the form.

A **sinus** is an air cavity within a bone. It is lined with mucous membrane and communicates to the exterior.

Axial skeleton

The axial skeleton includes bones on and around the midline (axis) of the body and comprises the skull, vertebral column, sternum and ribs.

Skull

The skull is the part of the skeleton in the head region. It provides bony protection to the brain, supports and protect most of the sense organs, forms passage for the entry of organs of respiratory and digestive systems, and forms the jaws along with teeth for mastication. The bones of skull are distributed in two groups. One, the cranial group of bones that forms cranium- the cavity within which the brain is lodged and the other, the facial group of bones that participate in the formation of the face and bound the oral and nasal cavities. Most of the bones of skull are flat bones and developed as membrane bones with the exception of a few ones forming the base of the cranium which are irregular and are developed as cartilage bones. The outer edges of most of the bones of the skull are serrated and are connected with each other by immovable joints appearing like suture lines and hence these joints are termed as sutures. All the bones of skull present numerous foramina, fissures and canals for the passage of nerves and vessels. Some of the bones of skull are excavated internally by air cavities termed as sinuses which are lined by mucous membrane and are interconnected with each other and they open into nasal chambers and hence are named as paranasal sinuses. The cranial group of bones consists of Frontal, Temporal, Parietal, Inter-parietal, Occipital, Sphenoid and Ethmoid bones. The occipital, sphenoid and ethmoid bones are single while the rests are paired. The facial group of bones include the Maxilla, Premaxilla Palatine, Pterygoid, Nasal, Lacrimal, Malar, Turbinate, Vomer, Mandible and Hyoid. The vomer, lacrimal and hyoid bones are single and the rests are paired.

Vertebral column

The vertebral column or back bone is a series of small irregular segmented bones extending backward over the dorsal median line from skull to the end of the tail. It consists of a flexible chain of the median irregular unpaired bones, the vertebrae. Most of these segmented bones remain free from each other in the chain throughout the life of the animal. These are called as true vertebrae or movable vertebrae. Some vertebrae especially those in the sacral region of the body get fused with the adjacent vertebrae forming a single peace of bony mass. These vertebrae are termed as false vertebrae or immovable vertebrae. The vertebral column as a whole is described of having five divisions named according to the part or region of the body of the animal in which the vertebrae are situated such as cervical, thoracic lumbar, sacral and coccygeal. The number of vertebrae in each region remains fairly constant in each species and is expressed in the form of vertebral formula which varies from species to species such as

Cattle	C-7, T-13, L-6, S-5, Cy- 15 - 20
Goat	C-7, T-13, L-6, S-4, Cy-16 - 18
Horse	C-7, T-18, L-6, S-5, Cy- 18 - 21
Dog	C-7, T-13, L-7, S-3, Cy- 18 - 23
Pig	C-7, T-14-15, L-6-7, S-4, Cy-20-23
Fowl	C-14, T-7, L+S- 14, Cy- 6

The vertebrae of one region are clearly distinguished from those of other regions. All typical vertebrae have a common architectural plan except a few regional variations. The bodies of the adjoining vertebrae are joined with each other by means of fibrocartilaginous disc called the intervertebral discs.

Structure of a typical vertebra

A typical vertebra consists of a body, an arch and the processes. The **body** is a solid cylindrical rod of osseous tissue over and around which the other basic structures like arch and the processes are attached. The cranial or anterior end of the body is considerably convex and the caudal or posterior end is correspondingly concave. The cranial end of one vertebra meet the caudal end of preceding vertebra and between them is interposed a disk of fibrocartilage- the intervertebral disc. The dorsal or superior surface of the body is flat and forms the floor of the spinal canal while the ventral or inferior surface is slightly convex or rounded and presents centrally the ventral or inferior spinous process which provides an area for attachment of muscles and ligaments. The **arch** is situated on the dorsal surface of the body and is formed of two lateral halves. Each half of the arch is made of two parts, the vertical- pedical and the horizontal- the lamina. The cranial and caudal edges of both, the left and right pedicals present notches- the vertebral notches, which when the adjacent vertebrae are in position circumscribe the intervertebral foramina for the passage of spinal nerves and vessels. The arch of each vertebra along with its dorsal surface forms a bony ring- the neural ring. A series of neural rings of all the vertebrae form the spinal canal and lodges within it the spinal cord.

The **processes** of the vertebrae are inconstant and variable in size, shape and development in different regions of the body. These are as under-

Oblique or articular process: These are four in number. Two of these, projects outward from the cranial edge and the other two from the caudal edge of the arch. They present articular areas called facets, facing upward on the cranial and downward on the caudal processes. The articular areas of the cranial processes of one vertebra articulate with the articular areas of the caudal processes of the preceding vertebra and form the synovial joints. The non articular area of these processes is roughened for the attachment of muscles and ligaments.

Transverse processes: These are two in number, each of them extending transversely outward from the arch or the junction of the body and arch of each vertebra. These processes vary in size and shape in different regions.

Dorsal spinous process: It is single projecting straightly upward or upward and backward from the middle of the dorsal part of the arch of the vertebra.

Ventral spinous processes: It is single extending downward in the form of a roughened elongated ridge on the ventral surface of the body of the vertebra.

Mammillary processes: these are paired small projections between the transverse and cranial articular processes appearing mostly in the cranial thoracic and caudal lumbar vertebrae.

Accessory processes: These are also paired small projections between the transverse and caudal articular processes. These processes mostly appear in the lumbar vertebrae in dogs.

The vertebral column as a whole

The vertebral column throughout its length presents different **curves** in different regions of the body. It is concave dorsally at the cervical region, concave ventrally in the thoracic and lumbar regions and strongly convex dorsally in the sacral region. The coccygeal part of the vertebral column is slightly concave dorsally. The caliber or the **diameter** of the neural canal which is formed by a series of neural rings of the vertebrae also varies in different locations of the vertebral column. It is widest at the first cervical i.e. atlas vertebra, reduced at the second cervical i.e. axis vertebra and again widens at the cervico-thoracic junction. Behind this it ones again become reduced till it reaches to the level of thoraco-lumbar junction. In the lumbar region it once again becomes wider and runes with the same caliber till it reach to the level of middle of the sacrum. Thereafter it reduces in size till the level of fifth or sixth coccygeal vertebra, where it totally disappears.

Ribs

The ribs are elongated, flat curved bony plates which form the skeleton of lateral walls of the thorax. They are arranged in pairs extending obliquely downward from the vertebrae on both side and joining with the sternum at the floor of the thorax. They are serially arranged in pairs and their number corresponds with the number of thoracic vertebrae. The first eight of these are termed as sternal ribs or true ribs because they reach to and articulate with the sternum individually by means of their cartilages. Whereas, the remaining five ribs are called as asternal or false ribs because they join each other at their ventral extremity by means of a common cord of cartilage that articulates on either side of the caudal end of the sternum. Each rib has a body and two extremities. The elongated body is, flattened and curved approximately in upper half of its length while its lower half is twisted and inclined inwards. The point at which the rib is most curved is called as angle of the rib and it bears a rough area for attachment of longissimus thoracis muscle. The lateral surface is convex and bears a wide groove close to its cranial border. The medial surface is smooth, concave and bears a distinct groove close to its caudal border. This is termed as subcostal groove. It runs downward up to the middle of the body of the rib and then disappears. This groove is meant for lodging the intercostal vessels and nerves. The cranial border is concave while the caudal border is correspondingly convex. Both the borders are thin and sharp and provide an area for attachment of intercostal muscles. The dorsal or vertebral extremity presents head, neck and tubercle. The head bears an articular area made up of two convex facets, the cranial and caudal costal facets separated by a nonarticular groove. These two facets articulate with the two adjacent thoracic vertebrae, except the first rib which forms articulation with the last cervical and first thoracic vertebra. The nonarticular groove provides attachment to the intraarticular ligament of the head of the rib. Neck is the constriction below the head and is roughened for the attachment of ligaments. Just caudal to the junction of head and neck is tubercle. At its dorsal surface it presents a transversely placed concave facet for articulation with the transverse process of the caudal of the two thoracic vertebrae with which the head of the rib articulates. This facet of the last two ribs is comparatively smaller and almost flat.

The ventral extremity of the rib is smooth and articulated with the costal cartilage.

Special characteristics of ribs: The first rib is shortest and least curved. The ventral extremity is greatly widened. The lateral surface presents rough area for attachment of scalenus medius muscle. .At the lower part of the cranial border is a smooth impression formed by the axillary vessels. Just dorsal to this is another impression made by dorsal root of brachial plexus. The tubercle of first rib is largest. The eighth, ninth and tenth ribs are longest and widest. Both in front and behind these, the length and width diminish gradually. The head and tubercle diminish in size from first to last rib.

Costal cartilages

The costal cartilages are elongated cylindrical rods of hyaline cartilage lying between the ribs and the sternum. The upper extremity of the costal cartilage forms an articulation with the rib and continues the corresponding rib to the sternum. While the lower extremity forms a joint with the sternum. The first eight costal cartilages form diarthroidal joints with the sternum and hence are called as costal cartilages of sternal ribs while the rests do not reach to the sternum, hence they are called the costal cartilages of asternal ribs.. They are longer, slender and pointed. They overlap and are attached to each other by elastic tissue to form the costal arch. The first costal cartilage is shortest. The dorsal end is wide and thick. The sternal end is small. The cartilages of other sternal ribs progressively increase in length and become more rounded.

Sternum

The sternum is medially placed central osseocartilaginous structure forming the floor of the thorax. It consists of seven sternebrae. It is elongated from before backward, flattened dorsoventrally and compressed laterily till about its middle. It is directed obliquely downward and backward. It has three parts namely- the cranial presternum or manubrium sterrni, the middle mesosternum or body and the caudal xiphi sternum. The dorsal surface is narrow in front and becomes gradually wider behind. It gives attachment to the dorsal sternal ligament running along the central line on this surface. Lateral to the ligament it provides attachment to triangularis sterni muscles. This surface forms the floor of the thorax. The ventral surface is extensive. It is strongly convex at the level of the first sternebra but more or less cocave behind the second sternebra. This surface presents attachment to the pectoral muscle and the rectus abdominis muscle. Both the surfaces present transverse marks indicating the lines of fusion of the adjacent sternebrae. The lateral borders are thick in front and thinner behind. Each border has eight concave articular facets for articulating with the corresponding costal cartilages. The first sternebra has two facets while the rests have one each. The cranial extremity of the sternum is formed by the cranial border of the first sternebra and it forms manubrium sterni. Behind this is the body. The caudal extremity is formed by xiphoid cartilage which is attached to the caudal border of the eighth sternebra.The xiphoid cartilage is thin flexible and heart shaped. Its dorsal surface is concave and it presents attachment to diaphragm close to its junction with last sternebra.. The part of the xiphoid cartilage behind the line of attachment of diaphragm forms the part of floor of abdomen and it presents on its ventral surface an area for attachment of rectus abdominis muscle and linea alba.

Appendicular skeleton

The appendicular skeleton comprises of the bones of fore limb (thoracic limb) and the hind limb (pelvic limb). The fore limb is connected with the axial skeleton through muscles while the hind limb is connected with the axial skeleton by a diarthroidal articulation at the hip joint.

Bones of fore limb

The fore limb has four segments namely- the **shoulder**, the **arm,** the **fore arm** and the **manus.** The shoulder is formed of the **shoulder girdle** which usually consists of three bones, the **scapula** (shoulder blade), **coracoid** and **clavicle**. However, in domestic animals only the scapula is well developed while the small coracoid is fused with the scapula. The clavicle is mostly absent or is a small rudiment embedded in the brachiocephalic muscle.

The arm is formed of a single bone, the **humerus** (arm bone). The fore arm is made up of two bones, the **radius and ulna**. The last segment the manus is composed of three parts the **carpus, metacarpus and digits**. The carpus is a group of small bones varying in number about six to eight in different species of animals. In ox these are six and are arranged in two rows between the radius and ulna above and the metacarpus below. The metacarpus has a large metacarpal and a small metacarpal. The digits are formed by phalanges and sessamoids. (For full description of the bones of fore limb refer the 'Anatomy of fore limb')

Bones of hind limb

The hind limb also has four segments. These include the **hip, thigh, leg** and **pes.** The hip (pelvis) is formed of the largest flat bones the **os coxae** (pelvic bones). The os coxae of the hind limbs of opposite side join each other at pelvic symphysis and articulate dorsally with the sacrum of the vertebral column. The os coxae of two sides along with the sacrum and first few coccygeal vertebrae form the pelvic girdle and encloses within it the pelvic cavity. The os coxae (pelvic bone) consists of three parts the **ilium, ischium** and **pubis**. The bodies of these three bones meet each other to form a large rounded cotyloid cavity the acetabulum which articulates with the head of the femur. The ilium and ischium forms the lateral walls of the pelvic cavity. The sacrum and first few coccygeal vertebrae form the roof while the pubes of the two sides join each other to form the floor of the pelvic cavity. The thigh is formed by a long bone the **femur.** The leg consists of two bones the **tibia** and **fibula** which are fused at their shafts. The pes has again three parts, as were in the case of manus of forelimb. However, these are named as **tarsus, metatarsus** and **digits**. The tarsus consists of five to seven small bones varying in different species and are arranged in two rows in between the tibia and fibula above and metatarsus below. The metatarsals and digits of the hind limb are similar in their number and form to those of metacarpals and digits of forelimb. (For full description of the bones of hind limb refer the 'Anatomy of hind limb').

2

Articular System (Syndesmology/Arthrology)

A branch of anatomy that deals with joints or articulations in the body is termed as arthrology or syndesmology. A joint is an articulation or union formed by two or more bones or cartilages with the help of connective tissue. To form a joint, the long bones meet at their extremities e.g. joints of fore limb and hind limb. Joints of flat bones are formed by their borders or edges e.g. joint of bones of skull, the cranial and facial bones. The short bones and irregular bones form a joint by uniting at any of their parts or surfaces e.g. intervertebral joints.

Classification of joints

Joints are classified on the basis of their structure i.e. the kind of tissue material by which the bones are united, the other constituent parts that help in uniting the bones and the kind of movement performed at that joint. On this basis, the following three major types of joints exist in the skeleton of animal body.

1. Fibrous joint or Synarthrosis
2. Cartilaginous joint or Amphiarthrosis
3. Synovial joint or Diarthrosis

Fibrous joint

In fibrous joints, the bony segments are united by the fibrous tissue. In these joints, the uniting medium holds the bones in such a manner that it prevents any movements at the joints. Thus, these are immovable joints. The fibrous layer of the periosteum of the uniting bones continue over the joint, completely covering the whole joint and the joint structure so that no intervening cavity i.e. synovial cavity remains in this joint. The uniting medium is ossified sooner or latter resulting in to synostosis or ankylosis. There are three types of synarthroses or immovable joints.

Suture: These are special type of joints formed in the skull. In these joints the opposing articular surfaces are united by a fibrous tissue called as sutural ligament. This ligament externally continues with the periosteum of the uniting bones and internally with the fibrous layer of the endosteum of these bones. These articulations are temporary and the uniting material and the bony segments of the joints get fused completely as the age of the animal advances after maturity. Depending on the type of edges of the opposing bones these joints are sub classified as **(a) Sutura serrata** when the edges of the opposing bones are irregular and interlocking e.g. the interfrontal suture. **(b) Sutura squamosa** when the edges are beveled and overlap e.g. joint between the squamous part of temporal and parietal bones. **(c) Sutura plana** or **sutura harmonia** when the edges of the opposing bones are plane or slightly roughened e.g. the internasal suture and **(d) Sutura foliata** when the edge of one bone fits into the fissure of the edge of the opposing bones e.g. the foliet suture.

Syndesmosis: These are the joints where the uniting medium is white fibrous or elastic tissue or a mixture of both e.g. the intermetacarpal joint.

Gomphosis: In these joints, a bone is inserted in to the socket formed in the opposing bone and these are united by the fibrous tissue e.g. the implantation of teeth in the alveoli.

Cartilaginous joints

In cartilaginous joints, the uniting material is fibrocartilage or hyaline cartilage or a combination of these two. These are also completely immovable joints. Sometimes, a kind of flexibility exists at these joints which depends on the thickness and pliability of the uniting medium i.e. the intervening cartilages or the shape of the articulating surfaces of the opposing bones of the joint. There are two types of cartilaginous joints.

Synchondrosis: These are joints where the intervening uniting medium is hyaline cartilage. These are temporary joints because the cartilage turns into bone before the animal reaches maturity or the stage of adult life. Most of these joints are fused by the time the growth of the bones ceases e.g. the epiphyseal plates between the epiphysis and diaphysis of long bone, basilar part of occipital bone with the body of basisphenoid bone.

Symphysis: These are the joints wherein the uniting material is fibrocartilage. These joints are invariably median in position e.g. the pelvic symphysis.

Synovial joints

The synovial joints are also termed as true joints or diarthroses which are characterized by the presence of a joint cavity or synovial cavity and a synovial membrane in the formation of these joints. These are fully movable joints. When a synovial joint is formed by two articular surfaces, it is called as simple joint while the one formed by more than two articular surfaces is called as composite joint. The following structures participate in the formation of these joints.

Articular surface: The articular surfaces are invariably smooth and of various forms. These are formed by a special kind of dense bone which is different than the ordinary compact bone. Some times, kind of small pits called as synovial fossae appear on the articular surfaces. These are nonarticular and rough in nature.

Articular cartilage: The articular cartilages are usually hyaline type of cartilages that cover the articular surfaces of bones of a joint. These are non-vascular, smooth, glossy and of varying thickness. In fresh state it appears bluish pink. They assist in reducing the friction and concussion of the opposite articular surfaces.

Articular capsule: The articular capsule or synovial capsule is a fibro membranous tube that is attached at its ends of the opposing articular surfaces. It consists of two layers, the external layer made of fibrous tissue and the internal layer made of a synovial membrane. The fibrous layer is attached to the rim of the articular surfaces or a little away from it and is called as **fibrous layer** of the **capsular ligament**. It protects the internal layer i.e. the **synovial membrane**. The thickness of capsular ligament greatly varies in different joints. In some joints it is extremely thick while in others it is very thin and sometimes it is totally absent. In such cases the synovial membrane is protected by the tendons of the muscles passing over it. **The synovial membrane** is thin and smooth. It is lined internally by endothelial cells which secrets the viscid, transparent lubricating fluid called as **synovial fluid** or **synovia**. The synovial membrane is richly supplied with vessels and nerves. Another structure, the **synovial sheath** is a sac like fold around the tendon with two layers. The outer layer forms a lining over the canal in which the tendon lies while the inner layer is adhered to the tendon. The two layers become continuous with each other along the fold termed the **mesotendon.**

Joint cavity: The articular cavity or joint cavity is a cavity formed between the articular cartilages of the opposing bones of the joint and is enclosed by the synovial membrane. It contains synovia to lubricate the joint.

Ligaments: These are white fibrous structures in the form of bands or strips binding the joints. Some times they may contain elastic tissue e.g. the nuchal ligament. When these ligaments are internally lined by membranes, these are called as **membranous ligaments** or **capsular ligaments** which protect the synovial cavity of the synovial joints. When these ligaments are in the form of round or flattened bands these are called as **binding ligaments** and they hold the bones in position e.g. the **collateral ligaments**.

Articular discs or menisci: These are thin plates of fibrocartilage or dense fibrous tissue placed in between the articular cartilages, dividing the joint cavity partially or completely into two compartments. They help in reducing the concussion and in allowing movements of the joints.

Marginal cartilage: These are ring like structures made of fibrocartilage encircling the rim of the articular cavity. It causes enlargement of joint cavity and prevention of fracture of the margin of the articular surfaces.

Movements of synovial (diarthrodial) joints

Various types of movements are performed at synovial joints. Basically there are three types of movements, the gliding movements, angular movements and rotary movements. Frequently different types of movements are combined to produce infinite variety of movements at one joint while there are a few others where only one type of movement can be performed.

Gliding movements: The gliding movement is the simplest form of movements occurring at a joint where the articular surfaces of the opposing bones are usually flat e.g. carpal joint and tarsal joint.

Angular movements: In performing these movements, the angle of the joint is either increased or decreased. There are four types of angular movements. These include flexion, extension, abduction and adduction.(1) **Flexion** occurs when the two opposing segments (bones) of a joint are brought together and the angle of the joint is reduced. (2) **Extension** occurs when the two segments of a joint move away from each other and the angle of the joint is increased. Example for these movements is the elbow joint or stifle joint. (3) **Abduction** occurs when a part of the body moves away from the midsagital plane of the body and the enclosing angle is increased where as, (4) the **Adduction** occurs when the part of the body moves closer to the body and the enclosing angle is reduced. The best example for these movements is when the limbs move away from the body or towards the body. These movements are performed at hip joint and shoulder joint.

Rotary movements: The rotary movements are those movements that are caused by rotation of one segment around the longitudinal axis of the other segment of the joint e.g. the atlantoaxial joint.

Circumduction: This type of movement is produced when one segment is made to circumscribe the conical space of the other segment of the joint. This type of movement seldom occurs in quadruped animals.

Classification of arthrodial joints

Based on the type of movements performed, the diarthrodial (Synovial) joints are classified as under.

Arthrodia (gliding joints): These are those joints which are formed by nearly plane articular surfaces and in which one segment glides over the other segment of the joint e.g. carpometacarpal and tarsometatarsal joints.

Enarthroses (ball and socket joint): These are the joints wherein the convex ball like head of one segment is received into glenoid cavity or cotyloid cavity of the other segment of the joint e.g. hip joint.

Gynglymus (hinge joint): These are the joints wherein the condyles of one segments are received into corresponding concavities of the other segment of the joint and they allow only fore and aft movements e.g. elbow joint.

Trochoid (pivot joint): In these joints one segment rotates around the axis of the other segment and the movement is restricted to rotation only e.g. atlantoaxial joint.

3

Muscular System (Myology)

A branch of anatomy that deals with muscles and their accessory structures is called as myology and the body system concerned with myology is called muscular system. The muscular system is composed of specialized cells called muscle fibres because of their shape in the form of fibre or spindle. The plasma of these cells contains myofibrils which are contractile elements that cause contraction of muscles in a definite manner under the influence of a stimulus which is a unique property of muscles. These cells together constitute the distinctive muscular tissue.

Classification of muscles

Based on their morphological and functional characteristics, there are three types of muscles in the body.

Smooth muscle: The muscular tissue in this type of muscles is constituted by masses of spindle shaped cells and they occur mainly in the walls of hollow visceral organs including glands, the vessels, eye ball and hair follicles. These are nonstriated muscles. Contraction in these muscles is weak but sustained and mostly consistent and rhythmic. The action of this muscle is involuntary i.e. not under the will.

Cardiac muscle: The muscle fibres of this muscle are arranged in irregular masses and they form cross striations. The ends of some fibres come in contact with the sides of others forming a kind of syncytium. This is a striated muscle and its action is involuntary. This muscle occurs only in the wall of the heart and the immediate proximal ends of the major blood vessels like aorta, venacava and the pulmonary veins.

Skeletal muscle: The muscle tissue of the skeletal muscle is arranged into distinct groups of muscle fibres of variable size called as individual muscle. It is composed of elongated cells or fibres lying parallel to each other. Each cell or fibre is unique in that it has several nuclei and when observed under microscope, it appears stripped or striated. Each cell or fibre of this muscle contains hundreds of thousands of microscopic fibrils each one of which has its own stripped appearance. These strips are formed of two different kinds of proteins that slide over each other making each cell to contract and in effect resulting into contraction of the individual muscle. Fibres of these muscles are closely associated with connective tissue. The fibres usually do not extend the entire length of the muscle and get attached to the fibres of connective tissue. Some of these fibres appear dark (red) and the others pale (white). Contraction of red fibres sustains for a longer period than the white fibres. Muscles which support the body usually contain more number of red fibres than the white fibres. The associating connective tissue forms a thin film around each fibre of the muscle and it is termed as endomysium. Several of such muscle fibres along with their endomysium constitute a bundle termed as fasciculus. Each of the fascicles is surrounded by greater amount of connective tissue which is termed as perimysium. Numbers of such fascicles are grouped into a large bundle of muscle which is again surrounded by a rather thick sheath of connective tissue, the perimysium. The connective tissue invested in the individual muscle continues with the connective tissue of the bone by which the skeletal muscle is attached to the skeleton. The connective tissue membrane that separates the muscles from each other and binds them together is termed as fascia. The consolidated mass of connective tissue at the end of each muscle forms tough rounded or flattened band or strip that is termed as tendon by which skeletal muscle is attached to the bone. The skeletal muscles are striated and voluntary and they act under the influence of a stimulus from nervous system.

Parts of skeletal muscle

The skeletal muscle has three basic parts, the origin, belly and the insertion. The **origin** is the attachment of the muscle on a stationary bone. The **insertion** is the attachment of the muscle on a movable bone. The **belly** is the fleshy middle portion of the muscle between the origin and the insertion. The origin is usually the first or proximal part of the muscle and it may be tendinous or muscular (fleshy) in structure. The insertion is usually the terminal or distal part of the muscle and it may also be tendinous or fleshy. The belly is the middle portion of the muscle and in majority cases it is fleshy except in certain muscles wherein the belly possesses tendinous fibres.

Attachments of skeletal muscle

The skeletal muscles are attached to the bones by way of tendons or by aponeurosis.

Tendon: The tendon is a flexible but elastic cord of strong fibrous connective tissue that connects muscle to the bone and it usually transmits the mechanical force of muscle contraction to the bone and pulls it on. It is capable of withstanding tension. The tendons are similar to ligaments, having both made of collagen tissue. The only difference is that the ligament joins one bone to another while the tendon connects muscle to the bone.

Aponeurosis: The aponeurosis is the sheet of purely white fibrous tissue which takes the place of a tendon in sheet like muscle having a wide area of attachment. These are histologically similar to tendons and are very sparingly supplied with blood vessels and nerves. Their primary function is to join the muscles to the body parts. It acts upon, whether it is bone or another muscle. The primary regions with thick aponeurosis are in the ventral abdominal region, dorsal lumbar region and the volar (palmer and plantar) regions of the fore limb and hind limb.

Some times, the tendon of muscle running over the joint is surrounded by the **synovial bursa**. It is a small fluid filled sac lined by synovial membrane with an inner capillary layer of viscus fluid. It provides a cushion between the bones and tendons and or muscles around a joint. It helps to reduce friction between the bones and allows free movement. These are present around most of the major joints of the body.

Etymology (Nomenclature) of skeletal muscles

The muscles, especially the skeletal muscles of the body are named on the basis of the location of the muscle, the direction of the fibres or the group of fibres (fascicles) of the muscle, the size of the muscle, the shape of the muscle, the action performed by the muscle and or on the basis of the number of heads of its origin. Accordingly, the muscles are named as below.

Location

Some of the skeletal muscles are named according to the structures especially the bones or bony parts where the muscle is attached. For example, the sternothyrohyoideus runs from sternum to the thyroid cartilage of the larynx and then to the hyoid bone. Similarly there are other muscles as zygomaticus that lies on the zygomatic (malar) bone, temporalis lies on the temporal bone and occipitohyoideus lies between the jugular process of the occipital bone and the thyrohyoid bone.

Direction

Rectus: The fibres run parallel to the midline (e.g. rectus abdominis)

Transverse: The fibres run perpendicular to the midline (e.g. Transversus abdominis)

Oblique: The muscle fibres run diagonal to the midline (e.g. Obliquus abdominis)

Size

Longus or longissimus means the longest among the group of muscles in a particular location e.g. Longissimus dorsi, longus colli etc.

Latissimus means the widest muscle in the location or group e.g. Latissimus dorsi

Magnus means a large and **major** means the larger e.g. Teres major

Minor means smaller e.g. Teres minor

Bravis means small e.g. Extensor bravis

Vastus means the great or greater e.g. Vastus medialis and vastus lateralis parts of the quadriceps femoris muscle of thigh.

Shape

Deltoid is a delta shaped muscle e.g. Deltoideus

Trapezius is a trapezoid muscle e.g. Trapezius

Rhomboideus is a rhomboid (diamond) shaped muscle e.g. Rhomboideus
Serratus is a saw toothed muscle e.g. Serratus cervicis, Serratus thoracis
Orbicularis is a circular muscle e.g. Orbicularis oris, Orbicularis oculi
Quadratus is a square like muscle e.g. Quadratus femoris

Gracilis is a slender gracious muscle e.g. Gracilis muscle of the thigh

Action

Flexor reduces the angle between the bones e.g. Flexor carpi radialis

Extensor increases the angle between the bones e.g. Extensor carpi radialis
Abductor moves the bone away from the midline e.g. Abductor digiti longus

Adductor moves the bone towards the midline e.g. Adductor muscle of the thigh

Levator elevates body part e.g. Levator nasolabialis

Depressor lowers the body part e.g. Depressor labi mandibularis

Sphincter decreases the size of the opening e.g. Sphincter ani externus

Tensor makes the body part rigid e.g. Tensor fasciae latae

Number of origin

Biceps is the muscle with two heads of origin e.g. Biceps brachii

Triceps is a muscle with three heads of origin e.g. Triceps brachii

Quadriceps is a muscle with four heads of origin e.g. Quadriceps femoris

The description of the skeletal muscle usually consists of (1) Name, shape and position (2) Origin (3) Insertion (4) Action and (5) Blood and Nerve supply. Based on their location in different regions of the body, the skeletal muscles are described as muscles of head and neck, muscles of thorax, muscles of abdomen and pelvis, muscles of the fore limb and the muscles of the hind limb. (See relevant chapters under respective regional parts of this book)

SECTION- B

SPLANCHNOLOGY

Splanchnology is the branch of anatomy that deals with the viscera of the body. Viscera are defined as prominent hollow or solid soft organs lying inside the visceral cavities of the body. The Hollow organs have multilayered wall. The three layers of the wall of visceral organs are known as tunics. These include the external viscus layer, the middle muscular layer and the inner mucous layer. The outer viscus layer is differently called as tunica serosa, tunica advantitia, tunica capsularis, tunica albuginia and tunica fibrosa in different organs. It laminates the visceral organs and then continues in the form of a lamina reaching to outer or parietal layer which is also differently called as peritoneum in case of intestine, pleura in case of lungs and pericardium in case of heart. This entire structure forms a sort of serous sac around the organs and protects them. The middle muscular layer is called tunica muscularis and is made of smooth muscles. Usually there are two layers of smooth muscles in the wall of the hollow visceral organs. The outer layer is longitudinal and the inner one is circular. The muscular layer, in addition to protecting and giving particular form to these organs, plays an important role in the movement of the wall of these organs. The movement of the wall of the visceral organs exerts pressure on the contents of the organs either by compression or propulsion. These actions are involuntary and are controlled by nervous system. The inner mucous layer is called the tunica mucosa. It consists of three sub layers as lamina propria mucosae, lamina muscularis mucosae and tela submucosa. The mucous layer provides viscous coating to the wall of the viscera. The solid organs are parenchymatous and have no cavity inside them. However, the parenchyma of the solid organs may or may not have tubular structures within them. The splanchnology includes the digestive, respiratory, urinary, genital and endocrine systems of the body. Most of the organs of these systems are placed in three major cavities called the coelomic cavities or visceral cavities of the body. These include the thoracic cavity, abdominal cavity and the pelvic cavity.

Thoracic cavity

The thoracic cavity is the cranial most of the three visceral cavities and it is second most in the size among the three cavities. It is compressed laterally, narrow in front and wide behind. The dorsal wall or roof of this cavity is formed by thoracic vertebrae and the muscles and ligaments connected with the vertebrae. The lateral walls are formed by the ribs and intercostal muscles. The ventral wall or floor is formed by the sternum, the cartilages of the sternal ribs and the muscles connected with them. The cranial aperture or the thoracic inlet is oval in form and it is bounded dorsally by first thoracic vertebra, ventrally by first sternebra and laterally by a pair of first ribs. In life, it is closed by the structures that enter and leave the thorax. The caudal wall or base of the thorax is a dome like convex structure formed by the diaphragm. A thin film of endothoracic fascia made of elastic tissue forms a longitudinal septum called mediastinum that extends vertically downwards from the dorsal wall to the ventral and caudal wall of thorax. It divides the thoracic cavity into two lateral chambers. Each of these chambers is lined by a serous membrane called pleura and the chambers are termed as pleural sacs that enclose lungs within them. The rest of the organs of the thorax i.e. the heart and major blood vessels lie in the mediastinum. The part of the mediastinum wherein the heart and pericardium lies is called middle mediastinum while the part cranial to it is cranial mediastinum and the one caudal to it is caudal mediastinum.

Abdominal cavity

The abdominal cavity is the largest of the three cavities. Cranially it is separated from the thoracic cavity by diaphragm while caudally it is continues with pelvic cavity. The line of demarcation between the abdominal and pelvic cavities is the pelvic brim or pelvic inlet. The abdominal cavity is ovoid in form and somewhat compressed laterally. Its long axis extends obliquely from the centre of the pelvic inlet to the sternal part of diaphragm. Its greatest dorsoventral diameter is at the level of the first lumbar vertebra and the transverse diameter is near the pelvis. It presents a roof, the floor, the two lateral walls and the cranial wall. The roof is formed by the lumbar vertebrae, the lumbar part of diaphragm and the sub- lumbar muscles. The lateral walls are formed by the the external and internal obliquus and the transversus abdominis muscles, the abdominal fascia, the central part of the ilia with their muscles, the cartilages of the sternal ribs and the parts of the caudal ribs below the attachment of diaphragm. The floor or the ventral wall is formed by the two rectus abdominis muscles, the aponeuroses of the external and internal obliquus abdominis and the transversus abdominis muscles, the abdominal fascia and the xiphoid cartilage. The cranial wall is formed by the diaphragm which is deeply concave resulting into greately increasing the size of the abdomen at the cost of the thorax.

Pelvic cavity

The pelvic cavity is the smallest of the three visceral cavities. It is continuous in front with the abdominal cavity. The line of demarcation between the abdominal and pelvic cavities is the pelvic inlet. The dorsal wall or roof of the cavity is formed by the sacrum and first three coccygeal vertebrae. The ventral wall or floor is formed by the pubic and ischial bones of the pelvis and the lateral walls are formed by parts of ilia and the sacro-sciatic ligaments. The pelvic inlet is bounded by base of the sacrum dorsally, the iliopecttineal lines laterally and the cranial borders of the pubic bones ventrally. The pelvic outlet is formed by the third coccygeal vertebra dorsally, the iscial arch ventrally and the caudal edges of the sacrotuberal ligament and the semimembranous muscles laterally. The outlet is closed by the perineal fascia consisting of the superficial and deep layers attached to the margin of the pelvic outlet, the anus and its muscles and the vulva in female and root of penis in male. The organs contained in the pelvic cavity include rectum, parts of urinary and genital organs, muscles vessels and nerves.

Peritoneum

The peritoneum is a serous membrane which lines the abdominal cavity and to some extent the pelvic cavity and covers the organs contained in them. In the male it is a completely closed sac but in female it has two small openings the abdominal openings of the oviduct or the fallopian tubes. The peritoneal cavity is a potential space formed between two layers, parietal and visceral which are normally in contact with each other. It contains a thin film of serous membrane. The parietal layer lines the boundaries of the wall of the cavity and then reflects over the organs contained in it forming the visceral layer. The double folds of peritoneum thus passing from the walls of the visceral cavity to the organs contained in it constitutes a pathway for the vessels and nerves supplying to the concerned organs. The folds that connect the stomach to other viscera is called omentum, the one that passes from the dorsal wall to the intestine is called the mesentery while the folds which are attached to the organs other than those of the gastro-intestinal tract (gut tube) are called as ligaments. However, these folds i.e. ligaments except the broad ligament of uterus does not transmit vessels and nerves.

4

Digestive System

The digestive system consists of organs concerned with prehension and digestion of food, absorption of digested food and expulsion of unabsorbed food. The digestive system extends from lips to the anus and consists of the primary and accessory organs of digestion. The primary organs include the mouth, pharynx and the alimentary canal (gastrointestinal tube) in that order of sequence. The accessory organs include the tongue, teeth, salivary glands, liver and pancreas. The alimentary canal extends from pharynx to anus and consists of the oesophagus, the stomach, the small intestine and the large intestine. The wall of the alimentary canal consists of, from within outward, the mucous membrane, the muscular layer and the serous layer forming the visceral peritoneum.

Mouth

The mouth is bounded dorsally (roof) by hard palate and behind that the soft palate, ventrally by the body of the mandible along with the mylohyoideus muscles and laterally by the cheeks. The entrance of the mouth cavity is bounded by the lips and it is called as rima oris, while its caudal opening into the pharynx is called as aditus pharyngis. The cavity of the mouth (cavum oris) is subdivided into two parts by the teeth and alveolar processes (the alveoli) of the mandible. The inner part i.e. the space within the teeth and alveoli is termed as mouth cavity proper, while the space between the cheeks and lips and the teeth and alveoli is called the vestibule of the mouth. The mucous membrane of the mouth cavity is continuous with the margin of the lips and the common integument and caudally it continues with the mucous membrane of the pharynx.

Hard palate

The hard palate forms the roof of the mouth cavity. It is bounded rostrally by dental pad, on the sides by alveolar arches of either side and is continuous caudally with the soft palate. The dental pad is formed by a thick pad of connective tissue on the body of the premaxilla (incisive) bone. It is covered by a thick layer of cornified epithelium. Dorsally the hard palate is attached to the bony palate formed by the palatine processes of the premaxillary (incisive), maxillary and the palatine bones. Its ventral surface, facing towards the mouth cavity (oral surface) is presented with about 15 to 19 transverse ridges covering the rostral two third of the palate. The caudal third of this surface of the palate is plane and presents the orifices of the palatine glands. The transverse ridges are straight and their free borders are serrated and caudally directed. A central median groove runs rostro-caudally along the whole length of the hard palate dividing it in to two equal halves. At the rostral end of the median groove and between the dental pad and first transverse ridge lies a diamond shape papilla named as papilla incisiva. This papilla is margined on either side by a fissure which presents the oral (palatine) opening of the naso-palatine duct (ductus incisivus). The nasal opening of this duct lies on the floor of the nasal cavity. The mucous membrane of the hard palate is more or less pigmented.

Lips

The lips are the two (upper and lower) musculomembranous folds that bound the opening of the mouth cavity. The upper and lower lips meet (unite) with each other laterally at the angles of union called the commissures which are situated at the level of the first cheek tooth. The external surface of the lips is covered by a thick skin with variable number of tactile and ordinary fine hairs. In bovine animals, the middle part of the external surface of the upper lip and the surface between the nostrils is bare and is termed the muzzle. In horse, the upper lip in its centre presents a deep furrow called as philtrum. The lower lip presents in its centre a rounded prominence called as chin. The internal surface is lined by mucous membrane which is usually pigmented. It bears number of small papillae which present the openings of the labial glands. A small fold of mucous membrane extending from the lips to the gums is called as frenum labis maxilaris (the upper one) and mandibularis (the lower one).

Cheeks

The cheeks form the lateral walls of the mouth cavity. These are continuous in front with the lips. These are attached to the alveolar border of the bones of the jaws i.e. maxilla forming the upper jaw and mandible forming the lower jaw. The cheeks are constituted externally by the skin, internally by the mucous membrane and between these two is a layer of muscles within which exists the buccal glands, vessels and nerves.

Tongue

The tongue is the chief organ of prehension. It is situated on the floor of the mouth, between the rami of the mandible and is supported by the slings formed by the mylohyoideus muscles because of which it has become highly protractile. It consists of a root, a body and the tip. The root is the caudal part and is attached ventrally and caudally to the hyoid bone, soft palate and pharynx. Its upper surface is free and slopes ventrally and caudally. The body is the middle part and has three surfaces. The dorsal surface (dorsum linguae) is rounded while the two lateral surfaces are flattened. The ventral surface is related to the geniohyoideus and mylohyoideus muscles. The tip or the apex is free and some what pointed. It has two surfaces the dorsal (upper) and ventral (lower) and a free rounded border. The dorsal surface (dorsum linguae) of the tongue is free throughout and remains in contact with the palate except at the glossoepiglottic space when the mouth is closed. The caudal part of the dorsum linguae is prominently raised and is sharply demarcated from the rest of the part by a transverse groove.

Structure of the tongue: The tongue consists of the outer layer of mucous membrane and the internal mass of the muscles and glands. It is richly supplied with the vessels and the nerves. The mucous membrane is intimately adhered to the underlying tissue mass of the muscles except at the lower part of the lateral borders of the body and the ventral surface of the tip. The mucous membrane is quite thick and dense on the dorsum while on the lateral borders it is thin. A thin fold of mucous membrane extending from the ventral surface of the free part of the tongue passes over the floor of the mouth. This fold is called as frenum linguae. The mucous membrane on the dorsum of the tongue presents various types of papillae. These include the filiform, fungiform, vallate, foliate and conical papillae. The **filiform papillae** are in abundance. These are fine, thread like projections. These papillae impart roughness to the tongue. These are located over the dorsum in front of the prominence and the sides of the tip of the tongue. The **fungiform papillae** are also numerous. These are larger, rounded (button like) at the free end and distinctly lying scattered between the filliform papillae on the dorsum and sides of the body and tip of the tongue. The **vallate (circumvallate) papillae** exist on the caudal prominence of the dorsum of the tongue. These vary in number from 8 to 17 and are arranged in rows on either side of the prominence of the dorsum. They are rounded and broader at their free ends than the attached ends and appear like sunk in the depressions binded by the annular walls. Their free surface is tubercular and bears small round secondary papillae. The **foliate papillae** are rounded eminences lying just rostral to the palatoglossal arches. The fungiform, vallate and foliate papillae are furnished with taste buds. The **lingual follicles** possessing lymphoid tissue are present in the caudal part of the dorsum and on each side of the glossoepiglottic fold. The lingual glands are present in the submucous tissue.

Teeth

The teeth are hard white or yellowish white structures implanted in the alveoli of the jaws formed by the maxilla (upper jaw) and mandible (lower jaw). They are organs of prehension and mastication. Domestic animals have two sets of teeth. The first set of teeth erupts during early life. These are termed as deciduous or milk teeth. These are temporary and after a specific time are replaced by the other set of teeth which are termed as permanent teeth. Based on their position in the alveoli and the function performed by them, the teeth are classified as (1) **Incisors**: These are most rostral in position and are used for cutting the food material. (2) **Canines**: These are next to and lateral to the incisors. These are used to seize and tear the food material (3) **Premolars** and (4) **Molars:** These teeth form the sides of the dental arch. They are adjacent to cheeks and hence are called cheek teeth and are used for grinding, chewing and mastication of the food material. The incisors, canines and premolars appear in both i.e. deciduous and permanent set of teeth. The molar teeth, however, erupt only in permanent set. The complete dentition of an animal is expressed in the form of dental formula. In this formula, the letters indicate the kind of teeth and the numerical in the upper and lower row indicate the number of teeth of that particular type of teeth in the upper and lower jaw. Thus the dental formula of permanent teeth in ox is as below.

$$2\left(I\frac{0}{4}\;C\frac{0}{0}\;M\frac{3}{3}\;\overset{\leftarrow}{\underset{\rightarrow}{}}\;P\frac{3}{3}\right) = 32$$

The individual teeth are designated numerically as first, second, third and so on in the respective type just as, I1, I2, P1, P2, M1, M2 etc. The incisors are present in almost all the domestic animals. However, these are absent in the upper jaw of the ruminants like ox, goat and sheep. Similarly, canine teeth are also absent in both the jaws of ox goat and sheep. In dog and cat these are prominent. The cheek teeth are flattened for grinding particularly in ruminants. Each tooth basically has two parts, the crown which lies above the gums and the root which lies embedded in the alveoli below the gums. The line of union of these two parts is constricted and is termed as neck of the tooth. The surfaces of the tooth are described as (1) the **occlusal or table surface** is one that is free and in opposition to the teeth of the opposing jaw. In ruminants, it is also called as **masticatory surface**. (2) The surface which is facing towards the vestibule is called the **vestibular surface**. (3) The vestibular surface of incisors and canine teeth is called **labial surface** because it is facing towards lips. Similarly the vestibular surface of the cheek teeth (premolar and molar) is called as **buccal surface** since it faces towards cheeks. (4) The surface that is facing towards the tongue is termed as **lingual surface** and (5) The surface of a tooth which is in contact with the neighboring tooth is called as **contact surface**.

Structure of the tooth: From within outward, the tooth consists of a soft structure the pulp in the centre, and it is covered by a hard yellowish white tissue the dentine. The outer layer covering the root is called cement while that of the crown is called the enamel. The pulp is filled with a soft gelatinous tissue and is supplied by the vessels and nerves of the teeth. Dentine is quite hard and forms the bulk of the tooth. Cement is harder than the dentine and in simple tooth it forms a thin layer covering the dentine of the root only. However, in the complex tooth it is quite thick and tends to fill in the spaces in the enamel folds of the crown in addition to forming the covering layer of the root. The enamel is the hardest tissue in the body and it strongly covers the dentine of the crown. It is usually bluish white in colour

Incisor teeth: In ox, these are absent in upper jaw. In lower jaw these are eight in number and are arranged in fan like manner. These are simple teeth and have no infundibula. The crown is white, short and shovel shaped. The occlusal surface of the crown is in the form of a sharp edge that separates the labial and lingual surfaces. Initially the entire crown is covered by enamel but as the age advances the enamel on the occlusal surface starts tearing that leads to expose the inner layer of dentine. The root is single and rounded. It is embedded in the alveolus on the alveolar border of the body of the mandible. It is so fixed in the alveoli as to allow a small amount of movement. Beginning from centre the first pair of incisor is called as central, the second as intermediate, third as lateral and the fourth as corner.

Canine teeth: These are absent in ox but it is considered that in herbivorous animals, the canines are converted into the last pair (corner) of incisors. However, in other species of animals especially in carnivores the canine teeth are prominent. The crown of the canine tooth is white or yellowish white rounded and tapering towards the table surface which is slightly curved inward. The root is single and rounded.

Cheek teeth: The cheek teeth (**premolars** and **molars**) are prismatic in form. The crown is quadrilateral in cross section except in the first and last cheek teeth which are triangular in cross section. The upper cheek teeth are embedded in the alveoli of the maxilla bone. They are slightly curved with the convexity towards the cheek. The buccal surface presents a central ridge and two grooves. The lingual surface presents a wide round ridge that separate the two grooves. The masticatory surface presents two prominent infundibula. It slopes obliquely downwards and outwards. The buccal edge is prominent and sharp. The first and last cheek tooth has three roots while the rests have three or four roots. The upper cheek teeth are longer on the outer side and the lower ones are longer on the inner side. The lower cheek teeth are implanted in the alveoli of rami of mandible. The lingual surface presents two or more grooves. The masticatory surface is oblique. It slopes upwards and inwards and its lingual edge is sharp. The first five cheek teeth have two roots and the sixth one has three.

The time of eruption of deciduous teeth and their subsequent replacement by permanent teeth has a definite correlation. However, there may be some variation based on the breed of the animal, nature of the food and assimilation of calcium. The status of the deciduous and permanent teeth in the mouth of the animal is used in practice for determination of the age of the animal. The tentative formula of eruption of teeth and the age of the animal in ox can be presented as below.

Eruption time of teeth in ox

Class of teeth	Position (number)	Age of animal	
		Deciduous	Permanent
Incisor	1st }	Birth to	18 month
	2nd }	2 weeks	2 years
	3rd }		3 years
	4th }		3-4 years
Premolars	1st }	1-4 weeks	1 year
	2nd }		1 and half to 2 years
	3rd }		2 and half to 3 years
Molars	1st }		18 months
	2nd }		1 to 1 and half years
	3rd}		2 to 2 and half years

Salivary glands

These are three pairs of large glands situated on the sides of the face and adjacent part of the neck. These are named as parotid, mandibular and sublingual salivary glands. Their ducts open in to the mouth.

The parotid gland is situated in the space between the ramus of the mandible and the wing of the atlas vertebra, overlapping the caudal part of the massater muscle. The parotid duct (Stenson's duct) arises from the ventral aspect of the medial surface of the parotid gland and opens on the papilla salivalis situated on the cheek at the level of the upper fifth cheek tooth.

The mandibular gland is the largest of all the salivary glands. It extends from the atlantal fossa to the basihyoid bone and is partly covered by parotid gland. The mandibular duct (Wharton's duct) extends from the middle of the concave border of the gland and opens on the caruncula sublingualis, a papilla situated on the floor of the mouth below the tip of the tongue at the level of and opposite to the corner incisor tooth.

The sublingual gland is situated beneath the mucous membrane of the mouth, between the body of the tongue and the ramus of the mandible. It consists of two parts the dorsal and ventral. The dorsal part (polystomatic sublingual gland) consists of fairly large number of glandular globes giving rise to equal number of small excretory ducts (the minor sublingual ducts) that open in to the lateral sublingual recess, The ventral part (monostomatic sublingual gland) has a single duct that opens either alongside or into the Wharton's duct.

Soft palate

The soft palate is a musculomembranous fold attached to the hard palate and the lateral walls of the oropharynx. It acts as active musculomembranous valve between the oropharynx and nasopharynx to assist in the digestive and respiratory functions. The dorsal border is attached to the hard palate while the ventral border is free and concave. It embraces the rostral surface of the epiglottis. The lateral free margins continue with the mucosal fold, the palatopharygeal arch which runs back on the lateral wall of the pharynx and meet the same arch of the opposite side on the caudodorsal side of corniculate cartilage of the larynx. From the middle of the lateral attachment of the soft palate extends the palatoglossal arch. The palatoglossal arches of the two sides along with the soft palate and the tongue forms the aditus pharyngis.

Pharynx

The pharynx is a musculomembranous sac common to digestive and respiratory passages. It is a funnel shaped organ with the broad rostral end continuing with the mouth and nasal cavities and the narrow caudal end opening in to the oesophagus. Air and food passages cross each other while passing through the pharynx. During respiration air passes from rostro-dorsal to caudo-ventral way and vise versa whereas during food intake the bolus takes its rout from rostro-ventral to caudo-dorsal way.

Alimentary canal

The alimentary canal begins at oesophagus, passes through the neck, thorax and abdomen and ends at the anus. During this long rout, it bears various organs like oesophagus, stomach, small intestine and large intestine.

Oesophagus

The oesophagus is musculomembranous tube like a hose pipe. It extends from pharynx, passes through the neck and then through the thorax and finally after piercing through the diaphragm it opens in to the stomach in the abdomen. During this course it takes several deviations in relation to trachea. At the beginning it lies dorsal to the larynx and trachea, then goes to the left of the trachea, then again gains the dorsal face of the trachea and then after termination (bifurcation) of trachea sleeps slightly to the right and finally to the left of the aorta. The wall of the stomach consists of muscles which contract in a wave like fashion that causes propulsion of food bolus through the oesophagus and pushes it into stomach.

Stomach

Stomach is a sac like structure lying mostly to the left of the median plane in the abdominal cavity just next to diaphragm. It is designed to store large volumes of food and to continue the process of digestion. The oesophagus that carries food from mouth to stomach opens in to stomach through a valve like sphincter called as cardia. On the interior surface of the wall of the stomach are several folds that help in fine grinding and digestion of food. They secrete HCL and digestive enzymes to breakdown the food and convert it in to partially digestible fluid form the chyle.. Ones this process is completed, the bulk of the chyle and the undigested part of the food propels and exits into the intestine through another sphincter the pylorus. The form of the stomach differs according to the nature of life and food of the animal species. The horse, dog and pig have simple stomach with single compartment (monogastric), whereas, ruminants have complex stomach with four compartments (polygastric).

Small intestine

The small intestine is a tubular musculomembranous structure that extends from the pylorus of the stomach and caudally joins the large intestine at the junction of the cecum and colon. It measures about 40 meters in length in ox, 25 meters in sheep and goat and 22 meters in horse. It consists of three parts, the duodenum, jejunum and ileum. The duodenum is the smallest of the three parts and presents a sigmoid (s shaped) flexure over which opens the bile duct of the liver and pancreatic duct from pancreas. It is attached to the peritoneum by a short fold the mesoduodenum. The jejunum being extensively long gets itself folded in to numerous close coils which are arranged in a festoon around the free border of the mesentery. There after it forms a U shaped series of loops along the fold of mesentery and then continues into a rather straight tube the ileum which runs behind for a short distance and opens into the large intestine at the ceco-colic junction. A large proportion of the digestion and absorption of the nutrients and the water occurs in the small intestine.

Large intestine

The large intestine connects small intestine to the anus. It consists of three parts the caecum, colon and rectum. It is adapted for retention and storage of fecal matter before its expulsion through the anus. Its main function is to absorb water from feces thus keeping hydration level of the body constant. For most of its length it is shorter and slightly broader than the small intestine. It lies mostly in the supraomental recess between the layers of the mesentery in the right dorsal part of the abdominal cavity related to the right surface of the rumen in ox. The ileum opens in to the large intestine at the junction of caecum with colon. The caecum is elongated blind sac. It opens in to colon at the ileo-caeco-colic junction. The colon begins as a direct continuation of caecum at the caeco-colic orifice. The greater part of it is arranged in double elliptical coils between the layers of mesentery. It directly opens into rectum, rather rectum is direct continuation of colon without clear demarcation between these two parts. The rectum begins at the level of the pelvic inlet and terminates in to the anus at the level of the pelvic outlet.

Anus

The anus is the terminal part of the alimentary canal. It is placed below the root of the tail forming a round projection with a central depression when contracted. Its lumen called anal canal is closed except during defecation by the contraction of the sphincter muscles lined internally by the folds of mucous membrane. It is covered externally by thin skin without hairs.

Liver

The liver is the largest gland in the body of the animal. It is situated obliquely on the abdominal surface of the diaphragm. It is held in position by the pressure exerted by other organs in relation to it in abdominal cavity and also by its attachment to diaphragm with the help of different ligaments. It appears like a large reddish brown mass divided into number of hepatic lobes that are so closely joined together that they are sometimes difficult to distinguish one from the other. However, in some species of animals the lobes of the liver are prominent and distinctly divided by deep fissures. The number of lobes of liver varies from species to species. All the lobes perform the same task and can compensate and share the workload of each other in diseased condition.The liver is an extremely important organ especially for metabolic activity in the body. It is responsible for protein, fat and carbohydrate metabolism, vitamin and mineral storage, digestion of food and detoxication of wastes. The secretion from the liver is carried by right and left hepatic ducts. These ducts after a short course unite to form a common hepatic duct which runs over the mesoduodenum and join the cystic duct from gall bladder to form the bile duct that opens into the duodenum.

Pancreas

The pancreas is a soft, elongated and flattened glandular (endocrine and exocrine) accessory organ of digestive system. It is situated transversely across the dorsal part of the abdominal cavity and lies in close association of the duodenum almost to the right of the median plane. It is mostly V shaped in almost all the species of animals. It consists of a body and two, left and right, lobes. The lobes are loosely united by interlobular connective tissue. Its endocrine part produces several important hormones including insuline, glucagon, somatostatin and pancreatic polypeptides which circulate in the blood. Its exocrine secretion, the pancreatic juice containing digestive enzymes is carried by pancreatic duct that opens into the duodenum alongside the bile duct.

5

Respiratory System

The respiratory system is a complex biological system comprised of several organs that facilitate the inhalation of oxygen and exhalation of carbon dioxide (breathing) in living organisms. The major functions of the respiratory system is providing oxygen to the body cells and removing carbon dioxide from the body. In addition to this, the respiratory system helps in controlling body temperature (especially in dogs), eliminating water (as vapour) and assisting in voice production. The organs of respiratory system extend from nose to lungs. These consist of two major parts, the upper respiratory tract and the lower respiratory tract. The upper respiratory tract is comprised of nose, nasal cavity, the part of mouth, and the part of pharynx. The lower respiratory tract is comprised of the larynx, trachea, bronchi and lungs.

Nose

The nose is the externally visible part of the respiratory system. It forms the part of the face of the animal extending from the transverse level of eyes to the rostral end of the head. Exteriorly it is formed by the bones, muscles, cartilages and the skin. Internally it encloses the nasal cavity which is lined by the mucous membrane. The dorsal part of the nose (roof of the nasal cavity) is termed as dorsum nasi. It is formed by the nasal and frontal bones of the skull. The lateral parts are formed by the incisive, maxillary, lacrimal and zygomatic bones. Covering these bones externally is a muscular layer formed by the facial muscles running over these bones and acting on the upper lip and nostrils. The muscular layer is externally covered by the skin. The skin on the nose bears fine hairs except at the tip of the nose that is formed by the nostrils. The rostral end of the nose is formed by nostrils which provide entrance to the nasal cavity. The nostrils are supported by cartilages which are the dorsal and ventral extensions of the cartilage of the nasal septum. The main aim of the nose is to support and protect the nasal cavity.

Nasal cavity

The nasal cavity is a hollow space within the nose. The main function of the nasal cavity is to warm, moisturize and filter the air entering the body before it reaches the lungs. It extends from external nares (nostrils) to the caudal nares (choanae).) The roof of the nasal cavity is formed by the nasal and part of frontal bones and the parietal (dorsal lateral) cartilages. Its floor is formed by the parts of incisive, maxillary and palatine bones and the parietal (ventral lateral) cartilages. The lateral walls are formed by parts of the incisive, maxillary, palatine, ethmoid and lachrymal bones and the parts of parietal (dorsal and ventral lateral) cartilages. The rostral osseous boundary of the cavity is demarcated by the rostral edge of the body of the incisive bones while the caudal boundary is formed by the cribriform plate of the ethmoid bone. The nasal cavity is divided into the left and right halves by the median nasal septum formed partly by the osseous and partly by the cartilaginous plate. The osseous part is the caudal and ventral portion and it is constituted by perpendicular plate of ethmoid bone and the vomer bone. The rest of the portion of the nasal septum is cartilaginous and it is formed by hyaline cartilage. The dorsal border of the nasal septum is attached to the frontal and nasal bones while its ventral border is received into the groove formed by the vomer. All the osseous and cartilaginous parts of the nasal cavity including the septum are lined by mucous membrane. The major part of the hollow space is occupied by two nasal conchae the dorsal and ventral conchae. These are the scrolls of turbinate bones which project in to the nasal cavity with the purpose of supporting the olfactory mucous membrane and increasing the respiratory surface area creating turbulence within the passing air. This helps in to filter and warm or cool the air passing through it. The conchae divide the nasal cavity into different meatuses. On either side of the nasal septum and between the septum and the conchae is a longitudinal space the common meatus. Branching out from the common meatus in the nasal cavity, there lies three meatuses, the dorsal, ventral and middle meatus. The dorsal meatus is the space between the roof of the nasal cavity and dorsal concha. The ventral meatus is a space between the ventral concha and the floor of the nasal cavity. The middle meatus is the space between the dorsal and ventral meatus. The nasal conchae and the septum are also lined by mucous membrane that continues in the paranasal sinuses which are the excavations in to the nasal, frontal, maxillary, lacrimal, and ethmoid bones that forms the skeleton of the nose and nasal cavity. The mucous membrane of the nasal cavity is lined by the ciliated epithelium. The mucous secreted by the mucosal glands trap the unwanted particles from the air passing through the nasal cavity and the cilia beating backward transport them down the pharynx for swallowing.

Larynx

The larynx is a hollow tubular organ situated below the pharynx lying partly between the rami of the mandible and caudally extending into the neck. Cranially it is connected to the pharynx at the level of division of pharynx in to nasopharynx and oropharynx. Rostrally it opens into pharynx and caudally into the trachea. It guards the entrance to the lower respiratory passage. It is an organ involved in breathing, sound production and protecting the trachea against food aspiration. The larynx houses the vocal cords which are essential for phonation. The vocal folds are situated just below where the pharynx divides into trachea and oesophagus. The larynx is made up of cartilages, ligaments, muscles and mucous membrane. The cartilage plates form the external skeleton of the larynx and it prevents collaps of this organ. The cartilages are fastened together by the ligaments and muscles. The mucous membrane of the larynx helps it to provide appropriate environment for passage of air through the tube of the larynx. The cartilages that constitute the skeleton of larynx are six in number. Three of them are paired and the remaining three are unpaired. The unpaired (single) cartilages are cricoid, thyroid and epiglottic while the paired cartilages include the arytenoid, corniculate and cuneiform. The articulations formed by laryngeal cartilages include the cricothyroid articulation, cricoarytenoid articulation and the thyrohyoid articulations. The muscles acting over the laryngeal cartilages and their joints are the extrinsic muscles and the intrinsic muscles. The extrinsic muscles assist the larynx to move rostrally or caudally. The intrinsic muscles help in narrowing or widening the rima glottis.

Trachea

The trachea or wind pipe is a cartilaginous and membranous tubular structure appearing like a hose pipe. It connects the pharynx and larynx to the lungs and is used as conduit for passage of air from larynx to lungs and vice versa in the act of breathing. It is formed of a series of 'C' shaped rings made of hyaline cartilage which are joined with each other by the fibro elastic membrane. These sheets of connective tissue are called as annular ligaments. The gaps between the free ends of the 'C' shaped rings of cartilage are filled in by smooth trachealis muscle. Thus, the complete series of these cartilage rings, the annular ligaments and the smooth tracheal muscles form the middle layer of the wall of the trachea throughout its length. This type of structural confirmation of trachea prevents it from collapse and also allows it to adjust in length and diameter due to traction during the movements of neck and at times of forceful breathing. The inner layer of the trachea lining it internally is formed by the mucous membrane with ciliated epithelium. It contains mucosal glands which secret mucous that traps the debris from the filtered air or from the exhaled air and moves it upward towards the oropharynx where it can be swallowed down the pharynx and oesophagus. This mechanism is called the muco-ciliary escalator. The outer layer of the trachea is formed by a serous membrane which is called as tunica advantitia in the neck and tunica serosa in the thorax. Beginning at the larynx, the trachea opens into the larynx through the cricoid cartilage which forms a complete ring around the cranial end of trachea. From here the trachea traverses through the neck lying median in position and running parallel to the oesophagus which lies to the left of the trachea throughout its cervical course. On entering the thorax it crosses the aortic arch and sleeps slightly to the right of the median plane. After reaching just dorsal to the base of the heart at the level of the fourth to fifth thoracic vertebra it bifurcates into bronchi.

Bronchi and bronchioles

Bronchus also known as principal bronchus or primary bronchus (pl-bronchi) is the part of respiratory system that connects trachea to the lung parenchyma. There are two principal bronchi- the right and left, that emerge from the bifurcation of the trachea at the level of fifth thoracic vertebra and enter the lungs through the hilus of the lung of the respective (right and left) side. After entering into the lungs, the primary bronchi divide into the smaller secondary or lobar bronchi which traverse to the respective lobe of the lung. Within the parenchyma of the lobes of the lungs, the secondary bronchi branch into still smaller tertiary or segmental bronchi. In the course of further branching, the bronchi divides into bronchioles, first into respiratory bronchioles and then into the alveolar bronchioles of about one mm diameter. The alveoli are thin walled sacs called the respiratory unit of the lung where gas exchange occurs. The primary bronchi contain the incomplete rings of cartilage and pseudostratified ciliated epithelium like that of the trachea. Hereinafter, in the course of branching, the amount of cartilage in the walls of the bronchi progressively decreases and eventually disappears by the time the bronchi divide into respiratory and alveolar bronchioles. From tertiary bronchi onward the mucous membrane changes from ciliated cuboidal epithelium with no goblet cells to nonciliated simple cuboidal epithelium with goblet cells. This extensive branching of respiratory channel is called the **Bronchial Tree.**

Lungs

Lungs are the principal organs of respiration. The primary function of the lungs is to extract oxygen from atmospheric air reached to them by way of bronchi and transfer it into the blood stream and simultaneously to extract carbon dioxide from blood stream and to release it in to atmosphere by way of the respiratory tract. This process of gas exchange occurs at the tiny respiratory units called alveoli of the lungs. The paired right and left lungs are situated in the thoracic cavity. Inside the thoracic cavity each lung is enclosed within a serous sac called the pleural sac. Each lung is roughly triangular conical in shape. Its base lies against the concave thoracic or cranial surface of the diaphragm while its apex lies close to the thoracic inlet. In fresh state, the lungs collected from the healthy animal appears yellowish pink in colour. They are light weight and float in the water. On squeezing they produce crepitating sound. On touching they are felt soft and spongy. After embalming, the lungs become hard and they present on their surfaces the impressions of the organs with which they are related inside the thoracic cavity including the ribs that form the wall of the thoracic cavity. The right lung is larger than the left. Each lung is subdivided into different lobes by means of deep fissures extending from the indented ventral border. The number of lobes, however, varies from species to species. The lobes of the lungs are defined by lobar (secondary) bronchi. The medial surface of each lung presents the hilus through which the principal bronchus, pulmonary vessels, lymphatics and nerves enter and leave the lungs. The hilus along with these structures is called the root of the lung and it holds the lung suspended inside the pleural sac which provides sufficient space for expansion of lungs during respiration.

6

Urinary System

Urinary system is relatively simple and consists of a pair of kidneys, a pair of ureters, the bladder and the urethra. The kidneys are the main organs that filter the blood and produce the urine while the rests of the organs of this system are simply accessory structures that are used for transport and storage of urine. For proper functioning of the metabolic processes of the body, it is essential to constantly maintain the chemical composition and volume of the tissue fluid. This is called the homeostasis. This particular task is performed by the urinary system and in particular by the kidneys.

Kidneys

The kidneys right and left, are bean shaped red brown relatively large glands situated in the abdominal cavity. These are placed retroperitoneal against the dorsal wall of the abdomen on either side of the spine. The right kidney is about half of its length ahead of the left kidney and it fits into the renal impression on the caudate lobe of the liver. An indentation at about the middle of the medial border is the hilus of the kidney through which pass the renal vessels, nerves and ureters. Both the kidneys are covered by a thin capsule formed of fibrous tissue which surrounds the parenchyma of the kidneys. The capsule can be easily striped away from the kidney. The function of the kidneys is to maintain the volume and composition of the plasma,regulate water, ion, and pH levels, retain nutrients and excrete fluid wastes, toxins and excess electrolytes. The kidneys achieve these functions through glomerular filtration, solute reabsorption, tubular secretion, water balance and acid-base regulation.

The renal capsule provides a stiff outer shell to maintain the shape and protect the inner soft parenchyma. Deep to the capsule is the soft, dense vascular cortex. Several cone shaped pyramids form the medulla deep to the cortex. The pyramids are aligned with their bases facing outward towards the cortex and their apices point inward towards the centre of the kidney. Each apex connects to a minor calyx, a small hollow tube that collects urine. The minor calyces merge to form three major calyces, which further merge to form the hollow renal pelvis at the centre of the kidney. The urine collected into the pelvis drains into the ureter that exits through the hilus of the kidney.

Ureters

The ureters are muscular tubes that transport urine from kidneys to the urinary bladder. The wall of the ureter consists of three layers. These include the outer fibrous coat, the middle muscular layer and the inner mucosal layer. The urine is propelled through the ureter because of the peristalsis (waving contraction) of the muscles in the muscular layer of the tube. The ureters open in to the wall of the urinary bladder near its neck.

Urinary bladder

The urinary bladder is a hollow muscular sac for temporary storage of urine. The form, size and position of the bladder vary according to the level of fullness of the bladder. When empty, it rests on the pubic bones and lies entirely in the pelvic cavity. In this state its wall is wrinkled and thick. When full and distended, the folds of the wall disappear and the wall becomes thinner. The base of the bladder extends on the floor of the abdominal cavity just in front of the pubic bones. Grossly the bladder is described as having a cranial broad blind end called the **fundus** (base), the intermediate main portion the **body** and the caudal narrow constricted end the **neck** of the bladder. The wall of the bladder is composed of an outer layer of fibrous connective tissue, the middle muscular level of smooth muscle and the inner mucosal layer lined by transitional epithelium. When the bladder is empty, the smooth muscles cause the wall along with the mucous membrane to form folds called '**ruguae**'. The ruguae and the transitional epithelium allow the bladder to stretch when filled with urine. The mucous membrane at the dorsal wall of the bladder near its neck forms a triangular area called **trigonum vesicae**. The angles of this area lie at the orifices of the two ureters and the urethra. The opening of the urethra is surrounded by a band of '**detrusor**' muscle forming an internal urethral sphincter. This sphincter is relaxed by involuntary control because of which the animal perceives the urge to urinate when the bladder is approximately half full.

Urethra

Urethra is a musculomembranous tube which conveys urine caudally from urinary bladder through pelvic cavity to the outside. The descriptive features of urethra vary according to the sex of the animal. The female urethra is a short tube opening into the floor of the reproductive tract at the junction of the vagina and vestibule. This opening is called the **external urethral opening**. The male urethra has two parts, the **pelvic part** and the **penile part**. The pelvic part of the urethra in male animal begins at the neck of the urinary bladder, passes caudally through the prostrate gland, continues behind on the floor of the pelvic cavity up to the level of ischial arch and then exits the pelvic cavity to continue as penile part. The penile part turns round the iscihal arch then enters the muscle of the penis running the length of the penis and opens into the external urethral orifice at the tip of the penis. The structure of the wall of urethra is same as that of the urinary bladder. The urethral muscle of the urethra runs the whole length of urethra and finally forms the sphincter called the external urethral sphincter at its opening to exterior at the tip of the penis. This sphincter is voluntarily controlled and is relaxed by the animal when a suitable time for urination is determined.

7

Genital System (Reproductive System)

Reproduction is the physiological process by which organisms produce offspring. Sexual reproduction involves production of gametes. The gametes are produced by the gonads. The rest of the process of converting the gametes into the offspring involves other reproductive organs. The male and female animals have different genital organs that contribute to reproduction. The organs of reproduction (genital organs) in male include a pair of male gonads the testes (sing.-testis), the epididymis, ductus deferens, the seminal vesicles, a prostate gland, a pair of bulbourethral glands (Cowper's glands), the male urethra, and the penis. In female the genital organs include a pair of gonads the ovaries, the fallopian tubes, the uterus, the vagina, the vulva and the mammary glands.

Male genital system

The overall function of the male genital organs is to continuously produce and store the male gametes the sperms, to maintain the continuous supply of semen, to detect estrus in female, and to inseminate and fertilize the female gametes. While the testes are the site for production of sperms, the epididymis, vas deferens and the accessory glands like prostate, seminal vesicles, and bulbourethral glands are responsible for the production of different secretions which mix together and are known as seminal plasma or seminal fluid. The seminal fluid provides a source of energy, buffers, antioxidants and other compounds needed for sperm survivability, maturation and motility. Once spermatozoa are mixed with the seminal fluid, the combined product is called the semen.

Testis

The testis is the male gonad. The primary function of the testis is to produce male gametes the spermatozoa (sperm) and the male sex hormone the testosterone. The testes are a paired organ lying close together separated by the septum of the scrotum and suspended vertically in the respective, left and right pouch of the scrotum. The testes are elongated and ovoid in form. These are attached to the body of the animal by the spermatic cord which enters the abdominal cavity through the inguinal canal. This particular arrangement is provided to keep the testes at a temperature 2 to 5 degree Celsius below the body temperature of the animal. This type of thermoregulation is critically essential for production of sperms in the testes. The outer surface of the testis is covered by a serous membrane called vaginal tunic. Beneath this tunic is a capsule of dense fibrous connective tissue called the tunica albuginea. From this tunic several strands of trabeculae enter into the parenchyma of the gland (testis). These trabeculae form the septa that divide the parenchyma into number of lobules (about 250 to 300) which are called the follicles. The spaces inside the follicles consist of seminiferous tubules which are supported by intralobular loose connective tissue. The seminiferous tubules are initially convoluted and latter become straight. The straight parts of the seminiferous tubules unite and form larger tubules called the tubuli recti. The tubuli recti from different lobes converge towards the cranial border of the testis and form the efferent ducts. In this way about 12 to 18 efferent ducts are formed. These efferent ducts pierce the tunica albuginea and open into the head of the epididymis. The convoluted seminiferous tubules are enclosed by a thick layer of basal lamina which is surrounded by 3 to 4 layers of smooth muscle cells (myoid cells) to support the basal lamina. The inside (lumen) of the tubules are lined by a layer of columnar epithelial cells. This layer consists of two types of cells. The majority of the cells are the spermatogenic cells. In between these spermatogenic cells are a few sertoli cells. The spermatogenic cells are arranged in four layers. These cells undergo the process of spermatogenesis and finally produce the spermatozoa, the male gametes (sperm cells). The sperms produced in the seminiferous tubules are transported through the tubuli recti and then the efferent ducts to the epididymis. The sertoli cells provide the mechanical and nutritive support to the spermatogenic cells. The interstitial tissue between the seminiferous tubules contains loose connective tissue, fibroblasts, vessels, nerves and lymphatics. Most importantly here lies the bunch of Leydig cells. These cells synthesize and secrete the hormones androgen and the cholesterol which generates testosterone, the primary male sex hormone that helps in developing and maintaining the functions of male reproductive organs.

Epididymis

The epididymis is a tubular structure attached to the caudal border of the testis. Its upper end is enlarged and is called the **head** of epididymis, the middle portion is the **body** and the lower end is the **tail** of epididymis. While travelling through the epididymis, the spermatozoa (sperms) obtain the capacity to be fertile, gain the ability to swim and are more concentrated for storage. The sperms are stored in the end portion the tail of the epididymis. The epididymis continues into the ductus deferens.

Ductus deferens

The ductus deferens (vas deferens) connects the epididymis with the pelvic part of the urethra. It begins at the tail of the epididymis, becomes part of the spermatic cord, gains entry into the abdominal cavity through the inguinal canal, runs caudally between the urinary bladder and the rectum and finally join the pelvic part of the urethra. During its course in the pelvic cavity, the wall of the ductus deferens is pierced by the ducts of the prostate, seminal vesicles and bulbourethral glands which pour the secretion of these glands into the ductus deferens. Inside the ductus deferens these secretions get them mixed with the sperms flowing through the ductus deferens and form the semen as described earlier in this chapter.

Accessory genital glands

The accessory genital glands (accessory sex glands) include the seminal vesicles, the prostate gland and the bulbourethral glands. The **seminal vesicle**s are paired elongated piriform glands which lie on each side of the caudal part of dorsal surface of the urinary bladder ventral to the rectum. The excretory duct of each of these glands passes under the prostrate gland and join the ductus deferens of the respective side before the later open in the urethra. The **prostate gland** is single and lobulated. It lies transversely on the dorsal part of the neck of the urinary bladder ventral to the rectum. It consists of two lateral lobes the right and the left and a transverse isthmus connecting the lateral lobes. The ventral or deep surface of the lobe lies in contact with the seminal vesicle of the corresponding side. Whereas, the dorsal surface of the globe along with the isthmus is covered by ventral surface of the rectum. The isthmus is a thin transverse band lying over the junction of the neck of the urinary bladder with the urethra. The secretion of the prostrate gland is carried by a series of 15 to 20 prostatic ducts which open into the urethra on respective side lateral to the seminal colliculus. The **bulbourethral glands (Cowper's glands)** are paired glands. These are situated on either side of the pelvic part of the urethra close to the ischial arch. These are ovoid in form some what depressed dorsoventrally and their long axis runs parallel to the urethra. The secretion of the bulbourethral glands is carried by about 6 to 8 ducts which open in series into the urethra on either side close to the median line of the urethra.

Penis

The penis is the external male genital organ and serves as an organ of copulation of male animals. It is cylindrical in form but in most of its length it is slightly compressed laterally. It extends craniad between the thighs from ischial arch to the umbilical region of abdomen. It is composed of the extra pelvic part of urethra which is essentially surrounded by sponge like erectile tissue richly invested by blood vessels that become filled with blood under pressure when the bull is sexually stimulated. The spongy erectile tissue is supported externally by the fascia and the skin. Grossly, the penis consists of three parts namely the root, body and glans. The **root** of the penis is attached to the ischial arch by two crura which converge and unite below the arch. The urethra passes over the ischial arch between the two crura, curves craniad and becomes incorporated into the substance of penis. The **body** of the penis begins at a junction of the crura and forms the bulk of the organ. In bovines it forms a 'S' shaped curve called sigmoid flexure just behind the scrotum. The glans of the penis is the tapering free end of the organ. It is pointed and twisted. It presents a groove in which the urethra opens and this opening is called the external urethral opening. The skin of the abdomen covering the penis extends beyond the length of the penis and forms a flap called **prepuce**. The **glans** is concealed inside this invaginated part of the skin. In the erectile condition the sigmoid flexure becomes unfolded, the penis lengthens and the glans emerges out from the prepuce.

Female genital system

Females not only contribute female sex cell (ovum / egg) for reproduction but also provides necessary support and environment in which the fertilized egg / embryo/ foetus develops. The overall functions of female reproductive system include (1) to produce female gametes (ova / eggs), (2) to produce hormones that are necessary for the control of activity of reproductive organs (3) to transport sperms through the female reproductive tract to the site of fertilization (4) to facilitate fertilization (5) to provide safe environment for embryo and foetus to grow and develop (6) to give birth to the offspring (7) to recycle for another pregnancy and (8) to nourish the offspring during early days of its life. These functions are performed by the primary and secondary organs of female reproductive system. The primary organs of reproduction are a pair of ovaries and they produce not only ova but also the hormones required for normal sexual behaviour of females. The secondary organs of reproduction are a pair of oviducts (fallopian tubes), the uterus, the cervix, the vagina and the vulva. The mammary glands are also considered as secondary sex organs as they are closely related to the completion of reproduction by the nourishment of young one.

Ovaries

The ovary is the female gonad homologous to male gonad the testis. It produces ovum (egg) the female gamete. It is a paired organ (gland) in most of the animals, but in birds only left ovary is present. Both the ovaries are ellipsoidal or oval in shape and their size is almost like that of almond. The size and shape of the ovary varies with the species and the stage of oestrus. The outer surface of the ovary is irregular because of the projection of the developing follicles and corpora lutea in the cortex. In bovines, both the ovaries are suspended from the mesovarium attached to the broad ligament of the uterus at the level of a little above the middle of the pelvic inlet in the abdominal cavity. The ovary is composed of the cortex and the medulla. The medulla contains vessels that nourish the follicles and other structures of the cortex. The cortex contains a stroma of connective tissue infiltrated by oocytes and the follicles at different stages of development. After the ovulation or rupture of the matured follicle, the ovum (egg) is released from the ovary and it is captured into the funnel like opening the infundibulum of the oviduct lying just below the ovary. The ovary secretes two hormones, oestrogens and progesterone that are vital for normal reproductive development and fertility. The oestrogens include the estradiol, estron and estriol. These substances are secreted by the granular tissue of the developing follicles of the ovary. These hormones work together to promote the healthy development of female sex characteristics during puberty and to ensure fertility. These are instrumental in the development of mammary glands and the other primary and accessory reproductive organs. In the event of ovulation, the fully developed graffian follicle ruptures, the egg migrates down the fallopian tube and the ruptured GF becomes the corpus luteum. This corpus luteum turns into the temporary gland for sometime and secretes the hormone progesterone. The progesterone prepares the body for pregnancy by causing the uterine lining to thicken. If the egg is not fertilized, the corpus luteum disappears.

Oviduct

The oviduct is a tube that connects the ovary to the uterus. There are two oviducts the left and the right oviduct which are suspended from the abdominal wall by mesosalpinx attached to the broad ligament of the uterus. Through these tubes the ovulated oocyte (egg) travels down to become fertilized by sperms present in this tube. The oviduct has three parts, the infundibulum, the ampulla and the isthmus. The **infundibulum** is funnel shaped enlarged cranial end of the oviduct. It is not directly connected to ovary. The margin of the tube at this end is irregular and is divided into several thin strips called the fimbrae. Some of these fimbrae get attached to the external connective tissue covering of the ovary, whereas, the rest of the part of the infundibulum opens into the peritoneal cavity through the opening called the ostium abdominale tubae. The **ampulla** is the longest part of the oviduct occupying about more than half of its total length, and also has the largest diameter. This part is the site for fertilization. It is distinguished by numerous mucosal folds. The **isthmus** is the caudal end of oviduct and is joined to the uterus (horn of the uterus) through the opening called the ostium uterinum tubae at the uterotuberal junction. The folded mucosa of the isthmus serves as the functional reservoir for sperms in the female tract. The sperms are released from the isthmus mucosa by the action of parocrine signals from an ovum travelling down the oviduct.

Uterus

The uterus is hollow muscular organ of the female reproductive system that is responsible for the development of embryo and foetus during pregnancy. It is incredibly distensible organ that can expand during pregnancy from around a size of a closed fist to large enough to hold a full term foetus. In general the size of uterus varies with the breed, age, and the stage of pregnancy. In adult bovines it is located almost entirely within the abdominal cavity. It is suspended in the body cavity by the broad ligaments which are attached to the pelvic and abdominal walls. The uterus consists of two long horns (cornua), a short body and a neck (cervix). The **horns** of the uterus extend cranially from the body of the uterus. Immediately after leaving the body of the uterus, both the horns run parallel and close to each other for some distance. In this part they are united by muscular and connective tissue and are commonly covered by peritoneal fold along with the body of the uterus. Because of this the horns appear shorter than their actual length whereas, the body of the uterus appears longer than its actual size. After this part, both the horns run outward and forward. As they run forward they tapper gradually and join the uterus so that the diameter of the horns and that of the body of uterus becomes almost equal. The free part of each horn forms spiral coil before joining the body of uterus of the respective side. The **body** of the uterus lies partly in the abdomen and partly in the pelvic cavity between the rectum dorsally and urinary bladder ventrally. It is cylindrical in shape but slightly compressed dorsoventrally. The cranial part of the body of the uterus from where the horns extend is wide and is called as fundus. The **cervix** is a sphincter like structure with a thick wall and narrow lumen. The lumen of the cervix is tightly closed except during oestrus and parturition. It forms a barrier between the uterus and the external environment. At the level of cervix, the ventral part of the uterus is almost completely fused with vagina whereas, its dorsal part projects into the cavity of the vagina in such a way that it encloses a deep groove between the dorsal wall of uterus and the vagina. This groove is called the fornix vaginae. The wall of the uterus consists of three layers the outer perimetrium made of connective tissue, the middle myometrium made of smooth muscle and the inner endometrium made of mucosa. It is studded with uterine glands. The endometrium of the uterine body bears numerous round button like elevations called caruncles. During pregnancy the caruncles attach to the cotyledons of the foetal membrane that surrounds the developing foetus. These attachments furnish sites for nourishing the foetus. The uterus plays many important functions in the reproductive process. (1) It is considered the organ of pregnancy because the foetus is housed, protected and nourished within this organ throughout the period of pregnancy. (2) The contractile muscles and secretary glands of the uterine wall assist in sperm viability and transportation to encounter and hopefully to fertilize the egg (3) The contractility of uterine muscles help to expel the foetus and foetal membranes during the calving process and (4) The secretary glands secret hormones such as prostaglandins which are required for maintaining preimplantation embryo.

Vagina

The vagina continues the female reproductive tract caudally behind the uterus. It constitutes the part of the female reproductive tract between the cervix and the vulva. It is the female copulatary organ. It extends from the ostium of the uterus to the external urethral opening. It is long and thin walled. It is located in the median position within the pelvic cavity between the rectum dorsally and urinary bladder with urethra ventrally. It is mostly retroperitoneal, but in some cases its cranial part may be covered by peritoneum. The cervix of the uterus projecting into the lumen of vagina restricts its cranial part to a ring like space the **fornix**. The part of the vagina extending from the external urethral opening to the vulva is called the vaginal **vestibule**. This part acts as a common passage for the urinary and reproductive tracts. It slopes down behind the ischial arch and opens into the vulva. The wall of the vestibule contains vestibular glands. Secretions from these glands keep the mucosa of the vestibule moist and facilitate coitus and parturition. At oestrus, the odour of these secretions sexually stimulates the male.

Vulva

The vulva is the external opening of the reproductive tract and is formed by two muscular folds the labia (lips) which meet with each other at the dorsal and ventral commissures surrounding the vertical slit called the vulval opening caudal to ischial arch. The dorsal commissure is rounded while the ventral commissure is pointed. The mucous membrane of the vagina continues over the vulva to line it internally and further behind this it terminates by joining the dermal layer that covers the external surface of the vulva.

Clitoris

The clitoris is the homologue of penis of male in the female animals. It lies within a fossa in the ventral commissure of the vulva and is largely covered by a mucosal fold which is a female equivalent of prepuce of male. The clitoris consists of a body and a glans (glans clitoris). The body has two crura, the right and the left. These are attached to the pelvic arch. The two crura come together to form the body. The glans is the only exposed part of the clitoris.

Mammary glands

The mammary glands are considered as the main external genital organ in female animals since these perform the major role of nourishing the offspring immediately after birth. The number, location and form of mammary glands vary from species to species. These are most developed in bovines where the glands of the opposite side join to form a single apparatus the udder. (The anatomy of udder is described in detail in the regional anatomy part).

SECTION- C

ENDOCRINE SYSTEM

The endocrine system is an organ system of the body which consists of a network of endocrine glands distributed throughout the body of the animal. The endocrine glands are ductless glands which secrete the substances called hormones and release them directly into the blood stream. In addition to being ductless, the endocrine glands are characterized by some other common features such as vascularity and presence of intracellular vacuoles and granules for the storage of hormones secreted by the cells of these glands. The hormones are biochemical substances secreted by the endocrine glands which are directly released into blood stream. The blood stream in turn transports these hormones across the entire body and delivers them at distant target cells of specific organs of the body. This is unlike the secretion of exocrine glands the secretions of which are released and carried away in the ducts of those glands at the target site. The hormones secreted by the endocrine glands accomplish various vital functions such as regulation of the growth of the body, metabolic activities and development and functioning of sexual activities. The main endocrine glands of the body are the pituitary, pineal, thyroid, parathyroid, adrenals, pancreas, testes and ovaries.

8

Endocrine Organs

Pituitary gland

The pituitary gland (hypophysis) lies at the base of the skull and is housed within a bony structure called the sella turcica in the body of the basisphenoid bone. It is a small pea shaped gland which is attached to the hypothalamus by the pituitary stalk. The pituitary gland has two distinct parts called the lobes. These are the anterior lobe (adenohypophysis) and the posterior lobe (neurohypophysis). The anterior lobe which is also called as anterior pituitary consists of five types of cells, each of which secretes different hormone or hormones. The types of cells, the hormones secreted by each type and the functions performed by them are narrated below.

1. The thyrotrophs secrete thyroxin called as Thyroid Stimulating Hormone (TSH). It stimulates production of thyroid hormone.

2. The gonadotrophs secrete leuteinizing hormone (LH) and Follicle Stimulating Hormone (FSH). The LH stimulates the production of oestrogen and progesterone by the ovaries in female and testosterone by the testes in male. The FSH stimulates the production of oestrogen and the growth of egg cells (oocytes) in the ovaries in female and sperm cells (spermatozoa) in the testes in male.

3. The corticotrophs secrete the Adreno-Cortico-Trophic Hormone (ACTH) which stimulates the production of cortisol and adrenogenic hormones by the adrenal cortex.

4. The somatotrophs secret Growth Hormone (GH). The GH is a growth promoting hormone which regulates the growth and differentiation of the skeletal system.

5. The lactotrophs secrete the Prolactine Hormone. The prolactine hormone is responsible for initiation of milk secretion by the acinar cells of the mammary gland.

The posterior lobe of pituitary which is also called as posterior pituitary is composed of the endings of the nerve cells located in specialized regions of the hypothalamus. These nerve cells produce two hormones the oxytocin and vasopressin. These hormones are carried down the nerves and are stored in the nerve ending that comprise the posterior pituitary. These hormones are released into the circulation in response to the nerve signals that originate in the hypothalamus and are transmitted to the posterior pituitary. The oxytocin causes contraction of uterus for parturition and milk secretion in females. The vasopressin increases reabsorption of water from the kidneys and raises blood pressure.

Thus the hormones secreted and released by the pituitary gland play an active part in controlling the activities of most of the other endocrine glands of the body. Hence, the pituitary gland is called as master gland of the endocrine system. However, some times the hormone secretion of the pituitary gland itself is controlled by the hypothalamus which lies just above the pituitary gland.

Pineal gland

The pineal gland is a small organ shaped like a pine cone (hens the name pineal). It is a rice grain sized gland located on the midline attached to the caudal end of the roof of the third ventricle between the two hemispheres tucked in a groove where the two halves of the thalamus join near the corpora quadrigemina. It is reddish grey in colour. The pineal gland is composed of the cells called pinealocytes and the glial cells. The pinealocytes secrete the hormone melatonin which affects the modulation of sleep pattern. The production of melatonin by the pineal gland is stimulated by darkness and inhibited by light. The pineal gland influences the pituitary gland secretion of sex hormones FSH and LH.

Thyroid gland

The thyroid gland is a pale or dark red butterfly shaped gland located on the cranial part of the trachea especially the first two tracheal rings or the laryngotracheal joint. It consists of two lateral flattened triangular lobes which are connected by a thin transverse strip of glandular tissue called isthmus across the ventral surface of the trachea. The lobes as well as the isthmus consist of numerous globular sacs called follicles. Each follicle is bounded by a single layer of epithelial cells (follicular cells) and a basement membrane surrounding a central lumen filled with a homogenous protein rich colloid (thyroglobulin). The colloid is a store of the thyroid hormones prior to secretion. When thyroid hormones are needed, the thyroglobulin is reabsorbed into the follicular cells from the colloid of the follicular lumen. In the cells, the thyroglobulin splits into its component parts including the two thyroid hormones, Thyroxin (T4) and Triiodothyronin (T3) which are released in to the circulation. Within the connective tissue, close to the follicles are 'C' shaped cells which are also called as parafollicular cells. They are found in clusters in the interfollicular space. These cells secrete the hormone calcitonin which acts to lower the plasma calcium level.

Parathyroid gland

The parathyroids are four small glands arranged in two pairs as cranial (external) and caudal (internal) closely associated with the left and right lateral lobes of the thyroid gland. The glands of the cranial pair are usually located cranial to the lobes of the thyroid gland. Each of these glands is yellowish brown flat ovoid or elongated in shape and appears like a lentil seed. Many times these are embedded in the surrounding connective tissue of the adjacent glands. The glands of the caudal pair are smaller than those of the cranial pair. These are located in the connective tissue close to the caudal edge of the lobes of the thyroid gland. These glands are often embedded in the tissue of the dorsal or tracheal surface of the isthmus of the thyroid gland; The parathyroid glands are quite easily recognizable from the thyroid gland as they have densely packed cells in contrast with the follicular structure of the thyroid. Two unique types of cells are present in the parathyroid glands. These are the chief cells and the oxyphil cells. The chief cells are small. They synthesize, secrete and release parathyroid hormone. These cells appear dark when loaded with parathyroid hormone and clear when the hormone has been secreted or when the cells are in their resting stage. The oxyphil cells which are lighter in appearance and increase in number with age have an unknown function. The main function of the parathyroid glands is to maintain the body's calcium and phosphate levels within a normal range so that the muscular and nervous systems can function properly. The parathyroid glands do this by secreting parathyroid hormone. The parathyroid hormone (parathormone) is a small protein that takes part in the control of calcium and phosphate homeostasis as well as bone physiology. Parathormone has the effects antagonistic to those of calcitonin.

Adrenal gland

The adrenal (suprarenal) gland is an important organ in adaptation to stress and to maintain homeostasis. It is a paired gland. Each is closely applied to the cranial pole of the kidney of the respective side. The right and left adrenal differs in shape, size and exact location in bovines. The right adrenal is somewhat triangular and is applied to the medial surface of the cranial pole of right kidney. It is slightly lighter in weight than that of the left adrenal. The left adrenal gland is nearly 'C' shaped. It is situated medial to the caudal vena cava approximately on the midline just behind the cranial mesenteric artery. The adrenal gland consists of the cortex and the medulla. The cortex is the outer larger part and it occupies about 80 to 90 per cent of the gland while the medulla is the inner smaller part occupying only 10 to 20 per cent of the gland.

The **adrenal cortex** is red to light brown in colour and is composed of three zones. All the three zones produce hormones derived from cholesterol which is abundant in these cells.

(1) **Zona Glomeruloza** is the outer zone. The cells of this zone secrete aldosteron which is concerned with electrolytes and fluid homeostasis which is required for maintaining the blood pressure.

(2) **Zona Fasciculata** is the middle zone. The cells of this zone secrete glucocorticoides which control metabolism of lipid, protein and carbohydrate.

(3) **Zona Reticularis** is the inner zone. The cells of this zone are concerned with sex hormones that supplements gonadal sex hormone secretion.

The secretion of all these hormones by the cells of three zones of adrenal cortex is controlled by ACTH of the anterior pituitary gland.

The **adrenal medulla** is in the centre of the adrenal gland. The cells of the adrenal medulla secrete the hormones adrenalin and noradrenalin. The secretion of these hormones by the cells of adrenal medulla is under control of the sympathetic nervous system.

Pancreas

The pancreas is an oblong shaped tubuloalveolar pinkish red gland. It is situated in the first curve of the duodenum. It is a mixed type of gland with duel functions the exocrine and endocrine. Consequently it has two types of tissues the exocrine tissue and endocrine tissue. The exocrine tissue occupies the greater part spread all over the gland. It is arranged in the form of numerous acinae surrounded by reticular fibres received from the connective tissue capsule of the gland. The cells of the exocrine part secrete digestive enzymes. This secretion is collected and carried through pancreatic duct that discharge this secretion into the duodenum of the small intestine.

The endocrine part of the gland consists of small irregular shaped clusters of cells. These clusters of endocrine tissue are scattered embedded in the connective tissue in between the acini of the exocrine tissue and appear like islands. Hence are called the islets of Langerhans. Each islet is composed of two to three thousand epithelial cells. These cells are arranged in compact structure that is richly supplied with capillary network. A thin layer of reticular fibres separate the islets from the surrounding exocrine tissue. There are four types of cells in the islets of Langerhans. Each of these secretes a different type of hormone.

1. The **alpha cells or 'A' cells**. These cells are located at the periphery of the islet. These constitute about 20 per cent of the total cells of the islet. These cells produce glucagon hormone which is said to be antagonistic to insulin.
2. The **beta cells or 'B' cells**. These cells are predominant (about 70 per cent of the cells of each islet) and are located in the centre of the islet. These cells produce the hormone insulin. This hormone regulates the amount of glucose in the blood by increasing the rate at which the glucose is converted to glycogen in the liver and also regulates the movement of glucose from the blood into the cells. The insufficient production of insulin by these cells leads to the condition diabetes mellitus wherein the glucose level in the blood increases.
3. The **delta cells or 'D' cells** are in low numbers and are scattered between other cells of the islet. These cells produce somatostatin. This hormone helps in regulating and fine tuning the insulin and glucagon producing cells.
4. The **gamma cells or 'F' cells** occur occasionally in a few species of animals especially in dogs. These cells secrete pancreatic polypeptides. This hormone helps to control water absorption from the intestines by stimulating the intestinal cells to release water and salts into the intestines.

Testis (See under the chapter Male Genital System)

Ovary (See under the chapter Female Genital System)

SECTION- D

BLOOD VASCULAR SYSTEM (ANGIOLOGY)

The blood vascular (cardiovascular) system, also called as circulatory system is an organ system that enables blood to circulate and transport the blood cells, nutrients, oxygen and carbon dioxide, hormones and the metabolic wastes from the cells and tissues of the body. While circulating through the blood, the nutrients, oxygen and the hormones are supplied to the cells and tissues while the carbon dioxide and the metabolic wastes are released in to the blood by the cells and tissues to carry and get them discharged from the body through the organs like lungs and kidneys. In order to keep the flow of the blood constant the circulatory system has been provided with the channels called the vessels and a pump called the heart. The vessels that carry the blood from the heart to the cells of different organs and parts of the body are called the arteries, arterioles and capillaries depending on their size. The vessels that carry blood back from the cells of different organs and parts of the body to the heart are called the veins and venules. The excess blood plasma recycled and filtered at the interstitial fluid is called lymph. The lymph is carried back from the tissues through a separate system of channels called the lymph vessels. The lymph vessels from all over the body join the large vessel called the lymph duct which pours the lymph in the blood circulation by opening into the cranial vena cava. The major organ that pushes the blood through the vessels constantly with a specific pressure is the heart.

9

Heart and Pericardium

Heart

The heart is a cone shaped thick walled and four chambered muscular organ. It lies obliquely craniocaudal in the middle mediastinum in between the left and right lungs and is covered by pericardium inside the thoracic cavity. The major part of heart (about 60 per cent) lies to the left of the middle mediastinum. The broad upper end is the base of the heart. It lies at the junction of the dorsal and middle third of the dorsoventral diameter of thorax at the level of about third to sixth rib and it faces craniodorsally. The narrow lower end is the apex. It lies just dorsal to the sternum at the level of about sixth rib and it faces caudoventrally. The surfaces, right and left are convex. They meet cranially at the right ventricular border and caudally at the left ventricular border. The right (cranial) border is strongly convex. It runs ventrally and caudally. The greater part of this border lies parallel to the sternum. The left (caudal) border is much shorter and nearly vertical. The surfaces of the heart are marked by grooves which indicate the division of the heart into four chambers the two atria dorsally and the two ventricles ventrally. The atria are separated internally by the interatrial septum. The ventricles are separated by interventricular septum. The circular coronary groove indicates the division of the heart in to atria dorsally and ventricles ventrally. It encircles the heart in its upper third part except at the level of the origin of pulmonary artery. The coronary groove is quite deep and wide. It provides passage for the coronary artery and vein. Apart from these, it is deeply filled with fat. The right (subsinuosal) interventricular groove and left (paraconal) interventricular groove indicates the line of separation between the two (right and left) ventricles by the interventricular septum. Both of these grooves run downward from the coronary groove towards the apex parallel to the respective borders and terminate just above the apex. The right and left ventricular grooves are occupied by the respective coronary vessels along with the fat.

Pericardium

The pericardium is the serous membrane that surrounds and protects the heart. It is composed of two layers the visceral and parietal which are separated by a thin cavity. The visceral layer is firmly attached to the wall of the heart and forms its outermost layer the epicardium. The parietal layer of pericardium is composed of inelastic connective tissue. The cavity between the two layers contains a little volume of fluid the pericardial fluid. It serves as lubricant for minimizing the friction during the possible movement of heart inside the pericardium. The pericardium is fastened with the wall of the thoracic cavity by the sternopericardiac ligament that extends from the parietal layer of pericardium and terminates onto the dorsal (thoracic) surface of the sternum in cattle and horse. The ligament called the phrenopericadiac ligament extends from the parietal layer of pericardium and terminates on the tendinous part of the diaphragm in dog and swine.

10

Major Blood Vessels

The great vessels that leave and enter the chambers of the heart include the Aorta, the Pulmonary Artery and the Pulmonary Veins.

Aorta

The Aorta is the main systemic arterial trunk. It begins as **ascending aorta** at the base of the left ventricle, passes craniad and dorsad between the pulmonary artery on the left and the right atrium on the right and then turns caudad inclining slightly to the left, thus describing a curve called the aortic arch with its convexity directed upward and forward and the concavity facing downward and backward. From here it proceeds caudad on the ventrolateral surface of the thoracic vertebrae and the longus colli muscle as the **descending aorta**. At its origin from the base of left ventricle, the caliber of the aorta is greatest forming the **bulbus aorta** and here it presents three dilatations called the **aortic sinuses.** As the descending aorta reaches the level of the seventh thoracic vertebra it continues behind as **thoracic aorta** running through the middle and caudal mediastinum between the left and right lungs. The thoracic aorta first lies to the left of the median plane and then gradually inclines inwards medially and becomes median in position when it reaches to the diaphragm. It then passes through the hiatus aorticus of the diaphragm and enter the abdominal cavity as **abdominal aorta**. From here it passes caudad below the bodies of the lumbar vertebrae and the psoas major muscle. After reaching at the level of the sixth lumbar vertebra, the abdominal aorta terminates in the iliac quadrification by dividing into two external and two internal iliac arteries.

Pulmonary artery

The pulmonary artery arises from the right ventricle at the conus arteriosus. It curves dorsad and caudad and divides behind the aortic arch into right and left pulmonary arteries. It is related cranially to the right appendix auriculi, caudally to left appendix auriculi and medially to the aorta with which it is enclosed in a common sheath of the visceral part of the pericardium Near its termination into left and right branches, it is connected to the aorta by the ligamentum arteriosum, the remnant of the foetal ductus arteriosus. The right pulmonary artery is a little longer than the left one. It passes under the bifurcation of the trachea to the hilus of the lung and inside the organ it accompanies the bronchial tree on its ventral surface.

Pulmonary veins

There are about 4 to 6 pulmonary veins and these are devoid of valves. The capillaries arise from the plexus around the alveoli of the lungs, unite to form large branches accompanying the arterial branches on the ventral face of the bronchioles and finally form the pulmonary veins which open into the left atrium.

11

Lymphatic System

The lymphatic system is a part of circulatory system and a vital part of the body's immune system. It is comprised of lymph vessels, lymph ducts, and lymph nodes that move the lymph from tissues to the blood stream and the organs such as the spleen, thymus and bone marrow that produce the lymphocytes and white blood cells. Lymph is very similar to blood plasma. During circulation through the body, the blood reaches to the capillaries at the interstitial spaces. The plasma of the blood is filtered through the capillary wall. The fresh oxygen along with nutrients, hormones and other necessary fluid matters from this plasma are released in to the interstitial fluid and about 85 per cent of the plasma along with the carbon dioxide and metabolic wastes, return into the circulation through the capillary walls. The remaining 15 per cent of the plasma along with the debris of other waste products and the lymphocytes constitutes the lymph which is returned to the circulation through an accessory route of lymphatic vessels and lymph nodes constituting the lymphatic system.

Lymph Vessels: The lymph vessels start as finger-like blind ending thin walled lymph capillaries in the interstitial connective tissue. These capillaries form a network and drain into the thicker walled collecting lymph vessels, lymph ducts and lymphatic trunks. Finally the larger lymph trunks and ducts empty their content the lymph into the cranial vena cava at the thoracic inlet. The lymph vessels contain numerous valves with one or two leaflets preventing the back flow of lymph through the lymph vessels. During its course in a centripetal direction through the lymph vessel, the lymph of each lymph vessel has to pass through at least one lymph node prior to its entry into the blood circulation. As a result there lies a chain of lymph nodes on the pathway of lymph vessels in the body.

Lymph nodes: The lymph nodes are spherical, bean shaped or oval glandular structures presenting a hilus on its outer surface through which the afferent and efferent lymph vessels, the blood vessels and the nerves enter and leave the node. These nodes are located at intervals along the lymph vessels. Many of the lymph nodes are grouped as clusters in various regions of the body.

Each lymph node is an organized collection of lymphoid tissue through which the lymph passes on its way to the blood. The afferent lymph vessel brings in lymph which percolates through the substance of lymph node and is then drained out by an efferent lymph vessel. The substance of the lymph node consists of lymphoid follicles in an outer circle of the gland called the cortex. The lymph follicle is a dense collection of lymphocytes. Next to cortex towards the centre is the medulla and between the cortex and medulla is a thin coat called the paracortex. The external surface of the lymph node is covered by the connective tissue capsule consisting of elastic and smooth muscle fibres. From the capsule extend number of trabeculae and septi into the parenchyma of the lymph node. These trabeculae form a meshwork of connective tissue inside the parenchyma. Around the trabeculae and septi inside the parenchyma are developed lymph sinuses which separate the lymphoid tissue from the connective tissue. The afferent lymph vessels drain the contents into the lymph sinuses of the cortex which after circulating through the lymphoid follicles in the cortex pass on the medullary sinuses. From the medullary sinuses the lymph is carried away by the efferent lymph vessels to finally empty the lymph in the blood circulation. The lymph nodes are mainly concerned with the immunological function in the body.

The gross morphology of the major lymph ducts that include the right lymphatic duct and the thoracic duct and the large lymph glands that include the spleen and thymus is described in the concerned regional anatomy sections.

SECTION- E

NERVOUS SYSTEM

The nervous system is the part of the animal body that coordinates its voluntary and involuntary actions and transmits signals to and from different parts of the body. It is responsible for coordinating the diverse activities of the animal body. It not only controls the maintenance of normal functions of different systems and parts of the body but also responds to cope up with the emergency situations. There are three basic functions that are performed by the nervous system. These are the sensory, interpretative and motor functions.

1. The sensory nerves collect information from inside the body and the outside environment. The nerves then carry this information to central nervous system.
2. The sensory information brought to the central nervous system is processed and interpreted in the brain.
3. The information on resultant reaction as per interpretation is carried and conveyed by motor output to the concerned tissue, structure, organs or parts of the body.

In order to perform these functions, the nervous system is organized in two parts (1) the Central Nervous System and (2) the Peripheral Nervous System. **The central nervous system** consists of brain and spinal cord while the **peripheral nervous system** consists of the nerves connected to brain i.e. the cranial nerves and the nerves connected to the spinal cord i.e. the spinal nerves inclusive of the **autonomic nerves and ganglia.**

12

Central Nervous System

Brain

The brain, a command centre of the body, is a complex organ. The substance of the brain is made of the grey matter and the white matter. The grey matter is often identified as cerebral cortex but other parts of the brain also contain the grey matter. Inside the brain, the grey matter is organized into large accumulations of neurons which are called the nuclei of the brain. Each nucleus is associated with a specific function. In addition to neurons, there is other type of cells the glial cells called neuroglia. The neurons are responsible for sending and receiving impulses or signals. The glial cells are nonneuronal and provide support and nutrition to neuronal cells, form myelin and facilitate signal transmission in the nervous system. The white matter is made of millions of nerve fibres that are coming from neurons and are going to establish communications with different parts of the brain and spinal cord. Since these nerve fibres are coated with myelin sheath around them these appear white and the area occupied by these nerve fibres become the white matter of the brain.

The brain has three basic components, the forebrain, midbrain and the hindbrain.

Fore brain: The forebrain (**Prosencephalon)** is the rostral portion of the brain. It consists of cerebrum (**Telencephalon**) and the thalamus, hypothalamus and pineal gland together constituting the interbrain (**Diencephalon).**

Mid brain: The midbrain (**Mesencephalon**) is the middle portion of the brain. It is in the centre lying between the interbrain and hindbrain. It consists of a cranial part of brain stem.

Hind brain: The hindbrain (**Rhombencephalon)** is the caudal most portion of the brain. It consists of remaining (caudal) part of the brain stem, the medulla oblongata (**Myelencephalon**) and the cerebellum and pons (**Metencephalon).**

Cranial nerves

Twelve pairs of cranial nerves emerge from the ventral (basal) surface of the brain, pass through the openings (foramina) of the skull and lead to the parts of head, neck, and the body trunk. The cranial nerves with their nuclei within the brain stem contain sensory and motor neuron components. The sensory fibre components have their cell bodies located in ganglia located outside the brain and the motor fibre components have their cell bodies located within the brain. Hence some of the cranial nerves are sensory nerves, some are motor nerves and some other nerves are mixed nerves with both, the sensory as well as motor fibres. The cranial nerves are named and numbered based on their location from the front to back of the brain. Thus the olfactory is the first and the hypoglossal is the twelfth cranial nerve. Accordingly the first to twelfth cranial nerves are numbered, named and classified (functional type) as below.

Sr. No. of Cr. Nerve	Attachment with brain	Name of the nerve	Type of the nerve
I	Fore brain	Olfactory	Sensory
II	Fore brain	Optic	Sensory
III	Mid brain	Oculomotor	Motor
IV	Mid brain	Trochlear	Motor
V	Hind brain	Trigeminal	Mixed
VI	Hind brain	Abducent	Motor
VII	Hind brain	Facial	Mixed
VIII	Hind brain	Vestibulocochlear	Sensory
IX	Hind brain	Glossopharyngeal	Mixed
X	Hind brain	Vagus	Mixed
XI	Hind brain	Accessory	Motor
XII	Hind brain	Hypoglossal	Motor

Spinal cord

The spinal cord is a vital link between the brain and the body. It is a mass of nervous tissue arranged in a cylindrical form of structure that is enclosed inside the vertebral canal extending from the level of the foramen magnum of the occipital bone of the skull to the level of last but one lumbar vertebra or the middle of the sacrum. It is a part of central nervous system that continues rostrally with the medulla oblongata without any natural line of demarcation between the two. Behind the medulla it descends down the vertebral canal inside which it is protected and surrounded by the bony vertebral column. Throughout its length it is cylindrical but compressed dorsoventrally with uniform diameter except at two places where it is enlarged. These enlargements are called as cervical (cervicothoracic) and lumbar (lumbosacral) enlargements from where the nerves for the fore limbs and hind limbs extend from the spinal cord. The caudal part of the spinal cord rapidly narrows to a point that is called conus medullaris. The conus medullaris is prolonged for a short distance by a slender filament of pia matter called the filum terminale.

The dorsal and ventral surfaces of the spinal cord are divided in the middle by a dorsal median groove and the ventral groove respectively. On either side of the dorsal median groove are the dorsal lateral grooves where the dorsal root fibres of the spinal nerves enter the cord. The ventral root fibres of the spinal nerves leave the cord a little lateral to the ventral median groove. The dorsal median groove is filled up by the dorsal median septum. The ventral median groove is narrow and deep and reaches to about the middle of the cord. The two halves of the cord are connected by commissures of grey and white matter. The grey commissure is a transverse band at the base of the dorsal median septum and is traversed by the central canal of the spinal cord. The white commissure is a bridge of white matter that connects the two ventral columns of the white matter. The central column opens rostrally into the caudal angle of the fourth ventricle of the brain and caudally it ends in the conus medullaris forming a slight dilation, the ventricularis terminalis..

The transverse section of spinal cord shows white matter in the periphery, grey matter inside and a tiny canal filled with cerebrospinal fluid at the centre. Surrounding the canal is a single layer of cells the ependymal layer. Surrounding the ependymal layer is the grey matter the area that appears like a letter ‘H’ or like a butterfly. The two wings of the butterfly are connected across the midline by the dorsal grey commissure and below it is the white commissure. The grey matter mainly contains the cell bodies of neurons and neuroglia. Each wing has four columns, the dorsal horn, intermediate column, lateral column and the ventral horn. The dorsal horn is comprised of sensory nuclei that receive and process incoming somatosensory information. From here the ascending projections emerge to transmit the sensory information to the mid brain and diencephalon. The intermediate column and the lateral horn comprise autonomic neurons innervating the visceral and pelvic organs. The ventral horn comprises motor neurons that innervate the skeletal muscles. The white matter of the spinal cord is arranged in the ascending and descending nerve tracts.

There are 37 pairs of spinal nerves that arise from the lateral aspect of the spinal cord and they are classified as eight cervical, thirteen thoracic, six lumbar, five sacral and five coccygeal. According to the attachment of these nerves to the cord the spinal cord is considered of having five regions as cervical, thoracic, lumbar, and sacral. As a result of unequal growth of the spinal cord and the vertebral column, correspondence between the two is unmatched and the spinal nerves have to travel a short distance caudad before they gain exit from the canal. The conus medularis reaches only up to the mid sacral level, and hence the rest of the sacral and all the coccygeal nerves occupy the whole vertebral canal before the exit of these nerves through their corresponding intervertebral foramen. As a result, a bundle of the spinal nerves along with the conus medularis and filum terminale in the middle of the bunch inside the sacral part of the vertebral canal appears like a horse tail and hence it is called the cauda equina.

The white matter is divided into three pairs of columns. The dorsal column lies on either side of the dorsal median septum and is laterally limited by the dorsal lateral groove. The ventral column lies on either side of the ventral median septum and is limited laterally by the ventral root fibres. The lateral column lies laterally between the dorsal and the ventral column. The columns of the left and right side are connected to each other through the white commisssure.

Spinal nerves

Each spinal nerve is attached to the spinal cord by two roots, a dorsal root which is a sensory root and a ventral root which is a motor root. The dorsal root is larger than the ventral root. The dorsal root fibres (motor fibres) enter the spinal cord at the dorsal lateral groove. On the course of this root, there is a ganglion called the spinal ganglion. This ganglion is located either near the inner opening of the interventricular foramen or inside that foramen. Beyond this ganglion, the fibres of the dorsal root join those of the ventral root. The spinal ganglia are external to dura matter. The ventral root fibres are efferent or motor. They contain less fibres than the dorsal root. The fibres of this root arise from the ventral horn cells of the grey matter, pass through the white matter, leave the spinal cord at its ventrolateral edge and then join the fibres of the dorsal root.

Immediately after leaving the spinal cord, the two roots join to form the spinal nerve. Each nerve gets exit through the intervertebral foramen, gives off a small meningeal branch which is joined by a bundle of nerve fibres from sympathetic trunk that enter the vertebral canal through the intervertebral foramen. Each spinal nerve, then divides into dorsal and ventral primary branches. The dorsal branches are distributed to the muscles and skin of the dorsal part of the body. The ventral branches supply in general to the muscles and skin of the ventral parts of the body including the limbs. Each nerve or its ventral branch is connected with its adjacent ganglion of the sympathetic by a communicating branch called the ramus communicans.

Meninges

Meninges are the fibrous membranes which enclose and protect the brain and spinal cord. There are three layers of meninges, the duramater, arachnoid and the piamater. The duramater is the outer most covering, the arachnoid is the middle layer and the piamater is the innermost layer closely adhering the brain and spinal cord. The meninges covering the brain are called the cranial meninges whereas those surrounding the spinal cord are called spinal meninges. However, the cranial and spinal meninges are continuous with each other at the foramen magnum.

13

Peripheral Nervous System

Peripheral nerves

The peripheral nervous system (PNS) is the part of the nervous system that lies outside the brain and spinal cord. It includes cranial nerves, spinal nerves and their roots and branches, peripheral nerves and neuromuscular junctions. In the peripheral nervous system, bundles of nerve fibres or axons conduct information to and from the central nervous system. The primary role of the peripheral nervous system is to connect the central nervous system to the bones, muscles and skin of the body trunk and the limbs and the organs to allow the complex movements and behaviour.

The **peripheral nervous system** is divided into the somatic nervous system and the autonomic (visceral) nervous system.

The **somatic nervous system** is associated with skeletal muscle voluntary control of body movents. It consists of afferent and efferent nerves. Afferent nerves are concerned with relaying sensation from the body to the central nervous system. The efferent nerves are responsible for sending out commands from central nervous system to the body, stimulating muscle contraction. This system is made up of nerves that connect to the skin, sensory organs and all skeletal muscles.

The **autonomic nervous system** is the part of peripheral nervous system that controls the visceral functions which occur below the level of consciousness. It consists of two divisions, the sympathetic nervous system and the parasympathetic nervous system.

The **sympathetic nervous system** is an aggregation of nerves, ganglia and plexuses through which the viscera, glands, blood vessels and the smooth muscles receive innervation. The most prominent feature of the sympathetic nervous system is a pair of ganglionated chain of sympathetic trunk extending from the cranial cervical ganglion at the base of the head, passing behind through the neck, thorax and abdomen on the ventrolateral surface of the vertebral column on either (left and right) side. Each sympathetic trunk is composed of a series of ganglia connected with each other by short nerve strands. Each of the thoracic and lumbar spinal nerves is connected with the respective paravertebral sympathetic ganglion of the sympathetic trunk by way of the white rami communicantes. Through these rami, it receives preganglionic nerve fibres (axons) whose cell bodies (neurons) are located in the intermediolateral mass of the gray horn of the spinal cord in the thoracic and upper lumbar region. Because of this, the sympathetic nervous system is also termed as thoracolumbar nervous system. The white rami communicantes conduct preganglionic fibres from spinal nerves to these ganglia. The gray rami communicantes (nonmyelinated fibres) pass from the sympathetic ganglia over the spinal nerves as post ganglionic fibres for peripheral distribution. The post ganglionic fibres extending from the paravertebral sympathetic chain ganglia run over the major blood vessels in the thoracic, abdominal and pelvic viscera. These fibres form the visceral (autonomic) plexuses along with the parasympathetic nerve fibres on the major blood vessels. Through these autonomic plexuses the sympathetic and parasympathetic nerve fibres are supplied to the thoracic, abdominal and pelvic viscera. The head region receives its sympathetic fibres from the cranial cervical ganglion as post ganglionic sympathetic nerve fibres which reach the cranial nerves by way of internal carotid nerve and then are distributed to various parts in the head region following the blood vessels or straight way joining the last four cranial nerves.

The **parasympathetic nervous system** is also involuntary and acts with the sympathetic system to maintain body homeostasis. The parasympathetic fibres begin in the central nervous system. The nerves supplying the head and neck are situated within four nuclei located within the brain stem. Each nucleus is associated with a cranial nerve. These nerves include the occulomotor, facial, glossopharyngeal and the vagus nerves. These nerves carry the parasympathetic fibres out of the brain. In addition to these, the visceral efferent fibres originating in the sacral part of the spinal cord also constitutes the parasympathetic nervous system. Because of this, the parasympathetic nervous system is also termed as the craniosacral nervous system. The parasympathetic preganglionic fibres leave the spinal cord as part of the ventral roots of the sacral nerves and participate in the formation of autonomic plexuses in the pelvic cavity.

After leaving the brain, the parasympathetic fibres from each nucleus synapse in a peripheral ganglion. These ganglia are typically located near to the target viscera. From these peripheral ganglia, the postganglionic parasympathetic fibres continue to the organs in the head and neck region. There are four parasympathetic ganglia located within the head region. These are the ciliary, otic, pterygopalatine and the submandibular. They receive fibres from occulomotor, facial and the glossopharyngeal nerves. The vagus nerve innervates the structures in the thorax and the abdomen. Most of these parasympathetic ganglia are associated with the sensory and sympathetic fibres also. However, these sensory and sympathetic fibres do not synapse in these ganglia. They merely travel through these ganglia.

The details of the autonomic (sympathetic and parasympathetic) nerves, ganglia and the plexuses in different regions of the animal body are described in the respective regional anatomy sections of this book.

SECTION- F

SENSE ORGANS AND COMMON INTEGUMENT

The sense organs are the organs of the body that respond to external stimuli by conveying impulses to the nervous system. The sense organs allow animals to sense changes in the environment around them and in their bodies so that they can respond properly. Animals can sense a wide range of stimuli that include the sense of vision, the sense of hearing, the sense of olfaction (smell), the sense of taste and the sense of touch including pain and pressure. In animals, there are two major groups of senses. These are the general senses and the special senses.

14

Organs of General and Special Senses

The sense organs are the organs of the body that respond to external stimuli by conveying impulses to the nervous system. The sense organs allow animals to sense changes in the environment around them and in their bodies so that they can respond properly. Animals can sense a wide range of stimuli that include the sense of vision, the sense of hearing, the sense of olfaction (smell), the sense of taste and the sense of touch including pain and pressure. In animals, there are two major groups of senses, the general senses and the special senses.

The general senses include the sense of touch, pressure, pain, and temperature that are distributed fairly evenly through the skin all over the body. Some of these are found in muscles and joints also.

The special senses include the sense of sight, hearing and balance, smell, and taste. The sense organs that include eye, ear, nose, tongue and skin (common integument) help to protect the body. These sense organs contain receptors that relay information through sensory neurons to the appropriate places within the nervous system. There are two types of receptors (1) the general receptors that are found through out the body because they are present in skin, muscles, joints and visceral organs and (2) The special receptors that include chemoreceptores (chemical receptors) found in the mouth (tongue) and nose, photoreceptors (light receptors) found in the eyes and the mechanoreceptors that are found in the ears.

Gross anatomical features of different organs of general and special senses are described under the "Anatomy of head and neck"

PART 1.2: ANATOMY OF HEAD AND NECK

SECTION-A
MUSCULO-SKELETAL COMPONENT

15

Skeleton of Head (SKULL)

The bones of skull (Fig 2-1) are divided into two groups, as cranial group of bones and facial group of bones. Most of the bones of the skull are flat bones and a few are irregular bones.

Cranial bones

The cranial bones form the cranium that encloses and protects the brain and organs of special senses e.g. eye and ear. These bones include the occipital, sphenoid, ethmoid, inter-parietal, parietal, temporal and frontal. The first four of these bones are single and the rests are paired.

Occipital

The occipital is a single bone (Fig 2 -1C) and is situated on the caudo- dorsal aspect of the skull. It consists of three parts, the lateral parts are called lateral occipital, the basal part is called the basi occipital and the dorsal (squamous) part is called the squamous occipital.

Lateral Occipital: It consists of two lateral parts, the right and the left lying on the respective side of the foramen magnum through which the brain continues behind into spinal cord. Each of the lateral parts consists of a condyle and a process called the paramastoid (jugular) process. The condyles articulate with the first cervical vertebra, the atlas. External to the condyle is a paramastoid (jugular) process which provides attachment for the muscles of the head and neck. Between the condyle and the jugular process is the condyloid fossa. Within the condyloid fossa is the hypoglossal foramen through which the XII cranial (hypoglossal) nerve exits from the cranium.

Basi occipital: The basal part is a wide, thick, strong bar of the bone that lodges the pons and medulla oblongata of the brain on its cranial surface. At its junction with the sphenoid bone, externally it presents a tubercle called the basilar tubercle which serves for muscular attachment. The lateral borders of the basi occipital forms the medial border of the foramen lacerum which serves

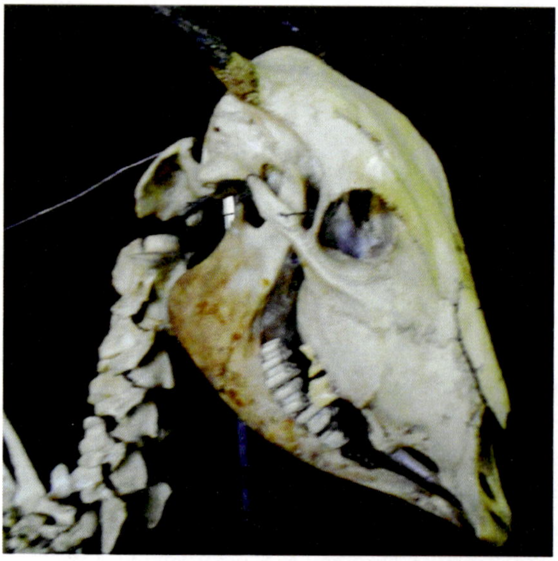

Fig. 2–1: Skeleton of Head and Neck of Ox

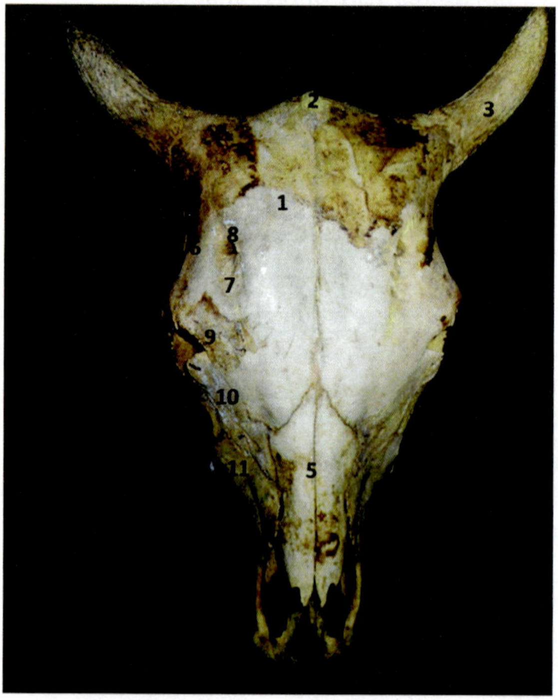

Fig 2-1 A. Skull of Ox; Dorsal View

1.Frontal bone; 2. Torus frontalis; 3. Cornual process; 4. Frontal suture; 5. Nasal bone; 6. Frontal crest; 7. Supraorbital canal; 8. Supraorbital foramen; 9. Orbital rim; 10. Lacrimal; 11. Maxilla; 12. Premaxilla; 13. Palatine fissure.

as passage for the cranial nerves IX (glossopharyngeal), X (vagus) and XI (accessory). The condyles of the lateral occipital and the dorsal border of the basi occipital form the foramen magnum.

Squamous occipital: The squamous part of the occipital bone is a quadrilateral plate of bone. Its external surface presents a strong protuberance for the attachment of ligamentum nuchae. The cranial surface of this bone is flat and smooth. It forms the roof of the cerebellar compartment of the cranial cavity. It meets the parietals and inter-parietal in front, lateral occipitals behind and the temporals laterally.

Sphenoid

The sphenoid bone (Fig. 2-1 C) is a single bone situated at the base of the cranium in front of the basi occipital. It has two parts, the basi sphenoid and the presphenoid.

Basi sphenoid: The basi sphenoid has a body, two wings and two sphenoidal processes. The body is cylindrical but flattened dorsoventrally. It is placed medially between the basilar part of occipital bone caudally and the body of presphenoid cranially. The external surface presents, closed to its junction with the wings, a groove called the vidian groove for the passage of vidian nerve. The internal or the cerebral surface presents a depression, the sella tursica, which lodges the hypophysis cerebri. The wings diverge outward from the body. Each wing is perforated in the middle by foramen ovale for the passage of ventral maxillary nerve and the middle meningeal artery. The cerebral surface presents a longitudinal groove leading to foramen orbitorotundum. The dorsal border of the wing forms the ventral border of the foramen lacerum. The ventral border forms a notch internally with which a similar notch on the wing of the presphenoid forms a foramen orbitorotundum for the exit of cranial nerves III (oculomotor), IV (trochlear) and VI (abducent). The external surface of the wing presents a pterygoid crest. The basi sphenoidal processes spring from the ventral part of the wings and extend ventrad and caudad. Its internal surface is concealed by the pterygoid and the palatine bones. The caudal border is thick and free.

Presphenoid: The presphenoid bone has a body and two wings. The external surface of the body is concealed mostly by the vomer and the pterygoid bones. The vidian groove is continued by vidian canal at the junction of the wing with the body, which opens into the pterygo-palatine fossa. The cerebral surface of the body presents rostrally a median ethmoidal spine, which joins the crista galli of the ethmoid. Caudally it has the optic groove which supports the optic commissure and the groove on either side leads to the optic foramen. The wing of the presphenoid at its junction with the body is pierced by the optic foramen.

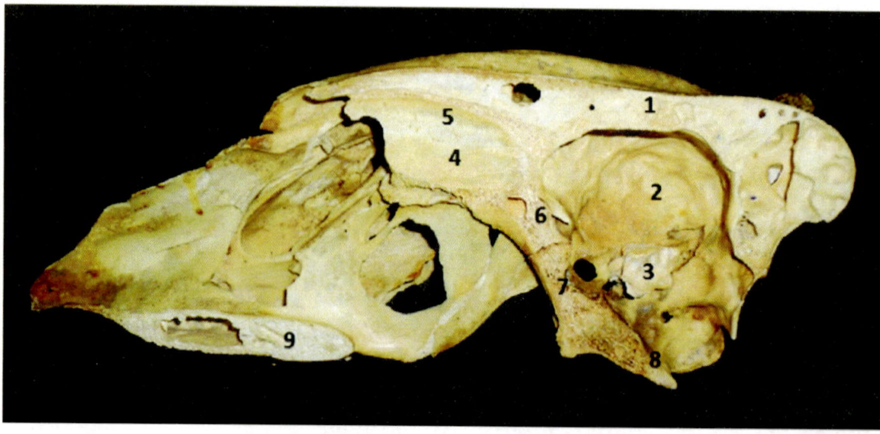

Fig. 2-1 B: Skull of Ox; Midsagital View

1. Frontal sinus; 2. Cranial cavity; 3. Internal auditory meatus on the petrous temporal bone; 4. Ethmoturbinate; 5. Dorsal turbinate; 6. Ethmoid; 7. Sphenoid; 8. Occipital bone; 9. Palatine sinus.

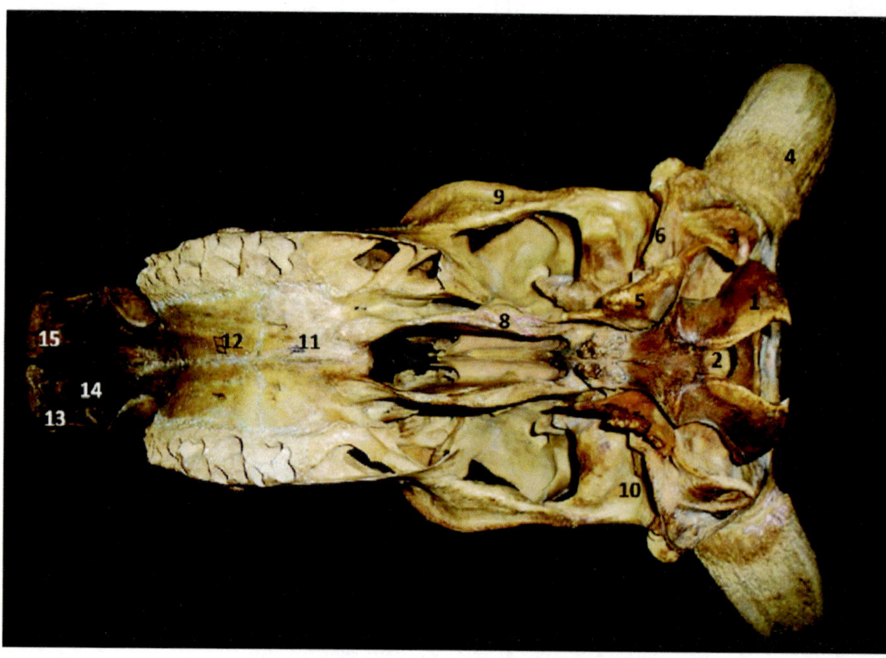

Fig. 2-1 C: Skull of Ox; Ventral View

1. Condyle of occipital bone; 2. Foramen magnum; 3. Paramastoid process; 4. cornual process; 5. Tympanic bulla; 6. Hyoid process; 7. Sphenoid bone; 8. Pterygoid bone; 9. Zygomatic process; 10. Glenoid cavity of temporal bone; 11. Caudal palatine bone; 12. Cranial palatine bone; 13. Premaxilla; 14. Palatine fissure; 15. Inter-incisive fissure;

The external surface of the wing forms a part of the wall of the orbit. Its cerebral surface lodges the cerebrum.

Ethmoid

The ethmoid (Fig. 2-1B) is a single bone. It is situated rostral to the presphenoid bone. It participates into the formation of the cranial, nasal and paranasal cavities. It consists of four parts, the cribriform plate, a perpendicular plate and two labyrinths.

The **cribriform plate** is horizontal sieve like partition between the cranial and nasal cavities. The cranial surface is divided by a median ridge, the crista galli, into two halves. Each half forms a deep ethmoidal fossa for the olfactory lobe of the cerebral hemisphere and lodges the olfactory bulb of the corresponding side within it. The numerous filaments of the olfactory nerve pass through the sieve like structure of the ethmoid fossa. The nasal surface of the ethmoid has the labyrinths attached to it.

The **perpendicular plate** forms the caudal part of nasal septum and is covered by mucous membrane. Caudally it rests on the groove of the vomer bone.

The **labyrinths** are conical masses covered externally by thin plates of bone called the lamina terminalis. Each of the labyrinths consists of a number of delicate scroll like plates of bone termed as ethmoturbinates. The largest of these is attached to the nasal bone and is termed as dorsal turbinate bone. The next in size is termed as the great ethmoidal cell and the rests are small turbinate cells.

Interparietal

The interparietal is a single bone. In foetus, the bones of the right and left side are separate but in the adult and the aged cattle these two are fused and become a single bone. This bone is situated between the parietals rostrally and the squamous occipital caudally. The interparietal is fused with the parietals shortly after birth.

Parietal

The parietal is a paired bone. It is situated on the dorso-caudal and lateral aspects of the cranium. Each of the parietals consists of two parts, the horizontal and the vertical.

The horizontal part is flat and quadrilateral The horizontal parts of the two sides, the left and right, unite with each other at the mid line and form the greater part of the roof of the cranium. The external surface of this part of the bone presents a strong crest in the middle for the attachment of nuchal ligament. The cerebral surface is marked by digital impressions.

The vertical part descends downward and forms the part of the temporal fossa. The junction of the two parts is marked externally by a prominent crest called the parietal crest which is continuous ventrally with the temporal crest and rostrally with the frontal crest.

Temporal

The temporal (Fig. 2-1 B) is a paired bone and it forms the lateral part of the wall of the cranium. It is situated between the occipital caudally, the parietal dorsally, the frontal rostrally and the basi sphenoid ventrally. Each temporal bone consists of two parts, the squamous and the petrous temporal.

The **squamous temporal** has a body and a zygomatic process. The external surface of the body is divided by the temporal crest into two parts. The area below the crest forms part of the temporal fossa and presents two or three foramina leading into temporal canal. The area above the crest is smaller and meets the occipital bone. The internal (cranial) surface is overlapped by the parietal and the sphenoid bones. The zygomatic process is wide above and narrow below. In the upper part of the process, rostrally it forms a part of the temporal fossa and caudally it presents an auricular area consisting of a condyle, a glenoid cavity and a post-glenoid process. Just above the glenoid process is the post glenoid foramen, which forms an external opening of the temporal canal. The lower part of the zygomatic process of the temporal meets the zygomatic process of the malar bone with which it forms the zygomatic arch.

The **petrous temporal** bone is situated on the caudolateral aspect of the cranium. It lies between the occipital bone above and the parietal bone below. The major parts of the organ of hearing are housed in this bone. It consists of two parts, the petrous and the tympanic. The petrous part is small and contains the internal ear (labyrinth). It is the hardest bone in the body and is made up of the dense compact tissue. The tympanic part is more extensive and comprises the external auditory process, the auditory bulla and the muscular and the hyoid processes.

The **petrous part** is pyramidal in form. Its rostral surface is free and faces the cerebral cavity. The caudal surface is slightly depressed. It presents an oblique groove which marks the junction of the condyloid and temporal canals. The lateral surface is concealed by squamous part of the temporal. The caudal surface and the lateral surface are separated by a strong projection called the mastoid process. The medial surface is free, irregularly concave and is marked by digital impressions. A sharp ridge called the petrosal crest separates the medial surface from the rostral surface. The opening of the internal meatus is placed in the ventral part of the petrosal crest. The temporal canal is formed by the opposition of a groove along the rostrolateral edge of this surface with a similar one of the squamous temporal.

The **tympanic part** is external and it consists of the following structures.

1. the **external auditory process** which is a curved plate of bone projecting through a notch on the squamous temporal
2. the **hyoid process** which is a rod of bone below the external auditory process
3. the **stylomastoid foramen** situated between the hyoid process and the paramastoid process
4. the **auditory bulla** whose cavity forms part of the middle ear
5. the **styloid process** of the petrous temporal which springs from below the bulla for muscular attachment
6. the **Gasserian fissure** which lies external to the styloid process and presents passage for chorda tympani nerve and
7. the **Eustachian tube** which is an osseous canal or a groove that lies internal to the styloid process.

Frontal

The frontal (Fig. 2-1 A) is a paired bone. The two frontals are very extensive, forming the entire roof of the cranium and about one half of the entire length of the skull. The fore head of the animal is formed entirely by the frontal bones. The characteristic appearance of the head of the ox is because of the anatomical characteristics of the frontal bones including the presence of the corneal process (horn core). The frontal bones are situated between the parietals caudally and the nasals rostrally. The parietal border of these bones forms with the parietal bones a large central protuberance, the highest point of the skull of ox.

Each of the frontal bones consist of the squamous part (the body), the orbital plate, the zygomatic (supra orbital) process and the cornual process (horn core).

The **squamous part** or the body of the frontal forms the basis of the fore head. Its external surface is smooth and convex and is covered by the frontalis muscle. Running parallel to the lateral border and just medial to the supraorbital process, the external surface presents a shallow supraorbital groove. In the middle of this groove is the supraorbital canal which leads to the supraorbital canal that passes through the substance of the frontal bone and opens into the orbital fossa. The frontal vessels run through this groove, foramen and the canal. The internal surface forms the part of the cranial and the nasal cavities. The bone consists of two tables or the plates, the cranial and the nasal. Between the two plates is enclosed the frontal sinus. The cranial plate is marked by digital impressions and presents the internal frontal crest to which the falx cerebri of the dura matter is attached. The nasal plate forms the roof of the nasal cavity along with the nasal bones. The cerebral and the nasal plates meet each other at the crista galli. The medial borders of the two frontals join each other mesially at the frontal suture. The lateral border has three parts, the temporal, orbital and lacrimal and participates into formation of the temporal and orbital fossa. The dorsal border articulates with the parietals. The ventral border articulates with the nasal bone at the nasofrontal suture.

The **supraorbital plate** forms the medial wall of the orbit. It presents the orbital opening of the supraorbital canal and above this is a depression for the cartilaginous pulley in fresh state where the tendon of the superior oblique muscle of the eye ball is deflected. The internal surface of this plate meet the sphenoid and ethmoid bones.

The zygomatic (supraorbital) process forms the part of the rim of the orbit. Its ventral face is related to lacrimal gland. It articulates with the zygomatic process of the malar bone to form the rim of the orbit.

The **cornual process** or the horn core of the frontal bone is a hollow conical osseous process projecting outward from the dorsolateral angle of the squamous plate (body) of the frontal bone. The length and the size and shape of this process vary according to the breed, sex and age of the animal. The external surface is rough and porous and is marked by number of grooves and foramina. In the fresh state it is covered by the corium of the horn that is made of the cornified epithelium of the skin. At the base of the horn core is a constriction called the neck. The interior is excavated to form a number of spaces divided by bony septa and is communicated interiorly with the frontal sinus.

Facial bones

The rest of the bones of the skull that mainly participate in the formation of the upper and lower jaws of the oral cavity and the nasal cavity are grouped as facial bones. These bones include the maxilla, incisive (premaxilla), palatine, pterygoid, nasal, lacrimal, malar (zygomatic), turbinate, vomer, mandible and hyoid. Of these, the vomer, mandible and hyoid bones are single and the rests are paired bones.

Maxilla

The maxillae (Fig. 2-1 A) are the largest bones of the upper jaw. These are also called as superior maxillary bones considering their major role in the formation of the upper (superior) jaw. These are situated on the lateral aspect of the face. Each bone consists of a body and three processes, the alveolar, zygomatic and palatine.

The **body** of the maxilla is irregularly triangular in outline. The bone has two tables (plates) between which the maxillary sinus is enclosed. The facial (lateral) surface presents, at about the level of first cheek tooth, the infraorbital foramen. It is the external opening of the infraorbital canal through which passes the infraorbital artery and the superior maxillary nerve. At about the level of the third or fourth cheek tooth, the external surface presents the facial tuberosity. Extending upward from this tuberosity is a curved facial crest. The internal surface of the maxilla forms the lateral part of the nasal cavity. It presents, at about its middle, the ventral turbinate crest. Immediately below this crest is the lacrimal groove for the passage of membranous nasolacrimal duct. The rostral border is oblique It articulates with the nasal bone and the nasal process of the premaxilla. The dorsal border articulates with the nasal and overlaps the malar and lacrimal bones.

The **alveolar process** forms the caudal border of the body of the maxilla. It is thick and presents six alveoli for the upper molar and pre molar teeth. Above the last alveolus is the alveolar tuberosity and behind the alveolar tuberosity is the maxillary tuberosity. The maxillary tuberosity forms the upper limit (proximal extremity) of the maxilla and has the maxillary sinus prolonged into it. Internal to the maxillary tuberosity is maxillary hiatus, a smooth depression in which are three foramina namely the maxillary, sphenopalatine and the caudal palatine. The maxillary foramen leads to the infraorbital canal which is an osseous tube that runs down between the two tables (plates) of the body of the maxilla and opens exteriorly into the infraorbital canal. The distal extremity of the body is pointed and is overlapped by the nasal process of the premaxilla.

The **zygomatic process** projects outward on the dorsolateral aspect of the maxillary tuberosity. It articulates with the malar bone and forms the part of the orbit.

The **palatine process** forms a large part of the bony palate. Its oral surface shows the palatine groove for the palatine artery and nerve. It is excavated to form part of the palatine sinus.

Incisive

The incisive bones (premaxilla) (Fig. 2-1 A) form the rostral part of the upper jaw. Each bone consists of a body and two processes, the nasal and palatine. The body is the rostral thick part of the bone. The labial surface of the body is convex and is related to the upper lip. The buccal surface is concave and is related to the dental pad. The internal edge of the body is sharp and concave and it marks the demarcation of the labial and buccal surfaces. It forms the lateral boundary of the incisive fissure.

The nasal process projects upward from the body and forms the lateral wall of the nasal cavity. The lateral surface of the nasal process is smooth and convex. The medial surface is concave and its caudal two third fits into the groove on the rostral edge of the body of the maxilla.

The palatine process is smaller than the nasal. It is thin plate of bone which forms the rostral part of the bony palate. Its nasal surface is grooved on its rostral part for the vomer bone and the nasal septum. Between the two processes is an elongated nasopalatine cleft or the palatine fissure.

Palatine

The palatine bones (Fig. 2-1 B) are very extensive. They are placed on either side of the caudal nares and form the caudal part of the hard palate. Each palatine bone is comprised of the horizontal and perpendicular parts.

The **horizontal part** forms caudal one fourth part of the bony hard palate. It presents two surfaces, the nasal and palatine. The nasal surface is nearly flat and smooth. It forms the lateral wall of the caudal nares. The palatine surface is mostly free and smooth. It is perforated in the middle by the rostral palatine foramen which is the ventral opening of the palatine canal. This canal continues downward as the palatine groove. The medial border of the bones of opposite sides meets each other at the median palatine suture. The nasal surface of the horizontal part is slightly concave and smooth.

The **perpendicular (vertical) part** forms the caudal part of the lateral wall of the nasal cavity. It articulates internally with the pterygoid bone and externally with the subsphenoidal process of the sphenoid, Along the rostral edge, it forms a notch in which it presents sphenopalatine foramen.

Pterygoid

The pterygoids (Fig. 2-1C) are thin plates of bone situated on either side of the caudal nares. The medial (nasal) surface forms the part of the lateral part of the caudal nares. The lateral surface is overlapped by the palatine and pterygoid processes of the sphenoid bone. The extreme upper part of this face forms a canal called the **vidian canal** with the sphenoid. The rostral border is irregular and meets the palatine bone. The caudal border forms lateral boundary of the caudal nares. The proximal extremity fits between the pterygoid process and the sphenoid bone. The caudal extremity is free and forms **hamulus pterygoideus** around which the tendon of the tensor palate muscle is reflected.

Nasal

The nasal bones (Fig. 2-1 A and B) are situated rostral to the frontal bones and the bones of the two sides together form the greater part of the roof of the nasal cavity. Each of the nasal bones is flat and curved from side to side and has two surfaces, two borders and two extremities. The facial (external) surface is convex from side to side but nearly straight from above downward. The nasal (internal) surface is correspondingly concave from side to side and nearly straight from above downward. The inner half of the nasal surface forms the dorsal meatus and immediately below it is the dorsal turbinate crest for the attachment of dorsal turbinate bone. The extreme upper part is excavated to a small extent to form a part of the frontal sinus. The medial border is rounded and meets the same of the opposite bone at the nasal suture. The lateral border is serrated and articulates with the frontal, maxillary and lacrimal bones. The lowermost part of the lateral border is free and forms the naso-maxillary notch with the premaxilla (incisive) bone. The dorsal (superior / proximal) extremities of the nasals of opposite side together form a projection which is received into a notch formed by the lower ends of the frontals. The ventral (inferior / distal) extremity presents two processes separated by a notch and the lower ends of the two bones together forms a trifid appearance.

Lacrimal

The lacrimal bones are situated on the rostral part of the floor of the orbit and extend rostrally downward on the face to meet the maxilla. The external surface of the bone has two parts, the orbital and the facial. The two are separated by the dentated orbito-facial crest which forms a part of the orbital rim. The orbital part forms the rostral part of the floor and medial wall of the orbit. Immediately behind the orbito-facial crest is the lacrimal fossa at the bottom of which is the upper opening of the lacrimal canal. On the floor of the orbit is a large and thin walled protuberance called the lacrimal bulla into which the maxillary sinus extends. The facial part of the external surface is extensive and smooth. The internal (nasal) surface is irregularly concave and presents the osseous lacrimal canal. The circumferential border is irregular and forms articulations with frontal, nasal and maxillary bones.

Malar

The malar or zygomatic (Fig. 2-1 A) bone is irregularly triangular and is situated between the lacrimal in front and maxillary bones below and behind. The lateral (facial) surface is convex and extensive. It presents facial crest, which is the continuation of the facial crest of the maxilla bone. The orbital surface is concave and smooth. It is separated from the facial surface by the rim of the orbit. It forms the part of the floor of the orbit. The medial surface is concave and faces the maxillary sinus. The rostral and caudal borders meet and form a pointed distal (lower) extremity. The proximal (upper) extremity bifurcates into frontal and zygomatic (temporal) processes. The frontal process meets the supraorbital process of the frontal bone to form the part of the rim of the orbit. The zygomatic (temporal) process is overlapped by the zygomatic process of squamous part of temporal bone and completes the zygomatic arch.

Vomer

The vomer is a single median bone. It extends from the presphenoid to the incisive (premaxilla) forming the caudal part of the septum nasi (nasal septum). It is composed of a thin, wide plate of bone that is grooved on the rostral edge to receive the perpendicular plate of the ethmoid bone and the septal cartilage. The lateral surfaces are covered by mucous membrane in life. The dorsal (superior) end presents a deep groove, the sulcus vomeris. It forms a partition between the caudal nares. The ventral (inferior) end lies in the groove formed by the palatine processes of the maxilla and premaxilla (incisive) bones. Its rostral edge (border) is beveled into which the cartilaginous septum is received to form the septum nasi. Thus it divides the nasal cavity into two chambers. The ventral edge (border) in its rostral third fits into the nasal crest of the maxilla. Caudal to this, the ventral edge is free and forms a slit like space through which the two chambers of the nasal cavity communicate with each other.

Turbinate

The turbinate bones, also called as nasal conchae (singular-concha), are delicate scroll like bones. These are two conchae, dorsal and ventral, on either side of the nasal cavity. These are attached to the lateral wall of the nasal cavity lying one in front of the other. Each of these bones is a thin cribriform plate covered by mucous membrane in fresh state.

The dorsal turbinate is smaller than the ventral one. It is wider in the middle and tapering at the extremities. The medial (septal) surface is free and flat. It is separated from the nasal septum by a small interval (space), called the common nasal meatus. The lateral surface is flat and free except at the place of attachment (turbinate crest) with the nasal bone. It communicates with the frontal sinus and is covered by the mucous membrane in fresh state. The space between the dorsal turbinate and the roof of the nasal cavity is called as dorsal meatus.

The ventral turbinate is larger but shorter than the dorsal one. It is attached to the turbinate crest of the maxillary bone by a basal lamina. This lamina is divided at its inner edge into two plates, which are rolled in opposite directions to enclose two cavities. The space between the dorsal and ventral turbinates is called the middle meatus, while that one between the ventral turbinate and the floor of the nasal cavity is called as ventral meatus.

Mandible

The mandible (Figure 2-1 D) is a single bone. It is the largest of the bones of the facial group of bones as well as those of the skull. It is made up of two halves which are not fused completely during the life. It consists of a body and two rami (singular- ramus).

The **body** of the mandible is formed by the incomplete fusion of the lower parts (ventral ends) of the two rami at the symphysis mandibulae. The lingual surface of the body is smooth and concave. It is covered by mucous membrane in life. The symphyseal surface is rough and irregular and is marked by projections and corresponding depressions. The labial surface is convex and more extensive than the lingual surface. The alveolar border presents eight alveoli for the lower incisor teeth. It separates the lingual and labial surfaces. The lateral border projects upward from the corner alveolus and continues on the ramus.

The **rami** (ramus) of the mandible diverge backwards from the body. Each ramus is bent so as to form two parts, the horizontal and vertical. The most prominent part of the curve is the angle of the ramus. The lateral surface is widest at the angle and narrow at either end. It is smooth and convex in the horizontal part and nearly flat in the vertical part. A rough elevation near the angle and the rough lines on the lateral surface of the ramus are for attachment of masseter muscle. It presents a fossa near its junction with the body. Placed in this fossa is the mental foramen which is the rostral (inferior) opening of the mandibular (inferior dental) canal. The medial surface of the horizontal part of the ramus has a faint longitudinal depression. Above this depression is a rough line called the myloid line for attachment of mylohyoid muscle. At its junction with the body, it presents a depression called the genial fossa for the attachment of geniohyoid and genioglossal muscles. The vertical part of the ramus on its medial surface presents an eminence for the attachment of internal pterygoid muscle. Approximately at the middle of this surface is the mandibular foramen which is the caudal (superior) opening of the mandibular (inferior dental) canal.

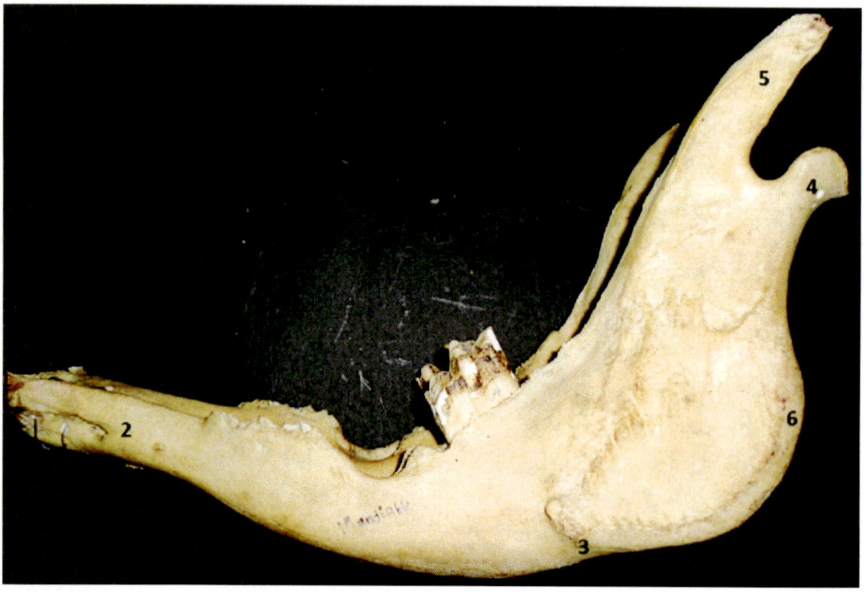

Fig. 2-1 D: Mandible of Ox; Lateral View

1. Incisivous part of body of mandible; 2. Mental foramen; 3. Groove for passage of vessels and nerve; 4. Condylar process; 5. Coronoid process; 6. Angle of jaw.

The alveolar border of the ramus presents interalveolar space in front and six alveoli behind. In the vertical part it serves for attachment of muscles. The ventral border of the horizontal part is convex and presents a smooth impression in its caudal part caused by the facial vessels. In the vertical part it is thin and concave.

The rostral extremity of the ramus continues into the body without any demarcation. The caudal extremity is called articular extremity and possesses a condyle placed caudally and a coronoid process rostrally. Between these two is a depression called the mandibular notch. The condyle is tubular and transversely elongated. It is situated below the summit of the corronoid process. It articulates with the zygomatic process of the squamous temporal bone at the temporomandibular joint. Between the two segments of this joint, lies the interarticular disc made of fibrocartilage. This is the only diarthrodial joint in the skull.

Hyoid

The hyoid is a osseo-cartilagenous structure placed between the rami of the mandible. It is attached to the styloid process of the petrous part of temporal bone by rods of cartilage, the tympanohyoid and supports the root of the tongue as well as the pharynx and larynx. It is composed of a body, the lingual process and four pairs of cornua.

The **body (basihyoid)** is a short transverse piece of bone that is compressed dorsoventrally. The dorsal surface is concave and smooth. It slopes ventrally and caudally. The ventral surface is flattened and roughened for muscular attachment. The rostral border presents medially the lingual process. The caudal border is concave and smooth.

The **lingual (glossal) process** is a short, blunt, conical process projecting rostrally from the middle of the rostral border of the body of the hyoid. It is embedded in the root of the tongue and gives attachment to mylohyoid, geniohyoid and hyoglossus muscles.

There are four pairs of cornua. These include the thyrohyoid, cerratohyoid, stylohyoid and the epihyoid.

The **thyrohyoid (thyroid) cornua** extend dorsad and caudad from the lateral parts of the body of the hyoid. They are compressed laterally. The rostral end articulates with the body forming a diarthrodial joint. The caudal end is prolonged by cartilage and is attached to the rostral cornua of the thyroid cartilage of the larynx.

The **cerratohyoid (small) cornua** are short rods of bone projecting dorsad and rostrad from either end of the body. Each is compressed laterally, but both the ends are slightly enlarged. The ventral end articulates with the basihyoid or the epihyoid.

The **stylohyoid (middle) cornua** are of the size of cerratohyoids. These are also compressed laterally. These are articulated with cerratohyoid at the distal end and with the epihyoid at the proximal end.

The **epihyoid (great) cornua** are the largest of all the cornua of the hyoid. These are directed dorsally and caudally. These are compressed laterally and narrow in the middle and enlarged at the ends. The rostral and caudal borders are sharp and concave. The dorsal border connects the articular and muscular angles. The articular angle unites with the hyoid process of the petrous temporal by a rod of fibro cartilage. The muscular angle is more extensive and, rough and flat.

Skull as a whole

The skull of ox (Figure 2-1 B) is clearly pyramidal in form. The frontal (dorsal) surface is formed by frontal, nasal and incisive bones. The frontal region is quadrilateral and the greatest width is at the transverse plane joining the orbits. The cornual processes project laterally from the lateral angles. The nasal region is short and convex from side to side. It is marked by a depression at about its middle of the rostral end. The incisive region is marked by a wide rostral part between the osseous nasal apertures. The lateral surface is triangular and presents a deep and narrow temporal fossa. It is bounded caudally by the temporal crest and is marked off from the orbit by pterygoid crest. The infraorbital foramen is situated at the level of the first cheek tooth on the lateral surface. The basal surface of the skull excluding the mandible comprises the cranial, choanal and palatine regions. The cranial region extends from occipital condyles and foramen magnum caudally to the vomer and pterygoid processes rostrally. Just in front of the foramen magnum is the basilar part of the occipital and the basi sphenoid bones. Rostral to these are the articular tubercle and mandibular fossa for articulation with the mandible. On either side of the basi sphenoid is the infratemporal fossa formed by the wing and root of the pterygoid process of the basi sphenoid bone. Rostral to this is the pterygoid crest. The choanal region presents the pharyngeal orifice of the nasal cavity which is divided into two cornua by the vomer bone. The palatine region covers almost half of the basilar surface of the skull. The nuchal surface is quite extensive and somewhat pentagonal in outline. It is separated from the frontal surface by a thick border which forms centrally the inercornual protuberance. Midway between the intercornual protuberance and the cornual process is the nuchal tubercle for attachment of nuchal ligament.

Cranial cavity

The cranial cavity (Figure 2- B) encloses the brain along with its meninges and vessels. It is ovoid in shape. It is formed by the cranial group of bones of skull those are described individually above in this chapter. The cavity has a roof, the floor, the lateral walls and the dorsal and ventral extremities.

The **roof** or the dorsal wall is formed by the frontal, parietal and the occipital bones. It extends from the ethmoidal fossa to the dorsal border of the foramen magnum. Projecting from the midline of the roof is the internal sagital crest which gives attachment to the falx cerebri. The **floor** is formed by the basilar part of the occipital and sphenoid bones. The **lateral walls** are formed by the vertical part of the parietal, temporal, and frontal bones and the orbital wings of the sphenoid. The ventral extremity is formed by the ethmoid bone. The dorsal extremity is formed by the occipital bone and the foramen magnum. The cavity has three compartments, the olfactory, cerebral and the cerebellar.

The **olfactory (ventral) compartment** is formed by sphenoid and ethmoid bones and supports the olfactory lobes and a part of the cerebrum. A sharp osseous crest called the crista galli separates the two ethmoid fossae that form the rostral limit of the cranial cavity. The olfactory lobes (bulbs) of the cerebrum of the brain are lodged in the ethmoid fossae. The dorsal limit of the olfactory compartment is formed by the osseous tentorium cerebelli, which gives attachment to the membranous tentorium cerebelli.

The **cerebral (middle) compartment** is the widest and largest of the three compartments. It extends dorsally from the osseous tentorium cerebelli to the level of junction of the sphenoid and occipital bones. The floor of this compartment is formed by the postsphenoid which is marked by a depression called the sella turcica or the pituatory fossa (hypophyseal fossa).On either side of the floor is a deep wide groove leading from the petrous temporal to foramen orbitorotundum. The lateral walls and roof of the middle compartment are marked by digital impressions.

The **cerebellar (dorsal) compartment** is formed at its floor by basi occipital, at the roof by squamous occipital and at the lateral walls by the petrous temporal bones. It lodges within it the cerebellum, pons and medulla oblongata. The medial wall of the petrous temporal is marked by the opening of the internal acoustic meatus.

Nasal cavity

The nasal cavity is a long osseous passage running vertically down along the face. It is divided into two, right and left, halves by a median septum nasi. Each half is called the nasal chamber. The **roof or the rostral wall** is formed by the nasal and frontal bones. It is nearly straight, extending from the dorsal ethmoturbinate and terminating at just below the naso-maxillary notch. The **floor or the caudal wall** is formed by the horizontal part of the palatine bone and the palatine process of the maxilla and incisive bones. The **lateral wall** is formed by the medial plate of the body of the maxilla, perpendicular part of the palatine and pterygoid, the nasal process of the incisive and the nasal bones. The **medial wall** that separates the right and left chambers is formed by the nasal septum which is a osseocartilaginous plate. It is constituted by the vomer and the perpendicular plate of ethmoid bones and the cartilage plate. Each chamber is occupied by the nasal and ethmoidal turbinate. The two chambers, however, communicate with each other at the dorsal one third over the horizontal part of the palatine. Running along the septal wall is the **osseous lacrimal groove** through which the membranous **naso-lacrimal duct** passes along this wall. The outer openings (orifices) of the nasal chambers are called the **external nares** and are bound by the nasal process and the body of the incisive and nasal bones. The inner orifices, the **internal nares** are circumscribed by the ventral surface of sphenoid, horizontal and perpendicular parts of the palatine and pterygoid bones. The walls of the nasal cavity and its contents are lined by mucous membrane. The mucous membrane of the nasal cavity continues into the paranasal sinuses.

Sinuses (Paranasal sinuses)

The sinuses (Figure 2-1 B) are the air spaces developed inside some of the bones of the skull, especially those which contribute into forming the facial region and more specifically those forming the walls of the nasal cavity. These are usually called as paranasal sinuses and they communicate directly or indirectly with the nasal cavity and all of them drain into the nasal cavity. They serve the purpose of lightening the weight of the head, humidifying and heating the inhaled air and presenting a crumple zone to protect vital structures in the event of injury or trauma to facial region. In forming the sinuses, the bones of the facial regions which are mostly the flat bones, are excavated in the form of several air cells (compartments) in between the two tables of the bones. All the sinuses are lined with mucous membrane with pseudostratified columnar ciliated epithelium containing a few serous gland cells in between them. The mucous membrane of the sinuses is in continuation of the mucous membrane of the nasal cavity. The sinuses are named according to the bones in which they exist. Accordingly these are the frontal, sphenoidal, maxillary, palatine and ethmoidal paranasal sinuses.

Frontal sinus: The frontal sinus is the largest of all the sinuses and is excavated in the frontal, parietal interparietal and squamous occipital bones. It extends from the caudal wall of the cranium down to the level of the interior margins of the orbit and laterally to the frontal crest and supra orbital process. Medially it is separated from its fellow by an imperforate bony septum. The cavity is divided into smaller spaces by partial septa. This sinus communicates with the middle meatus by narrow apertures at the ethmoidal meatus on either side of the nasal cavity. In the dry skull, the lacrimal part of maxillary sinus and the cavity of the rostral turbinate bone are observed to be communicating with the frontal sinus. But in fresh state these are found to be closed by mucous membrane.

Maxillary sinus: The maxillary sinus is formed in the body of the maxilla and is extended into the malar and lacrimal bones. Ventrally it extends to the facial tuberosity but in some subjects it may prolong up to the level of infraorbital foramen. Dorsally it extends to the level of lacrimal bulla. Rostrally, it is limited to a line joining the infraorbital foramen to the orbital rim. The caudal limit of the maxillary sinus lies at the base of the alveoli and the maxillary tuberosity. The maxillary sinus communicates freely with the palatine sinus and opens at the middle meatus of the nasal cavity.

Palatine sinus: The palatine sinus is formed in the palatine process of the maxilla and the palatine bone. It is separated from its fellow by a bony septum. The dorsal limit of this sinus lies at the horizontal part of the palatine bone. From here it extends ventrally to the level of about first cheek tooth. Laterally it communicates with the maxillary sinus. It drains out into a narrow opening in the middle meatus of the nasal cavity.

Sphenoid sinus: The sphenoid sinus is excavated in the body of the presphenoid bone. It is the smallest of all the paranasal sinuses and it opens into the ethmoidal meatus of the nasal cavity.

Ethmoidal sinus: The ethmoidal sinus is considered as the nasal sinus instead of the paranasal sinus. It is formed by the cavity of the ethmoturbinate bone in the nasal cavity. It communicates directly with the nasal sinus behind the caudal (internal) nares.

Orbital fossa (Orbit)

The orbital fossa (Figure 2-1 C) is a large, deep depression on the dorsolateral aspect of the facial part of the skull. It is approximately conical in shape with the apex on the deeper side and the base superficial in position. It firmly lodges the eye ball with its extrinsic muscles and periorbital structures within it. The long axis of the conical cavity if directed dorsad (upward), rostrad (forward) and laterad (outward). The opening of the orbit is guarded by the bony rim formed by the orbital parts of frontal, lacrimal and malar bones. The medial wall of the orbit is extensive. It is concave and smooth and is formed by the orbital wing of the frontal, lacrimal and the presphenoid bones. The lateral wall is formed by the zygomatic process of the frontal and the frontal process of the malar (zygomatic) bone. The dorsal wall (roof) is formed by the frontal and to a small extent by the lacrimal bone. It presents supraorbital foramen which to the supraorbital canal that traverses through the zygomatic process and the body of the frontal to open at the supraorbital groove on the external (dorsal) surface of the body of the frontal bone. The ventral wall (floor) of the orbit is formed by malar (zygomatic) bone and the zygomatic process of the temporal bone and to a small extent by the maxilla. On the floor, near the rim of the orbit is the lacrimal bulla that projects into the cavity In front of the bulla and near the margin is the lacrimal fossa for accommodating the lacrimal gland. Near the apex of the orbit is the optic foramen through which the optic nerve passes into the cranium. A little above this is the foramen orbitorotundum. The rim of the orbit is thin and rounded. Along the dorsal margin it is serrated. It is formed by the frontal, lacrimal and zygomatic bones.

Temporal fossa

The temporal fossa is partly a backward and outward continuation of the orbital fossa. It lies behind the orbit from which it is incompletely separated. The dorsal wall of this fossa is formed by the parietal and temporal bones. The ventral wall is formed by the supraorbital process. The frontal crest lies rostral to this fossa while the zygomatic process of squamous temporal lies caudal to the temporal fossa. The medial wall is concave and roughened and is formed by the temporal part of the frontal, parietal and the squamous temporal bones. The temporal fossa is marked off from the orbital fossa by the pterygoid crest of the sphenoid bone. About three to four foramina enter the temporal bone through the medial wall of the temporal fossa. Laterally this fossa is covered by the muscles in the fresh state.

16

Comparative Anatomy of Skeleton of Head

Horse

The skull of horse is also pyramidal in shape like that of ox but the base of the pyramid is less wide than that of the ox. It is shorter in length and narrower in width than that of the ox. The cranium is smaller externally, however, the cavity of cranium is larger than that of the ox. The nasal cavity is divided into two chambers by nasal septum. The floor of the nasal cavity is shorter and less concave than that of the ox. The left and the right nasal chambers are completely separated and do not communicate with each other. The horn core is absent.

The **occipital bone** is placed at the extreme caudal part of the skull, caudal condyloid foramen is absent, the basi occipital is longer and prismatic and the squamous occipital is crossed by a nuchal crest. The **sphenoid bone** has two parts, the pre and post sphenoid, as that in case of ox. The wing of the post sphenoid presents three notches, carotid, oval and spinosal for internal carotid artery, ventral maxillary nerve and spheno-spinous artery respectively. The foramen orbitale and the foramen rotundum are not united. There are no major differences in the **ethmoid bone** of ox and horse. The **frontal bones** are less expansive than those of ox. These are situated between parietals caudally and nasals rostrally. The supraorbital foramen perforates the root of the supra orbital process that joins the zygomatic process of the squamous temporal. The horn core is absent. The ventral borders of the frontal bones of the opposite sides form a projection which fits into the notch formed by the two nasal bones. The **temporal bone** in horse has three parts, the squamous, petrous and tympanic as against two parts, the squamous and petrous of the ox. The squamous part is much more developed than that of ox. It has three parts, the body, zygomatic process and the occipital (pyramidal) process. The later one arises from the caudal part of the squamous. The stylomastoid foramen is between the hyoid and the mastoid processes and the auditory bulla is smaller. The **interparietal** is a single bone as that of ox. The external (parietal) surface of this bone in horse is smooth, flat and quadrilateral. It presents a sagital crest medially for muscular attachment. The internal (cerebral) surface bears a three sided process which projects ventrally and rostrally into the cranial cavity between the cerebral hemisphere and the cerebellum. The **parietal bone** is placed entirely on the dorsolateral aspect of the skull and forms the roof of the cranium. The parietal crest is median in position in the dorsal part but it bifurcates ventrally to join the frontal crest on either side. The caudal border meets the occipital and curves inward and forms the parieto-temporal canal with the temporal. The **maxilla** is longe and narrow and is placed relatively higher than in ox. The zygomatic ridge is prominent. The infraorbital foramen is at the level of third cheek tooth and a small canal from this extends into the incisive bone. The palatine canal is formed between the palatine process of the maxilla and the palatine bones. At the junction of the maxilla and incisive bones is an alveolus for the canine tooth. The **incisive bone** has thicker body and it presents three alveoli for the upper incisors. The internal surface presents a groove. This with the similar one of opposite side forms foramen incisium. The nasal process is longer and presents at its junction with the maxilla an alveolus for the permanent canine tooth. The palatine process is wide and palatine fissure is narrow. **The palatine bone** like that of ox, has the horizontal and perpendicular (vertical) parts. The horizontal part in horse is not excavated. The vertical part is more extensive and the sphenopalatine foramen is formed entirely by this bone. It is excavated to form the sphenopalatine sinus. The medial border of the horizontal part meets its fellow at the median palatine suture. On the nasal aspect of which is the nasal crest. The **pterygoid bones** of horse are shorter and narrower. The **nasal bones** are larger and wider than those of ox. The dorsal ends of the two bones together form a notch into which the pointed ventral ends of the frontal bones are received. The ventral ends of nasal bones are pointed. The **lacrimal bones** of horse are smaller than those of ox. The facial part is less extensive and presents a small lacrimal tubercle near the orbital margin for the attachment of the lacrimal tendon of orbicularis oculi muscle. The lacrimal bulla is absent. The **malar (zygomatic) bone** of horse is almost similar to that of ox except that its upper extremity is not divided but it meets the zygomatic process of the squamous temporal. The facial surface is comparatively very small. The **vomer**, similar to that in ox is a median strip of bone with a beveled rostral border into which the cartilaginous septum is lodged. However, the caudal border of this bone in horse is firmly attached to the nasal crest and so the nasal chambers of the opposite sides are completely separated as against the incomplete partition formed in ox. The **turbinates (nasal conchae)** in horse are two as those of ox but the rostral turbinate is larger and longer in horse. The caudal turbinate forms only single roll and contains a large bulla. The body of the **mandible** is completely fused in the middle. The alveolar border of the combined body possesses six alveoli for the lower incisors and two for canines. The lingual groove is absent. The rostro-medial part of the condyle presents a depression called the fovea pterygoidiea for the external pterygoid muscle. The **hyoid bone** like that of ox, presents the body, a lingual (glossal) process and four pairs of cornua. The glossohyoid is longer with its free end pointed. The thyrohyoids are fused with the body. The body, thyrohyoids and glossohyoids form the spur. The epihyoid is fused with the lower end of the stylohyoid.

Amongst the **sinuses**, the maxillary sinus is the largest in horse as against the frontal sinus of ox. It is divided into the dorsal and ventral parts by an oblique septum. The **maxillary sinus** is formed by the maxilla, lacrimal, malar (zygomatic), caudal turbinate and the lateral masses of the ethmoid. The **frontal sinus** is formed by the frontal, lacrimal, ethmoid and rostral turbinate bones. It communicates with the maxillary sinus and caudal part of the rostral turbinate bone. The **sphenopalatine sinus** is formed by the presphenoid and vertical part of the palatine bones. It communicates with the internal part of the maxillary sinus. The **ethmoidal sinus** is the cavity in the large ethmoturbinate bone. It communicates with the maxillary sinus.

The **orbital fossa (orbit)** of the horse is placed more laterally. The lacrimal bulla is absent. The cavity of the orbit is formed by the orbital plate and supraorbital process of the frontal and the orbital wing of the maxilla. The complete rim of the orbit is smooth and rounded. The lacrimal fossa is deeper. At the apex of the orbit, rostral to the optic foramen is the ethmoid foramen. The foramen orbitale and the foramen rotundum are separate.

The **temporal fossa** is situated on the dorsolateral aspect of the cranium. It is shallow and wide. The right and left fossae are closer to each other than in ox and are separated by interparietal crest. Ventrally, the two fossae are separated above the sphenoidal notch. This fossa is formed by the occipital, interparietal, parietal, frontal and squamous temporal bones.

Dog

The skull of dog varies in shape, form and size as per the breed characteristics. Some of them have long and narrow skull (e.g. greyhound), while the others have short and broad skulls (e.g. bulldog, pug) and some others greatly differ from these. In most of the breeds of dog, the cranium is broad above and tapering below. The olfactory compartment of the cranium is very narrow. The olfactory fossae are deeper than those of other species and the crista galli recedes to the bottom. Roof of the cranium is formed by the parietal, interparietal and frontal bones. The cerebral and cerebellar compartments are prominently marked with the presence of sharp petrosal cleft and internal occipital protuberance. The size and form of the nasal cavity also differ with the breed of the animal. The rostral (external) nares are large and circular while the caudal (internal) nares are long. The ventral turbinate (concha) are extensive and occupy the most of the space at the rostral part of the nasal cavity. Dorsolateral to the caudal turbinate is the opening of the maxillary sinus.

The **occipital bone** is situated at the caudal part of the skull. The basi occipital projects from the base of the condyles. It is short and flat and the basilar tubercles are wide apart. It joins the bulla tympanica on either side. The paramastoid processes are short and do not descend below the level of the condyles. The nuchal crest is angular. The **interparietal** is wedged in between the two parietals. The external surface is almost absorbed into the sagital crest which has a variable growth depending up on the breed of the animal. The **parietals** are rhomboid in appearance. Each is situated on the dorsolateral aspect and forms the roof of the skull as that in the skull of horse. The **sphenoid,** as that in other animals, has two parts, the presphenoid and the postsphenoid. The **presphenoid** is very narrow and is excavated to form the sphenoidal sinus. The optic canal passes through the orbital wing of the presphenoid. The body of the **postsphenoid** is short. The temporal wings are extensive and articulate with the parietals. The hypophyseal fossa is shallower than in ox. The carotid notch with the similar one on the temporal forms the carotid foramen for the carotid artery. The foramen orbitale and the foramen rotundum are separate and have two different openings. The **ethmoid** is well developed. The ethmoidal fossae are deep. The crista galli is in the form of a faint ridge and it recedes deep into the ethmoidal fossae. The lateral masses of the ethmoid are very well developed and occupy about three fourths of the nasal sinus dorsally. The **frontal** bones are comparatively lower in position and are less extensive than those of ox and horse. The supraorbital process is short, blunt and does not reach the zygomatic. Hence, the orbital rim remains incomplete. The supraorbital foramen is absent. The frontal crest which is the continuation of the parietal crest curves laterally and terminates on the blunt end of the supraorbital process. Two ethmoidal foramina are present in the orbital plate. The squamous and the petrous parts of the **temporal** bones are fused with each other much earlier in life. The zygomatic process is strongly curved. At the base of this process, the condyle is absent and instead a glenoid cavity is formed. The bulla tympanica (auditory bulla) is very large and is fused with the basi occipital bone. The carotid foramen is internal to the Eustachian opening. The styloid and the hyoid processes are rudimentary. The size of the **maxilla** varies with the breed of the animal. The **maxilla** is short but its dorsal part extends very high. The facial crest and the alveolar tuberosity are absent. The maxillary tuberosity exists only in puppies. It is absent in adult dogs. The alveolar border (process) bears six alveoli. The incisive bone is very small. The body presents three alveoli for incisors. These increase in size from inside out. An alveolus for canine tooth is formed in the body of the incisive along with the maxilla. The nasal process wedges in between the nasal and maxillary bones. The **palatine** bones of dog are extensive. The horizontal part forms the caudal one third of the bony palate. The part that extends from the nasal surface meet its fellow to form the lamina transversalis which divides the olfactory and respiratory parts of the nasal mucous membrane. The vertical (perpendicular) part is very extensive. The pterygopalatine fossa is large. On the dorsomedial aspect of this plate is a depression in which two foramina are placed. These are the sphenopalatine and the caudal palatine foramina. The **pterygoid bones** of dog are short but wide and quadrilateral. These extend to the lateral wall of the caudal (internal) nares. The caudal border of the pterygoid is free and presents a distinct hook like hamulus. The **nasal bone** is long and narrow. The external (facial) surface is concave in its length and forms a central groove with its fellow. The internal (Medial) border projects into the nasal cavity to form the internal nasal crest which becomes very prominent caudally. The caudal parts fit into a notch formed by the frontal bones. The rostral ends of the opposite bones form an almost semicircular nasal notch. The **lacrimal bone** is very small. The facial surface does not extend beyond the orbital margin. The orbital surface is small and triangular. It presents an opening to the lacrimal canal. The **malar (zygomatic) bone** of dog, similar to that in ox, is situated between the lacrimal and the maxillary bones. The bulk of the zygomatic bone is formed by the temporal (zygomatic) process. It is very long and curved. The dorsal border is free and forms part of the orbital ring. It meets the zygomatic process of the temporal. It bears an eminence called the frontal process for the attachment of the orbital ligament. The **vomer** in dog is placed much higher. It spreads out laterally to join the palatine bone assisting in the formation of lamina transversalis. The proximal end is deeply notched. Caudally it is not in contact with the floor of the nasal cavity and does not divide the caudal nares. The **turbinate bones (nasal conchae)** are richly convoluted. They do not communicate with the sinuses of the skull. The caudal ends are narrow and deeply notched. The proximal part of the dorsal (ethmoidal) turbinate is wide. The distal part extends lower and terminates near about the same place where the ventral turbinate ends. The ventral (nasal) turbinate is short and very complex. The two halves of the **mandible** bone do not fuse completely even in old age. The body presents six alveoli for the incisors and two for canines. The incisor alveoli increase in size from first to third. The alveolar border is slightly concave in its length. The ramus of the mandible is relatively small. The horizontal part of ramus presents seven alveoli for cheek teeth. The external (lateral) face of the vertical part presents a deep masseteric fossa. At the angle of the ramus is the angular process. The coronoid process is extensive. Of the **hyoid bone,** the glossohyoid is absent. The epihyoid is as long as the stylohyoid. The stylohyoid is bent and twisted.

Amongst the **sinuses,** only frontal and maxillary sinuses exist in dog. The **frontal sinus** is confined to the frontal bone only. It is divided into a small medial and a much larger lateral sinus. Both of these and open into the dorsal (ethmoidal) meatus. The **maxillary sinus** is small and it communicates directly with the nasal cavity. It is bounded medially by the orbital plate of ethmoid and its lateral wall is crossed obliquely by the nasolacrimal canal.

The **orbital fossa (orbit)** communicates freely with the temporal fossa on the lateral surface of the skull. The caudal part of the orbital margin is absent. A distinct crest, the ventral orbital crest marks the limit between the orbital cavity and the pterygopalatine fossa. The preorbital region is somewhat triangular, concave lengthwise and convex dorsoventrally. The **temporal fossa** is extensive and covers a large portion on the lateral surface of the skull.

Sheep and Goat

The skull of sheep and goat is dorsoventrally triangular in shape. At the most caudal part of the skull is a transverse nuchal line. The **occipital bone** is extensive. It varies in shape from square to rectangular or even triangular in some cases. The basilar part, the condyles and the jugular process are similar to those of ox. However, the tubercles for muscular attachment are situated further caudad. The **sphenoid** bones form the rostral and middle parts of the floor and the lateral walls of the cranial cavity. The basi sphenoid unites caudally with the basi occipital. The hypophyseal fossa is deeper than that in ox. The oval foramen is slightly rostral in position and it is formed completely by the sphenoid. The presphenoid is partly covered by the vomer. The wings of the presphenoid are better developed. The **ethmoid** extends into the caudo-dorsal part of the nasal cavity. The cribriform plate is transverse in position. The ethmoidal fossae are shallow as compared to those of ox. The ethmoturbinate extend further rostral to a greater extent than that in ox. The **interparietal** is fused with the parietals. The **parietal** bones form almost one third of the roof and lateral walls of cranial cavity. They are more extensive than those in ox. The **frontal** bones are less extensive than those in ox. The cornual process varies in shape, size and direction as per the breed characteristics. The **temporal** bone has the squamous and petrous parts similar to that in ox but their fusion in the sheep and goat is latter than in ox. The tympanic bulla is larger, less compressed and more closely applied to the basilar part of the occipital. The styloid process is larger and less concealed. The squamous part is more extensive than in ox. The ventral border of the squamous part bears a notch through which the external acoustic meatus protrudes. The temporal crest is less developed. The **maxilla** forms about one half of the lateral wall of the face and almost two thirds of the hard palate. The facial surface of the maxilla is more convex than that in ox. The facial tubercle occurs dorsal to fifth cheek tooth. It is more dorsal in position than that in ox. The infraorbital foramen is above the second cheek tooth. The alveolar process occupies two thirds of the ventral border. It is convex and bears six alveoli. The zygomatic process is poorly developed. The palatine process is longer and narrower than in ox. The **incisive** bones are narrower and more pointed rostrally than those in ox. The palatine process is curved dorsoventrally as against the flattened process in horizontal direction in ox. The **palatine bone**, similar to that in ox, has horizontal and perpendicular parts. The horizontal plate forms only one sixth of the hard palate. The perpendicular plate forms more of the lateral walls of the internal nares (choanae) and the pterygopalatine fossa as compared to that in ox. The sphenopalatine foramen is elongate, oval to circular and more caudal in position than in ox. The **pterygoid bones** are elongated narrow plates of bone on the caudolateral part of the caudal nares. Laterally it forms the part of the pterygopalatine fossa immediately rostral to the foramen orbitorotundum. In the pterygopalatine fossa, the pterygoid bone is exposed more than the palatine bone. The **nasal bones** are convex longitudinally, with a transverse concavity near the rostral extremity. At the rostral extremity, the bones of the two sides form a single median projection which is not spine like as it is in the horse. The nasoincisive notch separates the nasal bone from the incisive and a portion of the maxilla. The **lacrimal bone** forms the rostral and medial parts of the orbit along with the lateral surface of the face. The facial and orbital parts are almost equal in size. The orbital rim is indented near the junction of the lacrimal with the zygomatic. Just dorsal to this junction is nasolacrimal fossa where a small foramen leads to the nasolacrimal canal. The lacrimal bulla is pyramidal and it covers almost one third of the floor of the orbit. The **zygomatic (malar) bone** forms the ventral part (floor) of the orbital fossa. A bony ridge from the facial tuber to the orbital rim divides the facial part of this bone into the dorsal and ventral parts. The **vomer** presents a deep groove in its dorsal border for the cartilage of the septum nasi. Only rostral one fourth of its ventral border is attached with the nasal floor while the rest of the ventral border is free allowing communication between the two chambers. The **turbinate bones (nasal conchae)** are more delicate than those in ox. There are three conchae in sheep and goat instead of two of the ox. The dorsal and ventral conchae are of almost same length. The middle one is, however, smaller and occupies the space between the dorsal and ventral conchae. It extends rostrally to the level of the third cheek tooth. It is indented dorsally and ventrally by the dorsal and ventral nasal conchae. The bony septum between the cavity of the dorsal concha and the sinus is incomplete. The **mandible** of sheep and goat is more or less similar to that of ox. The alveoli for the incisors are relatively larger than those of ox. The space between the rami is narrow. The ventral border of the horizontal part of the ramus is less convex. The lateral surface is less oblique than that in ox. The mental foramen lies midway along the interalveolar space. Near the junction of the body with the rami, is a ventral bony prominence from which a bony ridge extends caudally to the angle of the mandible. The ramus in its dorsal part curves laterally. The condyles are simple and the mandibular notch is shallow. The coronoid process is curved and is longer than that in the ox. Of the **hyoid bone**, the basihyoid is short and flattened. The glossohyoid is also short. The paired thyrohyoid is not firmly attached to the basihyoid. The cerratohyoid and epihyoid are relatively small.

Amongst the **sinuses,** the **frontal sinus** is limited to the frontal bone only. In some breeds of sheep and goat, it may extend to the lacrimal bone. The frontal sinus has two compartments, the lateral and the medial. The lateral frontal sinus is larger. It communicates with the nasal sinus and opens into the olfactory part of the middle nasal meatus. The medial nasal sinus is smaller and it opens into the middle meatus just caudal to the opening of the lateral nasal sinus. The **maxillary sinus** extends into the zygomatic and lacrimal bones. It is divided by the infraorbital canal into medial and lateral chambers. The lateral chamber is larger and extends caudally into the lacrimal bulla. The medial chamber is continuous with the palatine sinus. It opens into the middle meatus of the nasal cavity in common with the palatine sinus. The palatine sinus is formed into the hard palate. It extends from the alveolar process (border) between second cheek tooth and last cheek tooth to the median line of the palate in the horizontal part of the palatine. Whereas, in the vertical part, it extends from alveolar border of maxilla dorsally to the infraorbital canal ventrally. The **palatine sinus** communicates with maxillary sinus and the two sinuses open in common into the middle meatus of the nasal cavity. The **sphenoid sinus** lies in the ventral part of the presphenoid bone and communicates with the caudoventral part of the ethmoid sinus.

Pig

The skull of pig greatly differs in general gross outline from other species of animals. It also varies in different breeds of pig. The dorsoventral length of the skull is relatively more. The facial region is almost straight. The frontal region is flattened, slopes rostrally and lacks the external sagittal crest caudally. The lateral surface is triangular, temporal fossa is entirely lateral and its long axis is almost vertical. The cranial cavity is smaller although the cranium is greater in size. The nasal cavity is very long.

The **occipital bone** forms the caudal aspect of the skull. The squamous part is extensive, flattened and triangular. The base of the squamous part forms the highest part of the skull. The **sphenoid** has two parts, the basisphenoid and the presphenoid. The sella turcica on the body of the basisphenoid is limited caudally by the prominent dorsum sella which slopes caudally to join the basioccipital. Projecting rostrolaterally from the dorsum sella are paired caudal clinoidal processes. The hypophyseal fossa is formed by the presphenoid in association with the basisphenoid. The foramen orbitorotundum is formed by wings of the basisphenoid in association with the presphenoid. The dorsal border of foramen orbitorotundum is formed by caudal projection of the wing of the presphenoid. Medially this projection presents the rostral clinoidal process. The **ethmoid bone** in the immature subjects is usually fused with the vomer and the presphenoid. It is situated in the fundus of the nasal cavity. In addition to the lateral masses (labyrinth) and cribriform plates, it presents orbital plate. Each labyrinth has about twenty ethmoturbinates. Each of which possesses primary and secondary scrolls. However only about seven of these extend close to the midline and are well developed. These are called the endoturbinates. The rests are the ectoturbinates. The **interparietal bone** fuses with the occipital before birth. The interoccipital protuberance is absent. The **parietal bones** are extensive. A distinct temporal line on the external surface divides this part into the dorsal flat parietal plane and the lateral flat temporal plane. The medial planes of the bones of two sides unite in the middle and form the sagittal crest. The temporal plane forms a large part of the temporal fossa. Caudally it blends with the occipital and forms the distinct nuchal crest. The **frontal bones** have the squamous, nasal and the orbital parts. The external surface of the squamous part is mostly convex. The supraorbital foramina are placed midway between the orbital margin and the frontal suture. The supraorbital grooves extend rostrally from the foramina to the nasal region and from there to the maxilla. The nasal part fuses with the nasal bone. The orbital part is extensive. The **temporal bone**, as in other species, consists of squamous, tympanic and petrous parts. The occipital processes emerges from the caudal portion of squamous part. The temporal crest on the lateral surface forms the lateral limit of the temporal fossa. The cerebral surface of the squamous part is small and is divided by tentorial process of parietal bone into rostral and caudal parts. The temporal surface is small and convex and presents a prominent projection. The zygomatic process arises from the ventral portion of the temporal and joins the temporal process of the zygomatic to form the zygomatic arch. The bony orbit, however, remains incomplete because the zygomatic process of temporal bone does not join the zygomatic process of the frontal bone as it occurs in ox. The petrous part of the tympanic is relatively small and irregular. The crest forming the tentorium cerebelli is absent. **The vomer** is very long and reaches rostrally to the body of the incisive bone and caudally to the level of presphenoid. Its ventral sharp edge articulates with palatine proves of incisive. The middle half of this edge is received into a groove formed by the nasal crest of the palatine bone. It assists in extending the nasal septum caudally between the right and left nasopharyngeal meatuses. The **maxilla** is extensive and forms a considerable part of lateral wall of the nasal cavity. The facial crest extends onto the zygomatic process and is continued as a crest across the zygomatic bone. The **nasal bones** are relatively long. Approximately one fifth of its rostral part is free and extends into between the nasal cartilages. At its rostral end it forms nasomaxillary notch along with the incisive bone. The **incisive** bone has a body and three processes, the alveolar, nasal and palatine. The body of the opposite bones is incompletely fused and forms the interincisive fissure. The palatine surface of the body is marked by two or three transverse grooves similar to those of palatine bone. The alveolar process has three alveoli for incisors. The nasal process forms the nasoincisive notch in association with the nasal bone. The palatine processes of the bones of opposite side fuse medially.

The **palatine** bone has the horizontal and perpendicular parts similar to those in other species. Each of the **pterygoid bones** is narrow in the middle and wide at the ends. The lacrimal bone is irregular. Its orbital surface is concave. The facial surface is also concave and similar to that in other species. The nasal surface, however, is marked by a distinct ridge lateral to which is the maxillary sinus. The **zygomatic (malar) bone** is compressed mediolaterally. Its orbital surface is small and deeply grooved. Dorsally it presents the frontal process and ventrally the temporal process. Of the **turbinates (nasal conchae),** the ventral turbinate is larger and more complicated than the dorsal turbinate. It occupies major portion of the nasal cavity. The body of the **mandible** is formed by fusion of the two halves which diverge at a greater angle than that in ox and horse. The mental surface of the body slopes down and bears the prominence at the point of divergence of the bodies. It presents a pair of medial mental foramen and The labial surface presents the pair of lateral mental foramen. The alveolar border of the unified body of mandible presents six alveoli for the incisors. The rami of the mandible are almost same as that of horse except that the angle of the mandible thick and smoothly curved. Of the **hyoid bones**, the basi hyoid is broad rostrocaudally and short transversly. It bears lingual process on its ventral aspect. The thyrohyoids are wide and curved. The ceratohyoids are short, wide and flattened. The epihyoid is slightly longer than the ceratohyoid. The stylohyoid is very slender rod like.

In addition to these, the skull of pig has an additional bone called **the rostral bone**. This bone is situated in the most rostral part of the nasal septum. It is pyramidal in shape with its base directed rostroventrad and the apex is directed towards the nasal septum. Two pairs of projections extend from the caudoventral part of the base. Of these the medial pair extends directly towards the incisive bone while the lateral pair forms a base for the accessory nasal cartilage. The lateral surface of the rostral bone forms the medial wall of the nostrils.

Amongst the **sinuses**, the maxillary sinus is well developed and extends to zygomatic, lacrimal, ethmoid and ventral turbinate bones. The maxillary sinus opens into nasal cavity through an aperture called the nasomaxillary opening. The frontal sinus is the largest and most complicated amongst the paranasal sinuses in pig. It excavates the the frontal, parietal, occipital and temporal bones. It has two parts, the rostral and caudal. The rostral frontal sinus communicates with the nasal cavity through the ethmoidal meatus while the caudal frontal sinus opens directly into the nasal cavity. The lacrimal sinus is developed separately in pig. In some cases it may join the rostral frontal sinus to open into the nasal cavity. The sphenoid sinus is more complex in pig than in other species. It extends into the basisphenoid, basi occipital and the temporal bones. It communicates caudally with the fundus of the nasal cavity via the ventral ethmoidal meatus. In addition to these there are small independent excavations into the bones surrounding the lateral masses (labyrinths) of the ethmoid bone. These are called the ethmoidal cells. The conchal sinuses open directly in the nasal cavity.

Fowl

The skull of fowl is small and conical. Its rostral extremity is elongated. Generally it has most of the elements those are present in the mammalian skull. The constitution of head, placement of different segments of bones and their relations with the adjacent bones are almost same. Even then it is the most highly specialized skull amongst the vertebrate animals. The prominent features of the skull of fowl include the absence of teeth and paranasal sinuses, absence of sutures between different bones due to fusion of most of these bones of skull, pneumatisation of the bones by extension of air sacs, and above all these, the skull of fowl is kinetic in which the upper jaw is movable. It swings up and down and articulates with the cranium by a movable nasofrontal hinge joint. The quadrate bone, that is placed between the temporal above and mandible below articulates with these bones in diorthroidal joints. It also assists in the kinetic mechanism of the skull.

The cranium is composed of all the bones except the interparietal. The orbital fossae are relatively large and those of the opposite side are closer to each other . These are separated by a thin interorbital septum formed by the sphenoid and ethmoid bones. The bony rim of the orbit is comparatively small. The large optic foramen is placed at the caudal border of the septum.

The **occipital bone** has a single condyle (instead of two in domestic animals) that articulates with the atlas vertebra. This helps in rotating the head around the neck. The **interparietal is absent**. The **parietals** feel the space between the occipital and frontal bones. **Sphenoid** is triangular and forms greater part of the base of the cranium. The presphenoid has a body and a pair of wings. The post sphenoid has only body and no wings. It articulates with pterygoid and forms diorthroidal joint. The **ethmoid** has horizontal and perpendicular parts. The **frontal** has a strong supraorbital process which joins the zygomatic process of malar and temporal. The **temporal** has two parts. The caudal part contains the organ of hearing while the rostral part articulates with the quadrate bone. The **maxillae** are in the form of rudimentary bones placed on either side of the beak. The **incisive** (premaxilla) is a single bone formed by the fusion of two lateral parts. It forms the skeleton of upper jaw of the beak. **Palatine** forms the rostral boundary of the caudal nares and the part of the roof of the mouth. The **pterygoid** is in the form of a bony rod placed obliquely extending upward from sphenoid to quadrate bone. It forms caudal boundary of the caudal nares. **Nasal bones** are small, thin and pliable plate of bone. They form greater part of the roof of the nasal cavity. The rostral extremity is notched to form the caudal boundary of the rostral (external) nares. The medial border of the two nasal bones is separated by an interval, the internasal space which is filled in by the nasal process of the incisive bone. The **zygomatic** (malar) is slender, rod like bone lying below the orbit. It articulates rostrally with maxilla and caudally with the quadrate bone. The lacrimal is small and triangular plate of bone that forms the part of the orbital wing. The **vomer** is very slender. It separates the caudal (internal) nares and the nasal chambers. The **turbinate bones** (nasal conchae) are three in number, the dorsal, middle and the ventral. The middle turbinate is largest and ventral one is smallest. The **mandible** is formed of two halves fused medially. Each half of the bone consists of five parts. These are, the articular, angular, supra angular, splenial and dentary. The articular part forms the caudal part of the mandible and it is expanded. It bears a small facet for articulation with the quadrate bone. The angular is a slender strip of bone lying below the articular part along the caudal border s of the jaw. The supra angular is also slender and forms the caudal third or more of the upper border of the mandible. It bears a small coronoid process just in front of the articular facet for the quadrate bone. The splenial is a thin plate of bone placed along the medial surface of the mandible. The dentalis is the largest of the five parts of mandible and forms the rostral half of the lower jaw and the two of the opposite side unite in front. The **quadrate bone** is irregularly quadrilateral and is placed between the temporal and the mandible in front of tympanic cavity. It articulates dorsally with the pterygoid and ventrally with the mandible by diorthroidal joint. The **hyoid bone** in fowl is composed of three median segments and a pair of thin, long curved processes. The first median segment is rostral paraglossal (entoglossal) segment. It is a triangular arrow shaped piece of bone that is embedded in the tongue. Its caudal end articulates with the second median segment, the basihyal (body). It is slender rod like in shape and its rostral articulation with the paraglossal segment is movable. It articulates caudally with the third segment, the urohyal which is a long slender osseocartilagenous rod that rests on the larynx and laterally with the paired lateral processes by means of a transverse cartilaginous piece. Each of the lateral processes consists of the rostral longer rod of bone, the basi-branchial and the caudal shorter rod, the cerato-branchial. The two are connected by a cartilage. The cerato-branchial is continued by another piece of slender cartilage which lies behind the auditory opening.

17

Skeleton of Neck

Cervical vertebrae

The skeleton of neck (Fig 2-1) is formed by the cervical vertebrae. These are seven in number. Of these, the first and second cervical vertebrae are highly modified and deviate greatly from the general architectural plan of the vertebrae. The third, fourth and fifth cervical vertebrae are similar and confirm the general plan of the vertebrae. The sixth and seventh vertebrae have some special characteristics but do not deviate much from the general plan. The general plan of vertebrae and the vertebral column has been described in the chapter on skeletal system under Part I on systemic anatomy. Hence, only regional specific characters of the cervical vertebrae are described hereunder.

First cervical vertebra (Atlas)

The first cervical vertebra (Figure 2-2 A) is called the atlas vertebra because in man it supports the globe of the head. This is an atypical vertebra and it deviates greatly from the general plan of vertebrae. The body and the spinous process are absent. The arch forms a bony ring from which two large curved plates, the wings project laterally. The ring encloses the vertebral foramen. It forms a part of the vertebral canal through which passes the spinal cord.

The dorsal arch of the ring is dome shaped. Exteriorly it presents the median dorsal tubercle. The ventral arch is thicker, narrower and less curved than the dorsal arch and it posses exteriorly the median ventral tubercle, which presents attachment for the longus colli muscle. The internal surface of the ventral arch near its caudal border is transversely concave articular area called the fovea dentis on which the dens of the axis vertebra rests. Just cranial to this the floor of the ring is rough for attachment of ligamentum dentis. Exteriorly the dorsal and ventral arches of the ring possess two lateral masses.

The wings are extensive curved plates projecting ventrolaterally and caudally from the lateral masses. The dorsal surface of the wings is concave. Between the ventral surface of the wing and the lateral masses is a large depression

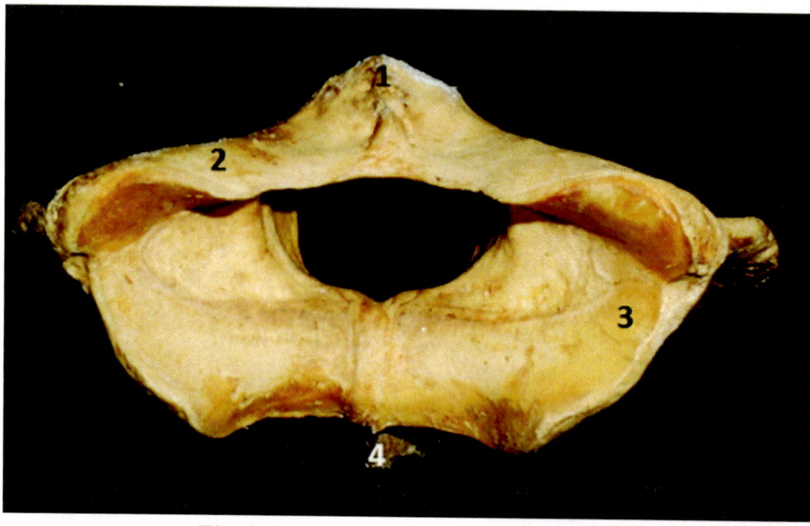

Fig. 2-2 A: First Cervical Vertebra (Atlas)
1. Dorsal tubercle; 2. Wing of atlas; 3. Articular facet; 4. Ventral tubercle

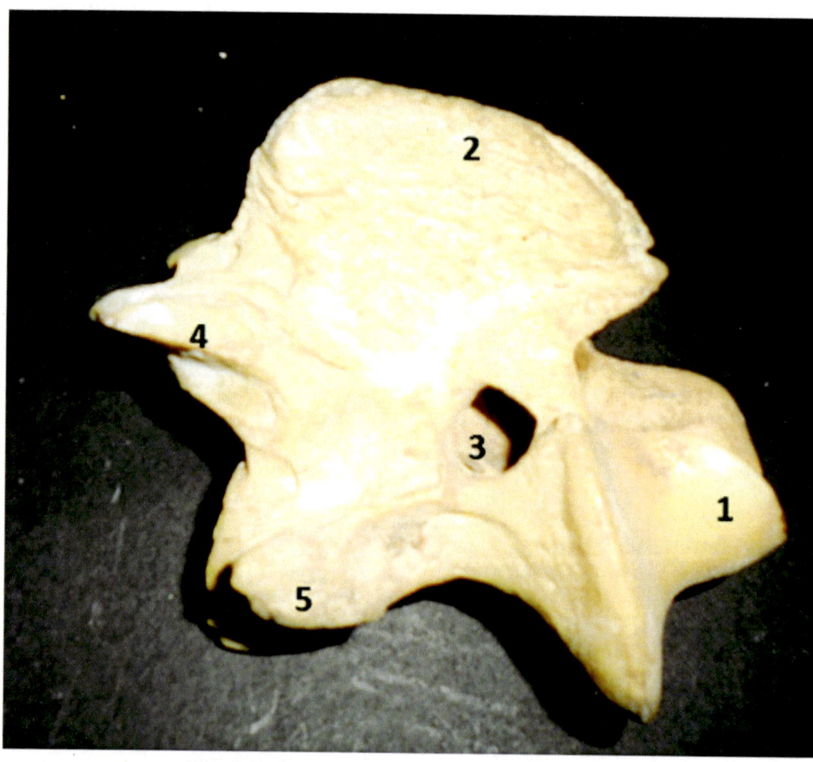

Fig 2-2 B: Second Cervical Vertebra (Axis)
1. Odontoid process; 2. Spinous process; 3. Intervertebral foramen; 4. Caudal articular process; 5. Transverse process.

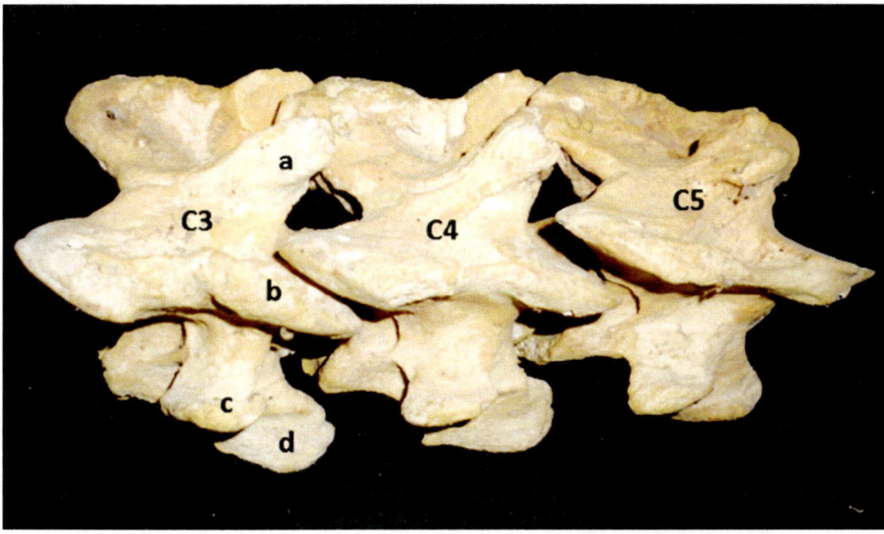

Fig. 2-2 C: Third, Fourth and Fifth Cervical Vertebrae
C3. Third cervical vertebra; a. Spinous process; b. Caudal articular process; c. Dorsal division of transverse process; d. Ventral division of transverse process; C4. Fourth cervical vertebra; C5. Fifth cervical vertebra.

(cavity) the atlantal fossa. At the bottom of this fossa are two foramina which open into the vertebral canal. The cranial of these provides passage for the first cervical spinal nerve and the caudal one provides passage for the vertebral vessels. Each wing is perforated by two foramina. One of these is called the alar foramen and the other is called the transverse foramen.

The cranial edge of the ring is notched above and below. On each side, it presents a deep articular cavity, the condyloid fossa for articulation with the occipital condyles. The caudal edge is rough and sharp in its upper part and presents one central and two lateral notches. The lower three fourths of this edge is extensive, nearly flat, smooth and articular for articulation with the axis vertebra. The right and left articular areas are continuous with each other across the ventral median line.

Second cervical vertebra (Axis)

The second cervical vertebra (Figure 2-2 B) is called the axis vertebra because its dentate process acts like axis around which the ring of the atlas moves in half rotation. It is also called as dentate vertebra because of the tooth like appearance of its process projecting from its cranial end. This is also an atypical vertebra because many of its features deviate from the general plan of vertebrae.

The body of the axis is longest among all the vertebrae of the vertebral column. The cranial end of the body presents centrally the dens or the odontoid process. The ventral surface of the dens is convex and articular for articulation with the atlas. The dorsal surface is concave and rough for the attachment of odontoid ligament. The two surfaces are separated by a sharp convex edge which is notched centrally. On each side of the root of this process, the cranial end of the body presents a nearly flat articular surface. This articular area continues with the ventral articular surface of the dens and these together articulate with the caudal part of the floor of the ring of atlas vertebra. The caudal extremity of the body is strongly concave to receive the convex cranial extremity of the third cervical vertebra forming the intervertebral joint. The pedicle of the arch of the vertebra on its caudal edge presents the notches on either (left or right) side. These notches along with the similar ones of the third cervical vertebra form the intervertebral foramina for the passage of the third cervical spinal nerves. The cranial notches, however, are converted into the oval foramina for the passage of second cervical spinal nerves.

The cranial articular processes are absent and the caudal pair resembles those of the succeeding vertebrae. The transverse processes are small, undivided and project backwards. The transverse foramen is in the form of an osseous canal with cranial and caudal openings. The spinous process (dorsal spine) is very large and strong. Its summit is narrow cranially but thick and wide caudally. It serves for the attachment of the nuchal ligament and muscles. The ventral spine resembles to those of the succeeding vertebrae.

Third, Fourth and Fifth cervical vertebra

The third, fourth and fifth cervical vertebrae (Figure 2-2 C) are typical vertebrae with most of their features similar to those described earlier as features of typical vertebra (This is described under part I- SystemicAnatomy). The bodies of these vertebrae are long with the convex cranial end and concave caudal end. The ventral surface of the body presents the ventral spinous process. This process is in the form of a sharp ridge that becomes prominent as it is traced behind and finally tuberculate as it reaches at its caudal end. The lateral surfaces of the body are slightly concave and with the ventral spinous process serve for muscular attachment. The dorsal surface of the body is flat and provides attachment to common vertebral ligament.

The arch of these vertebrae is very strong and the notches on the pedicles are deep. A foramen perforates the arch and communicates with the transverse foramen.

The facets on the articular processes are very large. The cranial and caudal oblique processes of the same side of the vertebra are connected by a bony plate. The transverse process is perforated by the transverse foramen. The series of these foramina of the cervical vertebrae constitutes the transverse canal for the passage of vertebral vessels and nerves. Each transverse process divides into the dorsal and ventral parts and provides rough area for attachment of muscles. The dorsal spinous process is in the form of a short, thick osseous rod that projects upwards and a little forward. The ventral spinous processes are well developed and serve for muscular attachment. Among the three, the body of the third is longest and it decreases in length from third to fifth. The dorsal spine gradually increases in height from third to fifth.

Sixth cervical vertebra

The sixth cervical vertebra (Figure 2-2 D) closely resembles to the preceding vertebrae with a few variations as under

1. The body is wider but shorter
2. The ventral division of the transverse process is more developed and it is plate like. It extends considerably below and behind the level of the body.
3. The dorsal spine of the sixth vertebra is longer than that of the fifth.
4. The ventral spine is totally absent in sixth vertebra.

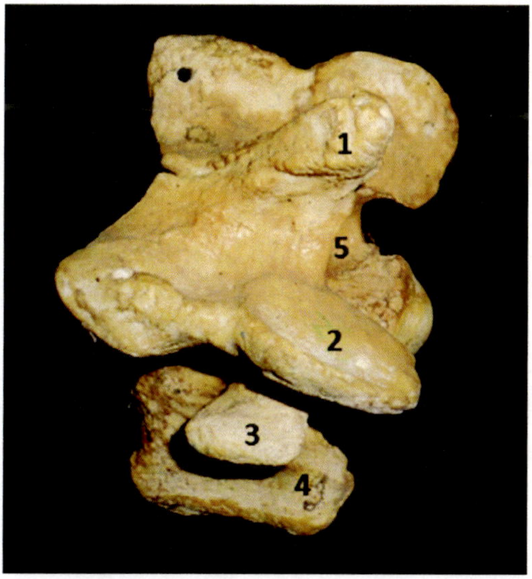

Fig. 2-2 D: Sixth Cervical Vertebra
1.Spinous Process; 2. Articular Process; 3. Dorsal division of transverse process; 4. Ventral division of transverse process; 5. Neural canal.

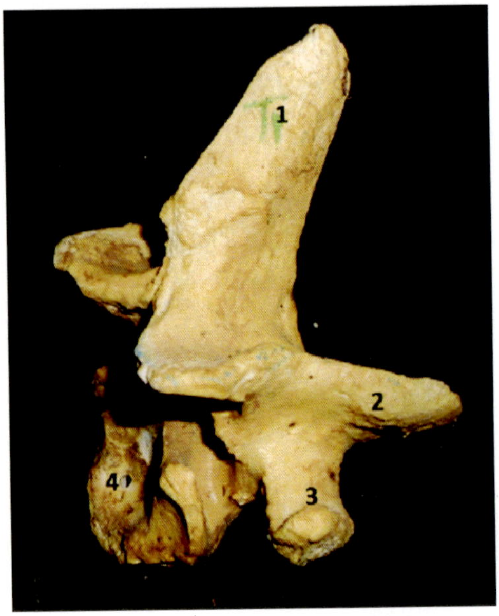

Fig. 2–2 E: Seventh Cervical Vertebra
1.Spinous process; 2. Cranial articular process; 3. Transverse process; 4. Costal facet.

Seventh cervical vertebra

The seventh cervical vertebra (Figure 2-2 E) has the following special features

1. The body of seventh cervical vertebra is shortest of all the cervical vertebrae.
2. The transverse process is single and undivided. The transverse foramen is absent.
3. The dorsal spinous process is well developed as a flattened plate of bone.

It is highest among all the cervical vertebrae and is inclined gently forward.

On either side of the caudal end of the body is a concave semicircular facet called the capitular facet that with similar one on the cranial end of the first thoracic vertebra forms the capitular cavity. This is for the articulation of the head of the first rib.

18

Comparative Anatomy of Skeleton of Neck (Cervical Vertebrae)

Horse

The **first cervical vertebra (atlas)** of horse is more or less similar to that of ox with a few variations as below

1. The wings of atlas are curved ventrad and laterad. These are thinner than in ox but their borders are thick.
2. The wings present an additional foramen, the transverse foramen in the caudal part.
3. A faint groove on the ventral surface of the wing connects the transverse foramen to the intervertebral foramen.

The **second cervical vertebra (axis)** of horse is also more or less similar to that in ox with the following variations.

1. The body of axis in horse is larger than that of ox
2. The dens is longer, narrower and more conical.
3. The cranial extremity presents an undulating saddle shaped articular area.
4. The dorsal spine is more massive and divides caudally into two ridges which terminate on the caudal oblique processes.
5. The transverse process is narrower.

The **third, fourth and fifth cervical vertebrae** in horse differ from those in ox in the following aspects.

1. The bodies of these vertebrae in horse are longer than those of ox.
2. A continuous plate of bone uniting the cranial and caudal oblique processes in horse extends to its full length only in the fifth cervical vertebra. However, in the fourth vertebra it covers only three fourth of the distance, while in third vertebra it reaches to only half way.

3. The dorsal spinous processes are ill developed.
4. The articular processes are better developed.
5. The transverse processes are bifid leading to formation of cranial and caudal divisions.

The **sixth cervical vertebra** in horse has a trifid transverse process, the third division of which is plate like bone extending below the level of the body caudally.

The **seventh cervical vertebra** in horse has a comparatively larger body and its dorsal spine is flattened, triangular and much smaller than that of ox.

Dog

The **first cervical vertebra (atlas)** of dog varies from that of ox and horse in following respects.

1. It is narrower in dog than in ox and horse.
2. Dorsal tubercle is absent.
3. Wings are horizontal
4. A notch represents the craniolateral foramen.
5. The caudal articular area is less concave.

The **second cervical vertebra (axis)** in dog differs in following respects.

1. The dens is rounded, very long, and reach almost to the occipital bone.
2. The cranial articular area is convex.
3. The dorsal spine is larger in size and it overhangs the ring of the atlas.
4. The cranial notches are deep and are never converted into foramina. The **third, fourth and fifth cervical vertebrae** are smaller in size and resemble more or less to those of horse.

The **sixth cervical vertebra** has an extensive transverse process with a plate like lower division and it is ridged on its medial surface.

The **seventh cervical vertebra** is easily distinguished by the shortness of the body, length of dorsal spine and the single undivided transverse process. The transverse foramen is absent.

Sheep and Goat

The cervical vertebrae in general are relatively longer in sheep and goat. The other differences are as below.

1. The first cervical vertebra (atlas) in sheep and goat has less developed dorsal prominence than that of ox.
2. The cranial articular cavities are often separated by a central ridge.
3. The wings are in the form of caudally directed blunt points.
4. The spinous process (dorsal spine) of the second cervical (axis) vertebra is not enlarged caudally.
5. The spinous processes of the third to seventh cervical vertebrae of sheep and goat are less developed than those in ox.
6. The spinous processes (dorsal spines) of the third to seventh cervical vertebrae increase in height from third to seventh cervical vertebra.
7. The arches of the third to seventh cervical vertebrae are separated dorsally by interarcuate spaces.

Pig

The **first cervical vertebra (atlas)** in pig is constituted by the ring and the wings similar to that in ox. However, there are some other deviations as below.

1. The ventral tubercle is long, compressed laterally and projects back under the second vertebra, the axis.
2. The wings are flattened and their caudal part possesses a tuberosity. The transverse foramen passes through the caudal border of the wing to its fossa and is not visible dorsally.
3. The internal surface of the ring of the atlas possesses on either side, a longitudinal projection that partially divides the cavity (vertebral foramen) into a small narrow ventral part and the large dorsal part. The ventral part receives the dens of the axis while the dorsal part provides the passage for the spinal cord.
4. In a fresh state, the gap between the left and right projections is filled in by the dentate ligament of atlanto- axial joint.

The **second cervical vertebra (axis)** has an elongated body and two elongated arches above the body forming the part of the vertebral canal, similar to that in ox. The other specialties are as below.

1. The spinous process (dorsal spine) is larger and is directed dorsally and caudally.
2. The dens is a thick cylindrical rod.

3. The transverse processes are very small.
4. The transverse foramen is often incomplete.

The **third to sixth cervical vertebrae** have the following specialties

1. All these cervical vertebrae are short and wide.
2. The long diameter of the body is in transverse plane.
3. The cranial articular surfaces are slightly convex from side to side with a little concavity dorsoventrally.
4. The caudal articular surfaces are slightly concave.
5. The ventral crest is absent.
6. The arches are wide transversely but the laminae are narrow resulting in larger space in the dorsal part of the vertebral foramen.
7. The pedicles of the arches are perforated by lateral vertebral foramina in addition to the usual intervertebral foramina. The transverse processes divide into two branches. Both of these increase in size from third to sixth.
8. The dorsal branch of transverse process extends laterally and caudally. It is short and thick at its free end.
9. The ventral branch of transverse process is in the form of quadrilateral plate which is directed ventrally. Each of these overlaps to the succeeding one. Thus a series of the lateral borders of the ventral division the transverse processes of the third to sixth vertebrae forms a deep and wide ventral groove.
10. The dorsal spine increases in height from third to sixth cervical vertebra. The cranial ones of these are inclines caudally while the caudal ones are inclined cranially.

The **seventh cervical vertebra** has a short, wide and flat body with a pair of small facets on its caudal margin for the head of the first rib. The spinous process (dorsal spine) of the seventh cervical vertebra is highest amongst the cervical vertebrae. The ventral division of the transverse process is absent.

Fowl

The cervical vertebrae in fowl are fourteen in number.

The **first cervical vertebra (atlas)** is a small ring like bone. The cranial articular surface of the ring is deeply concave for articulation with single occipital condyle. Caudally it presents three articular facets for contact with the axis.

The **second cervical vertebra (axis) possesses** the odontid process (dens) projecting cranially from the lower part of cranial end of its body, similar to that in other species. The cranial articular area is in the form of three facets for articulation with similar facets of the caudal articular area of the atlas. The dorsal and ventral spines are absent.

The rest of the **cervical vertebrae (third to fourteenth)** are more or less similar in characters.

1. The bodies of these vertebrae are rod like.
2. The cranial extremity of each vertebra is concave transversely and convex dorsoventrally.
3. The caudal extremity has convexity in transverse direction and concavity dorsoventrally.
4. The dorsal spine is small and the ventral spine is absent.
5. The articular processes are four in numbers (two pairs) and these are connected with the transverse processes.
6. The transverse processes are large and bear caudally directed slender projections.
7. The transverse foramen is absent.

19

Articulations of Head

Most of the bones of the skull are joined (articulated) with the adjacent bones by sutures. These are immovable joints (synarthroses). The uniting medium is a fibrous tissue and is called the sutural ligament. Most of these joints exist in the early life of the animals and as the age of the animal advances the adjacent bones fuse with each other.

The exception to this is temporomandibular joint which is diorthroidal joint formed between the ramus of the mandible and the squamous part of the temporal bone; and the joints of the hyoid bones The joints of the hyoid bones are amphiarthroses except the basi cornual joint which is an enarthrosis and the thyrohyoid articulation which is a diarthosis..

Temporomandibular articulation

The temporomandibular articulation (Figure 2-3 A) is formed between the condyles of the ramus of mandible and the articular facet of the squamous part of the temporal bone. A small disk of fibro cartilage is interposed between the articular surfaces of this joint to bring out the adaptations of the articular areas. This joint is fastened by two ligaments. The capsular ligament (joint capsule) is strong and tight. It is attached around the articular areas. The lateral ligament extends obliquely across the rostral part of the lateral surface of the capsule running between the zygomatic process and the neck of the ramus of mandible. The movements performed at this joint are the rotation and gliding during the opening and closing of the mouth and in transverse movements in grinding of the food.

20

Articulations of Neck

The articulations of the neck are between the bones of the cervical vertebrae. The atlanto occipital articulation and the atlanto axial articulation are the special vertebral articulations while the articulations between the rest of the cervical vertebrae are common vertebral articulations.

Atlanto-occipital articulation

Type of joint: This is a condyloid type of hinge joint (Ginglymus).

Articular surfaces: The atlanto-occipital joint (Figure 2-3 B) is formed between the condyles of the occipital bone and the condyloid cavities of the atlas vertebra.

Ligaments: The ligaments of this joint are

(1) The capsular ligament which surrounds the joint and is attached to the margins of the condyles and the cranial articular border of the ring of the atlas.

(2) The lateral occipito-atlantal ligaments. These are short right and left bands blended with the capsular ligament. These are attached to the jugular (mastoid) processes of the occipital bone cranially and the cranial margin of the wing of the atlas caudally.

(3) The dorsal occipito-atlantal ligament extends between the dorsal margin of the foramen magnum and the and the ring of the atlas.

(4) The ventral occipito-atlantal ligament extends from the ventral margin of the foramen magnum to the ring of the atlas.

(5) The synovial membranes are two in number, one for each condyle.

Movements: The movements performed at this joint are flexion and extension. Restricted lateral movements are also performed at this joint.

Atlanto-axial articulation

Type of joint: It is a pivot joint in which the atlas carrying the head with it rotates around the pivot formed by the odontoid process of axis.

Articular surfaces: The atlanto- axial joint (Figure 2-3 C) is formed between the atlas and the axis vertebrae. The caudal part of the floor of the ring of the atlas articulates with the ventral articular surface of the odontoid process of the axis vertebra.

Ligaments: The ligaments of this joint are

(1) The capsular ligament is very loose. It encloses the joint and the vertebral canal and is attached to the margins of the articular surfaces.

(2) The ligament of dens (odontoid ligament) is a short, flat, triangular band. It is attached to the dorsal surface of odontoid process of axis caudally and the floor of the ring of atlas cranially.

(3) The dorsal atlanto-axial ligament is elastic and membranous ligament which extends from the dorsal tubercle of atlas to the dorsal spine of the axis.

(4) The ventral atlanto-axial ligament is a thin fibrous band extending between the ventral tubercle of atlas and the ventral spine of the axis.

Movements: The movement performed at this joint is rotation.

The common vertebral articulations are formed between the bodies of the adjacent vertebrae (inter-central articulation) and between the articular processes of the arches of the adjacent vertebrae (inter-neural articulation).

Articulations of the bodies of vertebrae

(Inter-central articulations)

Type of joint: These are amphiarthroses formed between the bodies of the adjacent vertebrae (Figure 2-3 D).

Articular surfaces: These joints are formed by the concave caudal extremity of the preceding vertebra and the convex cranial extremity of the succeeding vertebra and in between these lies the inter-vertebral disc made of fibro-cartilage acting as uniting medium.

Uniting medium: The Inter-vertebral discs acting as uniting medium are interposed between the articular surfaces (concavity and corresponding convexity) of the bodies of the vertebrae. These discs are made of concentric rings of fibro cartilaginous material. This material is soft and pulpy in the centre and thick at the circumference of the disc.

Ligaments: The inter-central articulation is supported by the following ligaments.

(1) **Dorsal common vertebral ligament**: This is a ribbon like white fibrous band running along the floor of the vertebral canal. It extends from the floor of the vertebral foramen of the axis vertebra, runs behind covering the intercentral joints of the cervical vertebrae up to the seventh cervical vertebra and thereon continues in the thoracic part of the vertebral canal. During its course it is intimately attached to the dorsal faces of the bodies of the cervical and other vertebrae and the intervertebral discs.

(2) **Ventral common vertebral ligament**: This is a thin and indistinct ligament in the cervical region. It runs along the ventral surfaces of the vertebrae and the intervertebral discs. In the cervical part of the vertebral column it is supported by longus colli muscle.

Movements: These are amphiarthroses and hence the movements are restricted.

Articulations of the arch of vertebrae

(Inter-neural articulations)

Type of joint: These are diarthroses formed between the articular (oblique) processes of the vertebrae. These joints are abaxial in position.

Articular surfaces: The articular surfaces involved in these joints are the large, oval facets on the paired cranial and caudal articular (oblique) processes of the vertebrae.

Ligaments: The inter-neural articulations are supported and strengthened by the following ligaments.

(1) **Capsular ligament:** These ligaments wrap (enclose) within them the articular processes of the adjacent vertebrae together. The ligament lined by synovial membrane is firmly attached around the area of the facets of the articular processes. With this ligament, each cranial articular process of the vertebra is firmly held against the corresponding caudal articular process of the preceding vertebra.

(2) **Ligamenta flava**: These are membranous expansions of the yellow elastic tissue and they connect the arches of the adjacent vertebrae. These ligaments are externally covered by the muscles of the spine (vertebral column) and internally by the spinal dura mater.

(3) **Interspinous ligament:** These ligaments fill up the interspinous spaces. Each ligament is a narrow elastic band attached to the caudal border of the spinous process of one vertebra and the cranial border of the spinous process of the succeeding vertebra.

(4) **Nuchal ligament (Ligamentum nuchae) :** This is a powerful elastic apparatus that assists the extensor muscles of head and neck in suspending the head with the neck and the rest of the body of the animal. It extends from the occipital bone of the skull to the withers and further continues as thoracolumbar part of the supraspinous ligament. It consists of two parts, the funicular and lamellar.

- **Funicular part:** The funicular part of the nuchal ligament has two divisions, the right and the left. Both the divisions extend from the first thoracic spinous process, proceeds forward in close association with the fellow on the opposite side and terminate on the external occipital protuberance. In the lower cervical region, the right and the left divisions of the ligament unite and the combined ligament becomes broad. This broad part of the ligament is covered by the trapezius and the rhomboideus muscles.
- **Lamellar part:** The lamellar part of the nuchal ligament is thick and is made up of two divisions, the cranial and caudal. The cranial division is double. Its fibres proceed from the funicular part and become inserted to the dorsal spinous processes of the second, third and the fourth cervical vertebrae. The caudal part is single and its fibres arise from the dorsal spinous process of the first thoracic vertebra and are inserted on the dorsal spinous processes of the fifth, sixth and the seventh cervical vertebra.

Movements: The articular surfaces of these joints are flat and hence only gliding type of movements are performed at these joints.

21

Comparative Anatomy of Articulations of Head and Neck

Horse

Articulations of bones of skull

Most of the joints of the bones of skull are sutures similar to those in ox. However, in the adult horse many of the sutures are effaced. The ossification of the cartilage between the basilar part of the occipital and the sphenoid occurs quite earlier. The fusion of the mandibular symphysis takes place at about second to third month after birth. The **temporomandibular articulation** has an additional ligament which consists of elastic tissue. It connects the post-glenoid process to the caudal border of the ramys of the mandible.

Hyoidean articulations

In the hyoidean articulations, there is only one intercornual articulation in horse instead of the proximal and distal cornual articulations appearing in the ox. The middle cornu is generally lodged in the articulation between the great and small cornu.

Joints of cervical vertebrae

Articulations of cervical vertebrae

The **atlanto-occipital articulation**: The space between the foramen magnum and the atlas is wide, hence the membranous ligaments of this joint in horse are larger.

The **atlanto-axial articulation:** The ligament of the dens is better developed. The dorsal gap between the atlas and the axis is wide, hence the ligaments of this joint in horse are larger and better developed.

The **intervertebral articulations:** the intervertebral discs placed between the bodies of the vertebrae are thinner.

The **ligamentum nuchae** is less developed in horse than that in ox.

Dog

Articulations of bones of skull

In **the joints of skull,** the sutures remains fairly distinct throughout the life. The mandibular symphysis remains unossified.

In the **temporomandibular articulation**, the condyle of the mandible is fitted to the temporal articular surface and the fibrocartilage piece between the articular surfaces is thin. The mandible can move freely up and down but the lateral movement is restricted. The caudal ligament is absent.

The **hyoidean articulations** are similar to those of ox.

Articulations of cervical vertebrae

Atlanto-occipital articulation: The two synovial membranes communicate with each other and also with the atlanto-axial articulation.

Atlanto-axial articulation: The odontoid ligament is replaced by three separate branches. Two alar ligaments originate on either side of the dens and are attached to the foramen magnum on either side. The third ligament lies transversely on the dorsal surface of the dens and binds it to the atlantal arch ventrally.

Intervertebral articulations: The interspinous ligaments in the cervical region are replaced by the interspinous muscles. The funicular part of the ligamentum nuchae is reduced to a thin cord extending from the first thoracic vertebra to the axis.

Sheep and Goat

The articulations of the bones of skull and of the cervical vertebrae are more or less similar to those of ox.

Pig

Articulations of the bones of skull

The temporomandibular articulation allows retraction of lower jaw more freely because of the small size of the retroarticular process and comparatively larger longitudinal diameter of the temporal articular surface. The caudal ligament is absent. The transverse movement is limited.

Articulations of the cervical vertebrae

The **atlanto-occipital** and the **atlanto-axial** articulations resemble to those of dog.

The articulations of the rest of the cervical vertebrae are supported by the fibrous raphe and thin layers of elastic tissue which represent the ligamentum nuchae.

Fowl

Articulations of the bones of skull

The bones of skull are completely fused before the birth. Hence no sutures (articulations) are seen in the skull of fowl.

Articulations of the cervical vertebrae

The **atlanto-occipital articulation** is formed between a single occipital condyle and the cranial deeply concave articular surface of the ring of the atlas.

The **atlanto-axial articulation** is formed between the articular facets on the caudal surface of the ring of the atlas and the saddle shaped articular surface at the cranial end of the axis vertebra. At this joint, the long cranial odontoid process of the axis passes through the ring of the atlas and makes contact with the occipital condyle.

22

Muscles of Head

The muscles of the head (Fig. 2-3 A) are described in four groups viz (1) superficial muscles including the cutaneous muscle. The other muscles in this group of muscles are the muscles of lips, cheeks, nostrils, eyelids and external ear. (2) the orbital muscles (3) the mandibular muscles and (4) the hyoid muscles.

The cutaneous muscle on the head of the ox is well developed and extensive. In most of the regions of the head it is intimately adhered to the skin. The superficial fascia forms a continuous layer beneath the cutaneous muscle in this region except the natural orifices like nostrils, mouth, eyes and the external ear. The deep fascia forms a continuous layer particularly on the temporal, buccal, and the pharyngeal parts of the head. A part of the cutaneous muscle on the frontal region is called the frontalis muscle. The muscle fibres of this muscle blend with the muscles of the eyelids and the contraction of fibres of this muscle causes elevation of the superior eyelid and forms wrinkles to the skin on forehead.

The skeletal muscles of the head region are organized into different groups as per the organs and the sub region of the head on which they work. These groups of muscles are

(1) Muscles of facial region (lips, cheeks and nostrils).

(2) Muscles of palpebral region (eyelids)

(3) Muscles of auricular region (external ear)

(4) Muscles of temporo-mandibular region

(5) Muscles of hyoid region (hyoid bones)

(6) Muscles of ocular region (oculi)

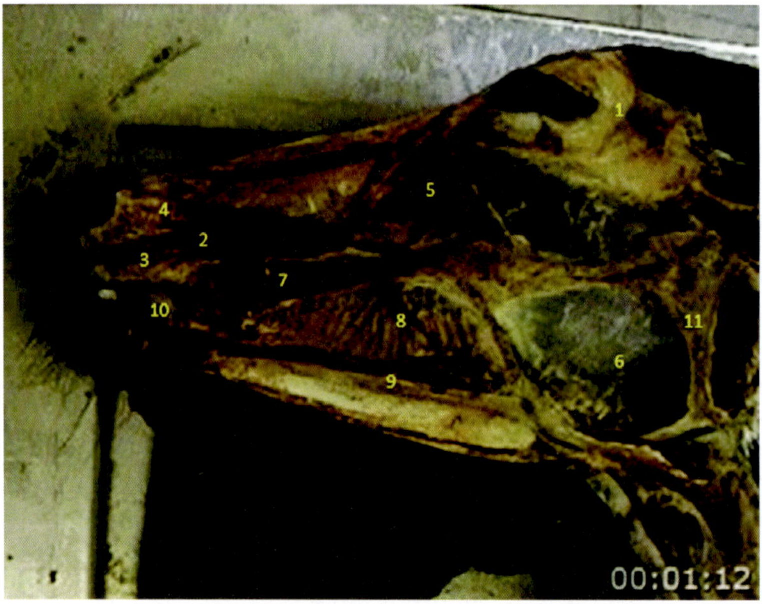

Fig. 2–3 A: Muscles of Head of Ox; Lateral aspect
1.Orbicularis oculi; 2. Levator labi superioris; 3. Dilator naris lateralis; 4. Depressor labi superioris; 5. Malaris; 6. Massater; 7. Zygomaticus; 8. Buccinator; 9. Depressor labi inferioris; 10. Orbicularis oris; 11. Parotido auricularis.

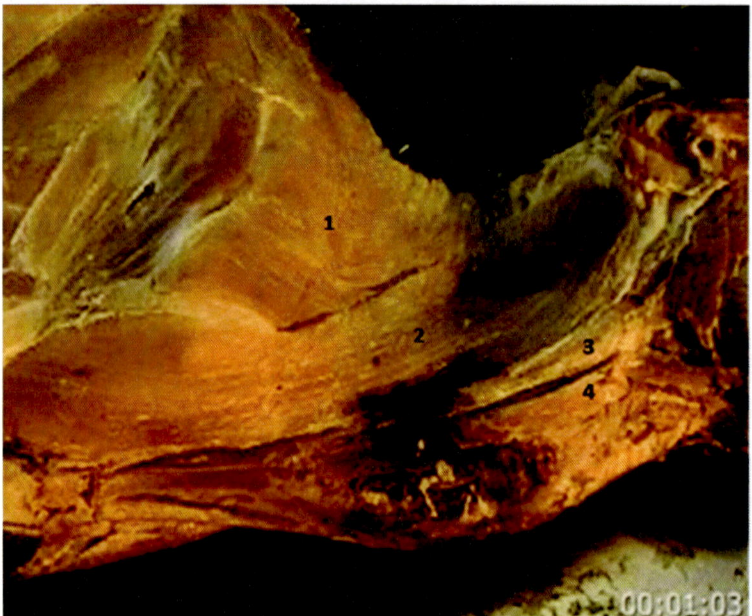

Fig. 2–4 A: Muscles of Neck of Ox; Lateral and Ventral group
1.Trapezius; 2. Brachiocephalicus; 3. Sternocephalicus; 4. Sternothyrohyoideus

Muscles of facial region

(Muscles of lips, cheeks and nostrils)

The muscles of the head are grouped into different groups as muscles of lips, cheeks, nostrils etc

Muscles of lips

Orbicularis oris

It is a sphincter muscle that surrounds the rim (rostral opening) of the mouth, except at the region covered by the muzzle. This muscle is covered externally by the skin and is lined internally by the mucous membrane. It blends with all other muscles of the face that converge to the angles of the mouth.

Action: To close the lips and help in suction and mastication.

Blood supply: Maxillary (superior) labial and Mandibular (inferior) labial arteries.

Nerve supply: Facial nerve, Superior and inferior maxillary nerves.

Levator nasolabialis

It is a thin and extensive muscle. It extends as a continuation from the frontalis muscle above and continues below up to the upper lip and the nostrils.

Origin: The nasal and frontal bones

Insertion: The nostrils and the upper lip, the nasal cartilage and the nasal process of incisive bone.

Action: To elevate the upper lip and to dilate the nostrils

Blood supply: Facial artery

Nerve supply: The facial nerve

Levator labii maxillaries (levator labii superioris)

It is a thin and flat muscle on the rostro-lateral aspect of the face. It extends from the facial tuberosity to the muzzle and is partly covered by the levator nasolabialis and malaris muscles.

Origin: Facial tuberosity.

Insertion: By several tendons to the upper lip.

Action: To elevate the upper lip and to draw it to a side.

Blood supply: The dorsal labial artery.

Nerve supply: The facial nerve.

Depressor labii maxillaries (depressor labii superioris)

It is a small fusiform muscle situated below the levator labii maxillaries on the side of the face. It extends from the facial tuberosity and runs down on the rostro-lateral aspect of the face and terminates into the upper lip'

Origin: Facial tuberosity

Insertion: Upper lip

Action: To compress (depress) the upper lip, may also assist in dilating the nostrils.

Blood supply: The maxillary (dorsal) labial artery

Nerve supply: The facial nerve.

Depressor labii mandibularis (depressor labii inferioris)

It is situated on the lower part of the lateral aspect of the face extending from the ramus of the mandible to the lower lip.

Origin: The alveolar border of the mandible in common with the buccinator muscle.

Insertion: The ventro-lateral aspect of the mandibular (lower) lip.

Action: To depress the lower lip.

Blood supply: The mandibular labial artery

Nerve supply: The facial nerve

Mentalis (levator labii mandibularis)

It is a small muscle lying between the ventral aspect of the mandible and the lower lip.

Origin: The ventral and lateral aspect of the body of the mandible up to the mental foramen

Insertion: Orbicularis oris in the lower lip.

Action: To elevate and to form wrinkles on the lower lip

Blood supply: The facial artery

Nerve supply: The facial nerve.

Zygomaticus

It is a strong, thin and narrow muscle situated on the side of the face extending from zygomatic arch to the upper lip.

Origin: The zygomatic arch and the adjacent masseteric fascia.

Insertion: The upper lip immediately above the commissure (angle of the lips) blending with the Orbicularis oris and the buccinator muscles.

Action: To retract the angle of the mouth.

Blood supply: The facial artery

Nerve supply: The facial nerve

Incisivus maxillaries

It is poorly developed muscle as a small fascicle situated in the maxillary (upper) lip.

Origin: The body of the incisive and the interalveolar space of the ramus of the mandible.

Insertion: The maxillary lip.

Action: To pull the lip towards the incisive bone.

Blood supply: The maxillary labial artery

Nerve supply: The facial nerve.

Incisivus mandibularis

It is poorly developed muscle as a small fascicle situated in the mandibular (lower) lip.

Origin: On the body of the mandible, ventral to the second and third incisors.

Insertion: In the mandibular lip blending with the orbicularis oris.

Action: Depression of the middle portion of the mandibular lip.

Blood supply: The mandibular labial artery

Nerve supply: The facial nerve.

Muscles of cheeks (mastication)

Buccinator

It is a broad, flat and thin muscle that forms the major portion of the cheek and lies on the side of the face. It is partly covered by the masseter muscle. Internally it is lined by the buccal mucous membrane. It extends from the maxillary tuberosity and the dorsal part of the alveolar border of the mandible to the angle of the mouth.

Origin: The alveolar border of the maxilla and the mandible from the angle of the mouth to the ramus of the mandible and the maxillary tuberosity.

Insertion: The orbicularis oris at the commissure (angle) of the mouth.

Action: It assists in mastication by retracting angle of the mouth and flattening the cheek.

Blood supply: The maxillary, mandibular and buccal arteries.

Nerve supply: The facial nerve.

Masseter

It is a short, wide muscle that extends from the zygomatic arch and a part of the facial surface of the malar (zygomatic) and the maxilla bones to the vertical part of the ramus of the mandible.

Origin: The facial tuberosity of the maxilla, the facial crest of the zygomatic bone and the ventral surface of the zygomatic arch.

Insertion: The lateral surface of the ramus of the mandible.

Action: To assist in rumination by moving the mandible rostrad and closing the jaw. The muscle of one side can move the jaw laterally outward on the corresponding side.

Blood supply: The facial, transverse, masseter, facial and the temporal arteries

Nerve supply: The masseter nerve.

Temporalis

It completely fills the temporal fossa and is situated on the lateral aspect of the cranium. It extends from the parieto-temporal crest to the vertical part of the ramus of the mandible.

Origin: The temporal fossa

Insertion: Coronoid process of the ramus of the mandible

Action: To close the mouth by retracting and raising the mandible.

Blood supply: The branches of deep temporal artery

Nerve supply: The deep temporal nerve branches of the mandibular nerve.

Pterygoideus medialis

It is situated on the medial surface of the ramus of the mandible. In its form and structure, this muscle resembles the masseter muscle but it is smaller than that muscle.

Origin: The pterygoid process of the basi sphenoid, the palatine crest and the lateral face of the perpendicular (vertical) plate of the palatine bone.

Insertion: The medial surface of the mandible ventral and caudal to the mandibular foramen and the angle of the mandible.

Action: It raises and closes the jaws when the muscle of either side act together, and moves the ramus towards the median plane when the muscle of one side acts.

Blood supply: Pterygoid branches from the maxillary artery.

Nerve supply: The medial pterygoid branch of the mandibular nerve.

Pterygoideus lateralis

It is a short, flat and triangular muscle which is situated in front of the temporo-maxilary joint and is partly covered by the pterygoideus medialis muscle. It extends from the pterygo-palatine fossa to the dorsal end of the ramus of the mandible.

Origin: The pterygopalatine fossa and the pterygoid process of the basi sphenoid bone.

Insertion: The rostromedial border of the mandibular condyle and adjacent part of the neck of the mandible

Action: The muscles of both sides acting together pushes the lower jaw rostrally while acting singly (one side only) the muscle causes lateral movement of the lower jaw to the opposite side.

Blood supply: The pterygoid branch of maxillary artery.

Nerve supply: The lateral pterygoid nerve of the mandibular nerve.

Digastricus

It is a long muscle extending from the jugular process of the occipital to the medial surface of the horizontal part of the ramus of the mandible. The muscle has two bellies, the rostral and the caudal with an intermediate tendon, the origin and insertion of both the bellies is common.

Origin: Jugular process of the occipital bone.

Insertion: Medial surface of the body of the mandible.

Action: To depress the lower jaw and open the mouth.

Blood supply: The external carotid and external maxillary arteries.

Nerve supply: The inferior maxillary and inferior buccal nerve.

Malaris

This is a broad, thin muscle which spreads out on the fascia over the buccinator and masseter muscles. It is located ventral and rostral to the eye.

Origin: The facial part of the lacrimal bone.

Insertion: The buccal fascia in the region of the dorsal border of buccinator.

Action: To elevate the caudal part of the cheek

Blood supply: The malar artery.

Nerve supply: The facial nerve.

Muscles of nostrils

Levator nasolabialis: Already described above under the muscles of lips

Lateralis nasi (dilator naris alaris)

This muscle is in two parts, the dorsal part and the ventral part. The dorsal part is named as dilator naris dorsalis (superioris) and the ventral part is named as dilator naris ventralis (inferioris).

Dilator naris dorsalis (medialis)

Origin: Alar cartilage of the nostril.

Insertion: Medial (Internal) wing of nostril. Action: To dilate the nostrils

Blood supply: The facial and infraorbital artery.

Nerve supply: The facial and infraorbital nerves.

Dilator naris ventralis

This muscle is in two layers, the superficial and deep layers.

Origin: The nasal process of incisive bone and the nasal lateral cartilage

Insertion: The lateral wing of the nostril.

Action: To assist in dilating the nostrils.

Blood supply: The facial and infraorbital arteries.

Nerve supply: The facial and infraorbital nerves.

Caninus (dilator naris lateralis)

It is located between the levator and depressor labii maxillaries. The muscle lies between the two portions of the levator nasolabialis.

Origin: The facial tuberosity.

Insertion: The lateral wall of the nostril

Action: To dilate the nostril.

Blood supply: The facial artery.

Nerve supply: The facial and nasal branches of the maxillary nerve.

Dilator naris apicalis

This muscle is situated in the muzzle beneath the pad of the nasolabial glands. It join the muscle of the opposite side at the median raphe.

Origin: The free border and the dorsal surface of the body of the incisive bone.

Insertion: The medial and ventral portion of the nostril.

Action: To dilate the nostril.

Blood supply: The nasolabial artery of the greater palatine.

Nerve supply: The facial nerve.

Muscles of palpebral and ocular region

(Muscles of eye lids and eye ball)

Muscles of eyelids

Orbicularis oculi

It is well developed flat, elliptical sphincter muscle around the eyelids. The muscle fibres are mainly attached to the skin and the palpebral ligament at the medial canthus of the eye.

Origin: The palpebral ligament originates as a narrow band of fibrous tissue originating at the facial part of the lacrimal bone.

Insertion: Skin and the palpebral fascia beneath and around the eyelids.

Action: To narrow and close the palpebral fissure.

Blood supply: The malar and supraorbital artery.

Nerve supply: The facial nerve

Cutaneus faciei

It is a thin muscle that covers the frontal and nasal regions and terminates in the upper eyelid.

Origin: In the area of the poll and the base of the horn.

Insertion: The fibres spread out over the forehead and converge with the orbicularis oculi.

Action: To wrinkle the skin of the forehead and elevate the upper eyelid.

Blood supply: The supraorbital artery

Nerve supply: The facial nerve.

Levator palpebrae superioris

It is the main elevator of the upper (superior) eyelid. It lies within the periorbita above the rectus dorsalis within the orbit.

Origin: The pterygoid crest

Insertion: The upper (superior) eyelid.

Action: To raise the upper eyelid.

Blood supply: The external ophthalmic artery.

Nerve supply: The oculomotor nerve.

Depressor palpebrae inferioris (malaris caudalis)

This muscle is a caudal portion of malaris muscle of cheek is located ventral to the lower (inferior) eyelid.

Origin: The masseteric fascia covering the rostral part of the massetor.

Insertion: The lower (inferior) eyelid close to the medial canthus of the eye, blending with the orbicularis oculi muscle.

Action: To depress the lower (inferior) eyelid and widen the palpebral fissure.

Blood supply: The malar artery.

Nerve supply: The facial nerve.

Muscles of eyeball

There are seven extraocular extrinsic (bulbar) muscles. Out of these, four are recti (singular-rectus) muscles, two oblique muscles and one retractor muscle of eyeball.

Recti muscles

These are named as rectus oculi dorsalis, rectus oculi ventralis, rectus oculi lateralis and the rectus oculi medialis. All the four muscles have a common place of origin and insertion with a slight difference of the side. They have similarity in action also, except the direction of the action.

Origin: All the four rectus muscles (dorsal, ventral, lateral and medial) arise in a common tendinous ring which is made of the fibrous tissue that surrounds the optic canal opening at the apex of the orbit. From their origin, these muscles pass straightway forward along the respective side of the eyeball. All the muscles, except the ventral, are thicker near their origin and reduce in thickness as they reach their point of attachment. The ventral muscle is thicker at the point of its origin.

Insertion: These muscles insert on the respective side (dorsal, ventral, lateral and medial) of the sclera in the fore part of the eyeball.

Action: The dorsal rectus is elevator, the ventral rectus is depressor, the lateral rectus is abductor and the medial rectus is adductor of the eyeball.

Blood supply: The external ophthalmic artery.

Nerve supply: The oculomotor nerve supplies to all except rectus lateralis which is supplied by abducent nerve..

Oblique muscles

The oblique muscles are two in number, the obliquus dorsalis and obliquus ventralis.

Obliquus dorsalis

It is the longest and narrowest of the bulbar muscles. It arises near the ethmoidal foramen on the medial wall of the orbit and passes rostrally, medial to the rectus medialis muscle on the globe of the eye. On reaching the root of the zygomatic process, it reflects almost at right angle around the trochlea from where it turns laterally and rostrally and passes between the dorsal and lateral rectus before terminating on the sclera of the eyeball.

Origin: The body of the sphenoid bone, near the ethmoid foramen.

Insertion: The sclera just caudal to the lateral rectus muscle.

Action: It elevates and rotates the eyeball outwards.

Blood supply: External ophthalmic artery

Nerve supply: The trochlear nerve.

Obliquus ventralis

This muscle arises from the depression behind the lacrimal fossa. It passes ventral to the rectus ventralis below the eyeball and inserts on the sclera between the lateral and ventral rectus muscles.

Origin: Lacrimal fossa on the orbital part of the lacrimal bone.

Insertion: Somewhere between the insertion of the lateral and ventral rectus muscles on the sclera of the eyeball.

Action: It depresses and rotates the eyeball inwards.

Blood supply: The external ophthalmic artery

Nerve supply: The trochlear nerve.

Retractor oculi

This muscle is enclosed within the recti muscles and envelopes the optic nerve. It consists of four bundles made of the muscle fibres extending from the fibrous ring around the optic foramen. These bundles of muscle pass forward along the eyeball and get attached to the caudal aspect of the sclera.

Origin: Fibrous ring around the optic foramen in between the recti muscles.

Insertion: Caudal aspect of the sclera of the eyeball.

Action: Retract the eyeball into the orbit.

Blood supply: The external ophthalmic artery

Nerve supply: The abducent nerve.

Muscles of auricular region

(Muscles of external region)

The auricular muscles may be subdivided into two sets, the extrinsic muscles and the intrinsic muscles. The extrinsic muscles arise on the head and the adjacent areas of the neck and move the external ear as a whole. The intrinsic muscles are confined to the auricle only.

Extrinsic muscles

Parotido auricularis

This is a thin wide ribbon like muscle situated on the parotid salivary gland. It is thin and wide at its origin and becomes somewhat narrow as it approach the conchal cartilage.

Origin: The fascia on the ventral and rostral part of the parotid gland.

Insertion: The the ventrolateral aspect of the base of the auricular cartilage of the

Action: To incline the ear ventrally and caudally.

Blood supply: The rostral auricular branch of the superficial temporal artery.

Nerve supply: The caudal auricular branch of the facial and the first and second cervical

Parietoauricularis It is a wide but thin muscle covering the Temporalis muscle.

Origin: The parietal bone, nuchal ligament and the nuchal surface of the occipital bones

Insertion: The medial face of the base of the concha.

Action: To adduct the concha and rotate it forwards (rostrally).

Blood and nerve supply: As above.

Cervicoauricularis

This is well developed muscle with three divisions, the superficial, medius and the profundus. It is situated over the caudal and lateral aspects of the base of the external ear.

Origin: The superficial division arises from the atlantal fascia and nuchal ligament just caudal to the intercornual protuberance. The medius division arises from the atlantoaxial fascia and the profundus from the cervical fascia just lateral to the occipital bone.

Insertion: All the divisions insert on the caudolateral aspect of the prominence of the auricular cartilage.

Action: To adduct the concha and direct its opening outward.

Blood supply: The rostral auricular branch of the superficial temporal artery.

Nerve supply: The auricular branch of the facial nerve.

Zygomaticoauricularis

It is a well developed muscle of almost uniform diameter from its origin to insertion.

Origin: From the zygomatic arch on the caudolateral aspect of the eye.

Insertion: Lateral prominence of the auricular cartilage.

Action: To erect the ear in the act of pricking.

Blood supply: The auricular branch of superficial artery.

Nerve supply: The facial nerve and the first two cervical nerves.

Intrinsic muscles

Scutuloauricularis

This muscle extends from the lateral surface of the scutiform cartilage to the rostral and medial sides of the conchal cartilage. It is composed of three layers, the superficial, middle and deep.

Origin: The superficial layer arises from the dorsal surface, the middle layer arises from the rostral half of the lateral surface, and the deep layer arises from the deep face of caudal half of the scutiform cartilage.

Insertion: The superficial layer inserts on the lateral surface, the middle layer to the medial surface and the deep layer to the rostral part of the medial surface at the base of the conchal cartilage.

Action: It assist the parietoauricularis in turning the opening of the ear forward.

Blood supply: The auricular branch of superficial temporal artery.

Nerve supply: The auricular branch of the facial nerve.

Antitragicus, Helicis and Transversus auricularis

These three are very small muscles and are comprised of a few muscle fibres but all of them are distinctly separate from each other. These are attached to the auricular cartilage.

Origin: At the junction of the two borders of the auricular cartilage.

Insertion: The antitragicus inserts on the caudal border, the helicis on the cranial border and the transversus on the convex surface of the auricular cartilage.

Action: To erect the external ear (concha).

Blood supply: The caudal auricular artery.

Nerve supply: The a uricular branch of facial nerve.

Muscles of hyoid region

The hyoid muscles are eight muscles which assist in the movement of the tongue, pharynx and larynx. Seven of these muscles are paired while the last one, hyoideus transversus is a single muscle.

Mylohyoideus

This is a thick, broad and flat muscle situated in the intermaxillary space and along the medial face of the ramus of the mandible. The two muscles (muscles of opposite side) together form a sort of sling to support the tongue.

Origin: The mylohyoid line on the medial face of the alveolar border of the ramus of the mandible.

Insertion: The median fibrous raphe, glossal process, body and the thyroid cornu of the hyoid bone.

Action: To raise the hyoid bone and elevate the tongue.

Blood supply: The sublingual artery.

Nerve supply: The inferior maxillary nerve.

Stylohyoideus

This is a ribbon like muscle extending from the muscular angle of the proximal extremity of great cornu to the thyroid cornu and the body of the hyoid bone. It has a long slender tendinous origin but a fleshy insertion.

Origin: The muscular angle of the stylohyoid bone.

Insertion: The lateral extremity of the basihyoid bone.

Action: To depress and retract the tongue by drawing the hyoid bone dorsally and caudally.

Blood supply: The facial artery.

Nerve supply: The stylohyoid branch of the facial nerve.

Occipitohyoideus

It is a small, thick, and triangular muscle which fills the space between the proximal extremity of the great cornu and the jugular process.

Origin: The lateral surface of the jugular process.

Insertion: The caudal border of the muscular angle of the stylohyoid bone.

Action: To draw the muscular angle of the stylohyoid bone caudally and to carry the rostral end of the stylohyoid bone ventrolaterally.

Blood supply: The caudal auricular artery.

Nerve supply: The stylohyoid branch of the facial nerve.

Geniohyoideus

It is elongated, fusiform muscle that extends from a little behind the symphysis of the mandible to the hyoid bone lying on the ventral surface of the tongue, deep to the mylohyoideus muscle. The muscles of the opposite side lie alongside to each other.

Origin: Oral surface of the body of the mandible near the mandibular symphysis.

Insertion: The basihyoid bone.

Action: To draw the hyoid bone rostrally and to protrude the tongue.

Blood Supply: The lingual and sublingual arteries.

Nerve supply: The hypoglossal nerve.

Ceratohyoideus (keratohyoideus)

This is a small triangular muscle that lies in the space between the thyrohyoid and ceratohyoid bones. It is covered mostly by the hyopharyngeus and partly by the hyoglossus muscles.

Origin: The caudal edge of the ceratohyoid and the border of the thyrohyoid bones.

Insertion: The dorsal edge of the thyrohyoid and a small attachment on the epihyoid.

Action: It elevates the thyrohyoid and pulls the larynx rostrally.

Blood supply: The lingual artery.

Nerve supply: The lingual branch of glossopharyngeal nerve.

Hyoideus transversus

It is a small unpaired bifid muscle which extends transversely between the two ceratohyoid bones.

Origin: The proximal extremity of small cornu and at its junction with the middle cornu.

Insertion: The body and small cornu of the hyoid bone.

Action: To elevate the root of the tongue.

Blood supply: The lingual artery.

Nerve supply: The glossopharyngeal nerve.

Sternothyrohyoideus and **Omohyoideus**: These muscles are described with the muscles of the ventral surface of the neck.

Muscles of tongue

(Lingual muscles)

The lingual muscles are of two types, the extrinsic and intrinsic.

Intrinsic muscles

The intrinsic are not the distinct muscles and are not attached to the bones. Instead, these are in the form of longitudinally, transversely and perpendicularly running muscle fibres blending with the extrinsic muscles and also with each other. These muscles arise and insert within the tongue itself. These muscles act jointly to shorten the tongue, lessen its width and thus change the shape and form of the tongue as per the need. The blood supply is through the lingual and sublingual branches of the linguofacial artery. The nerve supply is from the glossopharyngeal and the facial nerves.

Extrinsic muscles

The extrinsic muscles of the tongue arise from the bones, radiate from the point of their origin and enter the substance of the tongue and terminate there. A thin median connective tissue layer, the septum linguae separates the extrinsic muscles in to two opposite sets. There are four extrinsic muscles on each side.

Styloglossus

It is a long slender muscle lying along the ventrolateral surface of the tongue.

Origin: It originates in the form of a flat tendon from the rostral end of the stylohyoid.

Insertion: Rostrolateral part of the tip of the tongue.

Action: Retract and shorten the tongue. The unilateral action draws the apex of the tongue laterally.

Blood supply: The lingual and sublingual branches of the linguofacial artery.

Nerve supply: The glossopharyngeal nerve.

Hyoglossus

It is a wide and flat muscle. It lies lateral to the base of the tongue. It covers the genioglossus.

Origin: It arises from the basihyoid, the lingual process and the thyrohyoid.

Insertion: It blends with intrinsic musculature and terminates over the root of the tongue.

Action: To retract and depress the tongue.

Blood supply: The sublingual branch of the linguofacial artery.

Nerve supply: The glossopharyngeal and mandibular branch of the facial nerve.

Genioglossus

It is a flat muscle which lies parallel to the median plane on the ventral surface of the tongue. It is separated from the muscle of the opposite side by the septum lingue.

Origin: At the angle of the chin on the medial surface of the mandible just caudal to the symphysis of the body of the mandible.

Insertion: It converges with the fibres of the intrinsic muscle and terminates at the ventrolateral aspect of the tip of the tongue.

Action: The action of this muscle is composite. When the muscles of both sides are acting together, it depresses the tongue and a median groove is formed on the dorsum of the tongue. The caudal fibres pull the tongue rostrally, the middle fibres depress it and the rostral fibres retract the tip of the tongue.

Blood supply: The sublingual artery of the linguofacial trunk.

Nerve supply: The hypoglossal nerve.

Palatoglossus

It is a thin and narrow muscle extending from the soft palate to the root of the tongue.

Origin: It arises on the free border of the soft palate.

Insertion: It blends with the hyoglossus and then terminates on the root of the tongue.

Action: It narrows the isthmus fausium.

Blood supply: Sublingual branch of the linguofacial artery.

Nerve supply: The hypoglossal nerve.

Muscles of soft palate

Levator palati

It is a small thin muscle that extends from the tympanic part of the temporal bone, passes beneath the pterygo pharyngeus and expands above the glandular layer of the soft palate.

Origin: It arises from the styloid process of the petrous temporal bone.

Insertion: On the soft palate

Action: To raise the soft palate towards the roof of the pharynx and to close the caudal nares during deglutition.

Blood supply: The caudal palatine branch of the palato-nasolabial artery.

Nerve supply: The caudal palatine branch of the superior maxillary nerve.

Tensor palati

It is a thin muscle extending from the Eustachian tube and then running ventrally and rostrally to reach the hamulus of the pterygoid bone where it divides into deep and superficial parts. The deep part is attached to the bone while the superficial part forms aponeurosis with the soft palate.

Origin: The cartilage of the auditory (Eustachian tube) and the adjacent part of the temporal bone.

Insertion: In two parts. The deep part inserts on the lateral surface of the pterygoid bone. The superficial part forms aponeurosis with the soft palate.

Action: It tenses the soft palate which otherwise is arched in the relaxed condition.

Blood supply: The caudal palatine branch of the palato-nasolabial artery.

Nerve supply: The caudal palatine branch of the superior maxillary nerve.

Palatinus

This muscle is a small elongated bright red fasciculus lying along with its fellow on the median line of the soft palate.

Origin: It originates from the rudimentary caudal nasal spine on the choanal border of the bony palate.

Insertion: The muscles of the opposite side blend jointly with the oblique part of the palato-pharyngeus muscle and form aponeurosis on the ventral part of the palate.

Action: It raises the soft palate and dilates the isthmus fausium.

Blood supply: The caudal palatine artery.

Nerve supply: The vidian nerve.

Palatopharyngeus

It is situated in the caudal half of the soft palate. It extends downwards and backwards to the lateral wall of the pharynx lying lateral to the soft palate.

Origin: It arises in association with the muscle of the opposite side from the soft palate by aponeurosis.

Insertion: To the thyroid cartilage of larynx.

Action: It tenses the soft palate, shortens and elevates the pharynx and draws the pharynx and oesophagus towards the root of the tongue.

Blood supply: The caudal palatine artery.

Nerve supply: Caudal palatine branch of superior maxillary nerve.

Muscles of pharynx

The pharynx is attached by its muscles to the palatine, pterygoid and hyoid bones and to the cricoid and thyroid cartilages of the larynx. All of these muscles are constrictors except, the Stylohyoideus. These muscles are grouped as below.

Rostral constrictor muscles of pharynx

- Pterygopharyngeus
- Palatopharyngeus
- Stylopharyngeus caudalis

Middle constrictor muscles of pharynx

- Hyopharyngeus

Caudal constrictor muscles of pharynx

- Thyropharyngeus
- Cricopharyngeus

Dilator muscle of the pharynx

- Stylopharyngeus rostralis

Palatopharyngeus is described above under the muscles of the soft palate.

Stylopharyngeus caudalis is a very small short muscle. It arises from the medial face of the great cornu of the hyoid, passes along the lateral face of the palatopharyngeus and spreads out and terminates on the median raphe.

Hyopharyngeus arise from the thyroid cornu of the hyoid and its fibres spread out and terminate on the lateral wall of the pharynx.

Thyropharyngeus is placed behind the hyopharyngeus and arises from the external face of the wing of the thyroid cartilage of the larynx. The fibres pass toward and terminate on the median raphe.

Cricopharyngeus is a small muscle that lies behind thyropharyngeus. It arises from the external part of the cricoid cartilage of the larynx and the fibres run ahead to terminate on the median raphe on the pharynx.

Stylopharyngeus rostralis is a narrow strap like muscular band arising from the upper third of the great cornu of the hyoid. It descends on the side of the pharynx, where some of the fibres blend with those of the pterygopharyngeus, spread out along the wall of the pharynx and insert there.

Blood supply: The ascending pharyngeal artery and the ascending palatine arteries supply to all the above pharyngeal muscles.

Nerve supply: The glossopharyngeal, vagus, spinal accessory and the hypoglossal nerves along with the sympathetic nerve fibres through the cranial cervical ganglion supply branches to the pharynx and its muscles.

Muscles of larynx

Extrinsic muscles

Sterno- thyro-hyoideus Is described with the ventral cervical muscles.

Thyrohyoideus is a paired wide, thin strap like muscle that extends between the thyroid cartilage of the larynx and the body of the thyroid cornu of the hyoid bone.

Origin: Thyroid cornu of the hyoid bone.

Insertion: Oblique line on the lateral face of the thyroid lamina of the larynx.

Action: It elevates the larynx or depress the hyoid bone and draw the larynx towards the root of the tongue.

Blood supply: Laryngeal branch of the thyrolaryngeal artery.

Nerve supply: The hypoglossal nerve.

Hyoepiglotticus is a small paired muscle. The two muscles lie against each other on the median line, pass backward for a short distance and then terminate on the lower part of the epiglottis.

Origin: It arises from the ceratohyoid bone close to its junction with the basihyoid bone.

Insertion: The muscles of the two sides converge and terminate on the basal part of the oral surface of the epiglottis.

Action: It restores the epiglottis to its original respiratory position after deglutition.

Blood supply: Laryngeal branch of the thyrolaryngeal artery.

Nerve supply: The hypoglossal nerve.

Intrinsic muscles

Cricothyroideus muscle is paired and lies on the dorsolateral aspect of the larynx.

Origin: It originates on the caudal border and lateral surface of the arch of the cricoid cartilage of the larynx.

Insertion: The caudal border and adjacent part of the lateral surface of the caudal cornu of the thyroid cartilage.

Action: It tenses the vocal cord and shortens the larynx.

Blood supply: The laryngeal branches of thyrolaryngeal and external maxillary artery.

Nerve supply: Hypoglossal nerve.

Cricoarytenoideus dorsalis is a paired muscle. These muscles of the two sides together cover the entire dorsal surface of the lamina of cricoid cartilage.

Origin: The median ridge and one half of the lamina of the cricoid cartilage.
Insertion: Caudal tubercle (muscular process) of the arytenoid cartilage.
Action: It dilates the larynx as well as the glottis.

Blood supply: Laryngeal branch of superior maxillary artery.

Nerve supply: The hypoglossal nerve.

Cricoarytenoideus lateralis lies along with the thyroarytenoideus muscle on the medial surface of the lamina of the thyroid cartilage. It is a small triangular muscle lying between the thyroid and arytenoid cartilages.

Origin: Cranial border of the lateral part of the cricoid cartilage.

Insertion: Caudal tubercle on the arytenoid cartilage.

Blood supply: Laryngeal branch of superior maxillary artery.

Nerve supply: The hypoglossal nerve.

Thyroarytenoideus is a paired muscle that lies within the lamina of the thyroid cartilage. The muscle of each side is divided into two parts, the rostral called the vestibularis and the caudal part called the vocalis muscle.

The **vestibularis** muscle lies in the lateral wall of the larynx covered by the lamina of the thyroid cartilage.

Origin: The medial surface of the rostral part of the lamina of the thyroid cartilage and also from a part of cricothyroid membrane.

Insertion: The muscular process of the arytenoid cartilage.

The **vocalis** muscle lies medial to the lamina of thyroid cartilage and the lateral cricoarytenoideus muscle and lateral to the vocal ligament.

Origin: The body of the thyroid cartilage, medial to the part of the vestibularis muscle.

Insertion: It inserts into the muscular process of the arytenoid cartilage.

Action: It constricts the entrance to larynx in deglutition and relaxes the vocal cord.

Blood supply: Laryngeal branch of superior maxillary artery.

Nerve supply: The hypoglossal nerve.

Arytenoideus transversus is an unpaired muscle. It is the smallest of the intrinsic muscles of the larynx. It is placed across the concave dorsal surface of the arytenoid cartilage.

Origin: It arises from the median raphe and run over the lateral surface of the cricoid cartilage.

Insertion: It inserts on the muscular process of the arytenoid cartilage.

Action: Adduct the two arytenoid cartilages and narrow the glottis.

Blood supply: Laryngeal branch of superior maxillary artery.

Nerve supply: The hypoglossal nerve.

23

Muscles of Neck (Cervical Muscles)

Cutaneous muscle

In the cervical region of ox, the cutaneus muscle, **cutaneus colli** is poorly developed. It is in the form of a narrow strip on the ventral part of the neck. It arises from the ventral median connective tissue strip of the superficial fascia and extends cranially covering the cervical part of the deep fascia. The fibres of this muscle fan out dorsolaterally and form the aponeurosis with the cervical fascia and join the cutaneus facei.

Fascia

The major groups of muscles of the cervical region are covered by the thick superficial layer of fascia. The fascia is abundant and well developed in the cervical region of the ox. The fascia of the neck is in two layers, the superficial and deep. The superficial fascia is attached to the skin, whereas the deep fascia is again in two parts, the superficial and deep parts. The superficial part covers the superficial structures in the neck viz. the trapezius and brachiocephalicus muscles in the dorsolateral aspect and the jugular canal with jugular vein, and the rhomboideus muscles on the ventrolateral aspect of the neck. The superficial parts of the deep layer of cervical fascia of two sides meet at the median line both, dorsally and ventrally. The deep part of the deep fascia is attached to the vertebrae and the longus colli muscle on either side at the median line and covers the trachea, oesophagus, carotid artery etc before joining ventrally.

The skeletal muscles of the neck region are arranged in two groups, the ventral group and the dorsal or dorsolateral group of cervical muscles.

Ventral cervical muscles

This group of muscles consists of the muscles lying on the ventral and ventrolateral aspect of the neck. The muscles included in this group are as below (Figure 2-4 A)

Brachiocephalicus

This is a thin muscle that extends along the ventrolateral side of the neck from the head to the arm region of the fore limb. It lies beneath the skin and the cutaneus colli muscle. It is divided into two divisions, the dorsal division cleido cephalicus and the ventral division cleido brachialis.

Origin: The cleido cephalicus originates in two parts one from the occipital bone and the ligamentum nuchae (cleido occipitalis), and the other part from the temporal crest, and the mastoid process (cleido mastoideus). These two parts, after their origin combinely descend on the ventrolateral aspect of the cervical region and fuse with the rectus capitis ventralis muscle and form the ventral thick muscle the cleido brachialis which runs down to the craniolateral aspect of the arm region of the fore arm.

Insertion: The cleido brachialis division inserts on the musculospiral groove on the lateral surface of the shaft of the humerus.

Action: When the head and neck are fixed, it pulls up the fore limb craniad, when the limbs are fixed it depresses the head. The unilateral contraction of the muscle flexes the neck to the contracting side.

Blood supply: Superficial and deep cervical branches of the common carotid artery, the humeral and external thoracic artery.

Nerve supply: The ventral branches of the cervical spinal and axillary nerves.

Omotransversarius

It is located on the lateral surface of the neck, extending from the wing of the atlas to the shoulder. In its course, it runs along the deep face of the brachiocephalicus and in its caudal part it lies between the brachiocephalicus and the trapezius muscles.

Origin: On the wing of the atlas

Insertion: The fascia on the shoulder and through it, on the scapular spine.

Action: With the shoulder fixed, it moves the neck laterally. If the neck is fixed, it draws the shoulder and the fore limb craniad.

Blood supply: The vertebral and superficial cervical arteries.

Nerve supply: The cervical and accessory nerves.

Sternocephalicus

It consists of two divisions, the superficial and the deep. The superficial division of this muscle is called the **sternomandibularis** and the deep division is called the **sternomastoideus** (occipitalis). The sternocephalicus muscles of the opposite sides lie close to each other in the lower two thirds of the neck and then diverge from each other covering the lateral aspect of the trachea in the upper thirds of the neck.

Origin: Both divisions originate on the manubrium sterni and the first costal cartilage.

Insertion: The sternomandibularis inserts on the ventral border of the ramus of the mandible and the fascia covering the masseter muscle. The sternomastoideus inserts on the mastoid process of the temporal bone.

Action: When muscles of both sides acting together, it flexes the head and neck ventrally. Acting singly it causes turning the head to one side. The sternomandibularis assists in opening the mouth by depressing the mandible.

Blood supply: The common carotid artery.

Nerve supply: The ventral branches of the cervical spinal nerves.

Sternothyrohyoideus

This muscle lies on the ventral surface of the trachea. The muscles of the two sides lying close to each other completely cover the trachea ventrally and laterally except in the cranial third of the neck where the two muscles diverge laterally for their further course and insertion. The sternothyrohyoideus of each side divides into two parts after reaching near the base of the head. These two parts are named as the **sternothyroideus** and the **sternohyoideus.**

Origin: The sternothyrohyoideus muscle originates on the manubrium sterni.

Insertion: The strenothyroideus inserts on the lateral surface of the lamina of the thyroid cartilage of the larynx. The sternohyoideus inserts on the basihyoid bone medial to the insertion of the Omohyoideus.

Action: It retracts the hyoid bone, tongue and larynx and assists in deglutition.

Blood supply: The muscular branches of the common carotid artery.

Nerve supply: The ventral branches of the first two or three cervical spinal nerves.

Omohyoideus

This is a thin elongated muscle covered by the sternocephalicus and brachiocephalicus muscles. It extends from about the middle of the cervical region at its ventrolateral aspect obliquely upward and forward to the basihyoid bone.

Origin: The fascia covering the third and fourth cervical vertebrae and the cranial part of the serratus cervicis muscle.

Insertion: The ventral face of the body and the glossal process of the hyoid bone.

Action: To depress and retract the hyoid bone and root of the tongue.

Blood supply: The common carotid and vertebral arteries.

Nerve supply: The ventral branch of the first cervical spinal nerve.

Scalenus

This muscle is situated partly in the caudal part of the neck and partly on the craniolateral part of the thorax. It consists of two distinct divisions, the **scalenus ventralis** and **scalenus dorsalis**. The roots of brachial plexus emerge between these two parts.

Origin: The **scalenus ventralis** arises from the transverse processes of the third to seventh cervical vertebrae. The **scalenus dorsalis** arises from the transverse processes of fourth to sixth cervical vertebrae.

Insertion: The **scalenus ventralis** inserts on the first rib and the **scalenus dorsalis** inserts on the fourth rib.

Action: When the muscles of both sides are acting, the neck is flexed and when unilateral it inclines the neck on the corresponding side. If the neck is fixed, this muscle performs respiratory function by pulling the ribs cranially.

Blood supply: The dorsal inter costal and vertebral arteries.

Nerve supply: The ventral branches of cervical spinal nerves.

Rectus capitis ventralis major

It is a long flat muscle extending from sixth cervical vertebra to the base of the cranium lying along the ventrolateral aspect of the second to sixth cervical vertebrae. It forms the continuation of the longus colli muscle coming from the thoracic part of the vertebral column. It connects the entire ventral surface of the cervical vertebral column to the base of the skull.

Origin: The transverse processes of the third to sixth cervical vertebrae. **Insertion:** The muscular tubercle on the basilar part of the occipital bone. **Action:** To flex the head and to incline the head and cranial part of neck laterally.

Blood supply: The occipital and vertebral arteries.

Nerve supply: The ventral branches of second to fifth cervical spinal nerves.

Rectus capitis ventralis minor

This is a small but a strong fleshy muscle that lies dorsolateral to the longus capitis muscle. It crosses the lateral part of the ventral surface of the atlanto-occipital joint.

Origin: The ventral face of the wing of the atlas.

Insertion: The muscular tubercle on the basilar part of the occipital bone along with the longus capitis muscle.

Action: To assist the longus capitis muscle in the flexion of the head and lateral flexion of the cranial part of the neck.

Blood supply: The occipital artery.

Nerve supply: The ventral branch of first cervical spinal nerve.

Rectus capitis lateralis

This is a small muscle slender muscle that lies for the most part under the obliquus capitis cranialis muscle. It runs from the ventral arch and the ventral side of the wing of the atlas to the jugular process of the occipital bone.

Origin: The atlas vertebra.

Insertion: The jugular process of the squamous occipital and the muscular tubercle on the basi occipital bone.

Action: To flex the atlanto-occipital joint and place the head in oblique position.

Blood supply: The occipital artery.

Nerve supply: The ventral branch of the first cervical spinal nerve.

Longus colli

This is a long slender and strong muscle lying on the ventral surfaces of all the cervical and first five or six thoracic vertebrae thus having the cervical and the thoracic parts. The muscle of the two sides running in a V shaped form on ventral and partly on the lateral surface of the bodies of the vertebrae.

Origin: The bodies of the first six thoracic vertebrae and the ventral surfaces of the transverse processes of the cervical vertebrae except the atlas.

Insertion: The muscles arising in the thoracic part insert on the bodies and the transverse processes of the seventh and sixth cervical vertebrae, whereas the cervical part of the muscle inserts on the muscular process of the basioccipital bone.

Action: To flex the neck ventrally.

Blood supply: Common carotid, vertebral, occipital and intercostal arteries.
Nerve supply: Ventral branches of cervical spinal nerves except first and the ventral branches of first four or five thoracic spinal nerves.

Intertransversales colli

These are six segmental muscles. Each of these lie on the lateral aspect of the body of the vertebra and occupies the space between the articular and transverse process and pass from one vertebra to the next in the row in the cervical region of the vertebral column. It is however, not present in the first segment between the atlas and axis. Each muscle has two bundles the dorsal and ventral. The dorsal bundle, after arising at the transverse process of one vertebra runs forward and upwards and then gets attached to the articular process of the preceding vertebra. Whereas the ventral bundle occupies the intertransverse space and is attached to the adjacent transverse process. The muscle bundle from sixth to second cervical vertebra form a common mass of muscles with the strong tendon and is inserted to the wing of the atlas.

Origin: The transverse and articular processes of the cervical vertebrae except the first.

Insertion: In a common cord of muscle inserts on the lateral border of the atlas.

Action: To flex the neck laterally.

Blood supply: The vertebral artery.

Nerve supply: The ventral branches of the cervical spinal nerves.

Dorsolateral (lateral) cervical muscles

The muscles on the dorsolateral aspect of the neck (Figure 2-5 B) are arranged in four layers.

First layer

Trapezius

This is a wide, flat and triangular muscle with its base extending along the nuchal ligament in the cervical part and the supraspinous ligament in the thoracic part. Its apex lies ventrally covering the part of the shoulder. This muscle is very extensive and consists of two parts, the cervical part (**trapezius cervicis)** and the thoracic part (**trapezius thoracis**). However, there is no separation between these two parts. The part of the muscle lying in the cervical region is named as cervical part and the same muscle continues in the thoracic region as thoracic part of the trapezius muscle.

Origin: It originates on the funicular part of the ligamentum nuchae and the supraspinous ligament from the level of atlas or axis to the twelfth or thirteenth thoracic vertebra.

Insertion: The tuberous part of the scapular spine and the fascia of the shoulder and arm.

Action: The cervical part pulls the scapula dorsad and craniad while the thoracic part draws the scapula caudad and dorsad. It also causes inclination of the head and neck laterally.

Blood supply: The vertebral, deep cervical and dorsal intercostal arteries.

Nerve supply: The dorsal branch of the accessory nerve and the dorsal branches of the cervical and thoracic spinal nerves.

Brachiocephalicus

This muscle is described with the muscles of ventral group of cervical muscles.

Second layer

Rhomboideus

It is an extensive muscle extending from about the middle of the funicular part of ligamentum nuchae to the supraspinous ligament at the level of ninth or tenth thoracic vertebra. It has two parts, the **cervical part (rhomboideus cervicis**) and **thoracic part (rhomboideus thoracis).** There is no clear separation between the two parts.

The cervical part is thick and wide at its caudal portion and gradually narrows to about the middle of the neck. The thoracic part is thin and is irregularly quadrilateral.

Origin: The cervical part arises from funicular part of ligamentum nuchae and the supra spinous ligament at the level of the first three or four thoracic vertebrae. The thoracic part arises from the supraspinous ligament at the level of fourth to ninth thoracic vertebra.

Insertion: both the parts insert on the medial surface of the cartilage of the scapula.

Action: The cervical part draws the shoulder craniad and the thoracic part draws it dorsad.

Blood supply: The superior cervical and the dorsal scapular arteries.

Nerve supply: The branches of the cervical and thoracic spinal nerves.

Omotransversarius

This muscle is described with the ventral group of cervical muscle.

Third layer

Serratus cervicis

This muscle lies partly in the neck and partly in the thorax. It extends from the level of second cervical vertebra to the fifth rib. The caudal portion of this muscle is covered by the serratus thoracis muscle. It shows distinct serration ventrally in the thoracic region.

Origin: The transverse processes of the second to seventh cervical vertebra and the lateral surface of the first to fifth ribs.

Insertion: The cranial triangular area on the costal surface of the scapula and the adjacent part of the cartilage of the scapula.

Action: The serratus cervicis and the serratus thoracis muscles of the two sides together form slings which support and suspend the trunk between the two scapulae.

Blood supply: The superior cervical, ventral and intercostal arteries.

Nerve supply: Fifth to eighth cervical spinal nerves.

Fourth layer

Splenius

It is a thin flat triangular muscle lying on the lateral surface of the neck dorsal to the level of the cervical vertebrae.

Origin: It arises from the spinous processes of the first three or four thoracic vertebrae and from the nuchal ligament by aponeurosis right up to the third cervical vertebra.

Insertion: It inserts on the wing of the atlas and the transverse processes of the axis and the third cervical vertebra. It may also terminate on the occipital and the temporal bone.

Action: Acting together the muscles of either side extend the head and neck and acting singly it inclines the head and neck to the corresponding side.

Blood supply: The deep cervical, costocervical and the vertebral arteries.

Nerve supply: The dorsal branches of the cervical spinal nerves except the first two.

Longisimus capitis et atlantis

This is a long and thick strip of muscle located between the splenius and the complexus muscles in the neck. It extends from the level of first or second thoracic vertebra to the head. It consists of two divisions, the superior (**Longissimus capitis**) and the inferior (**Longissimus atlantis).**

Origin: The superior transverse process of the first or second thoracic vertebra and articular processes of the cervical vertebrae.

Insertion: The superior division inserts on the temporal bone by a thick wide tendon in common with the cleido temporalis and the splenius muscles. The inferior division inserts on the wing of the atlas in common with the Omotransversarius and intertransversalis colli muscles.

Action: Acting together, to extend the head and neck and acting singly to incline the neck to the corresponding side.

Blood supply: The superior cervical and vertebral arteries.

Nerve supply: The dorsal branches of the cervical spinal nerves except the first two.

Multifidus cervicis

This is a segmental muscle that lies in a series with the Multifidus thoracis. It consists of six muscular fasciculi lying over the laminae of the first thoracic and last five cervical vertebrae. This muscle lies between the complexus and longissimus capitis et atlantis externally and the lamellar part of the ligamentum nuchae and the superior division of the longissimus dorsi internally.

Origin: The oblique processes of the first thoracic and last five cervical vertebrae.

Insertion: The supraspinous ligament and the oblique processes of the last five cervical vertebrae.

Action: Acting together of the muscles of both sides extends the neck and acting singly it flexes the neck to the corresponding side.

Blood supply: The vertebral and superior cervical arteries.

Nerve supply: The dorsal branches of the last six cervical spinal nerves.

Complexus (semispinalis capitis)

This is the largest of the muscles lying dorsal to the cervical vertebrae. It is covered by the splenius and the Longisimus capitis et atlantis muscles lateral to the ligamentum nuchae. It is narrow at its origin from transverse process of ninth or tenth cervical vertebra. Thereafter it gradually increases in size and becomes a wide muscle till it reaches at the level of seventh cervical vertebra. From here onward it again reduces in size and becomes a narrow strong at the level of atlas vertebra.

Origin: The second, third and fourth thoracic spinous processes in common with the splenius muscle, the transverses processes of the first nine or ten thoracic vertebrae and the articular processes of the cervical vertebrae.

Insertion: The external protuberance on the squamous occipital bone.

Action: The muscles of the two sides acting together extend the head and neck.

Blood supply: The superior cervical and vertebral arteries.

Nerve supply: The dorsal branches of the cervical spinal nerves.

Rectus capitis dorsalis major

This is a narrow elongated fleshy and triangular muscle lying under the complexus lateralis muscle. It consists of two parts, the superficial and deep. The superficial part is longer and narrower. The deep part is three sided at its ventral aspect.

Origin: The spine (supraspinous process) of axis vertebra.

Insertion: The occipital bone near the external occipital protuberance and near the tendon of insertion of complexus muscle.

Action: To extend the head on the neck.

Blood supply: The descending branch of the vertebral artery.

Nerve supply: The dorsal branch of first cervical spinal nerve.

Rectus capitis dorsalis minor

This is a small muscle lying under the rectus capitis dorsalis major. It is located between the atlas and the occipital bone.

Origin: The dorsal arch of the atlas vertebra.

Insertion: The occipital bone lateral to the insertion of the funicular part of the ligamentum nuchae and the external occipital protuberance on the occipital bone.

Action: To extend the head on the neck.

Blood supply: The descending branch of the vertebral artery.

Nerve supply: The dorsal branch of first cervical spinal nerve.

Obliquus capitis cranialis

This is a short, strong quadrilateral muscle. It lies in the space between the atlas vertebra and the occipital bone. It is covered by the aponeurosis of the splenius and brachiocephalicus muscles.

Origin: The cranial border and ventral surface of the atlas vertebra.

Insertion: The mastoid and the jugular process of the occipital bone.

Action: To extend the head.

Blood supply: The descending branch of the vertebral artery.

Nerve supply: The first cervical spinal nerve.

Obliquus capitis caudalis

This is a thick, quadrilateral muscle that lies on the dorsolateral aspect of the atlas and axis vertebrae. It extends from the spine of the axis to the wing of the atlas.

Origin: The lateral surface of the spine and the caudal auricular process of the axis vertebra.

Insertion: The dorsal surface of the wing of the atlas.

Action: To extend or fix the atlantoaxial joint. In its unilateral action it rotates the head around the dens of the axis.

Blood supply: The descending branch of the vertebral artery.

Nerve supply: The second cervical spinal nerve.

24

Comparative Anatomy of Muscles of Head

Horse

The **cutaneous muscle** in horse is thin and incompletely developed in the superficial fascia. The cutaneous muscle of the facial region **(cutaneous fasciei)** is incomplete and poorly developed over the mandibular space and the massetor muscle. Rostrally it passes to the angle of the mouth and blends with the orbicularis oris. The cutaneous muscle of the cervical region (cutaneous colli) is situated along the ventral region of the neck.

The **frontalis** muscle is absent.

The **orbicularis** oris forms incomplete ring around the rima oris. The **levator nasolabialis** is less extensive and is divided into the superior and inferior branches. Between the two branches pass the dilator naris lateralis and levator labii superioris. The **levator labii superioris** extends from malar, lacrimal and the maxillary bones to the upper lip in a common tendon with the muscle of the opposite side. The **zygomaticus** is thin, short and weak. It arises from the fascia covering the massetor. The **incisivus maxillaris** muscle which is absent in ox exists in horse and it lies under the mucous membrane of the upper lip. It originates on the alveolar border of the incisive bone from the level of lateral incisor to the first premolar and it inserts to the upper lip. Its action is to depress the upper lip. The **incisivus mandibularis** which is also absent in ox exists in horse under the mucous membrane of the lower lip. It originates at the alveolar border of the body of the mandible from the level of lateral incisor to the first premolar and is inserted on the skin of the lower lip and the chin. Its action is to raise the lower lip. The incisivus maxillaris and the incisivus mandibularis muscles acting together cause the closing of rima oris. The **depressor labii inferioris** is thicker and extends further back. The **buccinator** is almost similar to that of ox.

The **orbicularis oculi** is thinner than that of ox. The **levator anguli oculi medialis (corrugator supercilii)** is well developed in horse. It extends from the fascia on the frontal bone and terminates in the upper eyelid at the medial canthus.

The **cutaneus faciei** is present as a separate muscle. It originates on the supraorbital process and inserts by blending with the orbicularis oculi. The **malaris** is very thin and smaller than that of ox.

The **massetor** is larger and stronger than that of ox. The **temporalis** is more cranial in position and is wide and short. The **pterygoideus** medius originates near the median plane. As a result, the lateral movement of the lower jaw is restricted.

The **occipito-mandibularis** which is absent in ox exists in horse. It is a short muscle extending from the jugular process of the occipital bone to the caudal border of the vertical part of the ramus of the mandible. It depresses the mandible leading to the opening of the mouth. The **digastricus** has a rounded tendon provided with the synovial sheath. The rostral bellies of this muscle are not connected by the transversus mandibularis as occurs in ox.

The mylohyoideus is thinner and less extensive. The **stylohyoideus** has a tendinous insertion. The tendon is perforated by the intermediate tendon of the digastricus. The **Geniohyoideus** is less developed. The **keratohyoideus** is inserted only to the upper border of the thyroid cornu. The **hyoideus transversus** is not unified. The **occipitohyoideus** is smaller and thinner.

The **parietoauricularis externus** arises from zygomatic arch and the parietal and frontal crest and is inserted to the scutiform cartilage. The **parietoauricularis internus** arises from the parietal crest and is inserted by an aponeurotic tendon to the scutiform cartilage.

The **cervicoauricularis externus** is a thin triangular sheet extending from the occipital crest and the ligamentum nuchae. Its base is at its origin and apex towards its insertion. The **cervicoauricularis medius** and **cervicoauricularis internus** also arise from the ligamentum nuchae along with the cervicoauricularis externus. The **scutoauricularis internus** arise from parietoauricularis externus and the caudal part of the medial surface of the scutiform cartilage. Its insertion is on the conchal cartilage.

Dog

The **cutaneous fasciei** is well developed. The **orbicularis oris** is rudimentary. The **levator nasolabialis** is widely expanded. The **levator labii maxillaris** terminates by numerous small tendons. Some of these are inserted around the nostrils and the remaining unites with those of opposite side before their insertion. The **dilator naris lateralis** is represented by a small triangular muscle lying inferior to the levator labii maxillaris. The zygomaticus is long narrow and it continues caudally with the zygomatico-auricularis. The **levator anguli oculi medialis** (**corrugator supercilii**) is well developed in dog. It extends from the fascia on the frontal bone and terminates in the upper eyelid at the medial canthus.

The masseter is very distinct thick muscle in dog. It originates on the zygomatic arch and extends beyond the caudal border of the ramus of the mandible. The temporalis is very strong and large muscle in dog. The lateral pterygoid is not distinctly separated from the pterygoideus medialis. The occipitomandibularis is comparatively stronger than in ox.

The Stylohyoideus is a slender muscular band much weaker than that in ox. The keratohyoideus is large. The occipitohyoideus and the hyoideus transversus are absent. The parotidiauricularis is comparatively larger but narrower. The parietoauricularis externus is extensive. The parietoauricularis internus and the cervicoauricularis externus are inserted to scutiform cartilage and also to the conchal cartilage.

Sheep and Goat

The muscles of head in sheep and goat are in general similar to those in ox. Only the special features about these muscles that deviate from those of ox are described below.

The **cutaneus muscle** is well developed and is adherent to the skin, similar to that in ox.

The **lateralis nasi** is less extensive than that of the ox and horse. The **caninus** is attached deeply to the incisive bone in the absence of the deep portion of the nasolabialis. The **levator nasolabialis** consists of single layer and it lies superficial to the levator labii maxillaris, caninus and depressor labii maxillaris. In goat, a small fascicle extending from the medial angle of the eye joins the lateral aspect of this muscle. The **levator labii maxillaris** is very prominent. It arises from maxilla near the facial tuber and inserts by means of tendinous bands to the skin between the nostrils. The **incisivus mandibularis** is more extensive in goat. It extends to the level of the angle of the mouth in sheep.

The **levator palpebrae superioris** is thin and it originates in the vicinity of pterygoid crest of the basi sphenoid and inserts in the form of a tendon on the superior eyelid. The **rectus lateralis** and **ventralis** in sheep originate on the ventral border of the foramen orbitorotundum while the rectus medialis and rectus dorsalis originate on the corresponding side of the optic foramen. The

obliquus dorsalis in sheep originates with two tendons which soon fuse with each other to form a single belly of this muscle. It then passes around the trochlear cartilage from medial to lateral side, underpass the rectus dorsalis and then inserts into the bulb of the eye. The **obliquus ventralis** after its origin on the lacrimal bone it passes ventral to rectus ventralis and then inserts between the insertion of the rectus ventralis and lateralis on the bulb of the eye. The **retractor bulbi** muscle originates on the dorsal wall of the foramen orbitorotundum and passes within the cone formed by the recti muscles. It does not attach at the limbus or the equator. The dorsal and medial portions of this muscle attach caudal to the equator.

The **zygomaticoauricularis** is broad at the origin and narrow at its insertion. The **frontoscutularis** is well developed and indistinct. Some fibres of this muscle are fused with interscutularis in goat. The **cervicoscutularis** is more developed in goat and ox than in sheep. The **cervicoauricularis profundus arises** from temporal line and the occipital.

The **masseter** has two layers in the goat and three layers in sheep. The **pterygoideus lateralis** in sheep inserts on the medial surface of the mandible from the base of the coronoid process to the junction of the ramus and the body of the mandible. The **mylohyoideus** has two distinct fleshy parts similar to that in ox, but in sheep and goat the medial part is more distinct amongst the two.

Pig

The **cutaneous faciei** is thin and firmly adheres to the skin. The **orbicularis oris** is little developed. The **levator nasolabialis** is thin and undivided. The **levator labii maxillaris** has a large pinnate belly. It arises on the preorbital fossa and inserts on the rostral part of the os rostri. A muscular strip connects it with incisive bone. The **zygomaticus** arises on the fascia over the masseter and inserts at the angle of the mouth. The **depressor labii mandibularis** separates from the buccinator near the angle of the mouth and terminates by a number of tendinous branches in the lower lip. The **caninus** is well developed. It arises on the preorbital fossa with the levator labii maxillaris and inserts by numerous tendons around the nostrils. The **dilator naris apicalis** consists of only a few fibres that cross over the os rostri. The **depressor labii maxillaris** arises on the facial crest and inserts by a strong tendon in the skin of the snout with the similar tendon of the opposite side. The **malaris** is absent and the other palpebral muscles present no special features.

The **masseter** is thick. The pterygoideus lateralis is large and distinct. The occipitomandibular part of the **digastricus** arises on the jugular process of the occipital bone and ends on the medial and ventral surface of the mandible.

The **mylohyoideus** consists of two distinct layers. The **transversus mandibulae** is one (superficial) of these. The **occipitohyoideus** and **ceratohyoideus** is small. The hyoideus transversus is absent. The **Omohyoideus** is thin. It arises on subscapular fascia close to the shoulder joint.

The **zygomaticoauricularis** is in the form of a slender strip of muscle and is uniform throughout its course. It originates on the zygomatic arch and inserts on the caudal border of the auricular cartilage. The **scutuloauricularis** is well developed. It originates on the dorsal surface of the scutiform cartilage and inserts on the medial aspect of the auricular cartilage. The **scutuloauricularis profundus** lie on the deep surface of the scutiform cartilage. The **frontoscutularis is** well developed. It originates on the frontal crest and inserts on the dorsal surface of the scutiform cartilage.

The **interscutularis** is well developed thick muscle. It originates on the frontal part of the temporal line and inserts on the dorsal surface of the scutiform cartilage. The **cervicoauricularis superficialis** is distinctly developed in pig. It originates on the nuchal crest of the occipital bone and the surrounding fascia. It inserts on the dorsal surface of the auricular cartilage. The **cervicoauricularis medius** is also well developed in pig with its origin on the deeper aspect of the fascia on the nuchal crest and insertion on the dorsal surface of the auricular cartilage. The **styloauricularis** is a thin sheet of muscle that lies over the rostral part of the parotid gland. It originates over the fascia on the rostral part of the parotid salivary gland and the angle of the mandible. Its insertion is at the base of the auricular cartilage. The **paratidoauricularis** is a small thread like strip of muscle lying on and embedded in the parotid salivary gland. It originates on the ventral part of the parotid gland and inserts in common with the styloauricularis at the base of the auricular cartilage.

Fowl

Muscles of head and neck of fowl have been described together under the next chapter on the comparative anatomy of muscles of neck.

25

Comparative Anatomy of Muscles of Neck

Horse

The **fascia** in the cervical region of horse has two layers, the superficial and deep. Each of these is also double layered. The superficial fascia contains the cutaneus muscle the **cutaneus colli.** The fascia of the two sides meets at the median line along the nuchal ligament and ventrally at the fibrous raphe.

The **brachiocephalicus** is undivided. It arises from the mastoid process, nuchal crest and wing of the atlas and the transverse process of the second, third and fourth cervical vertebrae. The **sternocephalicus** is also undivided. It arises from the cartilage of the manubrium sterni and inserts at the angle of the lower jaw. The dorsal border of this muscle forms the ventral border of the jugular furrow. The **sternothyrohyoideus** muscle consists of two separate but unequal parts, the sternothyroideus and the sternohyoideus. The **sternothyroideus** is and the **sternohyoideus** is larger. The first part inserts on the thyroid cartilage of the larynx and the second part inserts to the body of the hyoid bone. The **omohyoideus** is more extensive in horse than that in ox. It arises from the subscapular fascia near the shoulder joint and inserts at the body and the lingual process of the hyoid bone. The **scalinus** has two parts like those of ox, but the dorsal part in horse is smaller. It arises on the transverse process of the seventh cervical vertebra and inserts on the first rib. The ventral part is very extensive. It arises from the transverse processes of the third to sixth cervical vertebrae and inserts on the medial surface of the cranial border of the first rib. The **longus capitis** (**rectus capitis ventralis major**) arises from the transverse process of third, fourth and fifth cervical vertebrae and is inserted on the tubercle at the junction of basilar part of occipital bone with the basi sphenoid. It does not form aponeurosis either at the origin or at its insertion. The **rectus capitis ventralis** (**rectus capitis ventralis minor**) is smaller in horse than that in ox. The **intertransversarii cervicis** (**intertransversalis colli**) are smaller and present six fasciculi. The most cranial of these is separated from the common mass formed by the rest of these fascicles.

The **splenius** is more extensive, thicker flat and triangular. It arises from the spinous processes of the third, fourth and fifth thoracic vertebrae in the thoracic region and the funicular part of the ligamentum nuchae in the cervical region. It inserts on the occipital crest, mastoid process and the transverse processes of third, fourth and fifth cervical vertebrae. The **longissimus capitis et atlantis** is inserted to the mastoid process. The **semispinalis capitis** (**complexus**) is very extensive, large and triangular muscle in horse. It lies mainly on the ligamentum nuchae and is covered by the splenius. It originates over the spinous processes of the third, fourth and fifth thoracic vertebrae, the transverse processes of the first six or seven thoracic vertebrae and the articular (oblique) processes of the cervical vertebrae. Its insertion is on a rough area on the occipital bone just ventral to the nuchal crest.

Dog

The **cutaneus muscle** in the neck of dog is split in two layers. One of these is thin and the other is thick and extensive. The **sternocephalicus** is well developed. It extends from the manubrium sterni to the mastoid process of the temporal bone. The s**ternothyrohyoideus** is thick and has a single belly. It arises from the first sternal cartilage. The omohyoideus is absent. The **scalinus** is very long. Its dorsal division is very large and has two layers. The superior layer is short and terminates on the fourth rib. Its inferior layer is much larger and terminates on the seventh or eighth rib. The ventral division of the scalinus is small and terminates on the first rib. The **longus capitis** arises from the transverse processes of the second to sixth cervical vertebrae.

The **splenius** is extensive. The **semispinalis capitis** has two parts in dog like those in the ox and horse. One part arises on the supraspinous processes of the second to fifth thoracic vertebrae. Transverse processes of the last two cervical vertebrae and ligamentum nuchae. The other part arises from the transverse processes of the first three or four thoracic vertebrae and the oblique processes of the last five cervical vertebrae. Both the divisions insert by common tendon on the occipital crest.

Sheep and Goat

The **brachiocephalicus** in sheep and goat is similar to that in ox. The **sternocephalicus** is divided into sternomandibularis and sternomastoideus similar to that in ox. In sheep the **sternomandibularis** is poorly developed as compared to that in ox and goat. The tendon of insertion of the sternomandibularis in goat divides into two parts. One of these inserts on on the fascia on the masseter muscle and the other passes to the zygomatic arch for insertion. The **omohyoideus** in goat is in the form of a thin muscular band that join the sternohyoideus for insertion. In sheep, the omohyoideus lies deep to the sternomastoideus.

The **trapezius** and the rhomboideus in sheep and goat are similar to those in ox. The **rectus capitis dorsalis minor** and the **rectus capitis dorsalis major** inserts together near the tendon of insertion of the semispinalis capitis. The **splenius** in sheep and goat inserts on the transverse processes of the second to fifth cervical vertebrae. In goat, however, this insertion is through the fascia in this region. The rest of the cervical muscles of the sheep and goat are similar to those of ox.

Pig

The **cutaneus colli** muscle consists of two layers, the superficial and deep and these are distinctly separable. The **brachiocephalicus** has two parts, cleido occipitalis and cleido mastoideus. The first one originates on the nuchal crest and the mastoid process respectively. Both the divisions unite at their termination and insert on the clavicle. The sternocephalicus originates on the manubrium sterni and inserts on mastoid process by a round tendon. The sternothyrohyoideus arises on the manubrium sterni and at about the middle of the neck it divides in two divisions before termination. The omohyoideus is thin. It arises from the subscapular fascia near the shoulder joint and inserts on the body and the lingual process of the hyoid bone independently without any connection with the brachiocephalicus or with the muscle of the opposite side. The omotransversarius arises on the atlas or axis and is inserted on the scapular spine. The **scalinus** muscle is in two parts, the scalinus ventralis and scalinus dorsalis. The **scalinus ventralis** arises from the last four cervical vertebrae and ends on the first rib while the **scalinus dorsalis** arises on the transverse processes of the third to sixth cervical vertebrae and inserts on the third rib. The nerves of the brachial plexus perforate the scalinus ventralis. The **longus colli** muscle of the opposite sides is separated from each other and hence the parts of the bodies of the vertebrae remain uncovered by this muscle. The **intertransversarii** muscle is similar to that of ox. The **splenius** cervicis is thick and extensive. It inserts in three parts, the occipital, temporal and atlas. The **longissimus capitis et atlantis** is small while the semispinalis capitis is large. It has two parts, the superficial and deep (complexus). The **obliquus capitis caudalis** is relatively thin. The **rectus capitis dorsalis** muscles are thick and their fibres are fused with each other.

Fowl

The general organization of skeletal muscles in fowl is totally different than that in other domestic animals. The striated muscles associated with feather tracts constitute the **cutaneous muscle** in birds. **The constrictor colli** is the most superficial of the cutaneous muscles in the neck. The muscle fibres of this muscle are transversely oriented rather than the usual sheet form. Another cutaneous muscle of importance in fowl is the **cucullaris.** The **cranial part** of this muscle is attached to the skull and jaws while the **caudal part** is attached to the cervical vertebrae and the cervical fascia. The major muscles of the **head** are grouped as the **muscles of the jaws** and the **muscles of the hyoid apparatus.** The **cervical muscles** are grouped as the **axial** muscles and the **lateral cervical and the ventral cervical** muscles.

Jaw muscles

Depressor mandibulae

Origin: From the caudolateral surface of the skull

Insertion: On the caudomedial and ventral surface of the caudal process of mandible.

Action: To depress the mandible (lower law) and to elevate the upper jaw.

Adductor mandibulae externus

Origin: The superficial part arises from zygomatic process and the ventral and medial portions arise from the temporal fossa and optic process of the quadrate.

Insertion: All three portions insert on the dorsal and lateral surface of the mandible.

Action: To raise the mandible (lower jaw).

Pseudotemporalis superficialis

Origin: Medial to the origin of adductor mandibulae externus on postorbital region of the skull.

Insertion: Dorsal border of the mandible

Action: To raise the mandible (lower jaw).

Pseudotemporalis profundus

Origin: From medial and lateral surfaces of the orbital process of quadrate.

Insertion: The medial aspect of the ramus of the mandible.

Action: To swing the quadrate caudally so as to lower the elevated mandible and to raise the depressed mandible.

Pterygoideus

Origin: The palatine and pterygoid bones.

Insertion: The medial surface of the ramus of the mandible.

Action: To close the mouth by moving the opposite jaws towards each other so as to hold the object between the jaws.

Protractor quadratopterygoidei

Origin: From the orbitosphenoid bone and basitemporal plate of the brain case.

Insertion: On the medial surface of the quadrate and pterygoid bones.

Action: To raise the upper jaw by swinging the quadrate rostrad and protracting the palate.

The **blood supply** to all these muscles is through the branches of the **mandibular artery** and **nerve supply** through the **mandibular nerve.**

Muscles of hyoid apparatus

Extrinsic muscles

Intermandibularis

Origin: The medial surface of the mandible.

Insertion: On ventral median raphe.

Basibranchialis mandibularis (superficial and deep)

Origin: The lateral aspect of the caudal process of the mandible

Insertion: The dorsal surface of the rostral basibranchial bone.

Mandibularis epibranchialis

Origin: The medial and ventral surface of the mandible.

Insertion: The branchial element inserts on dorsal aspect of caudal mandibular salivary gland and the epibranchial element on the hyoid cornu.

Intrinsic muscles

These include the (1) Paraglossoceratobranchialis (2) Interceratobranchialis (3) Paraglossobasibranchialis lateralis and (4) Paraglossobasibranchialis medialis.

Action: All the extrinsic and intrinsic muscles of the hyoid apparatus are concerned with the movements of tongue and and the mechanism of swallowing.

Blood supply to all these muscles is through the **mandibular artery** and its branches while the **nerve supply** is through the **mandibular nerve.**

Axial muscles

Complexus

Origin: From the dorsal aspect of the transverse processes of first four or more cervical vertebrae.

Insertion: On the nuchal surface of occipital bone.

Action: Contraction of unilateral muscle rotates the head laterally and bilateral muscle contraction causes extension of the head.

Biventer cervicis

Origin: By aponeurosis from spinous processes of the most caudal cervical vertebrae and the succeeding thoracic vertebrae.

Insertion: One set of muscles insert by tendons over the mid cervical region and the other set of these muscles insert on the occipital bone on either side of the midline.

Action: Elevation of head and some times along with the elevation of neck.

Spinalis cervicis

Origin: Along with the preceding muscle.

Insertion: Caudal articular processes of cervical vertebrae up to about mid cervical region.

Action: Assists in elevation of head. Generally it elevates the neck along with the head.

Ascendentes

These are a series muscular slips oriented obliquely craniodorsally and are continuous from the base of the neck to the second cervical vertebra.

Origin: From the transverse processes of several thoracic and most of the cervical vertebrae.

Insertion: Each muscular slip passes obliquely on the presiding one or two vertebrae and inserts on the articular processes of those cervical vertebrae.

Action: Lateral flexion of the neck.

Lateral cervical muscles

Longus colli ventralis

These are a series of muscular slips and tendons of origin and insertion of muscles constituting a single fleshy unit.

Origin: The transverse processes of the cervical and thoracic vertebrae.

Insertion: On the cervical ribs of the cervical vertebrae and first few thoracic vertebrae.

Action: Ventral flexion of the neck.

Splenius capitis

Origin: From spinous processes of second to fourth cervical vertebrae.
Insertion: On the occipital bone along with biventer and some other muscles.
Action: Extension or unilateral turning of head.

Rectus capitis dorsalis

Origin: Two or three fascicles from the second, third and fourth cervical vertebra.

Insertion: On the caudal margin of the basitemporal plate of the skull.

Action: Ventral flexion of head.

Rectus capitis lateralis

Origin: From the third and fourth cervical vertebrae.

Insertion: Ventrolateral surface of the skull and primarily on the lateral surface of the occipital bone.

Action: To extend or to rotate the head around the axis.

Rectus capitis ventralis

Origin: The centra of first six cervical vertebrae.

Insertion: Basitemporal plate on the extensive area.

Action: Ventral flexion of the head.

Flexores colli brevis and profundus

Origin: From the ventral surface of the transverse processes of third, fourth and fifth cervical vertebrae.

Insertion: Ventral and lateral surface of the atlas vertebra.

Action: Flexion of first few cervical vertebrae assisting thereby in ventral flexion of the head.

SECTION-B

ORGANS AND GLANDS

26

Organs of Digestion

Mouth

The mouth is bounded dorsally (roof) by hard palate (2-5 B) and behind that the soft palate, ventrally (floor) by the body of the mandible along with the mylohyoide muscles and laterally by the cheeks (Fig. 2-5 C). The entrance of mouth cavity is bounded by lips and it is called as rima oris, while its caudal opening into the pharynx is called as aditus pharyngis or isthmus faucium. The cavity of the mouth (cavum oris) is subdivided into two parts by the teeth and alveolar processes (the alveoli) of the mandible. The inner part i.e. the space within the teeth and alveoli is termed as mouth cavity proper, while the space between the cheeks and lips and that between the teeth and alveoli is called the vestibule of the mouth. The mucous membrane of the mouth cavity is continuous with the margin of the lips and the common integument and caudally it continues with the mucous membrane of the pharynx.

Lips

The lips (Figure 2-5 A) are two (upper and lower) musculomembranous folds that bound the opening of the mouth cavity. The upper and lower lips meet (unite) with each other laterally at the angles of union called the commissures which are situated at the level of the corner incisor tooth. The external surface of the lips is covered by a thick skin with variable number of tactile and ordinary fine hairs. In bovine animals, the middle part of the external surface of the upper lip and the surface between the nostrils is bare but keratinized and is termed the planum nasolabiale (muzzle). It is kept cool and moist by the fluid secreted by the nasolabial glands that are lying in a layer underneath the skin. The muzzle is smooth and is marked by irregular lines mapping out the small polygonal areas over which are the openings of the ducts of the labial glands. The rest of the external surface of the upper lip presents long tactile hairs along with the ordinary fine hairs. The external surface of the lower lip presents in its centre a rounded prominence called as chin. The internal surface is lined by mucous membrane which is usually pigmented. It bears number of small papillae which present the openings of the labial glands. A small fold of mucous membrane extending from the lips to the gums is called as frenum labi maxilaris in case of the upper lip and frenum labi mandibularis in case of lower lip. The free border of each lip is bare and with the adjacent part of the internal surface it presents short blunt horny papillae which become larger, sharp and pointed towards the commissures of the lips.

Cheeks

The cheeks form the lateral walls of the mouth cavity. These are continuous in front with the lips. These are attached to the alveolar border of the bones of the jaws i.e. maxilla forming the upper jaw and mandible forming the lower jaw. The cheeks are constituted externally by the skin, internally by the mucous membrane and between these two is a layer of muscles within which exists the buccal glands, vessels and nerves. The skin of the face continues over the cheeks without any modifications. It is thin and elastic. The muscular layer is formed chiefly by the buccinator and partly by the levator nasolabialis, levator labii maxillaris, the zygomaticus and the depressor labii mandibularis. The buccal glands are arranged in three layers, the dorsal, middle and the ventral. The dorsal row consists of yellowish glands arranged in lobules and these extend from the angle of lips between the zygomaticus and buccinator muscles to the maxillary tuberosity. The middle row consists of scattered lobules placed on the deep surface of the buccinator. The ventral row consists of brownish lobules arranged from the angle of the lips to a short distance under the cover of the masseter. The mucous membrane is reflected upon the gums and is continuous behind with that of the soft palate. It presents large conical papillae directed caudally towards the isthmus faucium and are covered by horny epithelium. The largest of these are placed around the commissures of the lips. A large papilla called the papilla salivalis is situated on the mucous membrane of the cheeks at the level of the upper fifth cheek tooth and it presents the opening of the sternson's duct that carries the secretion (saliva) from the parotid salivary gland.

Roof of the mouth

Hard palate

The hard palate (Figure 2-5 B) forms the roof of the mouth cavity. It is bounded rostrally by dental pad, on the sides by alveolar arches of either side and is continuous caudally with the soft palate. The dental pad is formed by a thick pad of connective tissue on the body of the premaxilla (incisive) bone. It is covered by a thick layer of cornified epithelium. Dorsally the hard palate is attached to the bony palate formed by the palatine processes of the premaxillary (incisive), maxillary and the palatine bones. Its ventral surface, facing towards the mouth cavity (oral surface) is lined by thick mucous membrane. The submucous tissue which attaches it to the bony palate contains very rich venous plexus constituting erectile tissue. The central raphe extending through the length of the oral surface of the hard palate divides it into two halves. Each half presents about 15 to 19 transverse ridges covering the rostral two third of the palate. The caudal third of this surface of the palate is plane and presents the orifices of the palatine glands. The transverse ridges are straight and their free borders are serrated. At the rostral end of the median raphe and between the dental pad and first transverse ridge lies a diamond shape papilla named as papilla incisiva. This papilla is margined on either side by a fissure which presents the oral (palatine) opening of the naso-palatine duct (ductus incisivus). The nasal opening of this duct lies on the floor of the nasal cavity. The mucous membrane of the hard palate is more or less pigmented.

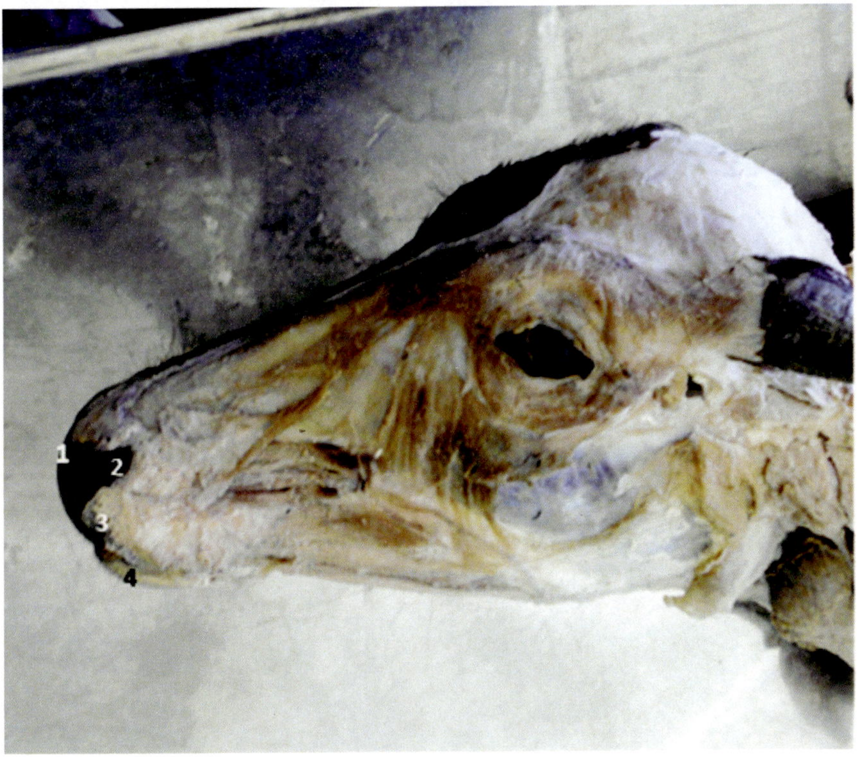

Fig. 2–5 A: Lips and nostrils of Ox
1. Muzzle; 2. Nostrils; 3. Upper Lip; 4. Lower Lip.

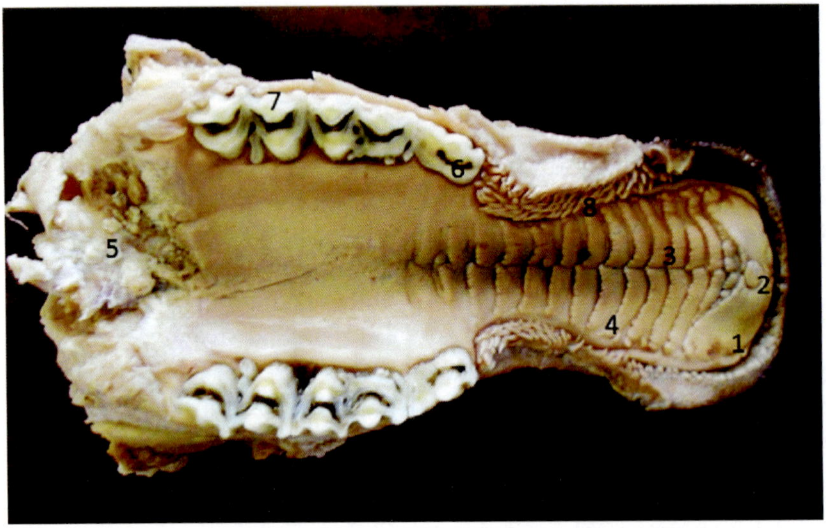

Fig 2-5 B: Roof of Mouth cavity of Ox
1: Dental pad; 2: Papilla incisiva; 3: Hard palate; 4: Ridges; 5: Soft palate; 6: Premolar 7: Molar; 8: Conical horny papillae.

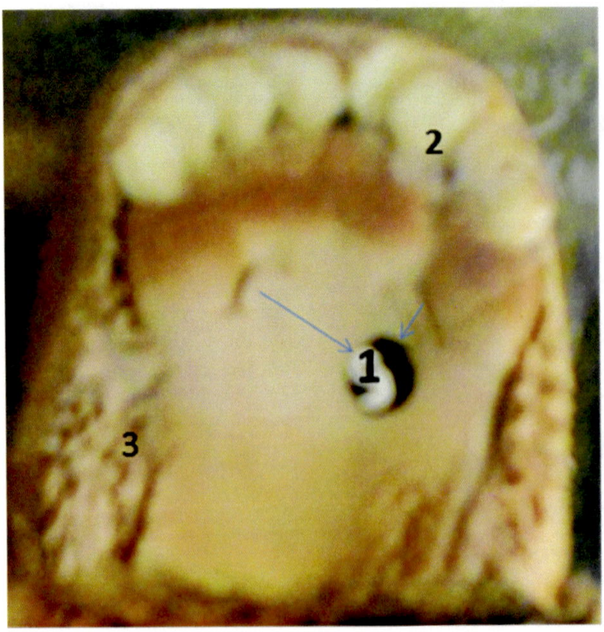

Fig 2-5 C: Floor of Mouth cavity of Ox
1.Caruncula subligualis; 2. Incisor teeth; 3. Conical papillae.

Soft palate

The soft palate is a musculo-membranous curtain that separates the mouth cavity from the oesophagus except in deglutition. It extends caudally downward from the hard palate to the epiglottis. Its rostral border is attached to the caudal border of the horizontal part of the hard palate and laterally it blends with the walls of the pharynx and isthmus faucium. The caudal border is concave and free. It presents two surfaces, the oral and pharyngeal. The oral surface faces ventrad and caudad and is covered with mucous membrane continuous with that of the hard palate. Numerous fine ducts of palatine glands open on this surface. On each side, a short thick fold of mucous membrane passes laterally and ventrally from the rostral border of the soft palate to the lateral border of the tongue. These folds are called the rostral pillars (palatoglossal arch) of the soft palate. The pharyngeal surface faces dorsad and caudad and is covered with the mucous membrane that is continuous with that of pharynx. The caudal free border is continued laterally on each side into the short fold of mucous membrane that passes to the lower part of the lateral wall of the pharynx. These folds are called as the caudal pillars (palatopharyngeal arch) of the soft palate. The space between the rostral and caudal pillars on each side bears a deep concave sinus called as tonsillar sinus. This sinus is occupied by a compact mass of lymphoid tissue which is called as tonsil. The part of this tonsil projects outward but is not visible in the mouth cavity.

Floor of the mouth

The floor of the mouth (Figure 2-5 C) is formed by the body of the mandible and the mylohyoid muscles. It is free only in its rostral part which is covered by the mucous membrane. Rest of the floor of mouth cavity is occupied by the tongue. Opposite the cheek teeth, the mucosa of the tongue is reflected onto the mylohyoid muscles forming a narrow groove which becomes shallower towards the caudal part of the mouth. The ducts of the dorsal part of the sublingual salivary gland open directly into this groove. On the mucosa covering the body of the mandible at the level of corner incisor tooth, there is a pair of leaf like papilla called as **caruncula sublingualis**. The duct of the mandibular salivary gland and that of the rostral part of the sublingual salivary gland open jointly or separately on the deep surface of this papilla. This papilla is wide, hard and serrated. Just behind this papilla is a median fold of mucous membrane passing to the ventral surface of the free part of the tongue. This fold is called the **frenum linguae.** On either side of the frenum linguae on the floor of the mouth is a linear series of papillae near which open the ducts of the sublingual salivary gland. Behind the last cheek tooth on each side of the mouth, a vertical fold of mucous membrane passes from lower to upper jaw. This fold of mucous membrane is called the plica pterygomandibularis and it contains the ligament of the same name.

Tongue

The tongue (Figure 2-5 D) is the chief organ of prehension. It is situated on the floor of the mouth, between the rami of the mandible and is supported by the sling formed by the mylohyoideus muscles because of which it has become highly protractile. It consists of a root, a body and the tip. The root is the caudal part and is attached ventrally and caudally to the hyoid bone, soft palate and pharynx. Its upper surface is free and slopes ventrally and caudally. The body is the middle part and has three surfaces. The dorsal surface (dorsum linguae) is rounded while the two lateral surfaces are flattened. The ventral surface is related to the geniohyoideus and mylohyoideus muscles. The tip or the apex is free and some what pointed. It has two surfaces the dorsal (upper) and ventral (lower) and a free rounded border. The dorsal surface (dorsum linguae) of the tongue is free throughout and remains in contact with the palate except at the glossoepiglottic space when the mouth is closed. The caudal part of the dorsum linguae is prominently raised and is sharply demarcated from the rest of the part by a transverse groove.

Structure of the tongue: The tongue consists of the outer layer of mucous membrane and the internal mass of the muscles and glands. It is richly supplied with the vessels and the nerves. The mucous membrane is intimately adhered to the underlying tissue mass of the muscles except at the lower part of the lateral borders of the body and the ventral surface of the tip. The mucous membrane is quite thick and dense on the dorsum while on the lateral borders it is thin. A thin fold of mucous membrane extending from the ventral surface of the free part of the tongue passes over the floor of the mouth. This fold is called as frenum linguae. The mucous membrane on the dorsum of the tongue presents various types of papillae. These include the filiform, fungiform, vallate, foliate and conical papillae. The **filiform papillae** are in abundance. These are fine, thread like projections. These papillae impart roughness to the tongue. These are located over the dorsum in front of the prominence and the sides of the tip of the tongue. The **fungiform papillae** are also numerous. These are larger, rounded (button like) at the free end and distinctly lying scattered between the filiform papillae on the dorsum and sides of the body and tip of the tongue. The **vallate (circumvallate) papillae** exist on the caudal prominence of the dorsum of the tongue. These vary in number from 8 to 17 and are arranged in rows on either side of the prominence of the dorsum. They are rounded and broader at their free ends than the attached ends and appear like sunk in the depressions binded by the annular walls. Their free surface is tubercular and bears small round secondary papillae. The **foliate papillae** are rounded eminences lying just rostral to the palatoglossal arches. The fungiform, vallate and foliate papillae are furnished with test buds. The **lingual follicles** possessing lymphoid tissue

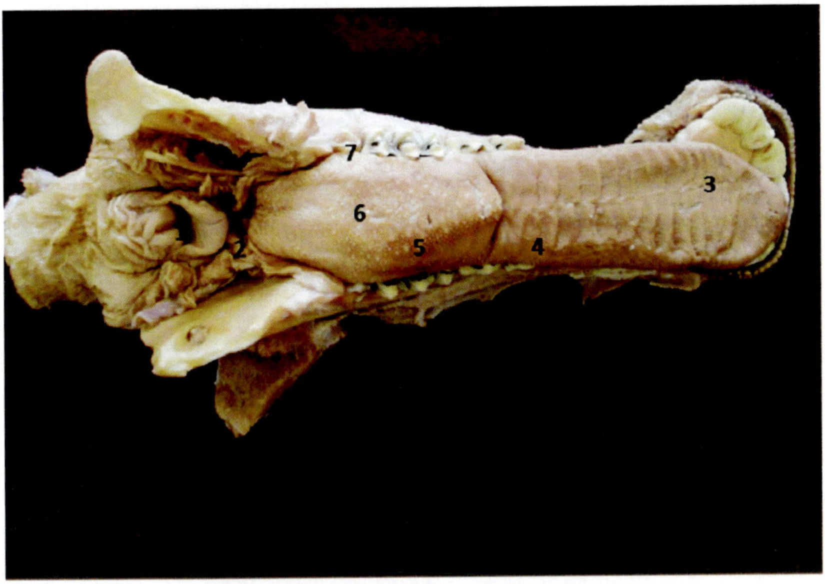

Fig. 2-5 D: Tongue of Ox (Dorsal view)
1. Pharynx; 2. Isthmus faucium; 3. Filiform papillae; 4. Fungiform papillae; 5. Circumvallate papillae; 6. Torus linguae; 7: Molar tooth.

are present in the caudal part of the dorsum and on each side of the glossoepiglottic fold. The lingual glands are present in the submucous tissue.

Teeth

The teeth are hard white or yellowish white structures implanted in the alveoli of the jaws formed by the maxilla (upper jaw) and mandible (lower jaw). They are organs of prehension and mastication. Domestic animals have two sets of teeth. The first set of teeth erupts during early life. These are termed as deciduous or milk teeth. These are temporary and after a specific time are replaced by the other set of teeth which are termed as permanent teeth. Based on their position in the alveoli and the function performed by them, the teeth are classified as (1) **Incisors**: These are most rostral in position and are used for cutting the food material. (2) **Canines**: These are next to and lateral to the incisors. These are used to seize and tear the food material (3) **Premolars** and (4) **Molars:** These teeth form the sides of the dental arch. They are adjacent to cheeks and hence are called cheek teeth and are used for grinding, chewing and mastication of the food material. The incisors, canines and premolars appear in both i.e. deciduous and permanent set of teeth. The molar teeth, however, erupt only in permanent set. The complete dentition of an animal is expressed in the form of dental formula. In this formula, the letters indicate the kind of teeth and the numerical in the upper and lower row indicate the number of teeth of that particular type of teeth in the upper and lower jaw. Thus the dental formula of permanent teeth in ox is as below.

$$2\left(I\frac{0}{4}\; C\frac{0}{0}\; P\frac{3}{3}\; M\frac{3}{3}\right) = 32$$

The individual teeth are designated numerically as first, second, third and so on in the respective type just as, I1, I2, P1, P2, M1, M2 etc. The incisors are present in almost all the domestic animals. However, these are absent in the upper jaw of the ruminants like ox, goat and sheep. Similarly, canines are also absent in the upper jaw of ox while in the goat and sheep they are totally absent. In dog and cat these are prominent. The cheek teeth are flattened for grinding particularly in ruminants. Each tooth basically has two parts, the crown which lies above the gums and the root which lies embedded in the alveoli below the gums. The line of union of these two parts is constricted and is termed as neck of the tooth. The surfaces of the tooth are described as (1) the **occlusal or table surface** is one that is free and in opposition to the teeth of the opposing jaw. In ruminants, it is also called as **masticatory surface**. (2) The surface which is facing towards the vestibule is called the **vestibular surface**. (3) The vestibular surface of incisors and canine teeth is called **labial surface** because it is facing towards lips. Similarly the vestibular surface of the cheek teeth (pre molar and molar) is called as **buccal surface** since it faces towards cheeks.(4) The surface that is facing towards the tongue is termed as **lingual surface** and (5) The surface of a tooth which is in contact with the neighboring tooth is called as **contact surface**.

Structure of the tooth: From within outward, the tooth consists of a soft structure the pulp in the centre, and it is covered by a hard yellowish white tissue the dentine. The outer layer covering the root is called cement while that of the crown is called the enamel. The pulp is filled with a soft gelatinous tissue and is supplied by the vessels and nerves of the teeth. Dentine is quite hard and forms the bulk of the tooth. Cement is harder than the dentine and in simple tooth it forms a thin layer covering the dentine of the root only. However, in the complex tooth it is quite thick and tends to fill in the spaces in the enamel folds of the crown in addition to forming the covering layer of the root. The enamel is the hardest tissue in the body and it strongly covers the dentine of the crown. It is usually bluish white in colour

Incisor teeth: In ox, (2-5 C) these are absent in upper jaw. In lower jaw these are eight in number and are arranged in fan like manner. These are simple teeth and have no infundibula. The crown is white, short and shovel shaped. The occlusal surface of the crown is in the form of a sharp edge that separates the labial and lingual surfaces. Initially the entire crown is covered by enamel but as the age advances the enamel on the occlusal surface starts tearing that leads to expose the inner layer of dentine. The root is single and rounded. It is embedded in the alveolus on the alveolar border of the body of the mandible. It is so fixed in the alveoli as to allow a small amount of movement. Beginning from centre the first pair of incisor is called as central, the second as intermediate, third as lateral and the fourth as corner.

Canine teeth: These are absent in ox but it is considered that in herbivorous animals, the canines are converted into the last pair (corner) of incisors. However, in other species of animals especially in carnivores the canine teeth are prominent. The crown of the canine tooth is white or yellowish white rounded and tapering towards the table surface which is slightly curved inward. The root is single and rounded.

Cheek teeth: The cheek teeth, **premolars** and **molars** (Fig. 2-5 B) are prismatic in form. The crown is quadrilateral in cross section except in the first and last cheek teeth which are triangular in cross section. The upper cheek teeth are embedded in the alveoli of the maxilla bone. They are slightly curved with the convexity towards the cheek. The buccal surface presents a central ridge and two grooves. The lingual surface presents a wide round ridge that separate the two grooves. The masticatory surface presents two prominent infundibula. It slopes obliquely downwards and outwards. The buccal edge is prominent and sharp. The first and last cheek tooth has three roots while the rests have three or four roots. The upper cheek teeth are longer on the outer side and the lower ones are longer on the inner side. The lower cheek teeth are implanted in the alveoli of rami of mandible. The lingual surface presents two or more grooves. The masticatory surface is oblique. It slopes upwards and inwards and its lingual edge is sharp. The first five cheek teeth have two roots and the sixth one has three.

The time of eruption of deciduous teeth and their subsequent replacement by permanent teeth has a definite correlation. However, there may be some variation based on the breed of the animal, nature of the food and assimilation of calcium. The status of the deciduous and permanent teeth in the mouth of the animal is used in practice for determination of the age of the animal. The tentative formula of eruption of teeth and the age of the animal in ox can be presented as below.

Eruption time of teeth in ox

Class of teeth	Position (number)	Age of animal	
		Deciduous	Permanent
Incisor	1st }	Birth to	18 month
	2nd }	2 weeks	2 years
	3rd }		3 years
	4th }		3-4 years
Premolars	1st }	1-4 weeks	1 year
	2nd }		1 and half to 2 years
	3rd }		2 and half to 3 years
Molars	1st }	18 months	
	2nd }		1 to 1 and half years
	3rd}		2 to 2 and half years

Isthmus faucium

The isthmus faucium is a wide tubular aperture through which the mouth cavity communicates with the pharynx. It extends from the rostral pillars of the soft palate to the epiglottis. It is bound dorsally by soft palate, ventrally by the dorsum of the tongue and on either side by the rostral pillars of the soft palate. The passage is small except during deglutition when it dilates enough to allow large boluses to pass from mouth to the pharynx. During this act much of the increased capacity of the isthmus faucium is due to elevation of the soft palate which simultaneously closes the respiratory passage by embracing the epiglottis.

Salivary glands

There are three pairs of large glands situated on the sides of the face and adjacent part of the neck. These are named as parotid, mandibular and sublingual salivary glands. Their ducts open in to the mouth.

The parotid salivary gland is situated in the space between the ramus of the mandible and the wing of the atlas vertebra, overlapping the caudal part of the masseter muscle. It is roughly triangular in shape with its base directed dorsally and the apex ventrally. Its external (lateral) surface is covered by fascia and the parotido auricularis muscle. It is crossed obliquely by the external jugular vein at its lower part. The internal (medial) surface is uneven and is related to several structures. These include the great cornu of hyoid bone, the masseter, digastricus and occipitohyoideus muscles, the tendons of brachiocephalicus and sternocephalicus muscles, the external carotid artery and its branches, the facial nerve and its branches and the pharyngeal lymph node and the mandibular salivary gland. The rostral border is closely attached to the masseter muscle and partly covers the parotid lymph node. The caudal border is concave and is attached to the surrounding structures. The base is notched and encircles around the base of the external ear. The apex is slightly bent and it fits into the angle of union of the external jugular and external maxillary veins. The parotid duct (Stenson's duct) arises from the ventral aspect of the medial surface of the parotid gland, crosses under the tendon of the sternocephalicus and gains the medial surface of the internal pterygoid muscle. Here onward it runs rostrally in the mandibular space below the external maxillary vein, winds round the ventral border of the ramus of the mandible, passes upwards in company with the facial vessels in front of the rostral border of the masseter muscle and pierces the cheek and opens on the papilla salivalis situated on the cheek at the level of the upper fifth cheek tooth.

The mandibular (submaxillary) gland is the largest of all the salivary glands. It is long, narrow curved and oval in form. It extends from the atlantal fossa to the basihyoid bone and is partly covered by parotid gland. The caudal extremity of this gland is rounded and is loosely attached to the fossa atlantis. Its rostral extremity is large and rounded and lies at the side of the root of the tongue underneath the mucous membrane of the floor of the mouth. Its external (lateral) surface is covered by the parotid gland, the digastricus and internal pterygoid muscles and the tendons of the brachiocephalicus and sternocephalicus muscles. The internal (medial) surface is related to the larynx, the rectus capitis ventralis major muscle, the carotid artery, the vagus and accessory nerves, and the sympathetic nerve trunk. The dorsal border is concave and thin and the duct leaves this border. The ventral border is convex and thick. The mandibular duct (Wharton's duct) extends from the middle of the concave border of the gland, extends forward crossing the digastricus and stylohyoideus muscles and then crosses under the hypoglossal nerve and gains the internal surface of the sublingual gland. It then runs forward under the mucous membrane of the mouth and opens on the caruncula sublingualis, a papilla situated on the floor of the mouth below the tip of the tongue at the level of and opposite to the corner incisor tooth.

The sublingual gland is situated beneath the mucous membrane of the mouth, between the body of the tongue and the ramus of the mandible. It consists of two parts the dorsal and ventral. The dorsal part (polystomatic sublingual gland) extends from the rostral pillar of soft palate to the symphysis of the mandible. It is long thin and pale yellow in colour. It consists of fairly large number of glandular globes giving rise to equal number of small excretory ducts (the minor sublingual ducts) that open in to the lateral sublingual recess, The ventral part (monostomatic sublingual gland) is shorter but thicker and lies ventral to the dorsal part. This part has a single duct that opens either alongside or into the Wharton's duct at the caruncula sublingualis. The whole of the sublingual gland is compressed laterally. Its external surface is related to the mylohyoideus muscle. The internal surface is related to the genioglossus and styloglossus muscles, the mandibular (Wharton's) duct and the branches of the lingual nerve. The dorsal border of the gland is under the mucous membrane of the floor of the mouth. The ventral border is related to the geniohyoid muscle.

Pharynx

The pharynx (Figure 2-6A) is a musculomembranous sac common to digestive and respiratory passages. It is a funnel shaped organ with the broad rostral end continuing with the mouth and nasal cavities and the narrow caudal end opening in to the oesophagus. Air and food passages cross each other while passing through the pharynx. During respiration air passes from rostro-dorsal to caudo-ventral way and vise versa whereas during food intake the bolus takes its rout from rostro-ventral to caudo-dorsal way. It is placed behind the soft palate, caudal nares and the isthmus faucium and is suspended obliquely caudad and ventrad by means of muscles with the pterygoid, palatine and hyoid bones dorsally and with the thyroid and cricoid cartilages of larynx ventrally. The cranial wide end of the funnel of the pharynx communicates with the mouth through the isthmus faucium and its caudal narrow tubular end communicates with the oesophagus. It is related dorsally to the base of the cranium and the suprapharyngeal lymph gland, ventrally to the larynx and laterally to the pterygoid muscle, great cornu of the hyoid bone, external carotid and external maxillary arteries, the glossopharyngeal, hypoglossal and rostral laryngeal nerves, the mandibular salivary gland and the para pharyngeal lymph glands. The cavity of the pharynx presents seven openings viz- two caudal nares situated at the rostrodorsal part communicating with the nasal cavity, the isthmus faucium below the caudal nares communicating with the mouth cavity, the aditus laryngis occupying the greater part of the floor and opening into the larynx, the aditus oesophagius opening into the oesophagus and two Eustachian orifices behind the caudal nares at the dorsocaudal part communicating with the Eustachian tubes.

The wall of the pharynx consists of muscles, aponeurosis and mucous membrane. The pharyngeal muscles form the muscular wall of the pharynx. These muscles are described separately as muscles of head and neck. The pharyngeal aponeurosis is the fibrous layer of the pharyngeal wall. It begins at the base of the cranium and passes beneath the muscular layer of the pharyngeal wall. The mucous membrane lines the cavity of the pharynx and is continuous with the mucous membrane of the mouth, nasal chambers, larynx, Eustachian tubes and oesophagus. Its rostral part is lined with ciliated epithelium and the ventral part is lined by the stratified epithelium. Lying between the muscular and the mucous layer is the submucous layer which contains numerous mucous glands.

Oesophagus

The oesophagus is a long musculomembranous tube like a hose pipe. It extends from pharynx, passes through the neck and then through the thorax and finally after piercing through the diaphragm it opens in to the stomach inside the abdominal cavity. From anatomical point of view, its two major parts, the cervical and thoracic are recognized. In its cervical course, it begins in the median plane dorsal to the cricoid cartilage of larynx and passes backwards and downwards on the dorsal surface of the trachea. At the level of the third cervical vertebra it inclines to the left surface of the trachea and continues in this position till the first rib where it becomes dorsolateral to the trachea again.. In its cervical course it is related at its origin to the rectus capitis ventralis major dorsally and cricoid cartilage of larynx ventrally. In the first segment of its cervical course, i.e. up to the level of the third cervical vertebra, it is related to the longus colli muscle dorsally and the trachea ventrally. In the second segment of its cervical course, the oesophagus lies to the left of the trachea and is related dorsally to the longus colli muscle, ventrally to the ventral cervical muscles especially the sternocephalicus and omohyoideus muscles, medially to the trachea and laterally to the left common carotid artery, the left vagosympathetic trunk, the left recurrent laryngeal nerve, the deep cervical lymph nodes and the scalinus and brachiocephalicus muscles. In addition to these, in calves and young animals the thymus gland is related to the oesophagus ventrally.

The wall of the oesophagus consists of striated voluntary muscles which contract in a wave like fashion that causes propulsion of food bolus through the oesophagus and pushes it into stomach. These muscles are arranged in two layers, the outer spiral and inner longitudinal. External to the muscular level is the fibrous coat and internal to the muscular coat is the mucous membrane. The mucous membrane is lined by the squamous stratified epithelium. In the upper cervical part of the oesophagus, its mucous membrane is extensively thrown in to longitudinal folds because of which the lumen of this part of the oesophagus appears to be contracted and almost closed. In the remaining part, its lumen is quite wide and varies in shape being oval, circular or slit like at different levels and at different times.

27

Organs of Respiration

Nose

The nose is the externally visible part of the respiratory system. It forms the part of the face of the animal extending from the transverse level of eyes to the rostral end of the head. Exteriorly it is formed by the bones, muscles, cartilages and the skin. Internally it encloses the nasal cavity which is lined by the mucous membrane. The dorsal part of the nose (roof of the nasal cavity) is termed as dorsum nasi. It is formed by the nasal and frontal bones of the skull. The lateral parts are formed by the incisive, maxillary, lacrimal and zygomatic bones. Covering these bones externally is a muscular layer formed by the facial muscles running over these bones and acting on the upper lip and nostrils. The muscular layer is externally covered by the skin. The skin on the nose bears fine hairs except at the tip of the nose that is formed by the nostrils. The rostral end of the nose is formed by nostrils which provide entrance to the nasal cavity. The nostrils are supported by cartilages which are the dorsal and ventral extensions of the cartilage of the nasal septum. The main aim of the nose is to support and protect the nasal cavity.

Nostrils

The left and right nostrils (Fig. 2-5 A) are placed obliquely dorsoventral one on each side of the muzzle. These are small, narrow and a little dilatable. They are somewhat oval or comma shaped. Because of their oblique position, they are closer together ventrally and slightly wide apart dorsally. Each nostril is bound by the medial and lateral alae or wings which meet above and below to form the commissures. The dorsal commissure is narrow while the ventral commissure is wide and round. Each nostril consists of cartilages, muscles and the skin. The alar and parietal cartilages form the basis of the nostrils. The alar cartilage has an oblong plate like portion the lamina and the narrow rod like portion the cornu. The lamina of the alar cartilage is attached to the rostral extremity of the dorsal parietal cartilage from which it curves downwards and outwards. The medial borders of the laminae of the alar cartilage of opposite sides are connected by fibrous tissue. The cornu of the alar cartilage begins from the lateral part of the lamina, curves outwards and upwards into the external wing, widens and bears at its termination a transverse bar of cartilage. The cornu along with its transverse bar looks like an anchor. The parietal cartilages are two, the dorsal and ventral. These are connected together by fibrous tissue. The two parietal cartilages along with the fibrous tissue fill in the space in the nasoincisive notch. The dorsal parietal cartilage is thin curved outward and downward from the rostral border of the nasal septum. The ventral parietal cartilage lies along the nasal process of the incisive bone. Its rostral part curves upwards and joins the cartilaginous prolongation of the caudal turbinate bone. The muscles dilator naris epicalis and lateralis, depressor labi superioris and inferioris and the nasal part of the levator nasolabialis cover the cartilages of the nostrils. The skin around these is smooth, moist and keratinized.

Nasal cavity

The nasal cavity (Figure 2-6 A) is a hollow space within the nose. The main function of the nasal cavity is to warm, moisturize and filter the air entering the body before it reaches the lungs. It extends from external nares (nostrils) to the caudal nares (choanae). The roof of the nasal cavity is formed by the nasal and part of frontal bones and the parietal (dorsal lateral) cartilages. Its floor is formed by the parts of incisive, maxillary and palatine bones and the parietal (ventral lateral) cartilages. The lateral walls are formed by parts of the incisive, maxillary, palatine, ethmoid and lachrymal bones and the parts of parietal (dorsal and ventral lateral) cartilages. The rostral osseous boundary of the cavity is demarcated by the rostral edge of the body of the incisive bones while the caudal boundary is formed by the cribriform plate of the ethmoid bone. The nasal cavity is divided into the left and right halves by the median nasal septum formed partly by the osseous and partly by the cartilaginous plate. The osseous part is the caudal and ventral portion and it is constituted by perpendicular plate of ethmoid bone and the vomer bone. The rest of the portion of the nasal septum is cartilaginous and it is formed by hyaline cartilage. The dorsal border of the nasal septum is attached to the frontal and nasal bones while its ventral border is received into the groove formed by the vomer. All the osseous and cartilaginous parts of the nasal cavity including the septum are lined by mucous membrane. The major part of the hollow space is occupied by two nasal conchae the dorsal and ventral conchae. These are the scrolls of turbinate bones which project in to the nasal cavity with the purpose of supporting the olfactory mucous membrane and increasing the respiratory surface area creating turbulence within the passing air. This helps in to filter and warm or cool the air passing through it. The conchae divide the nasal cavity into different meatuses. On either side of the nasal septum and between the septum and the conchae is a longitudinal

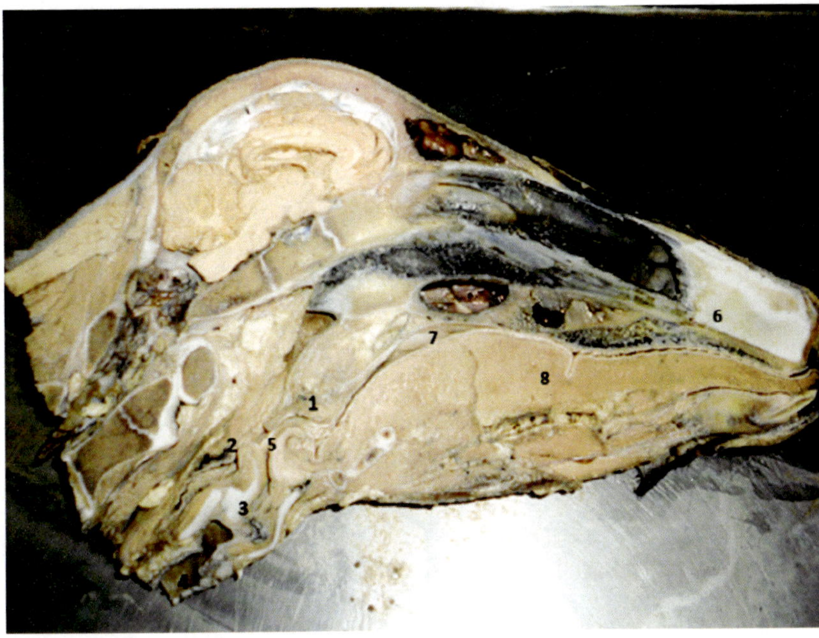

Fig. 2-6 A: Nasal cavity, Pharynx, esophagus, larynx and trachea of Ox 1.Pharynx; 2. Esophagus; 3. Larynx; 4. Trachea; 5. Epiglottis; 6. Nasal cavity; 7. Mouth cavity; 8. Tongue.

space the common meatus. Branching out from the common meatus in the nasal cavity, there lies three meatuses, the dorsal, ventral and middle meatus. The dorsal meatus is the space between the roof of the nasal cavity and dorsal concha. The ventral meatus is a space between the ventral concha and the floor of the nasal cavity. The middle meatus is the space between the dorsal and ventral meatus. The nasal conchae and the septum are also lined by mucous membrane that continues in the paranasal sinuses which are the excavations in to the nasal, frontal, maxillary, lacrimal, and ethmoid bones that forms the skeleton of the nose and nasal cavity. The mucous membrane of the nasal cavity is lined by the ciliated epithelium. The mucous secreted by the mucosal glands trap the unwanted particles from the air passing through the nasal cavity and the cilia beating backward transport them down the pharynx for swallowing. The mucous membrane of the rostral part of the nasal cavity or the vestibule contains small depressions which represent the openings of the nasal glands. This part is called the **respiratory region** while the caudal part which is covered by the thick and brownish olfactory mucous membrane is called the **olfactory region** of nasal cavity.

Lying along the ventral border of the septum nasi in its rostral third is a tube of cartilage named as **vomeronasal organ**. Its rostral opening is in common with the nasal opening of the ductus incisivus on the rostral part of the ventral meatus and caudally it is blind. The ductus incisivus is a mucous tube which extends from its nasal opening through the palate and opens in common with the vomeronasal organ in the fissure on either side of the papilla incisiva.

The rostral apertures of the nasal cavity are formed by the **rostral nares or the nostrils** while its caudal apertures are formed by the **caudal nares or the choanae**. The choanae are elliptical openings situated in the same plane as the floor of the nasal cavity at its caudal extremity and the two, left and right caudal nares are separated by the vomer bone.

Larynx

The larynx (Figure 2-6 A) is a hollow tubular organ situated below the pharynx lying partly between the rami of the mandible and caudally extending into the neck. Cranially it is connected to the pharynx at the level of division of pharynx into nasopharynx and oropharynx. Rostrally it opens into pharynx and caudally into the trachea. It guards the entrance to the lower respiratory passage. It is an organ involved in breathing, sound production and protecting the trachea against food aspiration. The larynx houses the vocal cords which are essential for phonation. The vocal folds are situated just below where the pharynx divides into trachea and oesophagus. The larynx is made up of cartilages, ligaments, muscles and mucous membrane. The cartilage plates form the external skeleton of the larynx and it prevents collapse of this organ. The cartilages are fastened together by the ligaments and muscles. The mucous membrane of the larynx helps it to provide appropriate environment for passage of air through the tube of the larynx. The cartilages that constitute the skeleton of larynx are four in number. Three of them are single unpaired and one is paired. The unpaired (single) cartilages are cricoid, thyroid and epiglottis while the paired cartilage is the arytenoid. The articulations formed by laryngeal cartilages include the cricothyroid articulation, cricoarytenoid articulation and the thyrohyoid articulations. The muscles acting over the laryngeal cartilages and their joints are the extrinsic muscles and the intrinsic muscles. The extrinsic muscles assist the larynx to move rostrally or caudally. The intrinsic muscles help in narrowing or widening the rima glottis.

Cartilages of larynx

The **cricoid cartilage** is the most caudal of the cartilages of larynx. It is situated just rostral to the first tracheal ring. It is shaped like a signet ring and presents a dorsal broad, thick quadrilateral part the lamina and the lateral narrow part an arch. The external (dorsal) surface of the lamina is marked by a median ridge. On each side of the ridge are two facets. Of these, the rostral facet articulates with the arytenoid cartilage of the corresponding side and the caudal facet articulates with the caudal cornu of the thyroid cartilage. The rostral border of the arch gives attachment to the crico-thyroid membrane while the caudal border gives attachment to the crico-tracheal membrane. The internal surface is lined by mucous membrane.

The **thyroid cartilage** is a shield shaped cartilage and is the largest of the cartilages of the larynx. It consists of a central part the body and the two lateral parts the laminae. The body is attached to the base of the epiglottis by the thyro-epiglottic ligament. The laminae form the sides of the larynx and enclose within them the cavity of the larynx. It presents two, rostral and caudal cornu on each side. The rostral cornu articulates with the thyroid cornu of the thyrohyoid bone and the caudal cornu articulates with the facet on the caudal part of the lamina of the cricoid cartilage. The rostral cornu presents below its upper border a thyroid foramen for the passage of the laryngeal nerve.

The **arytenoid cartilages** are paired and each is situated in front of the cricoid, partly medial and dorsal to the lamina of the thyroid cartilage. It is pyramidal in form. The apex is facing rostrally and the base caudally. Its base is concave and presents laterally a facet for the cricoid. The internal angles of the two opposite cartilages are connected by a transverse arytenoid ligament. The lateral angle of the base extends into a slender long vocal process.

The **epiglottis** is a leaf shaped cartilage placed above the body of the thyroid cartilage. Its base is attached to the thyroid cartilage. The apex is rounded. The dorsal and the ventral surfaces are covered by mucous membrane. It overhangs the aditus laryngis which it closes during deglutition.

Articulations, ligaments and membranes of larynx

The **cricothyroid articulation** is formed between the caudal cornu of the thyroid cartilage and the caudal facet on the lamina of the cricoid cartilage. This is a fibrous joint and it allows rotation of thyroid cartilage around the horizontal axis of the joint.

The **cricoarytenoid articulation** is formed between the rostral facet on the lamina of the cricoid cartilage and the facet on the lateral surface of the arytenoid cartilage on each side. It is a synovial joint and it allows gliding as well as rotation movement between two segments of the joint.

Thyrohyoid articulation is formed between the thyrohyoid bone and the thyroid cornu of the thyroid cartilage. This is a fibrous type of joint and the movement is restricted to a slight rotation of the thyroid cartilage around the horizontal axis.

The **ligaments** of these articulations are the fibroelastic bands extending between the cartilages of these articulations. These ligaments include the cricothyroid ligament, cricoarytenoid ligament, transverse arytenoid ligament, thyro-epiglottic ligament, hyoepiglottic ligament, vestibular ligament and the vocal ligament. The most prominent among these is the vocal ligament.

The **vocal ligament** is a strong elastic ligament which extends from the vocal process of the arytenoid cartilage to the dorsal surface of the body of the thyroid cartilage near its caudal border and close to the midline. Thus, ventrally the two vocal ligaments are attached close to each other in the thyroid cartilage.

The **mucous membrane** of the larynx is continuous rostrally with that of the pharynx at the aditus laryngis and caudally with that of the trachea. It is closely attached on the laryngeal surface of epiglottis and vocal processes of the arytenoid cartilages.

The **muscles of the larynx** have been described separately with the other groups of muscles under the chapter on muscles of the head.

Topographical relations of larynx

The larynx is externally attached to the body and thyroid cornu of the hyoid bone and the pharynx. It is related dorsally to the pharynx and oesophagus, ventrally to the skin, fascia and the sternothyrohyoideus and omohyoideus muscles and laterally to the parotid and mandibular salivary glands, and the internal pterygoideus, digastricus and stylohyoideus muscles.

Cavity of larynx

The cavity (lumen) of the larynx (cavum laryngis) extends from the aditus laryngis to the rima glottidis. It has three compartments. The rostral compartment extending from aditus laryngis to the vocal cords is called the vestibule of larynx. The lateral walls of this compartment are formed by the aryteno- epiglottic folds. Below this fold is a shallow depression called the lateral ventricle. Another small depression on the floor of the vestibule is the middle ventricle. A narrow part between the vocal cords and the vocal processes of the arytenoid cartilages is the middle compartment which is called the glottis. The portion of the laryngeal cavity behind the glottis and behind it and the trachea is the caudal compartment of the larynx. The **vocal cord** is a band of yellow elastic tissue placed behind the lateral ventricle of the larynx on each side. It extends from the junction of the body and lamina of the thyroid cartilage to the vocal process. In ox it is short and projects little into the cavity from its wall.As a result, the glottis in ox is wide.

Trachea

The trachea (Figure 2-6 A) or wind pipe is a cartilaginous and membranous tubular structure appearing like a hose (flexible pipe). It connects the pharynx and larynx to the lungs and is used as conduit for passage of air from larynx to lungs and vice versa in the act of breathing. It is formed of a series of 'C' shaped rings made of hyaline cartilage which are joined with each other by the fibro elastic membrane. These sheets of connective tissue are called as annular ligaments. The gaps between the free ends of the 'C' shaped rings of cartilage are filled in by smooth trachealis muscle. Thus, the complete series of these cartilage rings, the annular ligaments and the smooth tracheal muscles form the middle layer of the wall of the trachea throughout its length. This type of structural confirmation of trachea prevents it from collapse and also allows it to adjust in length and diameter due to traction during the movements of neck and at times of forceful breathing. The inner layer of the trachea lining it internally is formed by the mucous membrane with ciliated epithelium. It contains mucosal glands which secret mucous that traps the debris from the filtered air or from the exhaled air and moves it upward towards the oropharynx where it can be swallowed down the pharynx and oesophagus. This mechanism is called the muco-ciliary escalator. The outer layer of the trachea is formed by a serous membrane which is called as tunica adventitia in the neck and tunica serosa in the thorax. Beginning at the larynx, the trachea opens into the larynx through the cricoid cartilage which forms a complete ring around the cranial end of trachea. From here the trachea traverses through the neck lying median in position and running parallel to the oesophagus which lies to the left of the trachea throughout its cervical course. On entering the thorax it crosses the aortic arch and sleeps slightly to the right of the median plane. After reaching just dorsal to the base of the heart at the level of the fourth to fifth thoracic vertebra it bifurcates into bronchi.

In its cervical course, the trachea is related dorsally to the oesophagus up to the level of third cervical vertebra. There after for the rest of its course up to the thoracic inlet it is dorsally related to the longus colli muscle. Laterally it is related to the lateral lobe of the thyroid gland, carotid artery, vagus and the sympathetic nerves, recurrent laryngeal nerve, tracheal lymph duct and the cervical lymph glands. In this segment, the oesophagus lies to the left of the trachea. Ventrally it is related to the ventral cervical muscles. The sternocephalicus crosses it obliquely passing upwards and forwards to reach the angle of the jaw. The omohyoideus crosses the cervical part of the trachea in its upper third. The sternothyrohyoideus covers the ventral surface of the trachea. Thus, most of the exterior of the trachea in the cervical region is covered by the cervical muscles and the other structures leaving a very small area on its ventral surface in the upper third of the cervical course to be covered by the skin and the cutaneous muscle.

28

Organs of Central Nervous System

Brain

The brain, (Figure 2-7 A) a command centre of the body, is a complex organ. The substance of the brain is made of the grey matter and the white matter. The grey matter is often identified as cerebral cortex but other parts of the brain also contain the grey matter. Inside the brain, the grey matter is organized into large accumulations of neurons which are called the nuclei of the brain. Each nucleus is associated with a specific function. In addition to neurons, there is other type of cells the glial cells called neuroglia. The neurons are responsible for sending and receiving impulses or signals. The glial cells are nonneuronal and provide support and nutrition to neuronal cells, form myelin and facilitate signal transmission in the nervous system. The white matter is made of millions of nerve fibres that are coming from neurons and are going to establish communications with different parts of the brain and spinal cord. Since these nerve fibres are coated with myelin sheath around them these appear white and the area occupied by these nerve fibres become the white matter of the brain. The brain has three basic components, the forebrain, midbrain and the hindbrain.

Fore brain: The forebrain (**Prosencephalon**) is the rostral portion of the brain. It consists of cerebrum (**Telencephalon**) and the thalamus, hypothalamus and pineal gland together constituting the interbrain **(Diencephalon).**

Mid brain: The midbrain (**Mesencephalon**) is the middle portion of the brain. It is in the centre lying between the interbrain and hindbrain. It consists of a cranial part of brain stem.

Hind brain: The hindbrain **(Rhombencephalon)** is the caudal most portion of the brain. It consists of remaining (caudal) part of the brain stem, the medulla oblongata (**Myelencephalon**) and the cerebellum and pons **(Metencephalon).**

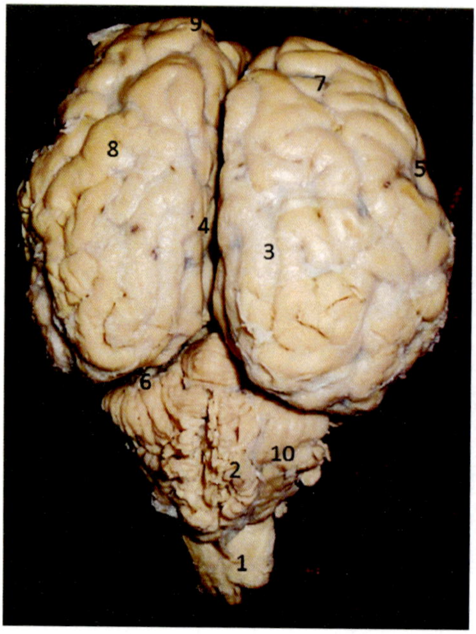

Fig. 2-7 A: Brain of Ox (Dorsal view)
1. Medulla oblongata; 2. Cerebellum;
3. Right cerebral hemisphere;
4. Longitudinal fissure; 5: Sylvian fissure;
6. Transverse fissure; 7. Sulci; 8. Gyri;
9. Olfactory lobe;
10. Lateral lobe of cerebellum.

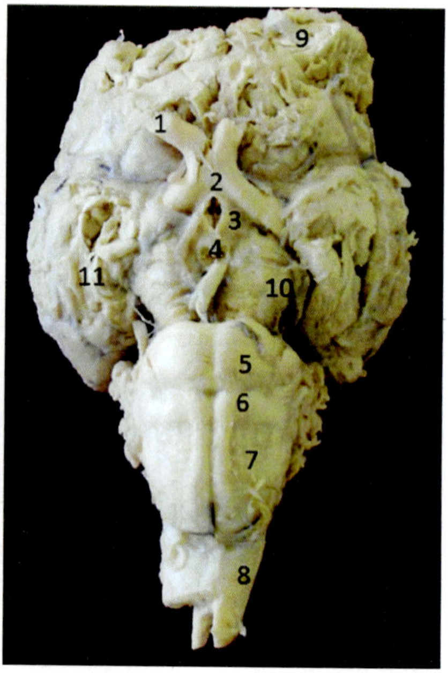

Fig. 2–7 B: Brain of Ox (Ventral view)
1. Optic nerve; 2. Optic tract;
3. Infundibulum; 4. Mammillary body;
5. Pons; 6. Corpus Trapezoideum;
7. Medulla oblongata; 8. Spinal cord;
9. Olfactory bulb; 10. Cerebral peduncles;
11. Pyriform lobe.

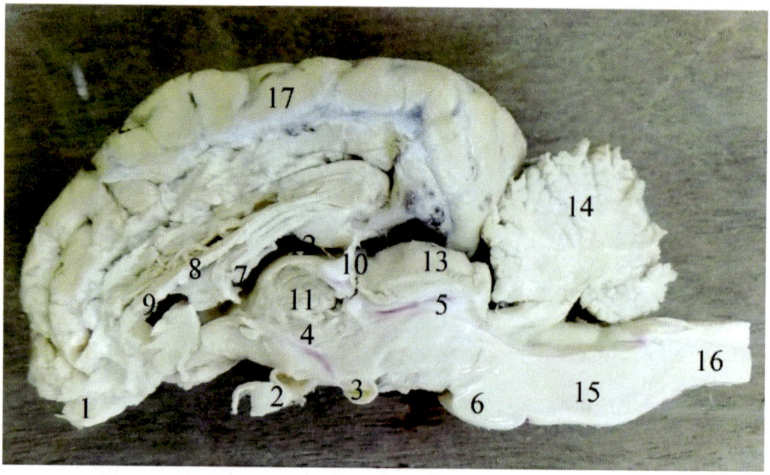

Fig. 2–7 C: Brain of Ox; Midsagital section, Medial view
1. Olfactory bulb; 2. Optic nerve; 3. Tuber cinerium; 4. Third ventricle; 5. Aqueduct of sylvius; 6. Pons; 7. Fornix; 8. Corpus callosum; 9. Genu; 10. Pineal body; 11. Thalamus; 12. Choroid plexus; 13. Superior colliculus; 14: Cerebellum; 15: Medulla oblongata; 16; Spinal cord; 17: cerebrum.

Hind brain

Brain stem

The brain stem (Figure 2-7 B) is the rostral continuation of the spinal cord into the brain. It forms the caudal most region of the brain. It consists of an elongated quadrilateral part, the medulla oblongata. Rostral to medulla is a transversely oriented pons and in front of the pons are four corporate bodies the corpora quadrigemina which forms the part of the mid brain. In addition, the hind brain consists of cerebellum that covers the dorsal surface of the pons and the part of the medulla.

Medulla oblongata

The medulla oblongata is oblong shaped quadrilateral structure. It is compressed dorsoventrally. It is wider towards its rostral end and narrower towards caudal end. Its ventral surface is convex transversely and presents a median fissure. The caudal portion of this median fissure is faint but it becomes deeper as it proceeds rostrally and ends into a small depression the foramen caecum. In front of the foramen caecum and just behind the pons is a transverse band of fibres called the corpus trapezoideum or the trapezoid body. The lateral ends of the trapezoid body furnish origin to the VII (facial) and VIII (vestibulocochlear) cranial nerves. On either side of the ventral median fissure are two longitudinally oriented fibre bundles called the pyramids. The pyramids are very prominent towards the rostral part just behind the pons but they gradually disappear as they reach the caudal end of the medulla where they cross over to the opposite side. This crossing over of pyramids is called as dicussation of pyramids. The pyramids are bounded laterally by the ventral lateral sulcus. The VI cranial nerve (abducent) arises at the angle formed by the trapezoid body and the lateral border of the pyramids. The root fibres of the XII cranial (hypoglossal) nerve originate in a linear series lateral to the pyramids.A prominent tubercle called the facial tubercle lies in the angle between the trapezoid body and the pyramids. This tubercle is laterally bounded by the dorsal lateral sulcus of the medulla.

The dorsal surface of the medulla is largely concealed by the cerebellum. It forms the greater part of the fourth ventricle. The dorsal median fissure runs in the middle of the dorsal surface. This is the continuation of the dorsal median fissure of the spinal cord and extends up to the middle of the dorsal surface of the medulla. At this place, the lateral lips of the dorsal median fissure which are called as restiform bodies diverge and form the lateral boundaries of a triangular depression that forms the caudal part of the fourth ventricle. The dorsal lateral grooves of the spinal cord wind outward and forward and then continue over the dorsal surface of medulla as the dorsal lateral sulcus. The roots of the IX (glossopharyngeal), X (vagus) and XI (accessory) cranial nerves arise from the lateral edges of the dorsal lateral sulcus of the medulla. The central canal of the spinal cord continues in the caudal part of the medulla and opens into the caudal angle of the fourth ventricle. The lateral surfaces of the medulla oblongata are narrow in the caudal part and become wider and rounded towards the rostral part. The recess between the medulla and the cerebellum is occupied by the choroid plexus of the fourth ventricle.

Pons

The pons is in the form of a protuberance projected transversely on the ventral surface in the centre of the brain stem. It occupies the position between the medulla and the cerebral peduncles. It is marked off from these structures ventrally by the cranial and caudal transverse grooves. Its lateral ends are convex in both the directions. It presents a median groove in the centre which lodges the basilar artery. Laterally, a large part of the pons curves dorsally and continues into the base of cerebellum and forms the middle cerebellar peduncles, The root fibres of V cranial (trigeminal) nerve arise from the lateral aspect of the ventral surface of the pons. The dorsal surface is blended on each side with the rostral cerebellar peduncles. The central free part of the dorsal surface forms the rostral portion of the floor of the fourth ventricle.

Cerebellum

The cerebellum lies caudal to the cerebral hemispheres. It overlies the pons and rostral part of the medulla oblongata and the fourth ventricle. It is globular in shape and compressed dorsoventrally. It is separated from the cerebral hemispheres by a great transverse fissure. Its dorsal surface is covered by tentorium cerebelli and the ventral surface covers the fourth ventricle forming its roof. The cerebellum is connected by three pairs of peduncles with the medulla, pons and mid brain. These three cerebellar peduncles, the rostral, middle and caudal peduncles on each side join the central white substance of the cerebellum the corpus medulare or medulla at its base. The cerebellum consists of three lobes, the median vermis and the two lateral hemispheres. The vermis is curved in a circular manner so that its two extremities are close together or even in contact with each other on the ventral surface. Its rostral extremity gives attachment to the rostral medullary vellum that extends from the area caudal to corpora quadrigemina while the caudal extremity joins the caudal medullary velum that extends from the medulla. The two vella complete the roof of the fourth ventricles. The vermis and the hemispheres of the cerebellum are externally separated from each other by circular fissures. The outer surface of the cerebellum is thrown into numerous folds and deep grooves called as gyri and sulci, the folds of piamater deep into the sulci.

The internal substance of the cerebellum consists of two major parts, the outer grey matter the cortex and the inner white matter the medulla. The grey matter consists of groups of nerve cells arranged in various nuclei. The white matter consists of the numerous fibre tracts by which the cerebellum is connected with different parts of brain.

Mid brain

The mid brain (Fig. 2-7 C) is relatively small part of the brain. It is situated between the medulla oblongata and pons caudally and the thalamus and hypothalamus rostrally. It is completely covered by the cerebral hemispheres. It is composed of **tectum**, **tegmentum, substantia nigra** and **cerebral crura**. The substance of the mid brain is traversed longitudinally by a narrow canal called the **cerebral (mesencephalic) aqueduct** that connects the fourth ventricle with the third ventricle.

Tectum

The tectum is the superior (dorsal) portion (lamina) of the mesencephalon. It consists of four large paired rounded bodies called the **corpora quadrigemina (colliculi).** These are arranged in two pairs, the rostral pair and the caudal pair which are separated by the transverse groove. The rostral colliculi are grey in colour and are placed at a higher level than the caudal colliculi. These are rostrally separated from the thalamus by a wide transverse grove. The caudal colliculi are pale in colour and smaller in size. These are caudally separated from the pons by a transverse furrow. The right and left colliculi are separated by a shallow longitudinal furrow. The rostral end oft his furrow widens and it forms a depression in which the pineal body is lodged. The IV cranial (trochlear) nerves emerge out from either ends of this furrow. Laterally each of the caudal colliculi is prolonged into medial geniculate body by a band of white fibres called the caudal brachium. Similarly, the rostral colliculi extend into lateral geniculate body by the rostral brachium.

Tegmentum

The tegmentum is situated, ventral to the mesencephalic aqueduct. It is closely related to the central grey area of the mesencephalon. The major structures contained in the tegmentum include the two large nuclei. One of these is the motor nucleus of the oculomotor nerve. It is situated in the rostral part of the tegmentum. This nucleus is composed of several subdivisions. The other nucleus is the motor nucleus of the trochlear nerve. It is situated in the caudal part of the tegmentum and lies ventromedial to the motor nucleus of oculomotor nerve.

Cerebral crura (cerebral peduncles)

The cerebral crura appear on the base of the brain as two large columns which emerge from under the pons on either side of the median line. The right and left crura are close together initially but diverge outward as they pass rostrally forward to enter the cerebrum. At the point of entrance into the substance of cerebral hemispheres, the lateral and ventral faces of each crus are crossed by the optic tract. The optic tract continues as optic nerve, the first cranial nerve that passes through the optic canal to reach the eye ball. The medial surface of both the crura forms the lateral boundaries of the inerpeduncular fossa. This fossa is pierced by numerous blood vessels and is called the caudal perforated substance. Just outside the point of divergence of the cerebral peduncles arises the III cranial (oculomotor) nerve.

Substantia Nigra

The substantia nigra is a dark substance of grey matter constituting the middle layer of the cerebral peduncles. Dorsal to this and forming the upper (dorsal) layer of the crus is the tegmentum while the lower (ventral) layer of the cruse is formed by the crusta. The substantia nigra presents a large dark nucleus between the pons caudally and the corpora quadrigemina rostrally. The majority of the cells of substantia nigra contain a varying amount of melanin granules that gives it a dark colour which is its characteristic appearance.

Cerebral aqueduct (mesencephalic aqueduct)

The cerebral aqueduct is a median longitudinal canal passing through the substance of the mesencephalon and hence it is also called as mesencephalic aqueduct. It runs under the corpora quadrigemina and connects the fourth ventricle with the third ventricle. The shape of the canal in transverse section varies at different levels of its length. Near its rostral opening into the third ventricle it appears T shaped, in the middle of its length it is oval in shape whereas, near its caudal opening into the fourth ventricle it is star shaped.

Fore brain

The fore brain (Fig. 2-7 C) (prosencephalon) constitutes the rostral portion of the brain. It consists of two major parts. The foremost part of the brain is the endbrain (telencephalon) that is comprised of the two **cerebral hemispheres** that enclose the lateral ventricles. The lateral ventricles communicate with each other by the median opening called the interventricular foramen (foramen of Moro). The remaining part of the fore brain is constituted by the rostral end of the brain stem the inter brain (diencephalon). It consists of the third ventricle and the structures surrounding this ventricle such as the **epithalamus, thalamus, subthalamus, hypothalamus** and the **pineal body.**

Epithalamus

The epithalamus is the dorsocaudal part of the diencephalon. It consists of rostral and caudal paraventricular nuclei, medial and lateral Habenular nuclei, stria medularis thalami, caudal commissure and the pineal body.

Thalamus

The thalamus plays an important role as relay and control station between brain stem and spinal cord on one side and the cerebral hemispheres on the other. It is a large ovoid mass situated obliquely across the dorsal face of the cerebral peduncles so that the left and right thalami meet in front at right angle. Medially they meet each other at the midline forming inter thalamic adhesion which obliterates the centre space of the third ventricle. The dorsal surface of the thalamus is convex and is separated from the hippocampus by the tela choroidea. Laterally it is separated from the caudate nucleus by a band of white matter the stria terminalis. The caudal part of the thalamus is in the form of a rounded ridge continuous laterally with the optic tract where the lateral geniculate body is blended with it. Behind the point of emergence of the optic tract in the angle between the thalamus and the cerebral peduncle is the medial geniculate body.

Subthalamus

The subthalamus is a part of diencephalon lying just ventral and beneath the thalamus and dorsal to the hypothalamus. Its prominent structure is the subthalamic nucleus. It connects to the globus palidus a basal nucleus of the telencephalon.

Hypothalamus

The hypothalamus is a part of the diencephalon that contains number of small nuclei with variety of functions. The most important function of the hypothalamus is to link the nervous system to the endocrine system via pituitary gland. The hypothalamus is located below the thalamus and subthalamus and just above the brain stem. It forms the ventral part of the diencephalon. Its rostral limit of the diencephalon is marked by the optic chiasma and the optic tract. However, the hypothalamus extends beyond this limit rostrally up to the preoptic area and is considered as rostral hypothalamic region. Beside this the other parts of the hypothalamus are the intermediate region and the caudal hypothalamic region. All these three regions of the hypothalamus contains some prominent and some minor nuclei.

Pineal body

The pineal body is a small ovoid or fusiform gland situated in a deep depression between the thalami and the corpora quadrigemina. It is attached to the caudal angle (quadrant) of the third ventricle by a hollow stalk in which is a small recess of the third ventricle. Immediately under the caudal part of the stalk is a short transverse band of white matter the caudal commissure of the cerebrum.

Cerebral hemispheres (cerebrum)

The cerebrum is the superior most and the largest part of the brain. It consists of two hemispheres called the cerebral hemispheres. The two hemispheres, left and right together form a large ovoid mass which is broad in the hind part and narrow in the front part. The left and right hemispheres are separated medially by the median longitudinal fissure except at a small area called the corpus callosum, the central white commissure that connects the two hemispheres above the rostral pair of the colliculi. The membranous fold called falx cerebri is lodged in this fissure. Each hemisphere has four surfaces. The dorsal surface is convex and it adapts to the roof of the cranium. The ventral surface is called the basal surface. It bears piriform lobe which is situated lateral to the cerebral crus and the hypothalamus. Just rostral to the piriform lobe on the ventral surface of the hemisphere lies a triangular area called the olfactory trigone. In the caudal part of the olfactory trigone is the olfactory tubercle. In the middle of the basal surface is a deep depression the lateral cerebral fossa which contains middle cerebral artery. The medial surface is flat and vertical. It forms the lateral boundary of the median longitudinal fissure of the cerebrum. The lateral surface is convex and it blends with the dorsal surface. The rostral extremity of the hemisphere is called the frontal pole. It is bilaterally compressed, convex and partially covered by the small oval rough body called the olfactory bulb. It is lodged in the ethmoidal fossa of the cranial cavity. The olfactory bulb is marked off from the hemisphere by the medial and lateral rhenal sulcus. The olfactory bulb continues caudally into a short fibre tract the olfactory peduncle which connects the olfactory bulb with the cerebral hemisphere. Rostrally, the olfactory bulb is connected to the fibres of the I st cranial (olfactory) nerve through the pores of the ethmoid fossa. The caudal extremity is called the occipital pole. It is wide and arched. On its ventromedial aspect it is flat and is separated from the cerebellum by a transverse groove that is lodged by a membranous fold the tentorium cerebelli. The exterior of each hemisphere is thrown into several ridges called as gyri which are separated by the grooves or fissures called the sulci. This particular arrangement of the external surface of the hemispheres increases the surface area of the cerebrum of the brain. The olfactory bulb, the olfactory peduncle, the olfactory tract and the olfactory tubercle together constitute the rhinencephalon.

Exteriorly each of the hemispheres is divided in to four lobes. These are the frontal, parietal, temporal and the occipital lobe. The **frontal lobe** is the most rostral part of the hemisphere. Its caudal limit is the central sulcus called the fissure of Rolando. This fissure separates the frontal lobe from the parietal and temporal lobes. The frontal lobe is associated with the control of voluntary muscles movements. The **parietal lobe** is immediately caudal to the frontal lobe from which it is separated by the central fissure. and from the temporal lobe by the lateral fissure. The parietal lobe is associated with the sensations including the sense of touch, perception, warmth and cold and the vibrations. The **temporal lobe** is ventral to the lateral fissure and rostral to the occipital lobe. It is separated from occipital lobe by imaginary line passing transversely through the widest part of the cerebral hemisphere. The temporal lobe is associated with the auditory processes and the olfaction. The **occipital lobe** is the caudal most part of the cerebral hemisphere. It is associated with the sense of vision.

The **interior** of the cerebral hemisphere consists of two major divisions. The outer greater layer which is grey area is called the cortex whereas, the inner small area which is white area is called the medulla of the cerebral hemisphere. The cortex is made of the nerve cells (neurons) and the medulla is formed of the white myelinated axons of the nerve cells. The cortex is arranged in two regions the neocortex (isocortex) and the allocortex. The neocortex is larger part and it consists of six layers called laminae. The allocortex is smaller part and has two layers or laminae.

Corpus Callosum

The corpus callosum is the great commissure that connects the two (left and right) hemispheres. It is an arched white structure curving rostrocaudad and is composed of commissural fibres. Its rostral end called genu continues with the lamina terminalis and closes the rostral part of the third ventricle. The caudal end is called the splenium which lies at a higher level than the genu. The dorsal surface of the corpus callosum is covered by a thin layer of grey matter that is called indusium griseum. The medial and lateral olfactory stria run along the respective side of the median line of the indusium griseum. The ventral surface of the corpus callosum forms the roof of the lateral ventricle. The fibres of the corpus callosum spread laterally in a radiating manner into the central white matter of the brain.

Fornix

The fornix is a 'C' shaped bilateral bundle of white nerve fibres that arch over the thalamus and the third ventricle. It consists of a body and two columns on each side. The body is formed by the fusion of the arches of two sides of the fornix. It is triangular in shape. The dorsal surface blends medially with the septum lucidium and on either side it forms the floor of the lateral ventricle. The lateral border is related to the choroid plexus and forms the internal boundary of the interventricular foramen. The rostral columns are two slender rounded bundles of fibres that emerge from the body in front of the interventricular foramen and diverge slightly as they curve ventrally and caudally to enter the mammillary body and they are crossed in front by the rostral commissure. The caudal columns are much larger bands which diverge widely from the caudal angles of the body of the fornix. Each column curves outward and caudad over the thalamus and is continued as the fimbria along the concave border of the hippocampus. The caudal columns give off fibres to form the alveus of the hippocampus and between them are transverse fibres which constitute the caudal commissure of the hippocampus.

Hippocampus

The hippocampus is a small subcortical area located in the medial temporal lobe of the cerebral hemisphere. It is a gyrus which curves from the deep face of the piriform lobe around the thalamus. Deeply it is separated from the dentate gyrus by the hippocampal fissure. A band of fibres of white matter called fimbria passes along the concave margin of the dentate gyrus from the hippocampus. The ventral surface of the hippocampus is covered with white matter called alveus which is derived from the caudal column of the fornix and the fimbria. The left and right hippocampus is connected to each other at their upper parts by hippocampal commissure. The hippocampus receives afferent fibres from the secondary olfactory cortex, the precommissural area and the hippocampus of the opposite side via the hippocampal commissure. The efferent fibres originate from the pyramidal cell layer and the alveus and continue into the fornix.

Mammillary body

The mammillary bodies are a pair of small round bodies located on the under surface of the cerebral hemispheres that as a part of the diencephalon forms part of the limbic system of the brain. These are located at the ends of the rostral arches of the fornix. They consist of two groups of nuclei, the medial mammillary nuclei and the lateral mammillary nuclei. They are connected to other parts of the brain and act as relay for impulses coming from the amygdaloid body and hippocampus via mammillo-thalamic tract to the thalamus.

Amygdaloid body

The amygdaloid body is subcortical structure located in the rostromedial part of the temporal lobe in front of the hippocampus of the cerebral hemisphere. It consists of several well defined nuclei and is connected with the precommissural area through the stria terminalis.. Some of the prominent pathways to amygdaloid body come from the temporal and frontal lobes of the cerebral hemispheres. The amygdaloid body is involved in a large number of functions ranging from motor activities, basic drives to memory and other cognitive processes.

Ventricles of brain

The ventricles of the brain (Figure 2-7 C) are a set of four interconnected cavities called ventricles inside the brain, where the cerebrospinal fluid (CSF) is produced. This set of ventricles is called the ventricular system of the brain and it is continued caudally into the central canal of the spinal cord. Within each ventricle is a region of choroid plexus, a network of ependymal cells that is involved in the production of cerebrospinal fluid. The same layer of ependymal cells also lines the central canal of the spinal cord. The ventricle system of the brain is responsible for the production, transport and removal of the cerebrospinal fluid which bathes the nervous tissue of the brain and spinal cord. The ventricular system of brain includes four ventricles.

Lateral ventricles

The lateral ventricles are two, the right and the left ventricles in the telencephalon. Each lateral ventricle is a cavity in the interior of each cerebral hemisphere, communicating with each other and with the third ventricle by the intervertebral foramen (foramen of Monro). Each of the lateral ventricle has three parts, a body and two cornua. The body extents caudad to the splenium and communicates with the third ventricle through the interventricular foramen situated below the fornix and between it and the thalamus, The rostral cornu is in front and it communicates with the olfactory bulb. The caudal cornu curves 'down, proceeds caudally and then turn to rostral to reach the pyriform lobe. The walls of the cavity (ventricle) consist of the roof, floor and the medial wall. The roof is formed by the corpus callosum, the floor is formed by two chief nuclei, the caudate nucleus in front and the hippocampus behind. The medial wall is formed by the septum lucidium. The hippocampus and the pyriform lobe on the floor of the ventricle are separated by an oblique groove which is occupied by the choroid plexus of the lateral ventricle.

Third ventricle

The third ventricle is the cavity of the diencephalon, a part of prosencephalon the fore brain. It is a narrow annular space around the internal extremities of the two optic thalami in the diencephalon. It communicates rostrally with the lateral ventricles through the interventricular foramen and caudally with the fourth ventricle through the cerebral (mesencephalic) aqueduct. The floor of this ventricle is formed by the structures of the interpeduncular fossa. The roof is formed by the lamina epithelialis of the tela choroidea and fornix. On the top of this lamina is located the choroid plexus of third ventricle. The rostral wall is formed by the lamina terminalis which is a thin layer of grey matter between the optic chiasma and the corpus callosum. A distinct rounded band of white matter called the rostral commissure extends across its caudal face between it and the rostral columns of the fornix. The fibres of the rostral commissure connect the pyriform lobe and the olfactory bulb to those of the opposite side. The cavity of the third ventricle presents three recess, the optic recess into the optic chiasma, the pineal recess in the stalk of the pineal body and the infundibular recess into the infundibulum.

Fourth ventricle

The fourth ventricle is the cavity of the rhombencephalon, the hind brain. It communicates caudally with the central canal of the spinal cord and rostrally with the third ventricle through the cerebral aqueduct. The floor of the third ventricle is formed by the medulla and the pons. The caudal part of the floor narrows to a point at its communication with the central canal of the spinal cord. This point is called as calamus criptorius. The lateral walls are formed by the restiform bodies and the rostral cerebellar peduncles. The roof is formed by the vermis cerebelli and the rostral and caudal medullary vela. The choroid plexus of the third ventricle is formed in association with the caudal medullary velum.

Cranial nerves

Twelve pairs of cranial nerves emerge from the ventral (basal) surface of the brain, pass through the openings (foramina) of the skull and lead to the parts of head, neck, and the body trunk. The cranial nerves with their nuclei within the brain stem contain sensory and motor neuron components. The sensory fibre components have their cell bodies located in ganglia located outside the brain and the motor fibre components have their cell bodies located within the brain. Hence some of the cranial nerves are sensory nerves, some are motor nerves and some other nerves are mixed nerves with both, the sensory as well as motor fibres. The cranial nerves are named and numbered based on their location from the front to back of the brain. Thus the olfactory is the first and the hypoglossal is the twelfth cranial nerve. Accordingly the first to twelfth cranial nerves are numbered, named and classified (functional type) as below.

Sr. No. of Cr. Nerve	Attachment with brain	Name of the nerve	Type of the nerve
I	Fore brain	Olfactory	Sensory
II	Fore brain	Optic	Sensory
III	Mid brain	Oculomotor	Motor
IV	Mid brain	Trochlear	Motor
V	Hind brain	Trigeminal	Mixed
VI	Hind brain	Abducent	Motor
VII	Hind brain	Facial	Mixed
VIII	Hind brain	Vestibulocochlear	Sensory
IX	Hind brain	Glossopharyngeal	Mixed
X	Hind brain	Vagus	Mixed
XI	Hind brain	Accessory	Motor
XII	Hind brain	Hypoglossal	Motor

Spinal cord

The spinal cord is a vital link between the brain and the body. It is a mass of nervous tissue arranged in a cylindrical form of structure that is enclosed inside the vertebral canal extending from the level of the foramen magnum of the occipital bone of the skull to the level of last but one lumbar vertebra or the middle of the sacrum. It is a part of central nervous system that continues rostrally with the medulla oblongata without any natural line of demarcation between the two. Behind the medulla it descends down the vertebral canal inside which it is protected and surrounded by the bony vertebral column. Throughout its length it is cylindrical but compressed dorsoventrally with uniform diameter except at two places where it is enlarged. These enlargements are called as cervical (cervicothoracic) and lumbar (lumbosacral) enlargements from where the nerves for the fore limbs and hind limbs extend from the spinal cord. The caudal part of the spinal cord rapidly narrows to a point that is called conus medularis. The conus medularis is prolonged for a short distance by a slender filament of pia matter called the filum terminale.

The dorsal and ventral surfaces of the spinal cord are divided in the middle by a dorsal median groove and the ventral groove respectively. On either side of the dorsal median groove are the dorsal lateral grooves where the dorsal root fibres of the spinal nerves enter the cord. The ventral root fibres of the spinal nerves leave the cord a little lateral to the ventral median groove. The dorsal median groove is filled up by the dorsal median septum. The ventral median groove is narrow and deep and reaches to about the middle of the cord. The two halves of the cord are connected by commissures of grey and white matter.

The grey commissure is a transverse band at the base of the dorsal median septum and is traversed by the central canal of the spinal cord. The white commissure is a bridge of white matter that connects the two ventral columns of the white matter. The central column opens rostrally into the caudal angle of the fourth ventricle of the brain and caudally it ends in the conus medularis forming a slight dilation, the ventricularis terminalis..

The transverse section of spinal cord shows white matter in the periphery, grey matter inside and a tiny canal filled with cerebrospinal fluid at the centre. Surrounding the canal is a single layer of cells the ependymal layer. Surrounding the ependymal layer is the grey matter the area that appears like a letter 'H' or like a butterfly. The two wings of the butterfly are connected across the midline by the dorsal grey commissure and below it the white commissure. The grey matter mainly contains the cell bodies of neurons and neuroglia. Each wing has four columns, the dorsal horn, intermediate column, lateral column and the ventral horn. The dorsal horn is comprised of sensory nuclei that receive and process incoming somatosensory information. From here the ascending projections emerge to transmit the sensory information to the mid brain and diencephalon. The intermediate column and the lateral horn comprise autonomic neurons innervating the visceral and pelvic organs. The ventral horn comprises motor neurons that innervate the skeletal muscles. The white matter of the spinal cord is arranged in the ascending and descending nerve tracts.

There are 37 pairs of spinal nerves that arise from the lateral aspect of the spinal cord and they are classified as eight cervical, thirteen thoracic, six lumbar, five sacral and five coccygeal. According to the attachment of these nerves to the cord the spinal cord is considered of having five regions as cervical, thoracic, lumbar, and sacral. As a result of unequal growth of the spinal cord and the vertebral column, correspondence between the two is unmatched and the spinal nerves have to travel a short distance caudad before they gain exit from the canal. The conus medularis reaches only up to the mid sacral level, and hence the rest of the sacral and all the coccygeal nerves occupy the whole vertebral canal before the exit of these nerves through their corresponding intervertebral foramen. As a result, a bundle of the spinal nerves along with the conus medularis and filum terminale in the middle of the bunch inside the sacral part of the vertebral canal appears like a horse tail and hence it is called the cauda equina.

The white matter is divided into three pairs of columns. The dorsal column lies on either side of the dorsal median septum and is laterally limited by the dorsal lateral groove. The ventral column lies on either side of the ventral median septum and is limited laterally by the ventral root fibres. The lateral column lies laterally between the dorsal and the ventral column. The columns of the left and right side are connected to each other through the white commissure.

Spinal nerves

Each spinal nerve is attached to the spinal cord by two roots, a dorsal root which is a sensory root and a ventral root which is a motor root. The dorsal root is larger than the ventral root. The dorsal root fibres (motor fibres) enter the spinal cord at the dorsal lateral groove. On the course of this root, there is a ganglion called the spinal ganglion. This ganglion is located either near the inner opening of the interventricular foramen or inside that foramen. Beyond this ganglion, the fibres of the dorsal root join those of the ventral root. The spinal ganglia are external to dura matter. The ventral root fibres are efferent or motor. They contain less fibres than the dorsal root. The fibres of this root arise from the ventral horn cells of the grey matter, pass through the white matter, leave the spinal cord at its ventrolateral edge and then join the fibres of the dorsal root.

Immediately after leaving the spinal cord, the two roots join to form the spinal nerve. Each nerve gets exit through the intervertebral foramen, gives off a small meningeal branch which is joined by a bundle of nerve fibres from sympathetic trunk that enter the vertebral canal through the intervertebral foramen. Each spinal nerve, then divides into dorsal and ventral primary branches. The dorsal branches are distributed to the muscles and skin of the dorsal part of the body. The ventral branches supply in general to the muscles and skin of the ventral parts of the body including the limbs. Each nerve or its ventral branch is connected with its adjacent ganglion of the sympathetic by a communicating branch called the ramus communicans.

Meninges

Meninges are the fibrous membranes which enclose and protect the brain and spinal cord. There are three layers of meninges, the dura mater, arachnoid and the pia mater. The dura mater is the outer most covering, the arachnoid is the middle layer and the pia mater is the innermost layer closely adhering the brain and spinal cord. The meninges covering the brain are called the cranial meninges whereas; those surrounding the spinal cord are called spinal meninges. However, the cranial and spinal meninges are continuous with each other at the foramen magnum.

Duramater

The cranial duramater closely adheres to the endosteum of the cranial bones. It is composed of two layers, the outer parietal layer and the inner visceral layer. The parietal layer is called the endosteal layer and it closely adheres to the endosteum of the cranial bones. The visceral layer is called the meningeal layer and it is in close contact with the middle layer of meninges the arachnoid.

The endosteal layer and the meningeal layers are close to each other except at the places where the cranial venous sinuses are located within them. The dura matter forms sheaths around the cranial nerves till they enter the foramina to enter or exit the cranial cavity. Another sheath of dura matter passes into the foramen magnum to continue with the spinal dura mater. The cranial dura mater presents three internal folds that lodge into the fissures separating the major parts of the brain. These folds are the falx cerebri, tentorium cerebelli and the diaphragm sellae.

Falx cerebri: The falx cerebri is a dorsal sickle shaped fold of dura mater which is situated in the great longitudinal fissure of the cerebrum that separates the two cerebral hemispheres. It is attached dorsally to the inter parietal and inter frontal crests, caudally to the inter occipital protuberance and rostrally to the crista galli. Its dorsal border is convex and here the two layers of dura mater are separated and enclose the dorsal longitudinal sinus. Its ventral border is concave and lies above the corpus callosum. Here again the two layers enclose the ventral longitudinal sinus.

Tentorium cerebelli: The tentorium cerebelli is the transverse fold of dura mater that occupies the transverse fissure between the cerebellum and the occipital lobes of the cerebral hemispheres. It is attached dorsally to the internal occipital protuberance and laterally to the petrosal crest. Its ventral border is concave, thin and free and forms an arch over the mid brain.

Diaphragm sellae: The diaphragm sellae is a thick horizontal fold of dura mater which surrounds the pituitary gland (hypophysis cerebri) and encloses the cavernous and inter cavernous sinuses. It is perforated dorsally for the infundibulum of the hypophysis. It separates the hypophysis from the ventral surface of the diencephalon.

The Spinal duramater is composed only of a meningeal layer and forms a very loose tube around the spinal cord. It is separated from the periosteum of the vertebral canal by a considerable **epidural space** which is occupied by connective tissue and fat. It furnishes sheaths around the spinal nerves up to the intervertebral foramina. The duramater and the arachnoid of the spinal meninges enclose a space which is called the **subdural space.**

Arachnoid

The arachnoid is a very thin delicate membrane situated between the dura mater and the pia mater. Its outer face is lined by endothelium and forms the inner wall of the subdural space. Its internal surface is also lined by endothelium and forms the outer boundary of subarachnoid space containing the cerebrospinal fluid (CSF). The arachnoid furnishes sheaths for nerves only for a short distance.

The arachnoid is connected to the pia mater by thin connective tissue trabeculae which pass through the subarachnoid space.

The cerebral arachnoid does not extend into the sulci on the outer surface of the brain. It closely adheres to the pia mater on the summits of the gyri. In certain locations the cerebral arachnoid is separated from the pia mater by a considerable distance to form the **subarachnoid cisterns**. Some of the major cisterns are as below.

The cisterna magna: The cisterna magna (cisterna cerebellomedullaris) is in the angle between the caudal surface of the cerebellum and the dorsal surface of the medulla oblongata. It communicates with the fourth ventricle through a central and two lateral openings and caudally with the subarachnoid space of the spinal cord.

The cisterna pontis is on the ventral surface of the pons.

The cisterna chiasmatis is located rostral to the optic chiasma, between the cerebral crura of the mesencephalon.

The cisterna basalis is at the base of the brain and is divided by optic chiasma into two parts.

The cisterna fossa lateralis is at the lower part of the lateral fissure.

The spinal arachnoid is continuous with that of the cerebral arachnoid at the level of foramen magnum and it forms a relatively wide tube around the spinal cord. The tubular extensions from the arachnoid cover the roots of the spinal nerves. Caudally the spinal arachnoid forms a cone shaped sac which confirms the cone formed by the spinal dura mater. The spinal arachnoid is connected to the spinal pia mater by the connective tissue trabeculae.

Piamater

The piamater is a very delicate vascular membrane which closely adheres to the brain and spinal cord.

The cerebral piamater accurately moulds itself on the brain by deeping itself into all the sulci and the fissures. Its external surface forms the inner boundary of the subarachnoid space and is lined by endothelium. From its deep surface thin trabeculae extend into the substance of the brain. The large folds of pia mater extend into two great fissures of the brain. One of these is the **tela choroidea**. The pia mater of choroid fissure of the lateral ventricles and the roof of the third and fourth ventricles is called as tela choroidea of the respective ventricle. The blood vessels of the pia mater modify in the tela choroidea and along with the ependymal layer form the plexus called the **choroid plexus** of the respective ventricles of the brain.

The spinal piamater is dense and thicker than the cerebral piamater. It sends a fold into the ventral longitudinal groove of the spinal cord and also helps to form the dorsal median septum.Along the mid ventral line it forms a thickening called the linea splendens in which runs the ventral spinal artery. It gives off strong longitudinal band between the dorsal and ventral roots of the spinal nerves on each side of the spinal cord. These bands are called as dentate ligaments. The lateral border of the spinal pia mater is serrated and is attached to the dura mater.

29

Sense Organs and Common Integument

Organ of vision (Eye)

The vision is by far the most used of the five senses and is one of the primary means that is used to gather information from the surroundings. The organ of vision or the bulb of the eye is contained in the bony socket called the orbit in the skull. The bulb of the eye (eyeball) is embedded in the fat of the orbit. Associated with the eyeball within the orbit are certain accessory structures viz. the muscles, fasciae, eyelids, conjunctiva and lacrimal apparatus.

Orbit

The orbit is the cavity or socket in the skull wherein the eyeball and its accessory structures (appendages) are situated. The orbit is continuous caudally with the temporal fossa. The axis of the orbit which is usually considered as running between the optic foramen and the middle of the socket is directed rostrad, laterad and dorsad. The medial wall of the orbit is formed by the frontal, lacrimal and the presphenoid (wing) bones of the skull. It is concave and smooth. The medial wall in its rostral part presents a fossa that is called the lacrimal fossa which accommodates the lacrimal sac along with the lacrimal gland. Caudal to the lacrimal fossa is a small depression for the attachment of obliquus ventralis muscle. The dorsal wall of the orbit is formed by the frontal and partly by the lacrimal bone. The supraorbital foramen, an opening of the canal perforating the root of the zygomatic process, is situated in the dorsal wall of the orbit. The ventral wall is slightly rough and is formed by the zygomatic bone, the zygomatic process of the temporal bone, the zygomatic process of the frontal bone and the part of the maxilla bone. The lateral wall (rim) of the orbit is formed by the zygomatic process of temporal bone and the temporal process of the zygomatic bone. Several foramina and/ or fissures for the passage of the vessels and nerves are located in the walls of the orbit. These include the optic, alar, oval, supraorbital, ethmoidal, lacrimal, maxillary, sphenopalatine, and the orbitorotundum foramen.

Extraocular (bilbar) muscles

The extraocular muscles are the three antagonistic pairs of striated muscles that are responsible for the movement of the eyeball within the orbit. These three pairs of muscles are

(1) The lateral and medial rectus muscles (rectus lateralis and rectus medialis)

(2) The dorsal and ventral rectus muscles (rectus dorsalis and rectus ventralis) and

(3) The dorsal and ventral oblique muscles (obliquus dorsalis and obliquus ventralis).

The recti muscles (lateral, medial, dorsal and ventral rectus muscles) originate from a common tendinous ring which is made of the fibrous tissue that surrounds the optic canal opening at the back of the orbit. From their origin, these muscles pass straightway rostrally to attach the sclera of the eyeball. The recti muscles have a straight path and they move the eyeball to their respective side. The lateral and medial rectus muscles move the eyeball horizontally outward and inward. The dorsal and ventral rectus muscles move the eyeball vertically upward and downward.

The dorsal oblique muscle originates from the body of the sphenoid bone, its tendon passes through a trochlea and then attaches to the sclera of the eye just caudal to the lateral rectus muscle. It depresses and abducts the eyeball and rotates it medially.

The ventral oblique muscle originates from the rostral aspect of the orbital floor and is inserted on the sclera of the eye just caudal to the ventral rectus muscle. It elevates and adducts the eyeball and rotates it laterally.

The oblique muscles have an angular path as against the straight path of the recti muscles.

Eyelids

The eyelids are two movable folds of skin situated in front of the eyeball and when closed, they cover the entrance into the orbit and protect the eyeball. The interval between the two, upper and lower, eyelids is called the palpebral fissure. The angles at which the upper and the lower eyelids meet are called the medial and lateral commissures or canthi (singular- canthus). The lateral commissure is rounded whereas the medial commissure is narrow and presents a 'U' shaped recess called the lacrimal recess. A round pigmented body, the caruncula lacrimalis lies in the lacrimal recess. The external surface of the eyelids is convex and is covered with short hairs. The internal surface is concave and is lined by a layer of mucous membrane called the palpebral conjunctiva which continues with the rostral part of the eyeball as the bulbar conjunctiva. The free margin of the eyelids is smooth, black and bears the smooth cilia. The attached margin bears the openings of the ducts of tarsal glands. The rest of the substance of the eyelids is made up of the muscle (orbicularis occuli) and the fascia. The central portion of the eyelids contains the dense connective tissue and the glandular tissue. This structure is called the tarsus. These tarsal glands open at the palpebral margins of the eyelids.

The eyelids are moved by two major groups of muscles, one group closes the lids and the other opens it. The closure of the lids is effected by contraction of the orbicularis occuli muscle. The levator palpebrae superioris muscle causes rising of the upper lid while the contraction of the muscle malaris causes moving the lower lid down, but it occurs rarely.

The third eyelid is formed at the medial commissure. It consists of a fold of conjunctiva called the membrana nictitans (nictitating membrane) which covers and encloses a curved plate of hyaline cartilage. On the deep face of the third eyelid is the harderian gland.

Lacrimal apparatus

The lacrimal apparatus is a group of structures in the orbit that are responsible for production and drainage of tears. It consists of (1) the lacrimal gland which secretes the tears and its excretory ducts which convey the fluid to the surface of the eye and (2) the puncta lacrimalia, lacrimal ducts, lacrimal sac, nasolacrimal duct and the periorbita by way of which the fluid is conveyed into the nasal cavity through the nasolacrimal duct.

The **lacrimal gland** is situated on the dorsolateral surface of the eyeball under the supraorbital process. It is flattened, oval and its orbital surface is convex and lobulated, while the bulbar surface is concave. It is well embedded in the fat. In some animals, the gland may be divided into two parts, one part lies ventral to the supraorbital process and the other part is associated with the superior eyelid. About six to eight large and equal numbers of small excretory ducts leaving the gland open up on the superior bulbar conjunctiva near the superior fornix. In addition, the excretory duct from the superficial gland of the third eyelid opens on the bulbar surface of the nictitating membrane. The secretion from the lacrimal glands, after gaining entrance to the eye, leaves it through the lacrimal duct, the lacrimal sac and the nasolacrimal duct.

The **puncta lacrimalia** are the small entrances at the free margins of the eyelids which converge to form the lacrimal ducts. The **lacrimal ducts** lead from the upper and lower eyelids to the lacrimal sac which is placed in the lacrimal fossa of the lacrimal bone. The lacrimal sac is the mucosa lined origin of the nasolacrimal canal that is surrounded by bone. The **nasolacrimal duct** extends from the orbital surface of the lacrimal bone, traverse through the maxilla and opens into the nasal cavity. The secretion of the lacrimal glands (tears) carried through the nasolacrimal duct is discharged into the nasal cavity. The **periorbita** is a conical fibrous sheath which encloses the eyeball with its muscles, vessels and nerves.

Eyeball

The eyeball (Figure 2-9 B) is situated in the rostral part of the orbit. It is protected in front by the eyelids and the conjunctiva, in the middle by the orbit and caudally by the orbital fascia, fat and muscles. It consists of three tunics that enclose three refractive media.

The tunics of the eyeball: The outermost tunic is the fibrous tunic and it consists of cornea and sclera. The middle tunic is a vascular tunic called the uvea. It is a nutrient layer and consists of the iris, ciliary body and the choroid. The innermost tunic is a nervous tunic. It is a layer of modified nervous tissue and it consists of retina.

Fibrous tunic

The fibrous tunic is composed of the anterior transparent avascular part the cornea and a posterior opaque vascular part the sclera.

Sclera: The sclera is a dense white fibrous membrane forming about four fifth of the fibrous tunic of the eyeball. Exteriorly it is attached to the fascia by a layer of loose, vascular connective tissue called as episclera. The external surface of the sclera along with the episclera provides insertion to the extraocular muscles of the eye. The internal surface is attached to the choroid coat by pigmented connective tissue tunic called the lamina fusca. The rostral border of the sclera is oval and it rostrally continues with the cornea. At this junction, the sclera appears to form a bevel in which the cornea is fixed. The optic nerve pierces the sclera in its caudal part.

Cornea: The cornea is a rostral continuation of the sclera. It forms the rostral one fifth of the fibrous tunic. It is oval, transparent, colourless and avascular. It consists of five layers of tissue. These are named from without inward the corneal epithelium, the external limiting membrane, the substantia propria, the internal limiting membrane and the endothelial membrane. The rostral (outer) surface of the cornea is convex and more so than the sclera. The caudal (inner) surface is concave and forms the rostral boundary of the anterior chamber of the eyeball. The corneoscleral junction is called the limbus. The corneal epithelium passes on to the conjunctiva at this junction. The curvature of the cornea and the rounded shape of the bulb of the eye are maintained by the presence of aqueous humor in the anterior and posterior chambers of the eye. Both these chambers are rostral to the lens and caudal to the cornea. The cornea acts as a window through which the light passes into the eye.

Vascular tunic

The vascular tunic lies internal to the fibrous tunic and comprises the chorioid, ciliary body and iris.

Chorioid: The chorioid is a thin membrane lying between the sclera and retina. It is loosely attached to the sclera by the lamina fusca except where vessels and nerves pass through. The internal surface is in contact with the pigmentary layer of retina. The chorioid is generally dark brown in colour but an extensive area above the layer of the optic papilla has a metallic luster with varying colour from iridiscent blue to green. This area is called the tapetum lucidum. Caudally it is perforated by the optic nerve. It is continuous rostrally with the ciliary body.

The tissue of the choroid is principally made up of blood vessels, with numerous pigment cells. It consists of four layers. The outermost of these is the lamina suprachoroidea which connects the choroid to the sclera. It is a loose, dark membrane composed of elastic fibres pigmented connective tissue. The next layer is the lamina vascularis. It is a vascular layer containing large blood vessels. It is the thickest layer of chorioid. The next inner layer is the lamina chorio capillaries. It is made up of capillaries embedded in a homogenous, pigmented matrics. The innermost layer of the choroid is the lamina basalis, which is thin and transparent. Between the second and third layer lies a network of fibroelastic tissue called the tapetum fibrosum which gives metallic luster to the eye.

Ciliary body: The ciliary body is the middle part of the vascular tunic and it connects the chorioid to the periphery of the iris. In meridional section, it is triangular in outline, with the base next to the iris. The ciliary body has three parts, the ciliary ring, ciliary process and the ciliary muscle. The ciliary process lies on the internal surface of the ciliary body, while the ciliary muscle is on its external surface. The **ciliary ring** is the caudal part of the ciliary body and it is thicker than the choroid. On its internal surface it presents numerous ridges called the **ciliary processes**. These are more than a hundred in number and form a circle of radial folds surrounding the lens and furnish attachment to the suspensory ligament of the lens. The internal surface of the folds is continuous with the lamina basalis of the choroid.

The **ciliary muscle** constitutes the outer surface of the ciliary body and it lies between the sclera and the ciliary processes. It forms a circular band of nonstriated muscle and its fibres are directed meridionally. They arise from the inner face of the sclera and ligamentum pectinatum iridis, runs backward along the sclera and are inserted to the ciliary processes and the ring, When the muscle contracts, it pulls the ciliary processes inwards, thus slackening the suspensory ligament of the lens and allows it to become convex. This is the mechanism of accommodation for near objects.

Iris: The iris is the muscular diaphragm placed in front of the lens and is visible through the cornea. It is pierced centrally by an opening the **pupil** which is elliptical in outline. The ciliary border is continuous with the ciliary body and the ligamentum pectinatum iridis of the cornea. The pupillary border surrounds the pupil. The upper margin bears small corpora nigra or granula iridis which are the masses of pigment cells. The rostral surface is dark brown in colour and is lined by the reflection of the corneal endothelium. It forms the caudal boundary of the anterior chamber. The caudal surface is dark. Its central part is in contact with the lens but peripherally it is separated from it by an annular space. It is lined by endothelium. The two chambers, the anterior and posterior, communicate through the pupil and contain aqueous humor secreted by the endothelium containing mostly water, very little sodium chloride and traces of albumen.

Nervous tunic

The nervous tunic, the innermost of the three basic layers or tunics of the eyeball consists of the **retina**. It extends from the entrance of the optic nerve to the margin of the pupil. It is composed of three parts. The posterior part called **para optica** is the main neural part containing the special neuroepithelium. This part terminates about the ciliary body where it ends in a circular line called the **ora ciliaris retinae**. Hereafter, the retina looses its neural character. This part of the retina which is over the ciliary body is called the **pars ciliaris** and the other one that is over the iris is called the **pars iridica retinae**. The entrance of the optic nerve is at the ventrolateral quadrant of the globe.. The entrance of the optic nerve into the posterior part of the retinal layer of the globe of the eye is an oval or round area which is called as the **optic papilla**. A round area lateral to the optic papilla is called the **macula**. Although, in the histological section of the retina, there appear ten layers, only three of these are said to be important from the functional point of view. It is these three layers that are composed of the neural cells of retina. These cells are called the **rods and cones.** These cells are bipolar and they are ganglion cells. The light stimulus has to pass through the pupil and then has to traverse through all the layers of retina before it can stimulate the rods and cones. The impulse of light, after stimulating the rods and cones are carried by the fibres of the optic nerve to the brain. The area of the retina through which the optic nerve fibres pass out of the globe is called the **area cribrosa sclera.** The fibres of the sclera form a sieve like structure to allow the nerve fibres of the optic nerve to penetrate the wall of the globe.

Chambers of eyeball

There are three chambers inside the globe of the eye. The first one is the **anterior chamber**. It is enclosed in front by the cornea and behind by the iris and the lens. It communicates through the pupil with the second chamber called the posterior chamber. The **posterior chamber** is in the form of a small annular space and it appears triangular in cross section. It is bounded in front by the iris, behind by the peripheral part of the lens and its ligaments, and externally by the ciliary processes. The anterior and posterior chambers are filled in by the aqueous humor. The third chamber is called the **vitreous chamber.** It is situated between the lens and the retina and it contains the vitreous body.

Refractive media of eye

The eye contains various refractive media within it, which effectively bend and refract the incoming light so that it is all focused upon a certain point on the retina. The refractive media of the eye are the cornea, aqueous humor, lens and the vitreous humor.

The **cornea** has already been described above.

The **aqueous humor** fills the anterior and posterior chambers of the eye. It is secreted by the ciliary processes and flown around the margin of the pupil and finally is deposited in the anterior chamber of the eye. This fluid has a different density than that of the sclera hence it can refract the light. It has alkaline reaction and consists of water and sodium chloride. The traces of glucose, urea and some proteins have also been detected in this fluid.

The **lens** (crystalline lens) is a biconvex transparent body that is situated in front of the vitreous body and in partial contact with the posterior face of the iris. The periphery of the lens is almost circular and is surrounded by the ciliary processes. The anterior face is convex and the posterior face is more convex and rests in the fossa of the vitreous body. It is enclosed in a capsule which is attached by the suspensory ligament to the ciliary processes. The central points of the anterior and posterior surfaces of the lens are the anterior and posterior poles and the line connecting these two poles is the axis of the lens. The lens substance consists of concentric laminae of lens fibres which are colourless and transparent. The lens is devoid of the vessels and the nerves.

The **vitreous body** is the semi fluid transparent jelly filled in the vitreous chamber situated behind the lens and between the lens and the retina. Several fine transparent fibres on the surface of the vitreous body are condensed and transformed into a vitreous membrane. This membrane is in contact with the posterior surface of the lens.

Mechanism of vision

The vision begins when light rays are reflected off an object and enter the eye through the cornea. The cornea refracts or bends the rays that pass through the pupil. The iris that surrounds the pupil, opens and closes to regulate the amount of light passing through the pupil. The light rays then pass through aqueous humor, lens and the vitreous humor which bend these light rays and focus them onto the retina. The photosynthetic cells of the retina (rod and cone cells) of the retina convert the light rays into electrical impulses. The optic nerve sends these impulses to the brain where an image is produced.

Organ of hearing and equilibrium (Ear)

The ear is the organ of hearing. It is also a part of the mechanism that controls the balance of the body (equilibrium). The ear consists of three major parts; these are the external ear, middle ear and the internal ear.

External ear

The external ear consists of the auricula or the pinna, a funnel like organ which collects the sound waves and the external acoustic meatus, which conveys these waves to the drum of the ear that separates the external ear from the middle ear.

The **auricula** (pinna) is attached by its base around the external acoustic process in such a manner as to be freely movable.. It has two surfaces, two borders, a base and an apex. The external surface is concave, faces outwards and presents four ridges. It is widest in the middle. The internal surface is convex. The rostral border is convex and its lower part is bent backwards. The caudal border is thin and convex. The apex is flattened and blunt and the base is strongly convex and is attached to the external auditory process. It overlaps the parotid salivary gland.

Structure: The external ear is comprised of a framework of cartilages (mainly three elastic cartilages), the integument and the muscles. The three elastic cartilages include the **auricular (conchal) cartilage** that determines the shape of the external ear. The base of this cartilage is coiled to form a tube which encloses the funnel shaped cavum conchae. The second one is the **annular**

cartilage. It is a quadrilateral plate curved to form three fourth of the ring. It embraces the external acoustic process and forms with the lower part of the conchal cartilage, the cartilaginous part of the external acoustic meatus. The last one is the **scutiform cartilage**. It is a quadrilateral plate situated in front of the base of the concha. Its superficial face is convex and the deep face is concave. Its rostral end is thin and rounded and the caudal end is thicker and wider. It gives attachment to the muscles of the ear. With the aid of these muscles, the auricula can be turned into different positions without turning the head. The **skin** on the convex surface of the auricula is attached to the cartilage by a considerable amount of the subcutaneous tissue except at the apex. The integument lining the concave surface is intimately adherent to the cartilage. About three to four cutaneous ridges run parallel to the borders of the conchal cartilage but do not extend to the apex of the cartilage. There are two sets of **muscles** of the ear. These are the **extrinsic muscles** and the **intrinsic muscles**. The intrinsic muscles are very small and are of little importance. But the extrinsic muscles are mainly responsible for the movement of the external ear. (The details of these muscles will be described under the chapter on regional anatomy of head and neck).

The **external acoustic meatus** leads inward from the bottom of the auricula and conducts vibrations to the tympanic cavity. It is directed downwards, forwards and inwards. It consists of a cartilaginous and osseous part. Its lumen at the inner end is one half of that at the outer end. In the meatus, the skin becomes thinner and it presents numerous ceruminous glands and is covered with fine hairs. In the osseous part there are no hairs and the glands are very few,

The vessels to the external ear are supplied from the rostral auricular artery, a branch of the superficial temporal; the caudal auricular artery a branch of the carotid artery and the occipital artery. The nerve supply is from the caudal auricular and auriculopalpebral branches of the facial nerve and from the first and second cervical nerves.

Middle ear

The middle ear comprises the tympanic cavity and its contents, the auditory (Eustachian) tubes and their diverticula called the guttural pouches.

Tympanic cavity is a space in the tympanic and petrous parts of temporal bone situated between the tympanic membrane and the internal ear. It is an air cavity lined by mucous membrane. It communicates with the pharynx by the auditory (Eustachian) tubes. It contains a chain of bones called the auditory ossicles by which the vibrations from the tympanic membrane are transmitted to the internal ear.

The cavity presents (1) a main part the **atrium** which lies internal to the tympanic membrane, (2) the **epitympanic recess** lying above the level of the tympanic membrane that contains the upper part of the malleus and greater part of the incus and the (3) relatively large **ventral recess** in the tympanic bulla.

The tympanic cavity has six walls. The **roof or tegmental wall** is crossed in its medial part by the facial nerve as the facial canal is deficient below and the nerve is covered by the mucous membrane. The **floor or jugular wall** is concave and thin. It is crossed by delicate curved ridges which radiate from the annular ring of the tympanic bulla. The **rostral or carotid wall** is narrow and is pierced by the slit like tympanic opening of the Eustachian tube. Above this and incompletely separated from it by a thin plate of bone is a semicanal for the tensor tympani muscle. The **caudal or mastoid wall** presents a tympanic antrum and mastoid cells but of no importance. The **lateral or membranous wall** is formed by the tympanic membrane. It is an oval disc which slopes downwards and inwards. It closes the medial end of the external acoustic meatus and thus forms the septum between the external and middle parts of the ear. The circumference of the tympanic membrane is attached in a groove called the sulcus tympanicus in a thin ring of bone called the annulus tympanicus which completely surrounds it. The handle of the malleus is attached to the internal surface of the tympanic membrane. The periphery of the membrane is thickened by fibrous tissue, the annulus fibrosus. The tympanic membrane consists of three layers, the outer thin cutaneous layer, a middle fibrous layer and an internal mucous layer. The **medial or labyrinthine wall** separates it from the internal ear. It presents an opening, the fenestra vestibule which is closed by the foot plate of the stapes. The fenestra cochlea is below it and is closed by a membrane which separates the tympanic membrane from the scala tympani of the internal ear.

The **auditory ossicles** form a chain of bones extending from the lateral to medial wall of the tympanic cavity. These are the malleus, incus, os lenticulare and the stapes. The **malleus** has a head, neck, handle and two processes. The head presents caudomedially a facet for the incus. The handle is attached to the tympanic membrane. The **incus** has a body and two processes. The body articulates with the malleus and the long processes articulate with the os lenticulare. The **os lenticulare** is a small nodule of bone articulating with the incus and the stapes. The **stapes** has a head, two crura and a base. The head meets the lenticulare and the base is attached to the fenestra vestibulii. The muscles of the middle ear are the tensor tympani and the stapedius. The blood supply is through stylo-mastoid artery and the nerve supply is through the tympanic plexus.

The **Eustachian tube (auditory tube)** extends from the tympanic cavity to the pharynx. Its upper end is at the internal aspect of root of the styloid process of petrous temporal bone and it communicates with the rostral part of the tympanic cavity by a small slit like tympanic opening. The tube, in its initial part is complete and its lumen is a capillary space. Further downward it is a groove and is completed below by a mucous membrane.

The **guttural pouches** are large mucous sacs each of which is a ventral diverticulum of the auditory tube. They are not present in domestic animals except the horse.

Internal ear

The internal ear houses the vestibulocochlear organ that maintains balance and receives sound from the middle ear. It has two parts, the osseous (bony) labyrinth, a series of cavities within the petrous part of the temporal bone and the membranous labyrinth, a series of communicating membranous sacs and ducts contained within the osseous labyrinth. The osseous labyrinth and the membranous labyrinth are separated by perilymph.

Osseous labirinth

The **osseous labyrinth** is excavated in the petrous part of the temporal bone, internal to the tympanic cavity. It consists of three parts, the cochlea, the vestibule and the semicircular canals. The **vestibule** is the central part of the osseous labyrinth. It communicates with the cochlea in front and semicircular canals behind. The lateral wall separates it from the tympanic cavity and inside it lies the fenestra vestibulii. Its medial wall corresponds to the external acoustic meatus. The caudal wall presents four openings of the three semicircular canals.

The **semicircular canals** are three in number and are behind and above the vestibule. They are at right angles to each other and are designated as dorsal (superior), caudal (posterior) and lateral. They communicate with the vestibule by four openings. Each canal is about three fourths of a circle, one end of which is slightly enlarged to form the ampulla

The **cochlea** is the rostral part of the bony labyrinth. It is in the form of a blunt cone, the base of which corresponds to the internal acoustic meatus and the apex or cupola is directed outward, forward and downward. It consists of a spiral canal which forms two and a half turns around a bony process called the modiolus. A thin plate of bone called the lamina spiralis projects from the modiolus and extends about half way into the canal. It divides the canal into two passages, an upper scala vestibule and the lower scala tympani. A membrane, the membrana basilaris extends from the free margin of the lamina to the lateral wall of the cochlea and thus completes the septum between the two scalae. The modiolus is traversed by a spiral canal along the attached border of the lamina spiralis and contains the spiral ganglion and vein.

Membranous labyrinth

The membranous labyrinth lies within the osseous labyrinth but does not fill it completely. It is attached to the osseous labyrinth by delicate fibrous strands which traverse the perilymphatic space. It consists of four parts.

The **utricle** is the larger of the two sacs and lies in the dorsocaudal part of the vestibule. It receives the openings of the semicircular ducts and the ductus utriculo sacularis which opens at its lower part into the ductus endolymphaticus.

The **saccule**s is the lower division and its lower part, the ductus reuniens, proceeds into the ductus cochlearis. A ductus endolymphaticus from the saccule is joined by the ductus utriculo sacularis. This duct traverses the aqueductus vestibulii and terminates under the dura on the caudal part of the internal face of the petrous temporal bone in a dilated end the saccus endolymphaticus.

The **semicircular ducts** correspond to the semicircular canals. The ampullae fill the osseous part but the rest of its extent occupies only about one sixth of the lumen.

The **cochlear duct** is a spiral tube situated in the cochlea. It begins in a blind end and ends in a second blind end attached to the cupola. The duct is triangular in cross section and has three walls. The vestibular wall or roof is formed by the membrane of Reissner which extends from the lamina spiralis to the outer wall of cochlea and separates the cochlear duct from the scala vestibule. The tympanic wall intervenes between the cochlear and scala tympani and is formed by the lamina spiralis and membrana basilaris. The outer wall consists of the fibrous lining of the cochlea.

Mechanism of hearing

The sound waves are collected by the auricula or pinna of the external ear and then are conveyed through the external acoustic meatus to the tympanic membrane of the middle ear. The tympanic membrane gets vibrated because of these sound waves. These vibrations are then passed on to a chain of bones called the auditory ossicles by which the vibrations from the tympanic membrane are transmitted to the internal ear. With the vibration of the stapes, the fluid between the osseous and membranous labyrinth particularly the cochlea of the internal ear is moved. It generates an impulse in the cells of the cochlea. From cochlea these impulses are carried by the nerve fibres of the vestibulo-cochlear nerve to the brain where the sound waves are differentiated and analyzed.

Organ of smell (Olfaction)

The organ of smell (olfactory apparatus) has two parts, the peripheral and the central. The **peripheral part** consists of the olfactory nasal mucous membrane on the turbinate bones, the adjacent part of the dorsal turbinate and the septum nasi. The epithelium of the olfactory mucous membrane is comprised of three types of cell. The basal cells rest on the basement membrane. They are short and triangular. The supporting cells are elongated, columnar tapering below and branched. The olfactory cells are bipolar cells situated between the supporting cells and have the form of long narrow rods with an enlarged lower part having a nucleus. The peripheral end of these olfactory cells pierces the limiting membrane and bears a tuft of fine cilia called the olfactory hairlets. The central process of these cells is the axon which is varicose and extends to the lamina propria where several fibres are gathered to form the olfactory nerve. The olfactory filaments pass through the cribriform plate of the ethmoid bone and enter the convex face of the olfactory bulb to form the olfactory glomeruli with the mitral cells.

The **central part** of the olfactory apparatus consists of the rhinencephalon, of the brain. It contains the two olfactory bulbs at the rostral extremity of the olfactory peduncle. The olfactory peduncles continue the olfactory bulbs and splits into three distinct tracts called the medial, lateral and the middle olfactory tracts. All the three tracts, after undertaking a short route disappear in the olfactory trigone. Just caudal to the olfactory trigone is the grey olfactory area.

Mechanism of smell

The odorant molecules mix with the air that is breathed in (inhaled). These molecules adhere to the cilia (hairlets) of the olfactory cells of the olfactory mucous membrane. This triggers the olfactory receptor neurons which in turn send signals to the olfactory bulb and from there to the grey olfactory area of the brain. It analyzes the pattern of impulse and identifies the substance whose molecules have struck to the cilia of olfactory cells.

Organ of test (Gustatory apparatus)

The organ of taste like that of olfaction also has two parts, the peripheral and the central.

The **peripheral part** of the gustatory apparatus is in the test buds which are situated in the foliate, fungiform and vallate papillae on the mucous membrane of the tongue, oral face of epiglottis and the soft palate. The taste buds are oval flask shaped masses which occupy the recesses in the epithelium. Each bud presents a small opening towards the surface, the gustatory pore. The taste bud consists of fusiform supporting cells grouped around central gustatory cells. The peripheral end of each gustatory cell bears a filament, the gustatory hair which projects through the gustatory pore. The central end of the gustatory cell does not end in axon, as in the case of olfactory cell, but remains within the taste bud where it has intimate contact with many fine terminations of nerves that pass into the taste bud through an opening in the basement membrane. The gustatory nerve though myelinated, looses its myelin sheath as its fibres enter the bud.

The central part of the gustatory organ is constituted by the gustatory nucleus which is a component of the solitary nucleus. The solitary nucleus is a series of nuclei forming a vertical column of grey matter embedded in the medulla oblongata. Taste information from facial nerve (rostral two third of the tongue), glossopharyngeal (caudal one third of the tongue) and the vagus nerve (a small area on the epiglottis).

Common integument (skin)

(Organ of Touch, Pressure and pain)

The common integument (skin) is the protective covering of the body and is continuous at the natural orifices with the mucous membrane of the digestive, respiratory and urogenital tracts. It acts as a special sense organ of touch through the tactile corpuscles. It regulates the temperature of the body and acts as an excretory organ. The thickness of the skin varies at different locations on the body and in different animal species. The skin is attached to the adjacent tissues by subcutaneous tissue. The skin consists of two layers, the epidermis and the dermis. The epidermis is an avascular squamous stratified epithelium mouled over the papillae of the dermis. The dermis consists of white elastic fibres with vessels, nerves and fat. It contains a few sweat glands, the sebaceous glands and the hair follicles.

Appendages of the skin: The appendages of the skin are modifications of the epidermis and comprise the hairs, hoofs, claws, horns and so forth.

Hairs: The hairs are extremely variable in colour and size in different breeds and individuals. They cover the entire surface of the body and are of two types, the ordinary hairs and the special hairs. The ordinary hairs determine the colour coat of the animal. The special hairs include the long hairs which are tactile hairs about the nostrils, lips, eyelashes, tragi of external ear and vibrissae of nostrils. The long hairs of the tail are brush type special hairs.

The part of the hair above the surface of the skin is the shaft while the part underneath the surface coat is the root which is embedded in a depression called the hair follicle. Most of the follicles have attached to them small smooth muscles called the arrectores pilorum. The contraction of these muscles causes erection of hair. The other appendages like the hoofs, claws, horns and other horny structures will be described under the regional anatomy sections.

30

Endocrine Glands in Head and Neck

Pituitary gland (Hypophysis cerebi)

The pituitary gland (hypophysis cerebri) lies at the base of the skull and is housed within a bony structure called the sella turcica in the body of the besisphenoid bone. It is a small pea shaped gland which is attached to the hypothalamus by the pituitary stalk. The pituitary gland has two distinct parts called the lobes. These are the anterior lobe (adenohypophysis) and the posterior lobe (neurohypophysis). The anterior lobe which is also called as anterior pituitary consists of five types of cells, each of which secretes different hormone or hormones. The types of cells, the hormones secreted by each type and the functions performed by them are narrated below.

1. The thyrotrophs secrete thyroxin called as Thyroid Stimulating Hormone (TSH). It stimulates production of thyroid hormone.
2. The gonadotrophs secrete leuteinizing hormone (LH) and Follicle Stimulating Hormone (FSH). The LH stimulates the production of oestrogen and progesterone by the ovaries in female and testosterone by the testes in male. The FSH stimulates the production of oestrogen and the growth of egg cells (oocytes) in the ovaries in female and sperm cells (spermatozoa) in the testes in male.
3. The corticotrophs secrete the Adreno-Cortico-Trophic Hormone (ACTH) which stimulates the production of cortisol and adrenogenic hormones by the adrenal cortex.
4. The somatotrophs secret Growth Hormone (GH). The GH is a growth promoting hormone which regulates the growth and differentiation of the skeletal system.
5. The lactotrophs secrete the Prolactine Hormone. The prolactine hormone is responsible for initiation of milk secretion by the acinar cells of the mammary gland.

The posterior lobe of pituitary which is also called as posterior pituitary is composed of the endings of the nerve cells located in specialized regions of the hypothalamus. These nerve cells produce two hormones the oxytocin and vasopressin. These hormones are carried down the nerves and are stored in the nerve ending that comprise the posterior pituitary. These hormones are released into the circulation in response to the nerve signals that originate in the hypothalamus and are transmitted to the posterior pituitary. The oxytocin causes contraction of uterus for parturition and milk secretion in females. The vasopressin increases reabsorption of water from the kidneys and raises blood pressure.

Thus the hormones secreted and released by the pituitary gland play an active part in controlling the activities of most of the other endocrine glands of the body. Hence, the pituitary gland is called as master gland of the endocrine system. However, some times the hormone secretion of the pituitary gland itself is controlled by the hypothalamus which lies just above the pituitary gland.

Pineal gland (Epiphysis cerebri)

The pineal gland (epiphysis cerebri) is a small organ shaped like a pine cone (hence the name pineal). It is a rice grain sized gland located on the midline attached by a short hollow stalk to the caudal end of the roof of the third ventricle between the two hemispheres tucked in a groove where the two halves of the thalamus join near the corpora quadrigemina. It is reddish grey in colour. The pineal gland is composed of the cells called pinealocytes and the glial cells. The pinealocytes secrete the hormone melatonin which affects the modulation of sleep pattern. The production of melatonin by the pineal gland is stimulated by darkness and inhibited by light. The pineal gland influences the pituitary gland secretion of sex hormones FSH and LH.

Thyroid gland

The thyroid gland is a pale or dark red butterfly shaped gland located on the cranial part of the trachea especially the first two tracheal rings or the laryngotracheal joint. It consists of two lateral flattened triangular lobes which are connected by a thin transverse strip of glandular tissue called isthmus across the ventral surface of the trachea. The deep surface of the gland is concave and is related to the trachea. The superficial surface is convex and the isthmus is flat. The lateral surface is related to the cervicohyoid muscle. The dorsal border lies on the oesophagus. The cranial border is almost straight and is related to the cricopharyngeal and cricothyroid muscles and the thyrolaryngeal artery. The caudoventral border is concave and lies on the trachea. The lobes as well as the isthmus consist of numerous globular sacs called follicles and is covered by a loose connective tissue capsule. A large number of trabeculae extend from the capsule and they pass in between the lobules of the gland. Each follicle is bounded by a single layer of epithelial cells (follicular cells) and a basement membrane surrounding a central lumen filled with a homogenous protein rich colloid (thyroglobulin). The colloid is a store of the thyroid hormones prior to secretion. When thyroid hormones are needed, the thyroglobulin is reabsorbed into the follicular cells from the colloid of the follicular lumen. In the cells, the thyroglobulin splits into its component parts including the two thyroid hormones, Thyroxin (T4) and Triiodothyronin (T3) which are released in to the circulation. Within the connective tissue, close to the follicles are 'C' shaped cells which are also called as parafollicular cells. They are found in clusters in the interfollicular space. These cells secrete the hormone calcitonin which acts to lower the plasma calcium level.

Parathyroid gland

The parathyroids are four small glands arranged in two pairs as cranial (external) and caudal (internal) closely associated with the left and right lateral lobes of the thyroid gland. The glands of the cranial pair are usually located cranial to the lobes of the thyroid gland. Each of these glands is yellowish brown flat ovoid or elongated in shape and appears like a lentil seed. Many times these are embedded in the surrounding connective tissue of the adjacent glands. The glands of the caudal pair are smaller than those of the cranial pair. These are located in the connective tissue close to the caudal edge of the lobes of the thyroid gland. These glands are often embedded in the tissue of the dorsal or tracheal surface of the isthmus of the thyroid gland; The parathyroid glands are quite easily recognizable from the thyroid gland as they have densely packed cells in contrast with the follicular structure of the thyroid. Two unique types of cells are present in the parathyroid glands. These are the chief cells and the oxyphil cells. The chief cells are small. They synthesize, secrete and release parathyroid hormone. These cells appear dark when loaded with parathyroid hormone and clear when the hormone has been secreted or when the cells are in their resting stage. The oxyphil cells which are lighter in appearance and increase in number with age have an unknown function. The main function of the parathyroid glands is to maintain the body's calcium and phosphate levels within a normal range so that the muscular and nervous systems can function properly. The parathyroid glands do this by secreting parathyroid hormone. The parathyroid hormone (parathormone) is a small protein that takes part in the control of calcium and phosphate homeostasis as well as bone physiology. Parathormone has the effects antagonistic to those of calcitonin.

Thymus gland

The thymus is a ductless gland and major lymphoid organ developed mostly in the later half of the foetal life (prebirth period) and it is extensively formed during the early life of the animal. It appears fully grown in the young animals but it undergoes gradual atrophy as the animal reaches to the adult stage. In the adult animal, hardly a small thoracic portion of this gland may be visible at the thoracic inlet or in the cranial part of the thorax. In the newborn animal, the thymus gland lies in the ventral part of the neck. In young animals, the gland extends more caudally reaching almost to the cranial part of the thorax. It is pale yellow in colour and is distinctly lobulated. The thymus gland consists of a thoracic and the paired cervical lobes. The thoracic lobe lies on the left side and it extends to the heart and apical lobe of the lung. The cervical lobes of the gland lie on the ventrolateral surface of the trachea in the caudal part of the neck and on its dorsolateral surface in the cranial half of the neck. In young animals the lobes extend to the larynx. On its deep surface, the gland is related to the trachea, common carotid artery and the vagosympathetic trunk. Superficially it is covered by the sternothyrohyoid and sternocephalic muscles. The dorsal border of the left lobe is related to the oesophagus. In the phase of atrophy of this gland, the thoracic lobe is the first to disappear. The atrophy of the cervical lobes is slow. The reduction in the size of the cervical lobes begins in the cranial part of the neck.

The gland is covered by an extensive loose connective tissue capsule that sends numerous trabeculae that pass between the lobules inside the gland. The parenchyma of the gland consists of a well developed cortex and medulla. The cortex contains large number of small lymphocyte like cells called the thymocytes. The medulla contains numerous primitive reticular cells. A few scattered primitive reticular cells of endocrine origin also appear in the cortex of the thymus.

31

Comparative Anatomy of the Organs and Glands in Head and Neck

Mouth

Horse

The mouth cavity (cavum oris) of horse is longer and narrower. The vestibule of the mouth cavity is less capacious than that of ox.

Dog

The form and size of the mouth cavity vary greatly in different breeds of dog. In some breeds the mouth is long and narrow while in others it is short and wide. Rima oris in general in all types of dogs is extensive.

Sheep and Goat

The mouth cavity is elongated and narrow. The rima oris is short. The buccal vestibule is capacious but the labial vestibule is small.

Pig

The porcine oral cavity is relatively long but variable. The variation in the length of the mouth cavity depends on the breed of the animal. The rima oris is extensive because the labial commissures are situated far caudad.

Fowl

In birds (domestic fowl), the mouth cavity (oral cavity) and pharynx form a common cavity, the oropharynx and there is no clear demarcation between the oral and the pharyngeal cavity. The caudal limit of the oral cavity lies at the level of the most caudal transverse row of papillae on the hard palate and the papillae on the base of the tongue.

Lips

Horse

The lips of the horse are thinner, narrower and more mobile than that of ox. The external surface of the upper lip does not possess the muzzle. Instead, there is a shallow median furrow that is called as philtrum. The labial commissures are placed at the level of first cheek tooth. The labial glands form compact masses near the commissures.

Dog

The lips of dog are thin and mobile and present numerous tactile hairs. The upper lip has a small central bare area which forms part of the muzzle and is marked by the central groove the philtrum. The lateral borders of the lower lip are flaccid and denticulated. The labial glands are small and scanty.

Sheep and Goat

The lips of the sheep and goat are thin and mobile. The upper one is marked by a distinct philtrum and is otherwise covered with hair. The planum nasale is restricted to the area between the nostrils.

Pig

The upper lip is thick and short and is blended with the snout. The loser lip is small and pointed. Both lips are hairy and bear sinus hairs at their margins.The part of the upper lip rostral to the incisor teeth is void of hair. The lips are not much motile. The labial glands are few and small.

Fowl

In birds, the Lips are absent but are functionally replaced by the hard keratinized epidermal beak which covers the rostral parts of the upper and lower jaws. The upper horny beak is short, narrow and pointed. It covers the fused premaxillary bones and extends caudolaterally on the maxillary bones. Caudally on either side it forms the ventrally directed operculum which partially closes the external nares. The dorsal part of the beak in midline is the culmen and the sharp ventral edge is the is the tomium. In the dermis of the upper beak are specialized sensory nerve endings. The lower horny beak covers the dentary bones of the mandible but the specialized sensory nerve endings are absent in the dermis of the lower beak. The keratin of the upper and lower beak is harder than that of the skin in the feathered parts of the body. The beak is, however, lost by wear and is continuously replaced.

Cheeks

Horse

The cheeks in horse are less capacious and flaccid. The buccal glands are arranged in two layers. The dorsal row of buccal glands lies on the outer face of the buccinator muscle near its upper border. The ventral row of the buccal glands is situated in the submucous tissue at the lower border of the buccinator muscle. The papilla salivalis is situated opposite the upper third cheek tooth.

Dog

The cheeks in the dog are loose and capacious. The mucous membrane is smooth and pigmented. The parotid duct opens into the cheek at the level of the second cheek tooth. About four or five ducts of the zygomatic glands open on the cheek at the level of the last cheek tooth. The zygomatic gland is the homologue of the dorsal buccal glands of the other domestic animals. The ventral buccal glands are situated in series with the ventral labial glands opposite the cheek teeth.

Sheep and Goat

The orifice of the parotid salivary gland that opens on the papilla salivalis in the cheek is placed at the level of the third or fourth cheek tooth. The rest of the characters of cheeks in sheep and goat are similar to those of ox.

Pig

The mucous membrane of the cheeks in pig is smooth. The buccal glands are compactly arranged in two rows opposite the cheek teeth. They extend from the angle of the lips to the masseter muscle which covers them in part. The parotid duct opens at the level of the fourth or fifth cheek tooth.

Fowl

The lateral walls of the oral cavity, the cheeks are much reduced. The paired triangular salivary glands are situated in the submucosa caudal to the junction between the upper and lower beaks. The duct of each gland opens close to the junction of the mucous membrane with the skin.

Hard palate

Horse

The hard palate of horse is longer and narrower than that of ox. The transverse ridges are eighteen in number and these cover the entire oral surface of the hard palate as against the rostral two third part appearing in ox. The ridges are curved and the concavity is directed backward. The dental pad is replaced by six alveoli for the upper incisor teeth. The fissures on the sides of the papilla incisivus do not contain the openings of the ductus incisivus as they are blind.

Dog

The hard palate in dog is widest between the fourth pair of the cheek teeth. It possesses eight to ten transverse curved ridges on each side of the median raphe. Caudal to the first pair of incisor teeth is the rounded or triangular incisive papilla which presents the opening of the incisivus ducts. The mucous membrane is usually pigmented.

Sheep and Goat

The hard palate in sheep and goat is narrow. Rostral to the palate is the dental pad. The transverse ridges on the oral surface of the hard palate are irregular, the right and left ridges alternate each other at the median raphe. The free edges of the ridges are smooth.

Pig

The hard palate of pig is long and narrow and the transverse ridges are twenty in number. Rostrally it bears the alveoli for upper incisor and canine teeth. Just behind the incisor teeth is a long prominence for incisive papilla. Rostral to the first pair of incisor, there is a round prominence.

Fowl

The hard palate in birds is incomplete and forms the roof of the oral cavity. In between the palatines and the vomer, caudal to the palatine processes lie the internal nares. On each side of the midline there is a space which is surrounded by the bones of the palate. The caudal part of this space is filled by the striated dorsal and ventral pterygoid muscles. The mucous membrane of the palate has a nonkeratinized stratified squamous epithelium. It is continuous with the epithelium of the nasal cavity at the nasal edge of the choanal slit. The choanal slit extends longitudinally in the midline in the caudal half of the palate. The rostral part of the choanal slit is narrow while its caudal part is wide. The narrow part of the slit is close to the dorsal surface of the tongue. The mucous membrane of the palate has several ridges and papillae. The ridges extend longitudinally on the palate. On the rostral third of the palate is a short medial ridge from which a long lateral ridge on each side of the midline extends caudally to the level of the junction of the rostral narrow and caudal wide parts of the choanal slit. When the mouth is closed, the lateral ridges of the palate are close to the lateral edges of the tongue. The papillae of the palate are arranged in short transverse rows close to the midline and medial to the lateral ridges. The submucosa of the palate contains the paired maxillary and palatine salivary glands and their ducts open in the angle at the junction of the medial and lateral ridges.

Soft palate

Horse

The soft palate of horse is long and more developed in horse than that in ox. It closes isthmus fausium along with the epiglottis and hence, oral breathing is not possible and in vomiting the vomit is expelled through the nose in horse. Instead of a compact tonsil, there is a loose mass of lymphoid tissue. The caudal pillars of the opposite sides unite over the beginning of the oesophagus.

Dog

The soft palate in dog is long and it is thick except at the margins. Normally it is in contact with the epiglottis. The tonsil is relatively larger, elongated and fusiform. It is completely concealed between the two folds of mucous membrane. The tonsillar sinus is also relatively larger. The caudal pillars of the soft palate are double. The upper fold passes to the dorsal wall of the pharynx and subsides there while the lower fold goes to the side of the epiglottis.

Sheep and Goat

The soft palate in sheep and goat is almost similar to that in ox.

Pig

The soft palate in pig is very thick. It is nearly horizontal in position and as a result of this it continues behind from the caudal border of the hard palate and extends to the middle of the oral surface of the epiglottis. More commonly it has a small median prolongation called as uvula. The oral surface presents a median furrow. On either side of this furrow is an oval raised area with numerous crypts containing the tonsillar tissue. Similar type of tonsillar tissue also occurs at the lateral wall of the isthmus faucium and the root of the tongue.

Fowl

The soft palate is absent in fowl.

Floor of mouth

Horse

The caruncula sublingualis is located opposite the canine tooth on each side. It presents the opening of the duct of the mandibular salivary gland only. The ducts of the sublingual glands do not open on this papilla. On either side extending from frenum linguae to the level of the fourth cheek tooth is a sublingual fold. This fold covers the sublingual gland. Several small short ducts from this gland open on the small papillae on the surface of the sublingual fold. The linear series of papillae on the floor is absent.

Dog

The caruncula sublingualis is placed in front of the frenum linguae opposite the lower first cheek tooth. The mandibular duct unites with the duct from the caudal division of sublingual salivary gland and opens over the sublingual caruncula. Some times the two open separately on this papilla.

Sheep and Goat

The anatomy of the structures of the floor of mouth is similar to that of the ox.

Pig

The caruncula sublingualis is absent. The mandibular duct opens directly on the floor of the mouth by the side of the frenum linguae.

Fowl

The mucous membrane of the floor of mouth cavity in birds has a stratified squamous epithelium. Most part of the floor is covered by the free part of the tongue. The frenum linguae extend rostrally to the ventral surface of the tongue but do not reach its apex. In the submucosa of the floor are large paired rostral submandibular salivary glands. These glands lie parallel to the rami of the mandible and their proximal parts lie close to the midline at the level of the apex of the tongue. The caudal parts of these glands are caudal to the level of the dorsal papillae of the tongue. The ducts of these glands open on the floor ventral to the tongue.

Tongue

Horse

The body and the root of the tongue in horse is narrow. The tip of the tongue is spatula shaped. The prominence on the caudal part of the dorsum of the tongue is absent. The vallate papillae are only two or three in number. These are arranged as one on each side of the median line and the third one when present lies behind the first two on any one of the two sides. In addition to the papillae appearing in ox, there is other type of papillae called the foliate papillae in horse. These are present as rounded eminence on the dorsolateral aspect of the tongue just in front of the palatoglossal arch on each side. These papillae contain test buds. The tongue of horse is not so protractile as in the ox and is not prehensile. The glossal muscles are less developed.

Dog

The tongue of dog is wide and thin rostrally and thick caudally. It is bright red in colour. The dorsum of the tongue presents median sulcus linguae. The filiform papillae appear on the entire dorsum. The fungiform papillae are present on the dorsum and on the sides of the tongue but are absent on the root of the tongue. The vallate papillae and the foliate papillae are similar to those in horse.

Sheep and Goat

The torus linguae though present is not prominent in sheep and goat. The filiform papillae are soft and the tongue is comparatively smooth. The fungiform papillae are more numerous in sheep and goat than those in ox. The vallate papillae are eight to seventeen in number in goat similar to those of ox. In the sheep the number is eighteen to twenty four.

Pig

The tongue in pig is long and narrow and its apex is thin. The vallate papillae are two or three in number. The fungiform papillae are small and they most numerous laterally. On the root of the tongue there are soft long and pointed papillae and these are directed caudally. The foliate papillae are also present in the pig. A prominent glossoepiglottic fold of mucous membrane is present and on either side of this fold is a depression. The frenum linguae is double. The caruncula sublingualis is very small and it is situated lateral to the frenum linguae.

Fowl

The tongue of the fowl is narrow and triangular and its apex is pointed in front. The muscular tissue is very little in the tongue of fowl. The root of the tongue is crossed by a row of pointed horny papillae whose apices are directed backwards.

Teeth

Dental formula of different species of domestic animals

Ox $2\left(I\frac{0}{4}\ C\frac{0}{0}\ P\frac{3}{3}\ M\frac{3}{3}\right) = 32$

Goat / Sheep $2\left(I\frac{0}{4}\ C\frac{0}{0}\ P\frac{3}{3}\ M\frac{3}{3}\right) = 32$

Horse $2\left(I\frac{3}{3}\ C\frac{1}{1}\ P\frac{3}{3}\ M\frac{3}{3}\right) = 40$ (42 when 4 premolars are present)

Dog $2\left(I\frac{3}{3}\ C\frac{1}{1}\ P\frac{4}{4}\ M\frac{2}{3}\right) = 42$

Cat $2\left(I\frac{3}{3}\ C\frac{1}{1}\ P\frac{3}{2}\ M\frac{1}{1}\right) = 30$

Pig $2\left(I\frac{3}{3}\ C\frac{1}{1}\ P\frac{4}{4}\ M\frac{3}{3}\right) = 44$

Horse

The incisors are present in both, upper and lower jaws. These are three on each side making 6 incisors in each jaw and 12 in the two jaws. The table surface of incisors present a deep rounded invagination the infundibulum which is filled in with cement. It helps in determining the age of the animal. The roots are firmly fixed in the alveoli and therefore do not allow any mobility unlike that in ox. The canines are four in number, one on each side of the jaws in males only. In mare these are absent or rudimentary. The cheek teeth of the upper jaw present double infundibula on the table surface. The first and last upper cheek teeth have three roots each while the remaining ones may have three or four roots each.

Eruption time of teeth in horse

Class of teeth	Position (number)	Age of animal	
		Deciduous	Permanent
Incisor	1st	1 to 4 weeks	2 and half years
	2nd	1 month	2 years
	3rd	6 to 9 months	3 years
Canine			4 to 5 years
Premolars	1st }	1-2 weeks	2 and half years
	2nd }		3 years
	3rd }		4 years
Molars	1st		1 year
	2nd		2 years
	3rd		3 and half to 4 years

Dog

The upper incisors are more developed and larger and stronger than the lower incisors. The crowns of the incisors are completely covered with brilliant white enamel. The size of the incisors goes on increasing from the central to corner one. The roots of the incisors are firmly fixed into the sockets of the alveoli. The canines are elongated, conical and curved outwards and backwards. The upper canines are larger and separated from the corner incisors by a space into which the lower incisors are received when the mouth is closed. Of the cheek teeth, the fourth premolar of the upper jaw and the first molar of the lower jaw are the largest and the rest of the cheek teeth goes on reducing the size both before and behind. The crowns of the upper molars are wide and quadrilateral and their table surfaces are tuberculate.

Eruption time of teeth in dog

Class of teeth	Position (number)	Age of animal	
		Deciduous	Permanent
Incisor	1st	1 month	4 to 5 years
	2nd	1 to 1 and half month	4 to 5 years
	3rd	1 to 1 and half month	4 to 5 years
Canine		2 to 4 weeks	5 to 6 years
Premolars	1st }	1 month	4 to 6 years
	2nd }	(lower jaw)	
	3rd }		
	4th]		
Molars	1st		4 years
	2nd		5 to 6 years
	3rd		6 years

Pig

The incisors are so placed that the medial incisor lies rostral to the intermediate incisor and much rostral to the lateral incisor. The vestibular surface of the crown is convex and is extensively covered by enamel. The lingual surface is slightly concave and the enamel covers only the margins of this surface. The rest of the part of this surface is covered by cementum. The upper incisors are separated from each other by spaces and there is a large interval between the third (lateral) incisor and the canine tooth. The crown itself continues as root and there is no distinct neck. The loser incisors lie in a horizontal plane and are close together. The roots of the incisors are long, round in cross section and are deeply implanted in the alveoli of the jaws. The canine teeth are well developed and project outward from the mouth especially in male animals. The crown of the upper canine is conical and it curves laterally dorsally and slightly caudally. The lower canines teeth are long, pointed and three sided. They are curved laterally and caudally. Cheek teeth: The cheek teeth (premolars and molars) increase in size from rostral to caudal on each side of the jaw. The occlusal surface of the premolars is sharp and cutting type while those of the molars are like crushing mounds. In the upper jaw, the first and second premolars have two roots, the third has three and the fourth has five roots. The molars of the upper jaw have six roots each. In the lower jaw, the first premolar has one root, the second and third has two roots and the fourth has three roots. The first and second molars have four roots and the third molar has five roots.

Eruption time of teeth in pig

Class of teeth	position (number)	Age of animal	
		Deciduous	Permanent
Incisor	1st	2 to 4 weeks	1 year
	2nd	2 to 3 months	4 to 5 years
	3rd	At the time of birth	8 to 10 months
Canines		At the time of birth	9 to 10 months
Premolars	1st }	1 to 4 weeks	1 to 1 and half months
	2nd }		
	3rd }		
	4th]		
Molars	1st		4 to 6 months
	2nd		8 to 12 months
	3rd		18 to 12 months

Salivary glands

Horse

The **parotid salivary gland** in horse is the largest of all the three salivary glands. It is yellowish grey in colour. Its medial surface is related additionally to the guttural pouch. The apex lies dorsally encircling the base of the ear. The base of the gland is on the ventral side and it is related to the external maxillary vein. The duct of the gland (Stenson's' duct) opens on the papilla salivalis at the level of upper third cheek tooth.

The **mandibular (submaxillary) salivary gland** is smaller than the parotid gland. The duct of the gland (Wharton's duct) passes between the hyoglossus and mylohyoideus muscles and gains the internal surface of the sublingual salivary gland before its opening at the caruncula sublingualis.

The **sublingual salivary gland** extends from the mandibular symphysis to the fourth or fifth lower cheek tooth. The ducts are numerous and open on the small papillae on the sublingual fold. The single duct extending from the ventral part of the gland as appears in ox does not exist in horse.

Dog

The **parotid salivary gland** in dog is very small and irregularly triangular with its base upwards. The apex overlaps the mandibular gland.

The **mandibular salivary gland** is larger than parotid. It is rounded in outline. The duct of the mandibular gland leaves the gland from its deep surface, crosses the Styloglossus muscle and opens on the floor of the mouth at a distinct papilla.

The **sublingual salivary gland** has two parts, the rostral and caudal. The rostral part is long and narrow and has numerous ducts which open directly into the mouth and some of these join the large duct.

The **zygomatic salivary** gland is an additional salivary gland in dog. It is situated at the rostral part of the pterygopalatine fossa. This gland is related dorsally to the zygomatic arch. It has four or five ducts that open in the mouth near the last upper cheek tooth.

Sheep and Goat

The **parotid salivary gland** in sheep and goat is rectangular in outline. Its dorsal angle embraces the ear and the cervical angle lies at the bifurcation of the jugular vein. The duct of the gland usually runs across the masseter muscle and opens at the popilla salivalis at the level of the fourth or fifth cheek tooth.

The **mandibular salivary gland** is roughly triangular in outline. The mandibular duct passes medial to the digastricus and hyoglossus muscles and along the monostomatic and polystomatic sublingual glands and open at the caruncula sublingualis.

The **sublingual salivary gland** in sheep and goat is similar to that in ox.

Pig

The **parotid salivary gland** is large and distinctly triangular in form. It extends very little onto the masseter muscle. Its dorsal angle does not reach to the base of the ear. The parotid duct open on the papilla salivalis at the level of fourth or fifth cheek tooth.

The **mandibular salivary gland** is small and oval in outline. It is completely covered by parotid. From its deep face a narrow process extends rostrad beneath the mylohyoid muscle along with the duct.

The **sublingual salivary gland** has an arrangement similar to that of ox.

Fowl

The salivary glands in birds are much developed and extensive. They form a continuous layer in the walls of the mouth and pharynx. The **maxillary, palatine, rostral lingual** and **rostral submandibular** glands and the glands at the angle of the mouth open into the oral cavity. The **sphenopterygoid, caudal lingual, caudal submandibular** and **laryngeal glands** open into the pharyngeal cavity. Majority of these glands are polystomatic. However, the maxillary glands and the glands at the angles of the mouth are monostomatic.

Pharynx

Horse

The pharynx in horse is large and narrow. The Eustachian orifice is larger. The caudal nares are larger. The aditus oesophagius is smaller.

Dog

The Eustachian orifices are smaller and slit like. The aditus oesophagius is small.

Sheep and Goat

It is similar to that in ox.

Pig

The pharynx in pig is long and narrow. It extends to the level of the second cervical vertebra. The nasopharynx and oropharynx are connected by the narrow interpharyngeal opening.

Fowl

The roof of the pharynx is divided by a short median longitudinal opening, the infundibular slit which is a common opening of the right and left auditory tubes. It leads dorsally to the infundibular cavity. The common duct of the auditory tubes opens onto the dorsal surface of the infundibular cavity between paired infundibular folds. In the submucosa of the roof are the sphenopterygoid salivary glands. The smooth muscle is present only in the caudal most part of the roof. The floor of the pharynx is formed by the root of the tongue. The mucosa of the roof and floor numerous papillae.

Oesophagus

Horse

In general the oesophagus in horse is longer, narrower and less dilatable than that in the ox. In its cervical course it slips to the left of the trachea at the level of fourth cervical vertebra as against third vertebra in ox. Similarly, it regains the position dorsal to trachea at the level of the sixth cervical vertebra as against the level of thoracic inlet in ox. The muscular coat of the wall of the oesophagus in its cervical course is of striated type. The mucous membrane has same features as those in ox.

Dog

The cervical part of the oesophagus in dog is proportionately wide and more dilatable throughout its cervical course except at its origin where there is a constriction. The fibres of the muscular coat are striated type. The course and relations of the cervical part of the oesophagus in dog is otherwise similar to that in ox and horse.

Sheep and Goat

The oesophagus in sheep and goat is in general similar to that in ox. It is dilatable and the diameter of the oesophagus gradually increases starting from its origin to its opening in the cardia of the stomach.

Pig

The oesophagus in pig originates from the oesophageal vestibule of the pharynx at the level of the caudal pharyngeal constriction. The course, relations and the structure of the wall of oesophagus in pig is similar to that in ox.

Fowl

The cervical part of the oesophagus in domestic fowl is shorter than the unextended vertebral column of the cervical region. Cranially it lies in the midline dorsal to the larynx and trachea. Caudal to fifth cervical vertebra it lies on the right side of the neck between the jugular vein, vagus nerve and the thymus gland dorsally and the trachea ventrally. After reaching just cranial to thoracic inlet it again shifts to median position. In its cervical course the oesophagus of the fowl is thin walled and extensible. It has relatively greater diameter in comparison to that in mammals. The diameter of the oesophagus in the cervical region is otherwise uniform except at cranial to thoracic inlet where it enlarges ventrally to form a saccular diverticulum called the **crop.** The crop is situated cranial to the clavicle and the pectoral muscles. The tunica adventitia of the crop is firmly attached to the skin. The muscular layer of the crop is formed by the striated muscle fibres. The mucous membrane on the internal surface of the oesophagus and crop is thrown into longitudinal folds and it is lined by stratified squamous epithelium similar to that in mammals.

Nostrils & Nasal cavity

Horse

The nasal cavity in horse is longer and cylindrical. The nostrils are much dilatable. The medial wing of the nostril has a cartilaginous base which forms a prominence dorsally. Extending from the prominence is a thick fold of skin which continues with a fold of mucous membrane. This fold is called the alar fold. The part of the nostril that lies ventral to the alar fold leads into the nasal cavity. The part that lies dorsal to the alar fold is called false nostril and it leads into a blind pouch of skin which is called the diverticulum. The cornu of the alar cartilage curves ventrolaterally. There is only one parietal cartilage on each side. The nasolacrimal orifice is visible on the floor of the true nostril behind the ventral commissure when the nostril is dilated. The ductus incisivus is blind at its dorsal end. The division of the nasal cavity into left and right chambers by the septum nasi is almost complete. The middle meatus is wider and is not divided caudally.

Dog

The nostrils appear as two commas closely opposed to each other by their convexities. The skin around the nostrils is keratinous, black and moist. The cartilaginous framework of nostrils is mainly formed by the parietal and septal cartilages. The cartilage of the septum extends rostrally beyond the body of the incisive bone and terminates in the snout. The lateral wing of the nostril is supported by the anchor shaped lateral accessory cartilage. The skin around and between the medial wings of nostrils is smooth and moist and forms **the nasal plane (planum nasi).** This part is mapped out by grooves which are characteristics of the individual animals

The length of the nasal cavity has a direct correlation with the length of the face which varies greatly in different breeds of dog. The nasal cavity is almost completely occupied by the turbinate bones. The middle meatus is short, narrow and divides caudally into two branches The caudal meatus is small in the middle. The lamina transversalis divides the nasal cavity into the upper olfactory and lower respiratory.

Sheep and Goat

The nostrils in sheep and goat are slit like in appearance. They are placed obliquely so that they are closer together ventrally and wide apart dorsally as is in the ox. The skin around and between the medial wings of nostrils is smooth and moist and forms **the nasal plane (planum nasi).** This part is mapped out by grooves which are characteristics of the individual animals similar to that in ox and dog. The median groove (philtrum) which divides the upper lip extends dorsally into the planum nasi. The serous secreting lateral nasal gland is located in the mucous membrane of the nasomaxillary opening and its duct opens into the nasal cavity close to the nostril. This gland is absent in ox.

Pig

In pig, the apex of the nose and the upper lip together form the **snout.** The nose is embodied within the skeleton of the face and it extends caudad to about the level of the eyes. The nostrils are situated in the snout and like in other species are bounded by medial and lateral wings and supported by the cartilaginous skeleton. These are round in shape. The dorsal and lateral walls of the nose are bony with the exception of a small rostral part of lateral wall which is cartilaginous. The dorsal and ventral parietal cartilages of the nose curve lateroventrally and laterodorsally respectively and meet to complete each side of the wall of the nose.

The skeleton of the snout and the nose is modified to form a prism shaped rostral bone called the os rostrale. The apex of the prism lies opposite to the rostral boundary of the nasal septum while its base underlies the skin between the two nostrils. The nostrils are further supported by the dorsal lateral and the lateral accessory cartilage. The nostrils in pig can not be dilated. The snout is covered by thin and sensitive skin which forms the planum rostrale. The surface of the skin is divided by shallow grooves into small irregular areas called the areolae. These surface markings are characteristics of individual animals and can be used for identification of the particular animal.

The nasal cavity in pig is relatively long and narrow. The nasal septum has osseous, cartilaginous and membranous part. The osseous part is formed by the vomer and perpendicular plate of the ethmoid bone. The dorsal border of the cartilage expands on each lateral side to form the thin lateral cartilages. Rostrally the ventral border is expanded on each lateral side to form the ventral lateral cartilage. The dorsal and ventral lateral cartilages curve to meet each other and complete the skeleton of the nasal cavity. A fold of mucous membrane forms the membranous part of the septum.

Fowl

The nostrils in bird are small elongated and narrow slit like openings in the upper beak. Each nostril is bounded by a sheet of horny skin, the operculum. The nasal cavity is roughly cone shaped, with the apex facing rostrally. The cavity consists of three compartments, the rostral compartment called the vestibule, the middle respiratory compartment and the caudal olfactory compartment. The vestibule contains the rostral concha (turbinate) and is lined by stratified squamous epithelium. The middle respiratory compartment contains the middle concha which is lined by the ciliated epithelium. The olfactory compartment contains the caudal concha and is lined by respiratory mucous membrane. The rostral nasal concha is cone shaped and its apex is pointed rostrally. It is not scroll like but 'C' shaped. The interior of the caudal concha is connected to the infraorbital sinus. The vomeronasal organ in young birds disappears. The nasolacrimal duct opens on the floor of the middle compartment of the nasal cavity.

Larynx

Horse

The larynx of horse has additional paired cartilage called the cuneiform cartilage. The cricoid cartilage is clearly ring shaped. The thyroid cartilage is incomplete ventrally. The epiglottis is long and pointed. Two additional cuneiform processes extend from the base of the epiglottis dorsad and caudad. The vocal cords are long and large. These cords project from lateral wall into the laryngeal cavity. The glottis is very narrow. The lateral ventricles are much deeper and each of these leads into a mucous sac, the laryngeal saccule.

Dog

The larynx of dog is very much similar but shorter than that of horse. The lamina of the cricoid cartilage is wider. The epiglottis is quadrilateral. The cuneiform cartilages are large. The laryngeal saccule is extensive and lies lateral to both, the true and false vocal cords.

Sheep and Goat

The constitution of the larynx in sheep and goat is almost similar to that in ox with some miner differences. The cranial border of the arch of the cricoid cartilage is set obliquely. The thyroid cartilage is relatively shorter and the laminae are relatively higher. The epiglottis is shaped like an obovate in sheep and like a cordate leaf in goat.

Pig

The larynx of pig is relatively long and extends from the level of a transverse plane through the occipital bone to the transverse plane through the fourth or fifth cervical vertebra. The lamina of the cricoid cartilage is long and narrow. The thyroid cartilage is very long. The rostral cornu of the thyroid cartilage is absent. The body of the thyroid cartilage is long and thickened ventrally to form the laryngeal prominence. The paired corniculate cartilages are fused with the apices of the arytenoid cartilages.

Fowl

The larynx in birds is formed by four cartilages, the median cricoid, procricoid and the paired arytenoid. The cricoid cartilage is unpaired. It consists of three parts, the median body and two lateral wings. The body is large gutter like plate which is concave dorsally. It becomes partly ossified in older birds but its shovel shaped rostral part remains cartilaginous throughout the life. The left and right thin plates of wings unite with the lateral part of the body by a thin line of flexible cartilage. The medial border of each wing articulates by synovial joint with the procricoid cartilage forming the crico-procricoid joint. The rostral border of the wing is thick and glides with the caudal border of the body of the arytenoid cartilage. The procricoid cartilage is median, dorsal and small. It is comma shaped with the body pointing rostrally and the tail caudally. The body presents two facets for articulating with the left and right arytenoid cartilages. The tail presents left and right facets which articulate with the left and right wings of the cricoid cartilage. The arytenoid cartilages are paired. Each of them consists of a body, a rostral process and a caudal process. The body articulates caudomedially with the procricoid at the procrico- arytenoid joint. The thyroid and epiglottis cartilages are absent. The cartilages of larynx are binded by different ligaments. These include five pairs of intrinsic ligaments, one unpaired ligament and one pair of extrinsic ligaments. The muscles supporting the cartilages and the joints include two paired intrinsic muscles, two paired extrinsic muscles, one unpaired extrinsic muscle and one paired dorsal mass of tangled muscle fibres intermingled with the caudal laryngeal salivary glands. The cavity of the larynx is compressed dorsoventrally. The inlet of the laryngeal cavity is a narrow slit. It is supported on either side by arytenoid cartilages. The inlet is continued caudally by laryngeal fissure which is a narrow groove extending caudally to the tuft of papillae at the caudal end of laryngeal mound. The laryngeal mound is an elevation carrying the opening into the cavity of the larynx.

Trachea

Horse

The cervical part of the trachea in horse is longer so also its calibre is more in horse than that in ox. The free ends of the cartilaginous rings overlap dorsally with the right end overlying the left one when the trachea is fixed in situ but the two ends fail to meet each other in the fresh state. The cervical course and relations of trachea in horse are similar to those in ox.

Dog

The cervical course, relations and the structure of trachea in dog is almost similar to that in ox and horse. However, the length of the trachea is relatively shorter.

Sheep and Goat

There is absolutely no difference in the trachea of sheep and goat and that of ox, except the length.

Pig

The cervical course, relations and the structure of trachea in pig is almost similar to that in other domestic animals described above. However, the length of the trachea is relatively shorter.

Fowl

The cervical part of trachea in fowl is relatively long and its diameter progressively increases in its cervical course as it passes down the neck. The tracheal rings are complete. The first and the last four tracheal rings are simple round rings of hyaline cartilage. The first tracheal ring lies immediately behind the cricoid cartilage of larynx. It is a simple ring. So also the last four rings of trachea which are in the thoracic part are also simple rings. The rest of the tracheal rings in the cervical region are like signet rings. The craniocaudal width of the rings progressively increases throughout the cranial third of the cervical part of the trachea and thereafter it progressively decreases as it passes down in the caudal third of its cervical course. The course and relations in cervical part of trachea is almost similar to that in other domestic animals.

SECTION-C

BLOOD VESSELS AND LYMPHATICS

32

Arteries of Head and Neck

Arteries of neck

Common carotid artery

The right and left common carotid arteries arise from the bicarotid trunk as it bifurcates on the ventral surface of the trachea at the thoracic inlet. In their course to reach the head, both of these, the right and left, common carotid arteries ascend through the neck along the ventrolateral aspect of the trachea and oesophagus respectively. During this course each of these arteries is accompanied by the vagosympathetic trunk dorsal to it, recurrent laryngeal nerve ventral to it and the internal jugular vein lateral to it. All these structures are enclosed in the carotid sheath. The external jugular vein is separated from the common carotid artery by the omohyoideus and sternocephalicus muscles. The right artery crosses the lateral surface of the trachea and passes along its dorsolateral surface and finally reaches to the lateral surface of the larynx and pharynx in front of the digastricus muscle ventral to the jugular process of the occipital bone. The left artery crosses the trachea and oesophagus and continues along its dorsolateral surface to the level of the third cervical vertebra. Here the oesophagus inclines towards the median plane and the artery follows the lateral surface of oesophagus till it reaches to the lateral surface of the larynx and pharynx just in front of the digastricus muscle and ventral to the jugular processes of the occipital bone. At this point the common carotid artery terminates by giving off the **occipital,** and **pharyngeal arteries** and then further continues as the **external carotid artery**. Along its course through the neck, the common carotid artery gives out several branches as below.

1. The **muscular branches** to the ventral cervical muscles both from the right and the left common carotid arteries in their upper and lower cervical course.
2. The **oesophageal branch** to the oesophagus from the left common carotid in its middle cervical course.

3. The **tracheal branch** to trachea from the right common carotid artery in its middle cervical course.
4. The **caudal thyroid artery** is branched off from the common carotid artery close to the caudal end of the gland. This artery is inconstant.
5. The **cranial thyroid artery** is given off close to the cranial end of the gland.
6. The **caudal laryngeal artery** arises from the common carotid artery on the lateral surface of the larynx. This is a small branch that runs caudally parallel to the caudal laryngeal nerve.
7. The **cranial laryngeal artery** may arise from the cranial thyroid artery or directly from the common carotid artery near the cricoid cartilage of the larynx. It accompanies the cranial laryngeal nerve passing through the thyroid foramen. It supplies the mucosa of the laryngeal vestibule.

The muscles and other structures in the dorsal and dorsolateral aspect of the neck region are supplied by three distinct branches, the **deep cervical artery**, the **vertebral artery** and the **superficial cervical artery** which arise from the **costocervical** or the **subclavian** branches of the **brachiocephalic trunk** near the thoracic inlet.

The **deep cervical artery** arises either separately or in common with the vertebral artery from the costocervical trunk. It passes dorsally and cranially between the transverse processes of the first thoracic or seventh cervical vertebrae or between the sixth and seventh cervical vertebrae. It ascends in the neck along the deep surface of the semispinalis muscle and supply the semispinalis, rhomboideus cervicis and the cervical part of the trapezious muscles.

The **vertebral artery** is the continuation of the costocervical trunk in the cervical region. It passes craniodorsally, reaches the transverse process of the sixth cervical vertebra, enters the transverse canal (a series of transverse foramina of the cervical vertebrae), ascends through this canal along with the vertebral vein and vertebral nerve, and gives branches to the intertransversarii muscles. During this course, opposite each intervertebral foramen it gives out a spinal branch that supplies the spinal cord and its meninges. A series of these branches inside the vertebral canal anastomose and form the dorsal and ventral spinal arteries. At the intervertebral foramen between the second and third cervical vertebra it enters the vertebral canal, passes on the floor of the canal and enters the cranial cavity, gives out a branch to join the condyloid branch of the occipital artery and finally join the rete mirabile cerebri on the floor of the cranial cavity.

The **superficial cervical artery** arises from the subclavian opposite the first rib, courses craniodorsally along the deep surface of the subclavious, brachiocephalicus, cervical part of the trapezious and the omotransversarius muscles. It then continues dorsally lateral to superficial cervical lymph nodes and finally ramifies in the deep face of the trapezious. In this course it supplies small branches to all the muscles and other structures that come in its way.

Arteries of head

The head region is supplied with blood through the branches of the **external carotid artery** which is the direct continuation of the common carotid artery after the latter reaches to the base of the head in front of the digastricus muscle ventral to the jugular process of the occipital bone. At this junction, before its continuation as internal carotid artery, two distinct branches, the pharyngeal artery and the occipital artery are branched off from the common carotid artery.

Pharyngeal artery

The pharyngeal artery (the ascending pharyngeal artery) arises from the termination of the common carotid artery or from the occipital artery. It passes medially and reaches the dorsolateral wall of the pharynx just caudal to the stylopharyngeal muscle and supplies branches to the dorsal and lateral walls of the **pharynx**, the **soft palate** and the **tonsil.**

Occipital artery

The occipital artery arises from the dorsal surface of the carotid sinus. It passes dorsad and medial to the jugular process of the occipital bone to reach the condyloid foramen where it divides into **rostral** and **caudal** branches. The **rostral branch** of the occipital artery enters the cranial cavity through the hypoglossal foramen, gives number of small branches to the lateral wall of the cranium and a large branch called the **condylar artery** which passes towards the hypophyseal fossa on the floor of the cranium. Here it gives out several small branches which form anastomosis with the terminal branch of the vertebral artery. From the anastomosis a branch passes through the intervertebral foramen of the atlas vertebra to the skin and muscles above and around the atlas vertebra. Another small branch from the anastomosis passes out through the alar foramen to supply the ventral straight muscles of the head. The **caudal branch** of the occipital artery passes ventrally along the margin of the atlanto-occipital joint and supplies the ventral straight muscles of the head.

External carotid artery

The external carotid artery is the direct continuation of common carotid artery on the deep face of the caudal belly of digastricus muscle. It runs cranially and dorsally between the digastricus and stylohyoid muscles towards the caudal border of ramus of the mandible, gives out several collateral branches during this course and reaches ventral to the temporomandibular joint. At this point it gives out the superficial temporal artery and then continues as the maxillary artery. During this course the external carotid artery gives out the following collateral branches.

1. The **linguofacial trunk** divides into lingual and facial arteries shortly after its origin from the external carotid.

    a. The **lingual artery** runs along the ventral border of the stylohyoid and styloglossus muscles and then on the lateral surface of the genioglossus muscle and finally terminates within the tongue. Inside the tongue it gives out the **dorsal lingual**, **sublingua**l and **deep lingual** arteries.

    b. The **facial artery** runs rostrally and ventrally over the medial surface of the of the digastricus and then along the medial surface of pterygoideus medialis, crosses the ventral border of the ramus of the mandible somewhat rostral to the mandibular angle and courses dorsally along with the facial vein, the ventral buccal branch of the facial nerve and the parotid duct and reach the rostral border of the masseter muscle. Here it gives out the **mandibular labial artery**, the **maxillary labial artery**, the **submental artery** and the **rostral lateral nasal artery** to supply the corresponding structures.

2. The **caudal auricular artery** arises from the upper border of the external auricular near the middle of its length. It passes upward and backward on the deep face of the parotid salivary gland and supplies the caudal auricular muscles.

3. The **masseteric artery** is a small branch which courses ventrally and rostrally and enters the caudal part of the masseter muscle.

4. The **superficial temporal artery** is the smaller of the terminal branches of the external carotid. It courses dorsally and rostrally and divides into the rostral auricular and transverse facial arteries.

    (a) The **transverse facial artery** passes through the parotid salivary gland and follows the course of the dorsal buccal nerve. It ramifies in the skin on the caudal part of the masseter muscle.

(b) The **rostral auricular artery** immediately divides into superficial and deep branches. The superficial branch crosses the zygomatic arch under the zygomaticoauricularis muscle with its satellite vein and the temporal branch of zygomaticoauricular nerve. The artery gives off several muscular branches and is continued caudally as the cornual artery.

(c) The **cornual artery** accompanied by the cornual vein and the cornual nerve courses along the frontal crest and reaches the neck of the cornual process where it divides into dorsal and ventral branches. Numerous branches of this artery branch off from it and enter the canals in the cornual process and supply the corium of the horn.

(d) The **lateral superior palpebral artery** arises from the superficial temporal artery caudal to the lateral angle of the eye and courses towards the superior eyelid.

(e) The **lateral inferior palpebral artery** arises caudal to the lateral angle of the eye and proceeds towards the inferior eyelid.

(f) The **lacrimal artery** arises from the terminal part of the superficial temporal reaches to the lacrimal gland and anastomoses with the lacrimal branch of the ophthalmic rete mirabile.

Maxillary artery

The maxillary artery is the direct continuation of the external carotid artery beyond the origin of superficial temporal artery in the vicinity of retromandibular fossa. It passes dorsally and rostrally through the pterygopalatine fossa and then reaches to the maxillary recess and divides into the greater palatine and infraorbital arteries. In this course, the maxillary artery gives out the following collateral branches

1. The **pterygoid arteries** are two small arterial branches arising from ventral surface of the internal maxillary a short distance away from its origin at the carotid sinus. These arteries run along the either side of the mandibular alveolar artery and supply the caudal part of the medial pterygoid muscle.

2. The **mandibular alveolar artery** is larger than the pterygoid arteries. It arises from the ventral surface of the internal maxillary next to the origin of pterygoid arteries. It passes ventrad and rostrad on the medial pterygoid muscle along with the mandibular alveolar vein and nerve and reaches to the mandibular foramen. In their further course, these three together enter the mandibular canal through the mandibular foramen and traverse the

entire length of the mandibular canal. After reaching the mental foramen, the artery divides into incisor and mental branches. The **incisor artery** continues forward in the incisor canal inside the body of the mandible and supplies the incisor teeth and the tissue surrounding their roots. The **mental artery** divides into several branches which are distributed to the structures of the chin and the lower lip. As the mandibular alveolar artery passes through the mandibular canal it gives out **dental branches** to the cheek tooth.

3. The **deep temporal artery** arises from the maxillary next to the origin of the mandibular alveolar branch and supplies the temporalis and further gives off the masseteric artery to supply the masseter muscle. Occasionally there may be two such arteries namely the **rostral and caudal deep temporal arteries.**

4. **The middle meningeal artery** arises from the dorsal border of the maxillary artery near the origin of the mandibular alveolar. It enters the cranial cavity through the foramen lacerum.

5. **The artery of the rete mirabile cerebri** is a single large or several small arteries arising from the maxillary artery near the origin of the ophthalmic artery. It enters through the cranial cavity through the foramen orbitorotundum meet similar artery or arteries of the opposite side and forms a complex arterial plexus around and over the pituitary gland at the hypophyseal fossa.

6. **The ophthalmic artery** is given off from the maxillary at the level of foramen orbitorotundum and enters the apex of the periorbita with the ophthalmic nerve. It distributes branches to the structures enclosed by the periorbita such as the **lacrimal branch** to the lacrimal gland and the **muscular branches** to the muscles of the eyeball. Thereafter the ophthalmic artery continues as the **nasociliary artery**. It gives off the **ciliary branches** to the eyeball and a long branch to third eyelid and then continues as **ethmoid artery** to supply the lateral masses of the ethmoid bone. It forms the ophthalmic rete mirabile in between the rectus muscles of the eyeball from which arises the **supraorbital artery** that passes through the supraorbital canal and supplies small branches to the mucous membrane of the frontal sinus and the musculature and skin on the surface of the frontal bone.

7. **The buccinator artery** arises from the ventral surface of the maxillary artery rostral to the origin of the ophthalmic artery. It passes rostrally and ventrally with the buccinator nerve and is distributed to the caudal part of the buccinator muscle and dorsal buccal glands.

8. **The malar artery** is a large branch arising from the maxillary artery or in a common trunk with the infraorbital artery in the rostral part of pterygopalatine fossa near the maxillary foramen. It passes dorsally and rostrally in the orbital fossa to the medial angle of the eye and the lateral aspect of the face. It gives off the following branches.

   (a) **Small branches** to the periosteum, periorbita and the mucous membrane of the maxillary sinus

   (b) **The muscular branches** to the obliquus ventralis

   (c) **The artery to the third eyelid** supplies to the nictitating membrane and the third eyelid.

   (d) **The medial inferior palpebral artery** arises slightly before the orbital margin and supplies the inferior eyelid.

   (e) **The angular artery of the eye** supplying the medial angle of the eye.

   (f) **The caudal lateral nasal artery** supplies the skin and muscles over the lateral surface of the nose.

   (g) **The dorsal nasal artery** is a continuation of the malar artery coursing along the dorsal surface of the nose and the muzzle.

The greater palatine (descending palatine) artery gives off the lesser palatine and sphenopalatine arteries and then passes through the palatine canal with the rostral palatine nerve to the oral surface of hard palate. It continues rostrally through the palatine groove to the rostral part of the palatine fissure where it enters the nasal cavity. The greater palatine artery supplies the mucosa of the hard palate, the dental pad and the mucosa of the floor of the nasal cavity. The **sphenopalatine artery** enters the nasal cavity with the sphenopalatine nerve through the sphenopalatine foramen and supplies the ventral turbinate body. The **lesser palatine artery** is a small vessel arising from the ventral surface of the greater palatine before it enters the palatine canal. It also supplies to the soft palate.

The **infraorbital artery** is the dorsal and larger of the two terminal branches of the maxillary artery. It enters the infraorbital canal through the maxillary foramen along with the infraorbital nerve and vein. While passing through the infraorbital canal it gives dental branches to the upper (maxillary)chick teeth. After reaching at the infraorbital canal it gets exit from the canal and divides into small branches spreading on the lateral surface of the face. Some of these branches anastomose with the lateral nasal artery supplying the maxillary lip and the nose.

Arteries of brain and spinal cord

The brain and spinal cord are supplied with blood mainly through a complex network of arteries called the rete mirabile cerebri situated on the floor of the cranium surrounding the sella turcica. This is formed by the branches of the **external carotid, maxillary, occipital** and **vertebral arteries.**

Rete mirabile cerebri

The rete mirabile cerebri is formed in two parts, the rostral and caudal parts and are called as rostral epidural rete mirabile cerebri and the caudal epidural rete mirabile cerebri respectively.

The **rostral rete mirabile cerebri** is situated rostral to the hypophyseal fossa and the pituitary gland. About two to four rete branches arise from the maxillary artery and enter the cranial cavity through the foramen orbitorotundum and perforate the dura mater to reach the cavernous sinus in front of the pituitary gland. These divide into number of fine branches and join similar branches from the arteries of the opposite side. The branches of the two sides intermingle and thus form the rostral rete mirabile cerebri.

The **caudal rete mirabile cerebri** is situated caudal to the hypophyseal fossa and the pituitary gland. It is contributed by the branches of the occipital and vertebral arteries. The condylar artery, a branch arising from the occipital artery passes through the hypoglossal foramen and divides into several fine branches. Similar branches from the vertebral artery which enters the cranial cavity through the floor of the foramen magnum join the branches of the condylar artery and form the network of arterial branches with similar branches from the arteries of the opposite side. This network is called the caudal rete mirabile cerebri.

The rostral and the caudal rete are connected with each other on the lateral sides of the hypophyseal fossa and pituitary gland. Thus the rostral and caudal rete mirabile cerebri join each other and distribute number of arteries to supply blood to different parts of the brain. These branches are primarily the branches of the emergent artery.

The **emergent arteries**, right and left, are the major vessels supplying the brain and it represents the internal carotid artery of the other species of animals. Each emergent artery emerges through the dorsal surface of the tuft of rete mirabile cerebri and leaves the hypophyseal fossa through a foramen in the diaphragm selli. After emerging through the dura mater at the base of the brain, each emergent artery divides into two **primary branches**, the **rostral** and **caudal** branches which diverge from each other and run in opposite directions.

The **rostral primary branch** is larger of the two. It passes rostrally and laterally, crosses the optic tract, continues in the same direction for a short distance, then curves inward in front of the optic tract and divides into the middle and rostral cerebral arteries. The **middle cerebral artery** passes outwards, gains the sylvian fissure and divides to supply the lateral aspects of the cerebral hemisphere. The **rostral cerebral artery** passes in front of the optic chiasma, gains the great longitudinal fissure. Here it is connected to its fellow by a small anastomotic branch and completes the rostral arc of the **circle of Willis**. It then divides into numerous branches to supply the medial aspect of the cerebral hemisphere. A small branch, the **internal ophthalmic artery** arises from this vessel, crosses the optic nerve and joins the external ophthalmic artery.

The **caudal primary branch** passes backwards as the caudal cerebral artery, inclines inwards, gives off the rostral cerebellar artery to the cerebellum and joins its fellow from the opposite side to form the basilar artery, thus completing the caudal arc of the circle of Willis. The **basilar artery** passes backwards in the central median sulcus of the pons and medulla oblongata and is continued on the spinal cord as the **ventral spinal artery**. During this course, the basilar artery gives off the **caudal cerebellar artery** and branches to the pons and medulla and the choroid branches to the **choroid plexuses**. The ventral spinal artery runs along the ventral median fissure of the spinal cord and is reinforced by branches from vertebral artery in the cervical region, intercostal arteries in the thoracic region, and the lumbar, sacral and coccygeal spinal arteries in the respective regions of the body.

33

Veins of Head and Neck

The venous blood from the head and neck is carried by two jugular veins (Figure 2-11 B), the internal and external jugular veins on each side. Both of these extend from the base of the head to the thoracic inlet and are located on the ventrolateral part of the neck. The internal jugular vein is smaller while the external jugular is larger one.

The **internal jugular vein** is formed by the union of the thyroid, laryngeal and occipital veins beneath the wing of the atlas between the mandibular salivary gland and the rectus capitis ventralis major muscle. It passes down the neck in company with the common carotid artery, vagus and sympathetic nerves enclosed within a carotid sheath, receives in its course the muscular venous branches, tracheal vein and the oesophageal vein and terminates by joining the external jugular vein just in front of the thoracic inlet.

The **external jugular vein** is the larger of the two jugular veins and is formed by the union of the superficial temporal and the maxillary veins just behind the caudal border of the mandible and on the deep face of the parotid salivary gland below the temporomandibular joint. It becomes superficial by emerging through the parotid gland, passes down the neck subcutaneously in the jugular furrow, receives the internal jugular vein forming a **common jugular vein** in front of the thoracic inlet. It receives along its course, the external maxillary vein, parotid veins, auricular veins, small veins from the muscles of the cervical region and the cephalic vein at its termination. While in the jugular groove it is bounded dorsally by the brachiocephalicus muscle, ventrally by sternocephalicus and medially by the sternomastoid part of the sternocephalicus muscle. The vein is covered by skin and fascia and is separated from common carotid artery, vagosympathetic trunk, recurrent laryngeal nerve and internal jugular vein by the upper border of the sternomastoid muscle.

The right and left common jugular veins unite and form the **jugular confluence** which joins the cranial vena cava ventral to the trachea slightly to the right of the median plane at the level of the cranial border of the first rib.

The major tributaries of the internal jugular vein

The **occipital vein** is a large vessel that is formed by a number of veins in the atlantal fossa. It joins the thyroid and laryngeal veins to form the internal jugular vein near the lateral border of the atlas vertebra.

The **thyroid vein** receives blood from thyroid gland and joins the **laryngeal vein** from the larynx near the termination of the maxillary vein and then continues as internal jugular vein.

The major tributaries of the external jugular vein

The **superficial temporal vein** is on the deep surface of the parotid salivary gland at the upper part of the caudal border of the mandible. It is formed by the small transverse facial and rostral auricular veins and joins the maxillary vein to form the external jugular vein.

The **transverse facial vein** is on the lateral surface of the mandible with the satellite artery and dorsal buccal nerve. It passes medial to the parotid salivary and parotid lymph gland to join the superficial temporal vein.

The **rostral auricular vein** is on the medial surface of the parotid salivary gland rostral to the base of the ear. It receives a tributary from the rostral auricular muscles, the cornual vein and an anastomotic branch from the vein within the periorbita.

The **internal maxillary vein** lies on the upper part of the medial pterygoid muscle and under cover of the temporalis muscle and the ramus of the mandible. It is the continuation of the sphenopalatine vein and joins the superficial temporal to form the origin of external jugular vein. It is ventral to the buccinator vein and is joined to it by a large anastomosis. The tributaries of the internal maxillary vein are the mandibular alveolar, pterygoid and deep temporal veins.

The **sphenopalatine vein** is formed in the maxillary recess by the infraorbital and caudal nasal veins. The infraorbital vein is in the infraorbital canal and receives the dental veins from the upper cheek teeth along its course. The caudal nasal vein receives blood from the ventral turbinate body and joins the infraorbital vein in the maxillary recess to form the sphenopalatine vein.

The **mandibular alveolar vein** is formed by several small veins from the chin, lower lip, and the incisor teeth. It passes through the mandibular canal receiving the dental veins from the lower cheek teeth along its course. After emerging from the canal at the mandibular foramen it crosses the medial pterygoid muscle and joins the ventral border of the internal maxillary vein.

The **pterygoid veins** are two small veins arising from the pterygoid muscles and joining the internal maxillary vein.

The **deep temporal vein** is a large vessel arising in the temporal fossa and passing downward on the rostral part of the temporomandibular joint. It joins the internal maxillary vein near its termination. It receives a large tributary from the masseter muscle which passes through the mandibular notch.

The **maxillary vein** is formed rostral to the medial angle of the eyelids by the union of angularis oculi and the dorsal nasal veins. It runs ventrad and rostrad along the rostral border of the malar muscle to the facial tuberosity and then continue along the rostral border of the masseter muscle. Hereafter it passes along the ventral border of the ramus of the mandible, and then between the sternomandibularis muscle and parotid salivary gland near the angle of the mandible and finally joins the external jugular just caudal to the angle of the mandible. The tributaries of the maxillary vein are as below.

(a) The **vena anguli oculi** is the continuation of the supraorbital vein which lies in the supraorbital groove covered by the cutaneous muscle and from which it receives tributaries and then join the frontal vein at the supraorbital foramen.

(b) The **dorsal nasal vein,** which is usually double, passes ventrad and caudad from the rostrodorsal part of the nasal cavity and joins the angularis oculi to form the maxillary vein.

(c) The **lateral nasal vein** is a small vein that passes from the lateral part of the nostril. It joins the maxillary vein just above the facial tuberosity.

(d) The maxillary labial vein extends from the upper lip and join the the maxillary vein.

(e) The **mandibular labial vein** lies on the deep surface of the buccinator muscle. It receives small tributaries from the lower lip and cheek and then joins the maxillary vein just before it passes between the insertions of the sternomandibular muscle over the caudal border and the angle of the mandible.

(f) The **buccinator vein** leaves the deep surface of the depressor labi mandibularis and passes upward along the caudal part of the buccinator muscle between the mandible and the masseter muscle. Near the maxillary tuberosity it passes between the buccinator artery and the nerve. It then crosses the caudal border of the mandible, turns backward between the pterygoid muscle and the mandible and finally join the dorsal border of the internal maxillary vein.

(g) The **superficial mandibular labial vein** is a small vessel along the lower border of the depressor labi mandibularis muscle.

The **lingual vein** lies along the ventral border of the styloglossus medialis and the mylohyoid muscle. It receives several tributaries from the tongue. At the caudal border of the mylohyoid muscle it passes ventrally between the digastricus muscle and the mandibular salivary gland to join the upper border of the maxillary vein. Near its termination into the maxillary, the lingual vein receives a small vein from the mandibular salivary gland.

34

Lymphatics of Head and Neck

The lymphatics of the head and neck region is comprised of the lymph nodes and the lymph ducts. The lymph nodes of the head are the parotid, pterygoid, mandibular, the lateral and medial retropharyngeal, and the rostral and caudal hyoid. The lymph nodes in the cervical region are the superficial and accessory superficial, cranial, middle and caudal deep cervical and the costocervical and subrhomboidal lymph nodes. The lymph from these lymph nodes is finally collected and carried to the common jugular vein by the tracheal and right lymphatic ducts.

Lymph nodes of head

Parotid lymph node

The parotid lymph node is large and elongated gland usually single but sometimes two small glands connected closely with each other by a fibrous tissue lying on the upper part of the lateral surface in the caudal half of the masseter muscle. It is ventral to the temporomandibular joint, partly or completely covered by the dorsal part of the parotid salivary gland and is situated lateral to the maxillary vessels and nerve. The afferent lymph vessels are received to this gland (node) from the muscles of head, ocular and auricular muscles, the parotid salivary gland, the gums, lips, appendages of the eye, ear, lacrimal gland, and from the bones of the head such as frontal, malar, nasal, maxilla, incisive, turbinate, mandible etc. The afferent from the parotid lymph node joins the tracheal duct of the corresponding side.

Pterygoid lymph node

The pterygoid lymph node is a small gland lying near the maxillary tuberosity, on the dorsal part of the lateral face of the pterygoideus muscle. Afferents of this node come from the hard palate and gums and the efferent from this node opens into the mandibular lymph node.

Mandibular lymph node is usually a single large gland on each side or may be two small glands (twins) on each side. It is located between the sternocephalicus muscle and the ventral part of the mandibular salivary gland and below the maxillary vein. It receives afferents from the lips, cheeks, hard palate, gums, sublingual salivary gland, skin and some of the muscles of the head, and the mandible, hyoid, nasal and incisive bones. The afferents from the parotid and pterygoid lymph nodes are also received by the mandibular lymph node it being the lymphocentre of this group of the lymphatics. The efferent from this node joins the retropharyngeal lymph node.

Lateral retropharyngeal lymph node (atlantal lymph node)

The lateral lymph node is usually one large lymph node accompanied by one to three small lymph nodes in a group. It is situated ventromedial to the wing of the atlas vertebra, caudoventral to the origin of digastricus muscle and dorsal to the carotid artery. It is laterally related to the vagus, sympathetic and the accessory nerves. It receives afferents from the tongue, mucous membrane of the oral cavity, gums, lips, hard palate, muscles of the hyoid apparatus and most of the muscles of the neck. The efferent from this node joins the tracheal lymphatic trunk.

Medial retropharyngeal lymph node

The medial retropharyngeal lymph node is situated medial to the stylohyoid bone on the dorsolateral face of the pharyngeal muscles. Afferent lymph vessels for this lymph node are received from the tongue, floor of mouth tonsils, gums, hard palate and soft palate. Some of the afferents are also received from the cervical muscles and the rostral hyoid lymph node. The efferent from this lymph node joins the lateral retropharyngeal lymph node.

Rostral hyoid lymph node

The rostral hyoid lymph node is situated on the thyrohyoid bone at the insertion of the stylohyoideus muscle. It receives afferents from the tong and the efferent from this node joins the lateral retropharyngeal lymph node. This lymph node is inconsistent in appearance.

Caudal hyoid lymph node

The caudal hyoid lymph node is small lymph node located on the dorsal end of the stylohyoid bone or in the angle between the bone and the occipitohyoideus muscle. It receives afferents from the mandible and the efferent from this node joins the lateral pharyngeal lymph node.

Lymph nodes of neck

Superficial cervical lymph node

The superficial cervical lymph node (Figure 2-12 B) is an elongated gland situated on the scalenus muscle at the cranial border of the supraspinatus muscle. The dorsal two thirds of this gland is covered by omotransversarius and the ventral third by brachiocephalicus muscle. Afferents to this node are received from the skin of the neck, shoulder, part of the ventral and lateral surfaces of the thorax to the extent of tenth or twelfth rib and from the skin and subcutis, muscles, tendons and fascia of the fore limb and shoulder girdle. The efferent of the accessory superficial cervical lymph node also joins this lymph node as afferent. The efferent vessel from the right superficial cervical lymph node descends over the scalenus muscle and opens in the right tracheal trunk near its termination. The efferent from the left node join either the left tracheal trunk or the thoracic duct,

Accessory superficial cervical lymph node

The accessory superficial cervical lymph node is a group of small lymph nodes dorsal to the superficial cervical lymph node along the border of the supraspinatus muscle and covered by the trapezius and omotransversarius muscles. Its afferents come from the muscles and fascia in its vicinity. The afferent opens into the superficial cervical lymph node.

Cranial deep cervical lymph node

The cranial deep cervical lymph nodes vary from four to five in number and are usually small in size. These nodes lie along the course of the common carotid artery usually cranial and caudal to the thyroid gland. The most cranial of these nodes are covered by the omohyoideus muscle and the caudoventral angle of the parotid salivary gland. These receive afferents from the larynx, trachea, pharynx, oesophagus, thyroid, thymus, and the muscles of the neck in the adjacent part of these nodes. It may also receive afferent from the lateral retropharyngeal lymph node. The efferent lymph vessels from these nodes join the tracheal trunk or may open into the middle deep cervical lymph node.

Middle deep cervical lymph node

The middle deep cervical lymph nodes are small in size and they vary in number, size and position. Usually these nodes lie on either side of the trachea in the middle third of the neck. The series of these nodes may extend cranially to the group of the cranial deep cervical lymph nodes and caudally to the extent of a group of caudal deep cervical lymph nodes. The afferents for these nodes come from the trachea, oesophagus, thymus and the ventral cervical muscles. The efferent from these nodes either join the tracheal trunk or they may open in the caudal deep cervical lymph node.

Caudal deep cervical lymph nodes

The caudal deep cervical lymph nodes vary in number from three to five. These are placed near the thoracic inlet, dorsal and ventral to the common jugular vein. One of these lies above the manubrium sterni, one under the axillary vein and others dorsal to the insertion of the sternohyoideus and sternocephalicus muscles. The afferents for these nodes come from trachea, oesophagus, thymus, ventral cervical muscles. The afferents from the middle deep cervical, axillary, costocervical and occasionally from the cranial deep cervical lymph nodes also join these lymph nodes. The efferent vessels from caudal deep cervical lymph nodes usually empty in the tracheal trunk but in some cases they may join the terminal part of the thoracic duct (left) or the common jugular vein (right).

Costocervical lymph node

The costocervical lymph node lies just in front of or medial to the first rib above the common carotid artery and the vagosympathetic nerve trunk and is covered by the scalenus ventralis muscle. The right node lies lateral to trachea while the left node lies lateral to oesophagus. It receives afferents from the trachea, oesophagus, cervical muscles, shoulder and the costal pleura. The efferent from the right gland opens into the right tracheal trunk and that from the left gland opens into the thoracic duct near its termination.

Subrhomboid lymph node

The subrhomboid lymph node is a large gland lying embedded in a mass of fat above the shoulder joint in front of the cranial angle of the scapula. It is covered by the cervical part of the rhomboideus muscle. Its afferents come from the muscles of the neck and shoulder. The efferents open into the costocervical lymph node which finally terminates into the tracheal lymph duct and the right lymphatic duct.

Large lymph ducts of head and neck

The lymph from the lymph nodes of the head and neck is collected and carried to the common jugular vein through a common trunk called the tracheal lymph duct and the right lymphatic duct.

Tracheal lymph duct

The right and left tracheal lymph ducts are the continuation of the efferents of the retropharyngeal lymph nodes of the corresponding side. In case of more than one efferent from this node, they unite before their further course and form a single trunk for each side. Each tracheal lymph duct extends from the retropharyngeal lymph node and passes down the neck on the lateral aspect of the trachea under the omohyoideus, gains the company of the internal jugular vein under cover of the sternocephalicus muscle. During its course through the neck, each tracheal lymph duct receives the efferents of the cranial, middle and caudal cervical; costocervical and prescapular lymph glands. On reaching the lower part of the neck, the left duct either opens into the common jugular vein or joins the thoracic lymph duct just before its termination. The right tracheal duct continues for a short distance as **right lymphatic duct** which opens either into the right common jugular vein or the jugular confluent.

35

Comparative Anatomy of Blood Vessels and Lymphatics of Head and Neck

Arteries

Horse

The **common carotid artery** in horse has a similar origin, course and distribution as that in ox except that it has no relation with the internal jugular vein since this vein is absent in horse. Each common carotid artery at its termination in front of the digastricus gives out internal carotid artery in horse in addition to the occipital and pharyngeal arteries given off by the common carotid artery in ox.

The **internal carotid artery** which is absent in ox is present in horse. It is considered as chief source of blood for the brain in horse. It passes over the guttural pouch and enters the cranial cavity through the foramen lacerum and gains the cavernous sinus. The internal carotid arteries of the opposite sides are connected by a large transverse branch called the **intercarotid artery** that lies behind the pituitary gland (further course of this artery will be described with the blood supply of the brain in horse).

The **external carotid artery** which is a direct continuation of the common carotid artery after its termination in front of the digastricus muscle is related to guttural pouch during its course along with other structures described in ox.

The **maxillary artery** arises as one of the collateral branches of the external carotid artery as against its direct continuation in ox. The external maxillary artery in horse terminates over the levator labii maxillaris muscle by dividing into angular artery and the rostral nasal artery.

The **superficial temporal artery** terminates by dividing into rostral auricular and transverse facial arteries. It does not give out the palpebral, lacrimal and frontal branches and the branches to the horn core in absence of horns in horse.

The **transverse facial artery** is longer and it communicates with the caudal deep temporal and external maxillary arteries.

The **internal maxillary artery** in its course runs in three parts. The first part is the longest of the three and it undertakes the course upwards on the guttural pouch. The second is intrarosseous part and the third is infraorbital part.

The **blood supply to brain** is through two sources, the **internal carotid artery** and the **basilar artery.** Each internal carotid artery leaves the cavernous sinus, penetrates the dura mater, gives off the caudal communicating artery, passes forward along the side of the pituitary gland and divides at the optic chiasm into the **middle cerebral** and **rostral cerebral arteries**. The caudal communicating branch passes backwards and anastomoses with the caudal cerebral branch of the basilar artery. The basilar artery is formed by the union of the cerebral branches of the occipital arteries of the two opposing sides inside the cranium caudal to the pituitary gland. The anastomosis of the two rostral cerebral arteries in front of the pituitary gland and that of the two caudal cerebral and caudal communicating branches behind the pituitary gland encircles the pituitary gland and is called as the **circle of Willis**.

Dog

The right and left **common carotid arteries** arise independently from the brachiocephalic artery instead of the origin from the bicarotid trunk. The bicarotid trunk is absent in dog. The course and branching of the right and left common carotid arteries in the neck is almost identical. Both the arteries terminate with division into **occipital, internal carotid** and **external carotid** arteries at the level of the basihyoid bone. The origin, course and distribution of collateral branches of the common carotid artery of dog is almost similar to that of ox. Out of the three terminal branches, the occipital is smaller and some times it originates from the external carotid. The caudal meningeal artery, a branch of the occipital enters the cranium through the mastoid foramen and anastomoses with the middle meningeal artery.

The internal carotid artery enters the cranial cavity through the carotid foramen penetrates the dura mater and assists in the formation of circle of Willis.

The external carotid artery undertakes the course and distribution similar to that in ox.

The internal maxillary artery is similar to that in horse. It passes through the sphenoidal canal during the intraosseous course.

The **blood supply to brain** and spinal cord is mainly from two sources, the **internal carotid** and the **basilar artery.**

Sheep and Goat

The **common carotid artery** in the cranial part of the neck passes between the caudal belly of the digastricus and stylohyoid muscles and gives out the occipital artery and then continues as the external carotid artery.

The **caudal thyroid artery** is present in sheep but may be absent in goat.

The **ascending palatine artery** may arise directly from the common carotid artery at the level of cranial laryngeal and ascending pharyngeal artery.

The **external carotid artery** is the continuation of the common carotid beyond the origin of the occipital artery.

The **lingual artery** arises singly from the external carotid artery while the facial artery is absent. The **transverse facial artery** compensates the absence of the facial artery.

The **superficial temporal artery** is the last collateral branch of the external carotid artery before its continuation as **maxillary artery**.

The **blood supply to brain** in sheep and goat is mainly through the internal carotid artery and the branches of the maxillary artery by formation of the **epidermal rete mirabile cerebri** like that of the ox. Rest of the formation and distribution of the rete mirabile cerebri is similar to that of ox.

Pig

The **common carotid artery** accompanies the internal jugular vein like that in ox. It terminates by dividing into the occipital, internal carotid and external carotid artery in the cranial deep aspect of the jugular furrow.

The **external carotid artery** is one of the terminal branches of the common carotid artery and not in the form of direct continuation of the common carotid artery. The rest of the description about the course, branching and disposition of the branches of this artery is same as of the ox.

The **blood supply to brain** is through the **intercarotid plexus** which is formed by the internal carotid and basilar arteries of the opposing sides. A network of fine arterial branches is formed on the right and left side of the pituitary gland contributed by the internal carotid artery, basilar artery and the meningeal arteries of the corresponding sides. These networks (anastomoses) of the two sides are joined rostral and caudal to the pituitary gland. From this formation, a number of fine arterial branches are distributed to different parts of the brain.

Fowl

The **common carotid artery** in fowl is a short trunk arising from the brachiocephalic artery within the thoracic inlet. It passes cranially parallel to the jugular vein and the vagus nerve up to the level of the cranial border of the first rib and divides into an internal carotid artery and a common trunk of the vertebral and vagus artery.

The **vertebral artery** passes through the transverse canal formed by the series of the transverse foramina of the cervical vertebrae as the ascending vertebral artery along with the vertebral vein and the cervical sympathetic nerve trunk. After reaching at the base of the skull the ascending vertebral artery terminates into an end to end anastomosis formed with the descending branch of the deep occipital artery. During its course through the transverse canal, the ascending vertebral artery supplies a series of branches to the axial musculature, the cervical spinal nerves, meninges and the spinal cord.

The **vagus artery** along with the vagus nerve, jugular vein and the thymic chain ascends through the neck to the base of the skull. During its course it supplies branches to the oesophagus, crop and the intermediate part of the trachea.

The **internal carotid arteries** of the right and left side are wide apart in their initial course in front of the thoracic inlet lying on the corresponding side of the neck. Then each of them curves with its convexity to the front and gains the median line thus coming close and parallel to each other in their course ascending the neck, the right passing above the trachea and the left above the oesophagus. Thus the right and left internal carotid arteries ascend side by side below the longus colli from thirteenth to the second cervical vertebra from where they diverge and reach to the angle of the jaw on the respective side. At this place each of the internal carotid arteries gives off the external carotid artery and reaches a shallow parabasal fossa at the base of the skull. Here it divides into two terminal branches, the external ophthalmic and cerebral carotid arteries.

The collateral branches of these arteries in the head region are described in two groups, the extracranial and intracranial arteries. The **extracranial** group includes the external carotid, occipital mandibular, caudal auricular, descending oesophageal, descending tracheal, maxillary, submandibular, rostral auricular, facial, pterygopharyngeal and external ophthalmic arteries.

The **intracranial** arteries supply blood to brain. These include the internal carotid artery and the cerebral carotid artery. These arteries form the intercarotid anastomosis just caudal to the hypophysis cerebri. This anastomosis distributes branches for different parts of the brain.

Veins

Horse

The **internal jugular vein** is absent in horse. There is only one jugular vein on each side and it corresponds with the external jugular vein of ox. The left and right jugular veins unite and form the jugular confluent at the thoracic inlet. Each **jugular vein** is formed by the union of the superficial temporal and internal maxillary veins.

The **superficial temporal vein** is formed by the rostral auricular and transverse facial veins.

The internal maxillary vein is the continuation of the buccinator vein.

The collateral tributaries of the internal maxillary artery are the linguofacial vein, the mandibular dental veins, the pterygoid vein and the middle meningeal vein.

The jugular vein of each side undertakes the course through the neck similar to that followed by the external jugular vein in ox. The tributaries of the jugular vein in horse are the masseteric vein, the caudal auricular vein, the occipital vein, the external maxillary vein, the thyroid vein, the parotid vein, the tracheal vein, the oesophageal vein, and the muscular veins from the muscles of the neck.

The external maxillary vein in its course receives the transverse facial vein; a common trunk of maxillary dental, sphenopalatine, greater palatine, and ophthalmic veins; the lingual vein and the sublingual vein.

Dog

The jugular veins in dog are similar to those in ox.

The **internal jugular vein** is formed in the tympano-occipital fissure by the union of ventral petrosal vein and the sigmoid sinuses and rarely with the vein of the hypoglossal canal. It initially lies in association with the internal carotid artery and then it continues down the neck along the common carotid artery inside the carotid sheath. In the lower cervical region it joins the external jugular vein. The tributaries of the internal jugular vein are the laryngeal, pharyngeal, thyroid, tracheal and oesophageal veins.

The **external jugular vein** begins by the union of linguofacial and maxillary veins caudal to the mandibular salivary gland or at the transverse plane through the cricoid cartilage of the larynx and the axis vertebra. Its further course is through the jugular canal and its lateral surface is directly under the skin and the cervical fascia. It receives the omobrachial and cephalic veins in front of the cranial border of the shoulder and then the superficial cervical vein just before the internal jugular vein merges with the external jugular vein in front of the thoracic inlet.

The linguofacial vein is formed by the union of lingual and facial veins ventral to the mandibular salivary gland receives a small tributary from this gland, emerges through the caudal border of this gland and join the maxillary vein.

The maxillary vein begins ventral to the alar canal as an extension of the ophthalmic vein.

Sheep and Goat

The internal jugular vein is absent in the sheep and goat.

The **external jugular vein** is formed by the union of linguofacial and maxillary veins near the caudoventral border of the parotid salivary gland on the lateral surface of the mandibular salivary gland. It descends down the neck inside the jugular furrow which is bounded dorsally by the cleidomastoideus and ventrally by sternomastoideus muscles. In the caudal part of the neck it lies deep and courses under cover of the brachiocephalicus whereas in the cranial part of the neck it runs subcutaneously under the superficial cervical fascia and the cutaneous colli. It joins the cranial vena cava either independently or by a common trunk with its fellow of the opposite side. The tributaries of the external jugular vein in sheep and goat are the occipital vein, the cranial thyroid vein, the caudal thyroid vein and the variable number of the muscular branches from the muscles of the neck. Since the internal jugular vein is absent, the tracheal and oesophageal tributaries also join the external jugular vein in sheep and goat.

The **linguofacial vein** of sheep and goat is relatively more slender than the maxillary vein and runs rostrally along the ventral and lateral borders of the mandibular gland between the pterygoideus medialis and digastricus. In the goat it passes beneath the insertion of the sternomandibularis.

The **maxillary vein** courses craniodorsally under the parotid salivary gland towards the caudal border of the ramus of the mandible, piercing the pterygoideus medialis.

Pig

The **internal jugular** in pig accompanies the common carotid artery inside the carotid sheath throughout its cervical course similar to that in ox. During this course it is joined by the ventral cerebral vein, occipital vein, cranial thyroid, middle thyroid and caudal thyroid vein, and the variable number of tributaries from the muscles of the neck. It join the external jugular vein of the same side in the lower cervical region in front of the thoracic inlet similar to that in ox.

The **external jugular** vein emerges through the ventral surface of the parotid salivary gland and undertakes the same course as that in ox. It join the internal jugular artery of the same side first and then join the common jugular canal at the thoracic inlet. The tributaries of the external jugular vein include the muscular branches from the muscles of the cervical region, the cranial and middle thyroid veins, the superficial vein and the cephalic vein.

Fowl

The blood from the head and neck in fowl is drained out by the **right and left jugular veins.** The right jugular vein is the larger of the two. These are not the satellites of the carotid arteries. The jugular veins are superficially placed on the corresponding sides of the trachea, while the carotid arteries are placed on the median line under the longus colli muscle. The two jugular veins are connected by an oblique or transverse branch just below the base of the cranium. The jugular vein joins the subclavian vein of the corresponding side at the inlet of the thorax and a combined trunk of these two join the cranial venacava of the corresponding side. There are two, the right and left cranial venacava in fowl.

Lymphatics

Horse

The pterygoid lymph node is absent in horse. The **parotid lymph node** is represented by a chain of two or three nodules placed on the medial surface of the parotid salivary gland. The **mandibular lymph node** is in the form of an elongated mass situated in the intermaxillary space between the digastricus and omohyoideus muscles and a little above the maxillary artery. The nodes of the opposite sides meet rostrally but caudally they are wide apart. The **pharyngeal lymph node** is in the form of elongated mass containing a group of large number of loosely united small glands placed on the lateral wall of the pharynx and larynx below the guttural pouch and internal to the digastricus muscle. The lateral retropharyngeal lymph node lies below the internal carotid artery and is covered by the upper end of the mandibular salivary gland. **The cranial deep cervical lymph node** in horse is placed along the carotid artery and on the larynx, thyroid gland, trachea and oesophagus. Some of these are covered by the caudoventral angle of the parotid salivary gland and some others lie between the mandibular salivary gland and the thyroid gland. The **middle deep cervical lymph node** lies below the carotid artery on the trachea and on the course of the tracheal lymph duct. The **caudal deep cervical lymph node** lie at the thoracic inlet below the trachea and is covered by the sternomaxillaris and cervical cutaneous muscles. This lymph node receives afferents from the cranial and middle deep cervical, prescapular and axillary lymph nodes. The efferents from these nodes on right side open into the right lymphatic duct and the left one opens into the tracheal duct. The **tracheal lymph duct** and the **right lymphatic ducts** in horse are similar in formation, course and termination to that of ox.

Dog

The **pterygoid lymph node** is absent in dog. **The parotid lymph node** is usually single but some times there may be two small glands. The **mandibular lymph nodes** are usually two or three on each side and are placed subcutaneously between the mandibular salivary gland and the masseter muscle. The **retropharyngeal lymph node** lies on the dorsal wall of the pharynx medial to the sternocephalicus and the mandibular salivary gland and lateral to the rectus capitis ventralis muscle. The **cranial deep cervical lymph node** in dog is absent but when present they are in the form of small nodules. The **middle deep cervical lymph nodes** are absent. The **caudal deep cervical lymph nodes** may also be absent but when present they lie on the ventral face of the trachea near the thoracic inlet. The **tracheal lymph duct** and the **right lymphatic duct** in dog has the same formation, course and termination as that in ox.

Sheep and Goat

The locations of the lymph nodes of the sheep and goat resemble in general to those of ox.Amongst the lymph nodes of sheep and goat there may be variations in the number of lymph nodes. When a single gland is present it is larger in size. When more than one, usually two or three, these are smaller and oval in shape. The afferents and efferents of these lymph nodes also resemble to those in ox.

Pig

The lymph nodes of the head and neck in pig resemble in general to those of other domestic animals described earlier. Only a few variations exist. The **pterygoid lymph node** is absent. The **accessory mandibular lymph nodes** are found ventral to the linguofacial vein. They are located caudal to the mandibular salivary gland on the sternomastoideus muscle and are covered completely by the parotid salivary gland. The afferents to these accessory lymph nodes come from the mandibular area that includes the muscles and skin, the tongue mucous membrane of the floor of the mouth tonsils and cheeks and the rostral third of the nasal cavity, upper lip, and from the ventral part of the neck.

The efferents from these lymph nodes join **the dorsal and ventral superficial cervical lymph nodes**. In the cervical region, in addition to the dorsal and ventral superficial cervical lymph nodes, there is **middle superficial cervical**

lymph node. These are two inconsistent groups of small lymph nodes. Of these, the dorsal group is located along the course of the superficial cervical vein to its termination into the external jugular vein. The second group is located dorsal to the course of the external jugular vein and it is covered by the cleido mastoideus and cleido occipitalis muscles. The afferents to the dorsal group are received from the dorsal superficial cervical lymph nodes and from adjacent structures. The afferents to the ventral group are received from the dorsal group and from the caudal group of the ventral superficial cervical lymph nodes. The efferents from both the groups either join the tracheal trunks or to the caudal deep cervical lymph nodes.

The **tracheal trunks** originate from the medial retropharyngeal lymph node. These may be a single or two large ducts on each side which courses along the common carotid artery and internal jugular vein and receive the efferents of the cranial, middle and caudal deep cervical lymph nodes. The tracheal lymph ducts open into the common jugular vein or the brachiocephalic vein.

Fowl

The main drainage of lymph from head and neck in fowl is through the lymph vessels accompanying the jugular vein. Usually there are two such vessels, one coursing dorsal and the other ventral to the jugular vein. These lymph vessels are formed by the union of the lymph vessels of rostral cephalic vein and the caudal cephalic vein. The jugular lymphatics themselves receive tributaries directly from the skin at the regular intervals, the muscles of the neck, the thymus, thyroid, trachea, oesophagus and crop. The jugular lymph vessels open into the jugular vein cranial to its junction with subclavian vein.

SECTION-D

NERVES

36

Nerves of Head (Cranial Nerves)

The nerves of the head connect the central nervous system i.e. brain with the structures like skin, muscles, glands, blood vessels, organs of special senses etc. so as to monitor or control their functioning. These nerves are the cranial nerves and their branches. There are twelve pairs of cranial nerves.

Olfactory nerve (Cranial nerve I)

The olfactory nerve is the first cranial nerve and is known as the nerve of sense of smell. It consists of fibres which are the axons of olfactory cells of olfactory part of nasal mucous membrane. These fibres are nonmedulated and they form number of small bundles which are enclosed into connective tissue sheaths derived from the meningeal layers of the brain. These nerve fibres bundles pass caudally upward through the cribriform plate of the ethmoid bone and enter the cranium to join the olfactory bulbs of the brain. Besides the olfactory nerve bundles there are two more nerves that extend from the nasal mucous membrane, traverse through the cribriform plate and join the parts of the brain. These include the vomeronasal nerve that is formed by the nerve fibres arising on the vomeronasal organ and terminating on the accessory olfactory bulb of the brain. The other one is the terminal nerve that after reaching the brain joins the olfactory trigone.

Optic nerve (Cranial nerve II)

The optic nerve is the second cranial nerve and is known as the nerve of the sense of vision. This nerve is composed of nonmedulated fibres which are axons of the ganglion cells of retina of the eyeball. The nerve fibres from the cells of the retina converge at the optic papilla and form a consolidated nerve called the optic nerve. It pierces through the choroid and sclera, emerges from the ventrolateral quadrant of the eye, and passes caudally and medially to the optic foramen. On entering the cranium the two nerves decussate at the base of the brain and form an optic commissure. From the optic commissure, the optic tract passes into the lateral geniculate body and the dorsal quadrigeminal body (caudal colliculus). The optic nerve at its entrance to the optic foramen in the orbit is flexuous and embedded in fat. It is surrounded by retractor oculi muscle. It is also enclosed in the fibrous sheath derived from the meninges of the brain.

Oculomotor nerve (Cranial nerve III)

The oculomotor nerve is the third cranial nerve and is the motor nerve for the muscles of eyeball. It arises from the ventromedial aspect of the cerebral peduncle (intercrural fossa) turns sharply rostrad and laterad crossing over the caudal primary branch of the emergent artery (caudal communicating artery) of the rete mirabile cerebri, passes through the cavernous sinus along with the ophthalmic nerve and ophthalmic branch of the trigeminal nerve. It leaves cranium through the foramen orbitorotundum, enters the orbit, pierces the periorbita and divides into the dorsal and ventral branches to supply all muscles of eyeball except the dorsal oblique, lateral rectus and the retractor muscles. The ventral branch, along with the muscles of the eyeball, also supplies motor fibres to the ciliary ganglion.

Trochlear nerve (Cranial nerve IV)

The trochlear nerve is the fourth cranial nerve and it is the motor nerve for some of the muscles of eyeball. It is the finest of all the cranial nerves. The motor fibres constituting this nerve arise from the mid brain and emerge in the area of the rostral medullary velum. It then passes rostrad and laterad along the lateral border of the trigeminal nerve and leaves the cranium through foramen orbitorotundum. After reaching the orbit, the nerve supplies motor nerve fibres to the dorsal oblique muscle of the eyeball.

Trigeminal nerve (Cranial nerve V)

The trigeminal nerve is the fifth cranial nerve and is a mixed type of nerve constituted by the sensory and motor nerve fibres. It is the largest of all cranial nerves. It is connected to the lateral aspect of the pons by a large sensory root and a small motor root. The sensory root possesses a ganglion named as trigeminal ganglion or the Gasserian ganglion along its intracranial course close to the cranial opening of the foramen ovale. The motor root courses separately rostrad and passes under cover of the ganglion and then joins one of the three branches of the trigeminal ganglion before leaving the cranium. The convex face of the trigeminal ganglion gives out three branches, the ophthalmic, maxillary and the mandibular.

The **ophthalmic nerve** is entirely sensory. It leaves the cranium through the foramen orbitorotundum and enters the periorbital fossa at the apex of the periorbita. It gives off cornual, frontal, and lacrimal branches and continues as nasociliary nerve.

- The **cornual nerve** is thin and wide. It passes dorsad on the deep surface of the periorbita, pierces it, turns caudad on the temporal muscle and reaches the frontal crest about midway between the supraorbital process and the neck of the cornual process. The nerve continues caudad ventral to the frontal crest with the cornual artery and vein and divides into three branches which are distributed to the corium of the horn and adjacent skin. The nerve is closest to the surface of the about an inch rostral to the horn process.
- The **lacrimal nerve** is medial to the cornual nerve. It is wide and thin and reaches the widest part of the lacrimal gland dorsal to the eyeball. Some fibres from this nerve cross the gland and supply the skin of the upper eyelid.
- The **frontal nerve** passes dorsad and medially medial to the lacrimal nerve and enters the orbital opening of supraorbital canal. It passes through this canal along with the frontal artery and vein and after getting exit through the supraorbital foramen distributes branches to the skin around the foramen and the adjacent part of the frontal region.
- The **nasociliary nerve** is wide, flat and thick. It is the continuation of the ophthalmic nerve. It passes between the rectus dorsalis and retractor oculi and then between the rectus dorsalis and rectus medialis muscles of the eyeball. It crosses the rectus medialis and turns sharply ventrad and caudad to reach the ethmoid foramen. It enters the ethmoid foramen and continues as the ethmoid nerve. Before its continuation as ethmoid, the nasociliary nerve at its bent gives off several small ciliary nerves and the large infratrochlear nerve. The **ciliary nerves** are the sensory fibres from the ciliary body of the eyeball. The **infratrochlear nerve** passes rostrad below the trochlea for the dorsal oblique muscle to reach the medial canthus of the eyelids. Here it supplies the skin and conjunctiva of this part, the third eyelid and the lacrimal duct and lacrimal sac.
- The **ethmoid nerve** enters the cranial cavity through the ethmoid foramen at the ventral margin of the ethmoid fossa. It leaves the cranium through the cribriform plate of the ethmoid fossa and enters the nasal cavity. Here it supplies sensory fibres to the mucosa of the nasal septum and the dorsal turbinate.

The **maxillary nerve** is the largest of the three branches of the trigeminal and is purely sensory like the ophthalmic. It emerges out of the cranium through the foramen orbitorotundum, enters the pterygopalatine fossa and divides into the infraorbital and the sphenopalatine nerves.

- The **infraorbital nerve** runs towards the orbit, reaches to the floor of the orbit and then to the maxillary hiatus. Here it enters the maxillary foramen, passes down the infraorbital canal of the maxillary bone along with the infraorbital artery and vein. It gets exit from the infraorbital canal through the infraorbital foramen and divides into three branches, the external nasal, lateral nasal and the maxillary labial nerves. The **external nasal nerve** supplies to the dorsal part of the nose. The **lateral nasal nerve** supplies the skin of the lateral part of nostril and the nasal vestibule. The **maxillary labial nerve** supplies the skin and mucous membrane of the upper lip. All three branches distribute nerve fibres to the skin of the face rostral to the infraorbital foramen. The infraorbital nerve, while passing through the infraorbital canal gives out dental branches to the maxillary (upper) cheek teeth.
- The **sphenopalatine nerve** after getting separated from the infraorbital, divides into the caudal nasal and greater palatine nerves. The **caudal nasal nerve** enters the nasal cavity through the sphenopalatine foramen and is distributed to the ventral turbinate bone. The **greater palatine nerve** passes through the palatine canal with the great palatine artery. It continues rostrad in the palatine groove with the artery and supplies the mucous membrane of the hard palate. The greater palatine nerve before entering the palatine canal, gives out a slender branch called the **lesser palatine nerve** which is distributed to the structures of the soft palate.

The **mandibular nerve** is a mixed nerve. Its sensory root arises from the trigeminal ganglion and is immediately joined by the motor root of the trigeminal nerve. The mixed nerve thus formed leaves the cranium through the foramen ovale of the temporal wing of the sphenoid bone. It runs ventrad and rostrad on the medial surface of the lateral pterygoid muscles and then enters the mandibular foramen on the vertical ramus of the mandible. Through this foramen, the mandibular nerve runs down the mandibular canal, gains exit through the mental foramen on the lateral surface of the lower part of the horizontal ramus of the mandible, turns rostrally and continues as the mandibular labial nerve distributing number of filaments to the mandibular (lower) lip. During its course before entering the mandibular foramen, passing through the mandibular canal and after gaining exit through mental foramen, the mandibular nerve gives out following branches.

- The **buccinator nerve** arises from the rostral border of the mandibular nerve immediately after its exit through the oval foramen. It passes rostrad and ventrad across the medial surface of the pterygoid muscle and internal maxillary artery. Ventral to the orbit, the nerve turns ventrad along the rostral border of the buccinator vein and then turns rostrad into the cheek under the buccinator muscle and is distributed to the mucosa of the cheek.
- The **parotid nerve** is given off just before the buccinator nerve enters the cheek. It passes ventrad along the rostral border of the masseter muscle, between the insertions of the sternomandibular muscle and then caudad with the ventral buccal nerve and parotid duct above the external maxillary vein and enters the ventral part of the parotid salivary gland.
- The **deep temporal nerve** has a short common trunk of origin with the masseteric nerve from the rostral border of the mandibular nerve close to oval foramen. It passes dorsally into the temporal fossa and supplies the temporalis muscle.
- The **masseteric nerve** passes laterally along the rostral surface of the temporomandibular articulation and through the mandibular notch to enter and supply the masseter muscle.
- The **superficial temporal nerve** leaves the caudal border of the mandibular nerve a little below the foramen ovale. It passes caudad to the caudal border of the mandible a little below its neck, and divides into **transverse facial nerve** which supplies the masseter muscle and the **subzygomatic nerve** which turns laterad and rostrad under the parotid lymph gland to join the buccal nerve.
- The **pterygoid nerves**, one or two in number, arise in the angle between the buccinator and mandibular nerves. They are short and small nerves distributing the pterygoid muscles.
- The **lingual nerve** is the last branch of the mandibular nerve before it enters the mandibular canal. It passes rostrally on the lateral surface of the pterygoid muscle to the root of the tongue. Here it passes medial to the mylohyoideus muscle and along the ventral border of the styloglossus muscle to about the middle of the length of the tongue and divides into the superficial and deep branches. The **superficial lingual** nerve passes rostrad between the sublingual salivary gland and the floor of the mouth to distribute branches to these structures. The **deep lingual nerve** runs dorsad into the substance of the tongue and terminates into small branches supplying the dorsum and the fungiform papillae of the tongue.

- The **mandibular alveolar nerve** is the continuation of the mandibular nerve after entering the mandibular canal through the mandibular foramen. While running down the mandibular canal this nerve gives out **dental branches** to the mandibular (lower) cheek teeth. It gains exit through the mental foramen and divides into the mental and incisor nerves. The **mental nerve** continues rostrally over the lower lip as the **mandibular labial nerve** to supply the structures of the lower lip and the **incisor nerve** passes through the incisor canal of the incisive bone to supply the incisor teeth.

Abducent nerve (Cranial nerve VI)

The abducent is the sixth cranial nerve and is a motor nerve for some of the muscles of the eyeball. It arises from the angle formed between the ventral lateral pyramid of the medulla oblongata and the pons. It passes forward across the pons, pierces the dura mater, accompanies other nerves in the cavernous sinus, leaves the cranium through the foramen orbitorotundum and enters the orbital fossa at the apex of the periorbita. Here it supplies the rectus lateralis and the retractor oculi muscles and the nictitating membrane of the eyeball.

Facial nerve (Cranial nerve (VII)

The facial is the seventh cranial nerve and is a mixed nerve. It arises from the corpus trapezoideum on the lateral surface of the medulla oblongata immediately behind the pons. It passes laterally across the trigeminal nerve and in front of the acoustic nerve and enters the internal acoustic (auditory) meatus with that nerve. At the bottom of the acoustic meatus, the facial nerve gets separated from the acoustic nerve, bears a small ganglion known as geniculate ganglion and enters the facial canal. The facial nerve leaves the cranial cavity through this facial canal which opens at the stylomastoid foramen. The facial nerve after gaining exit through this foramen turns rostrad under cover of the parotid salivary gland and divides into the dorsal and ventral buccal nerves. During its course it gives off number of branches within the canal and outside the canal. The branches given out by this nerve inside the canal are known as intraosseous branches and those outside the canal are the extra osseous branches.

Intraosseous branches

These are mostly the branches arising from the geniculate ganglion of the facial nerve.

- The **great superficial petrosal nerve** arises from the geniculate ganglion in the facial canal, passes backward, reaches the cranial cavity by the internal auditory meatus, meets here some of the branches of the sympathetic system and forms the vidian nerve.

- The **vidian nerve** leaves the cranium through the foramen lacerum basis cranii, passes in the vidian groove and canal and supplies the levator palati and azygos uvulae muscles of the soft palate.
- A **small superficial petrosal nerve** is formed by the fibres from the geniculate ganglion that unite with the filaments from the tympanic plexus and join the otic ganglion.
- The **stapedial nerve** is given off from the facial nerve to supply the stapedius muscle within the canal.
- The **chorda tympani nerve** arises from the facial nerve in the facial canal, crosses the tympanic cavity and emerges out of the styloid foramen, gains the company of the lingual branch of the trigeminal nerve and supplies gustatory fibres to the rostral two thirds of the mucous membrane of the tongue. It also supplies secreto- motor fibres to the mandibular and sublingual salivary glands through the submandibular ganglion.

Extraosseous branches

- The **digastricus nerve** arises from the facial near the stylomastoid foramen. It passes downwards and supplies the caudal belly of the digastricus, occipitohyoid and the stylohyoid muscles.
- The **caudal, middle and the rostral auricular nerves** arise from the facial immediately after its exit through the stylomastoid foramen. These nerves supply the (auricular) muscles of the external ear.
- The **ventral buccal nerve** is the ventral terminal branch of the facial nerve. It passes downwards in the substance of the parotid salivary gland and then turns rostrad on the lower part of the masseter muscle and gives branches to the masseter, sternomandibularis and the depressor labi mandibularis muscles and then terminates in the ventral part of the orbicularis oris muscle.
- The **dorsal buccal nerve** is the dorsal terminal branch of the facial nerve. It passes rostrally in the substance of the parotid salivary gland between the masseter muscle and the parotid lymph gland and continues rostrad to the lateral surface of the face. It supplies the malar and zygomatic muscles, the muscles of the nostril and those of the cheek above the level of the labial commissure.

Vestibulocochlear nerve (Cranial nerve VIII)

The vestibulocochlear is the eighth cranial nerve and it is a known as the nerve of sense of hearing and equilibrium. It is also called as acoustic or auditory nerve. The nerve receives afferent fibres from the internal ear. It is attached to the medulla oblongata at the lateral part of the corpus trapezoideum just caudal to the facial nerve. It has two roots, the vestibular and cochlear. It passes outward along with the facial to the internal acoustic meatus. Here it divides into two branches, the upper vestibular and the lower cochlear nerves. In the internal acoustic meatus this nerve is connected to the geniculate ganglion of the facial nerve by filaments and presents the vestibular ganglion. The peripheral processes of the ganglion cells are distributed to the maculae of the utricle and the saccule and the cristae of the ampullae of the semicircular canals of the internal ear. The cochlear nerve gives off filaments to the saccule and passes through the modiolus and joins the spiral ganglion. The peripheral processes of the cells of this ganglion pass through the lamina spiralis and are distributed to the organ of corti in the cochlea.

Glossopharyngeal nerve (Cranial nerve IX)

The glossopharyngeal is the ninth cranial nerve and it is a mixed nerve. It arises from the lateral surface of the medulla oblongata in a series of filaments caudal to the acoustic nerve. These filaments pass outwards and converge into a bundle which pierces the dura mater and gains exit from cranium through the foramen lacerum. Immediately after emerging through the foramen, the nerve bears a ganglion named as **petrosal ganglion** and then turns downward medial to the great cornu of the hyoid bone and divides into two branches, the glossal (lingual) and the pharyngeal. The **pharyngeal branch** receives parasympathetic fibres from the vagus nerve and the sympathetic fibres from the cranial cervical ganglion and forms the **pharyngeal plexus** on the lateral surface of the pharynx. This plexus supplies nerve fibres to the muscles and the mucosa of the pharynx. The **lingual branch** passes along the great cornu of the hyoid bone and disappears under the hyoglossus muscle. It gives branches to the soft palate, isthmus faucium and the tonsil and finally terminates by supplying the ordinary and gustatory fibres to the mucous membrane of the caudal one third of the tongue.

Vagus nerve (Cranial nerve X)

The vagus is the tenth cranial nerve and is a mixed nerve. It is the longest and most widely distributed cranial nerve. It contains the afferent and efferent fibres of the larynx and parasympathetic fibres to the heart, lungs and the abdominal organs. It is attached to the lateral aspect of the medulla oblongata by several filaments in a series with those of the glossopharyngeal in front and the spinal accessory behind. The filaments of the nerve converge in a bundle of nerve trunk that passes outwards, pierces the dura mater and emerges out of cranium through the foramen lacerum. In the foramen the vagus nerve bears a jugular ganglion which is connected to the spinal accessory and hypoglossal nerves and the petrosal ganglion of the glossopharyngeal nerve. Outside the foramen, the vagus nerve passes downwards on the caudal surface of the bulla tympanica, crosses the lateral surface of the rectus capitis ventralis minor muscle behind the cranial cervical ganglion. Here it turns caudad, crosses the pharyngeal lymph node above the cervical sympathetic trunk and reaches the dorsal border of the common carotid artery. At the level of the axis vertebra, the vagus nerve is joined by the cervical sympathetic trunk and becomes the vagosympathetic trunk. Here, the vagosympathetic trunk, the recurrent laryngeal nerve and the internal jugular vein together with the common carotid artery are enclosed in a common sheath called the carotid sheath. From here downward, the vagosympathetic trunk along with other structures in the carotid sheath passes down the neck along the trachea on the right side and the oesophagus on the left side of the neck up to the thoracic inlet. The course of the vagus nerve beyond this level will be described under the chapter on nerves of thorax in part three. The collateral branches given off by the vagus nerve in the head and neck region are as below.

- The **auricular branch** from the jugular ganglion enters the aquiductus fallopius, leaves the bone at the base of the concha and supplies branches to the lining membrane of the external ear. It gives communicating branches to the cranial and middle cervical ganglia.

- The **pharyngeal branch** arises from the vagus above the pharynx and associates with the sympathetic branch from the cranial cervical ganglion to form the autonomic plexus. From the plexus, motor fibres are supplied to the pharyngeal constrictors, the mucous membrane of the pharynx and the cervical part of oesophagus.

- The **cranial laryngeal nerve** arises from vagus at about the level of the division of carotid artery and immediately after origin bears the ganglion named as nodose ganglion. From this ganglion numerous sensory fibres are supplied to the mucous membrane of the larynx and external laryngeal branch for the cricothyroid muscle of the larynx.

- The **caudal laryngeal** or the **recurrent laryngeal nerve** is given out by the vagus after it reaches the thorax. From its point of origin from vagus, the recurrent laryngeal nerve ascends the neck along the common carotid artery to reach the larynx and supplies the motor fibres to all muscles of the larynx except the cricothyroid,

Spinal accessory nerve (Cranial nerve XI)

The spinal accessory nerve is the eleventh cranial nerve and it is the motor nerve. It has two roots of origin, the medullary and the spinal. The spinal root is formed by several fibres from the lateral surface of the spinal cord as caudad as the fourth or fifth cervical vertebra. These fibres converge and form a root that passes forward between the dorsal and ventral toots of the spinal nerves and enters the cranial cavity through the foramen magnum. In the cranial cavity it joins the medullary root which is formed by the fibres arising from the lateral surface of the medulla oblongata. The nerve thus formed pierces the dura matter and leaves the cranium through the foramen lacerum. It passes backwards ventral to the wing of the atlas vertebra where it divides into dorsal and ventral branches. The dorsal branch passes backward on the deep surface of cleido occipital and cervical part of trapezious muscle and finally end in the thoracic part of the trapezious muscle. The ventral branch passes downward across the oesophagus and trachea and enters the deep surface of the sternomastoid and sternomandibular muscles caudal to their insertions.

Hypoglossal nerve (Cranial nerve XII)

The hypoglossal is the twelfth cranial nerve and it is a motor nerve for tongue. The root fibres of this nerve arise from the ventral surface of the spinal cord in a series lateral to the caudal half of the pyramid. The filaments converge into three or four bundles which perforate the dura mater and unite to form the nerve. It leaves the cranium through the hypoglossal foramen. The nerve passes downward on the caudal surface of the tympanic bulla, crosses the occipital artery obliquely opposite the atlantooccipital joint. It then passes between the vagus and spinal accessory nerves, turns ventrad and rostrad, passes over the glossopharyngeal nerve and the great cornu of the hyoid bone. It gains the lateral face of the hyoglossus and divides into several branches to supply the muscles of the tongue.

37

Nerves of Neck (Cervical Spinal Nerves)

There are eight pairs of cervical spinal nerves in ox. The first of these emerges out through the lateral vertebral (alar) foramen of the atlas vertebra. The second through the lateral vertebral foramen (at the cranial border of the arch) of the axis vertebra and the eighth nerve emerges through the intervertebral foramen between the last cervical and first thoracic vertebra. The third to seventh nerves emerge through the corresponding intervertebral foramen. Each of these nerves divides into dorsal and ventral branch immediately after their exit from the vertebral canal through respective foramina. The dorsal branches are larger than the ventral except for the first and last two and most of them divide in to medial and lateral branches. They supply the dorsal (dorsolateral) cervical muscles, skin and the cervical part of the nuchal ligament. The ventral branches are distributed to the ventral cervical muscles and skin, The ventral branches of the last two cervical nerves are large.

- The **first cervical spinal nerve** after its division into dorsal and ventral branches, the dorsal branch supplies the dorsal muscles of the head which includes the obliquus capitis caudalis, the rectus capitis dorsalis major and the caudal auricular muscles and the adjacent skin including that covering frontal eminence. The ventral branch passes downward through the alar foramen. It receives ramus communicans from the cranial cervical ganglion and continues down to the sternothyrohyoideus and supplies the sternohyoideus, sternothyroideus and the omohyoideus muscles.

- The **second cervical spinal nerve** is larger than the first, emerges from the vertebral canal through the intervertebral foramen of the axis vertebra. The dorsal branch supplies the obliquus capitis caudalis and then turns backward and upward, passes over the caudal part of this muscle, runs between the complexus muscle and ligamentum nuchae and finally terminates in the skin on the dorsal part of the neck. The ventral branch gives fibres to the spinal accessory nerve and becomes subcutaneous at the ventral border of the cleido occipital muscle and the wing of the atlas and divides into caudal cutaneous auricular and the cutaneous branches. The caudal cutaneous auricular nerve passes upward and forward to the base of the ear and divides into several branches supplying the skin on the convex surface of the conchal cartilage. The cutaneous branch passes downwards and supplies the skin over the jugular vein and that of the mandibular space.

- The **third, fourth and fifth cervical spinal nerves** are similar in their course and distribution. The dorsal branches of these nerves supply the longus colli, intertransversarii, semispinalis and complexus muscles and the skin over the dorsal and dorsolateral aspect of the neck. The ventral branches of these nerves supply the rectus capitis ventralis, brachiocephalicus and sternocephalicus muscles and the skin covering the ventral and ventrolateral aspect of the neck.
- The **sixth cervical spinal nerve** contributes fibres from its dorsal branch to run with those of the preceding nerves. The ventral branch, in addition to sending fibres to pass with those of preceding nerves, participates in the formation of the phrenic nerve and the brachial plexus.
- The **seventh and eighth cervical spinal nerves** are small and usually do not share nerve supply to the skin from their dorsal branches. The ventral branches of these nerves contribute mainly to the formation of the phrenic nerve and the brachial plexus.
- The **phrenic nerve** is the motor nerve of the diaphragm. The origin of this nerve is from the ventral branches of the fifth, sixth and seventh cervical spinal nerves. The fibres from these nerves cross the superficial surface of the scalenus ventralis muscle, enter the thorax ventral to the brachial artery and continue backward in the mediastinal space to reach the diaphragm. The further course and distribution of the phrenic nerve will be described in the next part on anatomy of thorax under part three.

The **brachial plexus** is formed by anastomosis of ventral branches of the last three cervical and the first two thoracic spinal nerves. Some times the fifth cervical nerve may also supply a branch to this plexus. The plexus appears as two wide bands placed between the thoracic wall and the medial face of the shoulder. The details on the formation and distribution of this plexus will be described under the chapter on nerves of thorax.

Cervical sympathetic nerves

The cervical part of sympathetic nervous system (fig. 2-8A) is comprised of three cervical sympathetic ganglia, the cervical sympathetic trunk and the ansa subclavia. These are situated bilaterally on the left and right side of the neck. The ganglia are-the cranial cervical, middle cervical and the caudal cervical. The sympathetic trunk connects all the three ganglia while the ansa subclavia connects the middle cervical and the caudal cervical ganglia.

Cranial cervical sympathetic ganglion

The cranial cervical sympathetic ganglion is elliptical in shape and measures about 15 to 25 mm in length, about 4 to 6 mm in width and about 2 to 3 mm in thickness. It is located at the base of the cranium, ventromedial to tympanic bulla and lies on the lateral surface of the muscle rectus capitis ventralis minor. The gland is partly covered by the suprapharyngeal lymph node. Its lateral surface is crossed by the glossopharyngeal nerve and caudal meningeal artery. The nerve fibres emerging from the proximal end of this ganglion extend into the foramen lacerum and join the last four cranial nerves through which the sympathetic nerve fibres are supplied to the organs and glands of the head and neck. The nerve fibres emerging from the distal end of this ganglion constitutes the cervical sympathetic trunk.

Middle cervical sympathetic ganglion

The middle cervical sympathetic ganglion is a small, elongated and slightly cylindrical ganglion. It is about 10 to 12 mm long and 2 to 4 mm in diameter. The right ganglion lies on the lateral surface of the trachea and the left ganglion on the lateral surface of the oesophagus at the level of sixth cervical vertebra. The ganglion of both (right and left) sides is covered by the muscle scalenus ventralis. The ganglion is connected cranially with the cranial cervical sympathetic ganglion through the cervical sympathetic trunk and caudally with the caudal cervical sympathetic ganglion through the remaining part of cervical sympathetic trunk and the ansa subclavia. Sympathetic fibres from this ganglion are supplied to heart through the middle cervical sympathetic cardiac nerve and to the larynx and trachea through the recurrent laryngeal nerve. Fibres to oesophagus are also supplied from this ganglion.

Caudal cervical sympathetic ganglion

The caudal cervical sympathetic ganglion seldom exists separately. It is usually fused with the first thoracic sympathetic ganglion forming the cervicothoracic ganglion. When separate, it is small quadrilateral and lies on the ventrolateral surface of the muscle longus colli at the level of seventh cervical vertebra. When fused with the first thoracic, it becomes part of the cervicothoracic ganglion extending from the level of seventh cervical to second thoracic vertebra lying on the lateral surface of longus colli muscle medial to the head of first two ribs.

Cervical sympathetic trunk

The cervical sympathetic trunk is a cord of sympathetic nerve fibres emerging through the cervical and thoracic sympathetic ganglia. It begins at the distal end of the cranial cervical sympathetic ganglion, descends for a short distance and joins the vagus nerve forming the vagosympathetic trunk on the lateral surface of the muscle rectus capitis ventralis minor at the level of atlantoaxial joint. For its further course down the neck, the vagosympathetic trunk descends along the common carotid artery on the ventrolateral aspect of trachea on right side and oesophagus on left side of the neck. At the level of sixth cervical vertebra, the vagosympathetic trunk dissociates from the common carotid artery and thereafter the sympathetic trunk itself dissociates from the vagus at the level of sixth cervical vertebra to join the proximal end of the middle cervical sympathetic ganglion. Here the sympathetic trunk leaves the distal end of the middle cervical ganglion and proceeds caudally along the longus colli muscle to join the caudal cervical sympathetic ganglion which is a part of the cervicothoracic ganglion.

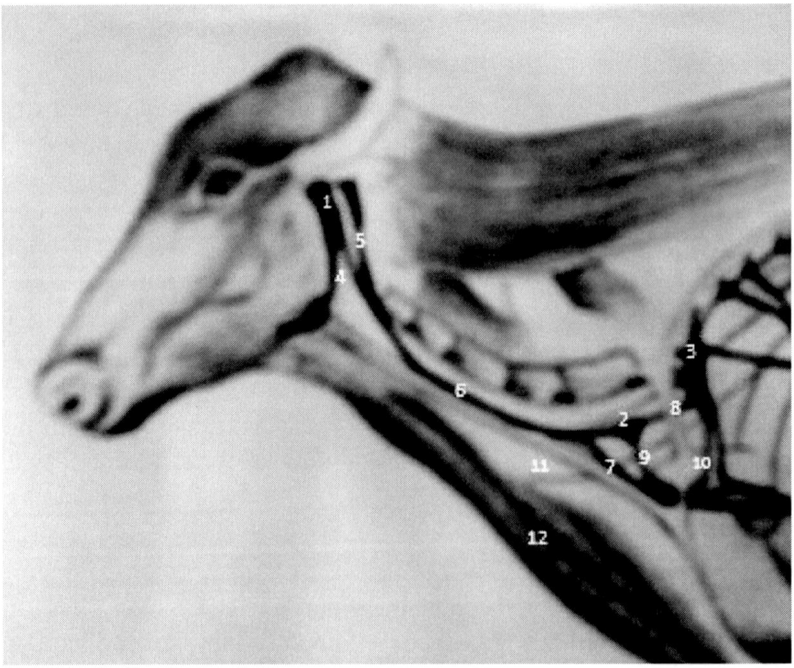

Fig. 2-8A Cervical sympathetic trunk (Left)

1. Cranial cervical sympathetic ganglion 2. Middle cervical sympathetic ganglion 3. Cervicothoracic ganglion, 4&8 Cervical sympathetic trunk, 5&7 Vagus nerve, 6. Vagosympathetic trunk, 9&10. Decending & ascending limb of ansa subciavia 11. Cesophagus, 12. Trachea

Ansa subclavia

The ansa subclavia is also the part of sympathetic trunk that connects the middle cervical sympathetic ganglion to the caudal cervical sympathetic ganglion or the cervicothoracic sympathetic ganglion. It leaves the proximal end of the middle cervical sympathetic ganglion, descends caudally parallel to the vagus nerve, turns round the brachiocephalic artery and then ascends to join the proximal end of the cervicothoracic sympathetic ganglion medial to the first rib.

38

Comparative Anatomy of Nerves of Head and Neck

Horse

The **optic and oculomotor nerves** in horse are thinner than those in ox. The **oculomotor** nerve leaves the cranial cavity with the ophthalmic and abducent nerves through the orbital foramen and the trochlear nerve leaves the cranial cavity through a small foramen immediately above the orbital fissure in horse as against the foramen orbitorotundum in ox. The ophthalmic branch of the **trigeminal nerve** leaves the cranium through the orbital fissure, the maxillary branch through the foramen ovale and the mandibular branch through the foramen rotundum. As against this, the ophthalmic and maxillary branches in ox emerge through the foramen orbitorotundum and the mandibular branch through the foramen ovale. The **lacrimal nerve**, a branch of the ophthalmic, runs rostrad on the rectus dorsalis and levator palpebrae superioris and ramifies chiefly in the lacrimal gland and the upper eyelid. One of its branches communicates with the orbital branch of the maxillary nerve, penetrates the periorbita, gains the temporal region behind the supraorbital process, forms a plexus with the branches of the frontal and auriculopalpebral nerves and divides to distribute fibres to the skin of the temporal region. The continuation of the **maxillary nerve** as infraorbital nerve gives out the caudal maxillary alveolar and middle maxillary alveolar branches to supply the molar and premolar teeth and before emerging through the infraorbital foramen gives out the rostral maxillary alveolar branch for the incisor and canine teeth.

The **facial nerve** on emerging through the stylomastoid foramen, gets under cover of the parotid salivary gland, passes forwards between this gland and guttural pouch and then passes between the origin of superficial temporal and maxillary arteries medially and superficial temporal vein laterally. It then crosses the caudal border of the ramus of the mandible just below the temporomandibular joint. Here it receives a branch from the auriculotemporal nerve and divides into dorsal and ventral buccal branches.

The **glossopharyngeal nerve** after leaving the cranial cavity through the jugular foramen (foramen lacerum) descends and curves forward over the guttural pouch. It then passes between the guttural pouch and the medial pterygoid muscle, crosses the external carotid artery, passes beneath the hyoglossus muscle and gains the base of the tongue with the lingual artery.

The jugular ganglion of the **vagus nerve** is smaller than that of ox. Beyond the jugular ganglion, the vagus nerve is intimately related with spinal accessory nerve for a short distance and then separate. The vagus descends behind the guttural pouch to the cranial cervical ganglion and joins the cervical sympathetic trunk constituting the vagosympathetic trunk.

The **spinal accessory nerve**, after separating from the vagus, crosses the upper extremity of the mandibular salivary gland. And the deep face of the brachiocephalicus, passes backwards along the superior border of this muscle, supply branches to the brachiocephalicus and sternocephalicus near the shoulder and terminates into the trapezious muscle near its insertion.

The **hypoglossal nerve** after emerging through the hypoglossal foramen runs ventrad and caudad between the guttural pouch and the capsule of the atlantooccipital joint for a short distance. It gives off a branch which crosses the lateral face of the pharynx and larynx, receives a communicating branch from the ventral division of the first cervical spinal nerve and supplies the muscles on the rostral face of the trachea.

The **cervical spinal nerves** in horse almost resemble to those of ox and there no major differences between these two species.

Dog

The first four cranial nerves in dog are more or less similar to those in ox. The fifth cranial, the **trigeminal nerve** divides into three major nerves, the ophthalmic, maxillary and mandibular like those in ox. The **lacrimal nerve**, a branch of ophthalmic nerve after emerging from the orbit divides into branches smaller branches which join similar branches of the frontal and zygomatic nerves and form the auricular plexus. In some cases the lacrimal nerve may arise from the maxillary nerve. The rest of the branches of ophthalmic are similar to those of ox. The **zygomatic nerve** arises from the maxillary nerve. The rest of the branches of the maxillary nerve are the pterygopalatine, greater palatine, lesser palatine, and caudal nasal nerves. The **infraorbital nerve** enters the infraorbital canal through the maxillary foramen gives out the **caudal maxillary alveolar** branch supplying branches to caudal molar teeth and the **middle maxillary alveolar** branch to supply the rostral molar teeth. The infraorbital nerve before emerging from the infraorbital canal gives out the **rostral maxillary alveolar** nerve that passes through the incisor canal and supplies branches to the incisor and canine teeth.

The **facial nerve** after emerging out of the stylomastoid foramen courses rostrad and laterad inside the parotid salivary ganglion and divides into its terminal branches, the auriculopalpebral nerve and the dorsal and ventral buccal nerves. The **auriculopalpebral nerve** courses rostrad and dorsad to the auricular cartilage of the external ear and divides into the zygomatic and rostral auricular branches. The zygomatic branch passes over the zygomatic arch and supplies the eyelids and the rostral auricular branch contributes to the formation of rostral auricular plexus. The dorsal buccal nerve receives a connecting branch from the ventral buccal nerve and forms a plexus over the masseter muscle. From this plexus extends a branch that passes through the orbicularis oris and terminates into the muscles of the lateral nasal region. The ventral buccal branch after giving a connecting branch to dorsal buccal branch for the plexus terminates into the ventral portion of the orbicularis oris muscle.

The cervical part of the **vagus nerve** in dog is more intimately united with the sympathetic trunk forming the vagosympathetic trunk. The **hypoglossal nerve** gives off a long branch that unites with the ventral branch of first cervical spinal nerve and supplies the muscles on the rostral face of trachea. The origin, course and distribution of **cervical spinal nerves** in dog is similar to that in ox.

Sheep and Goat

The gross disposition and distribution of the cranial and cervical spinal nerves in pig is more and less similar to that in ox.

Pig

The gross disposition and distribution of the cranial and cervical spinal nerves is more or less similar to that in ox.

Fowl

There are twelve pairs of cranial nerves in fowl similar to that in other domestic animals. Their origin, course and distribution also resembles to that in other domestic animals to a great extent except a few differences that occur due to absence of pons in the brain of fowl. The olfactory nerve in fowl, although originates in the form of several filaments from the olfactory mucous membrane of the nasal cavity as is in the other animals, it consolidates in a solid trunk of the nerve which passes along the dorsomedial aspect of the orbital cavity and enters the cranium through a large olfactory foramen instead of the cribriform plate of the ethmoid of other animals. The optic nerve and the optic chiasm is relatively large in fowl.

The **trigeminal nerve**, like that in other animals, divides in ophthalmic, maxillary and mandibular branches. The **ophthalmic nerve** enters the orbit, reaches to the apex of the cone of eye muscles and then passes towards the interorbital septum, gives off a ciliary branch for ciliary ganglion and then reaches to the rostral part of the orbit. Here it divides into two branches, the lateral and medial. The medial branch enters and supplies the nasal chamber. The lateral branch becomes superficial, innervates the integument of the frontal region, the upper eyelid, conjunctiva, the glands in the orbit, and then reaches to the tip of the upper beak. The maxillary and the mandibular branches of the trigeminal nerve leave the cranium together through the maxillary sinus. The **maxillary nerve** gets separated from the mandibular, gives off a branch that resembles the infraorbital nerve of the domestic animals and breaks up into several branches to the upper beak. The **mandibular nerve** after leaving the company of the maxillary outside the cranium divides into two branches. One of these passes through the lower mandibular bone and reaches its lower extremity. The other branch supplies the skin around the mandible and reaches the tip of the lower jaw.

The **facial nerve** is small and is distributed to the muscles of the face, jaws, tongue and erecter muscles of the feathers of the crest.

The **cervical** part of the **vagus nerve** leaves the cranium in the form of two or three separate filaments and then constitutes a single trunk after coursing for a short distance outside the cranium. The rest of the branching and distribution of this nerve is more or less similar to that in other animals. The recurrent laryngeal nerve supplies the crop in addition to the larynx.

The **hypoglossal nerve** is more or less similar to that in other domestic animals except for an additional branch given off to pass along the jugular vein to pass towards the chest. The two terminating branches, the dorsal and ventral of the hypoglossal nerve supply the corresponding surface of the tongue.

The origin, course and distribution of the **cervical spinal nerves** in fowl is same as in other domestic animals. However, their number differs. The fowl has fifteen pairs of cervical spinal nerves.

SECTION-E

APPLIED ANATOMY

39

Applied Anatomy of Head and Neck

Teeth

Estimation of age from appearance of teeth

The teeth are used as a tool for estimation of age of animal. The time of eruption and the stage of wear of incisors are usually considered as parameters for this purpose. The time of eruption of the incisor teeth in ox has been described under the chapter on gross anatomy of head. The eruption time of incisors in other species is described under the chapter on comparative anatomy of head and neck. To differentiate the deciduous teeth from the permanent teeth is important criteria in this process. The deciduous teeth are smaller, their neck is visible just above the gum line and these are usually whitish in colour. The permanent teeth are larger, their crowns are slightly wider and the neck which separates the crown from the root is concealed inside the gums. These are usually yellowish in colour. In ox, all the four incisors (deciduous) are erupted at the age of 4 years.

The permanent teeth start wearing from fifth year onward. The process of wearing commences on mesiolabial side of the masticatory surface. When the entire masticatory surface is in wear, the outer and inner enamel rings are completely separated by yellow dentin and that particular tooth is considered as leveled. In the process of wearing, the gum starts receding and the neck of the tooth is exposed. In ox, usually the wearing begins at I-1 at the age of 6 years, this is followed by I-2 at 7 years, I-3 at 8 years and I-4 at 9 years. Up to the age of 14-15 years usually all incisors fall off but those remained are reduced to small round pegs.

Wearing of molars can also be considered for estimation of age of animal but is seldom practiced because of difficulty in observing the clear status of those teeth.

Estimation of age of animal on the basis of horn rings

Apart from the teeth, the horn rings is also indicative of the age of the animal in horned cattle. In this case the age of the animal is determined from the following formula.

Age of animal = Number of horn rings + 1

Paranasal sinuses

Trephination of paranasal sinuses

The paranasal sinuses are an intricate network of air sacs inside the bones of head. There are six pairs of sinuses, the frontal, maxillary, dorsal conchal, ventral conchal, middle conchal and the sphenopalatine. All of these communicate with each other and with the nasal passage either directly or indirectly. Emphyemia and tumor of these sinuses occurs some time in large animals, Frontal sinus is most affected in cattle and maxillary sinus in horses. Removal of tumor is a difficult process but removal of the fluid or the pus from the sinuses in the cases of emphyemia is done by the process of trephination of the sinuses. For this purpose, thorough understanding of the structural relationships of all the sinuses is essential to plan the best approach to the affected sinus. Detailed anatomy of paranasal sinuses has been described under the chapter on skeleton of head and their structural differences are mentioned in under the chapter on comparative anatomy of skull.

In the process of trephining of frontal sinus, the outline of frontal sinus is drawn on the head of the animal. A transverse line is drawn from the middle of one orbital arch to the other on the fore head and the site for opening the sinus is determined on this line at a distance of about 6 to 8 cm from the midline. A hole is drilled through the rostral wall of the frontal sinus taking care to avoid the supratrochlear and supraorbital neurovascular bundles as well as the sub compartments of the sinus.

The trephining of maxillary sinus is made just dorsal and caudal to the facial tuberosity taking care to avoid any injury to the roots of the cheek teeth which project into the maxillary sinus.

Salivary glands

Ligation of parotid duct

Stenosis of parotid (Stenson's) duct is the most common affection of salivary glands in cattle. The duct of parotid gland is obstructed by a part of the bolus from mouth during mastication. This causes distension of the parotid duct and it leads to enlargement of the parotid gland.

The parotid salivary gland can be palpated in the retromandibular space (the space between the ramus of mandible and the wing of atlas vertebra) over the caudal part of the masseter muscle. The duct emerges from the distal extremity of the gland and courses along the ventral border of the masseter muscle and the medial surface of the ventral border of the ramus of the mandible, turns upward along the cranial border of masseter with the facial artery and vein and opens in the cheek at the buccal vestibule opposite the fifth cheek tooth (the anatomy of salivary gland is described under the chapter on organs and glands of head and neck).

As a remedy, ligation of the parotid duct is performed under local anaesthesia. An incision of about 6 cm is given in the skin along and parallel to the rostral border of the masseter muscle under septic conditions and then along the duct at the site of the calculus, any object causing obstruction is removed and then the duct and skin over it are sutured separately.

Lymph nodes

The parotid and mandibular lymph nodes are often examined for diagnosis of localized infection in the mouth cavity including teeth of the animal. The parotid and mandibular lymph nodes are particularly examined by palpation for judging the size and consistency of these lymph nodes and for collection of lymph from them. The **parotid lymph node** is superficial in position. It is large and movable on the cranial border of the parotid salivary gland. The **mandibular lymph node** is on the lateral side of the mandibular salivary gland. The palpable part of the mandibular salivary gland is pendant near the midline in the caudal mandibular space. The lymph node is small and firm. It is covered by sternocephalicus muscle. It can be palpated by grasping the mandible and the sternocephalicus with the thumb on the lateral surface and rolling the sternocephalicus back and forth with the finger tips until the lymph node is felt upon the mandible.

Muzzle prints as a tool for identification of individual cattle

The muzzle (planum nasolabiale) is the bare area in the middle of the upper lip extending from the edge of the upper lip to the tip of the nostrils and the surface between the nostrils. It is smooth and is kept cool and moist by the clear fluid secreted by the underlying subcutaneous nasolabial glands. A wet and moist muzzle is a sign of healthiness of the animal. A dry muzzle indicates some thing wrong with the health of the animal.

The surface of the muzzle is marked by irregular grooves outlining small polygonal areas on which the openings of the glands are visible. These openings cause distinct elevations of the polygonal areas in which the glands open. This results into a characteristic design on the muzzle. Each design thus created on the muzzle of the bovine animal is specific for that individual animal. As the animal gets older, the muzzle becomes larger. However, the pattern of ridges and grooves remains unaffected. These individual specific designs are used as a means of positive identification of the bovine animals by recording their prints (Muzzle Prints).

There are two methods for recording the muzzle print.

The first method is the ink method. It is similar to the procedure used by police in making fingerprints. In this method, the black ink (Stamp pad ink or India ink) is applied on the muzzle and this is immediately followed by pressing a white index card or paper against the muzzle. The print of the specific design of the muzzle is marked on the index card or the paper.

The other method is to take a black and white picture of the muzzle with a close-up lens of the camera.

In addition to this, a third method called the Biometric Identification System for cattle is being developed by the scientists on the basis of the muzzle designs.

Sites for some commonly used nerve blocks

Site for nerve blocks for extirpation of eyeball

The extirpation or removable of eyeball is indicated in the cases of injury to eyeball or in the cases of cancer of eyeball. The surgical process is performed under three nerve blocks, the supraorbital, auriculopalpebral and retrobulbar.

Site for supraorbital nerve block

The supraorbital nerve block is performed by injecting the anaesthetic solution in the supraorbital foramen. This foramen lies in the middle of the supraorbital groove and leads to the supraorbital canal through which the supraorbital nerve passes. The site is identified first by pressing the supraorbital groove by fingers on the frontal bone and then locating the supraorbital foramen in the groove. The needle is inserted directly into the foramen. This nerve block desensitizes the upper eyelid.

Site for auriculopalpebral nerve block

The auriculopalpebral nerve block is performed by injecting the anaesthetic agent into the temporal fossa from the zygomatic arch. This nerve block desensitizes the lower eyelid.

Site for retrobulbar nerve block

The retrobulbar nerve block is performed by passing a finger from lateral canthus of the eye into the orbit. A long needle is inserted along the finger behind the eyeball to inject the anaesthetic solution. The incision is given at the medial and lateral canthus of the eye.

Lingual Nerve Block

The lingual nerve block is indicated for removal of foreign body from the tongue, Ranula (cyst) and cut or lacerated wound on the tongue.

The tongue is innervated by three nerves. (1) The lingual nerve, a branch of trigeminal (5th cranial) nerve (2) The chorda tympani, a branch of facial (7th cranial) nerve and (3) The lingual branch of hypoglossal (12th cranial) nerve. The first two are sensitive nerves while the third one is the motor nerve. In order to achieve complete desensitization of tongue, all of these three nerves need to be blocked.

To block the lingual nerve, a long needle is inserted into the medial surface of the tongue up to the level of 5th cheek tooth.

To block the lingual branch of hypoglossal nerve, the needle is inserted about 2 cm deep in the groove formed by styloglossus and hyoglossus muscles towards the base of the tongue.

Cornual nerve block

The cornual nerve block is applied for desensitizing the horn core in cattle. The horn and the skin around the base of the horn are innervated by the cranial branch of the lacrimal nerve which is a branch of ophthalmic division of trigeminal nerve. The cornual nerve passes through the periorbital tissue dorsally and runs along the frontal crest to the base of the horn. This nerve block is performed in the cases of horn cancer and dehorning.

Site of the cornual nerve block is midway between the base of the horn and the lateral canthus of eye on the ventrolateral border of the frontal crest where the nerve is superficial.

Infraorbital nerve block

The infraorbital nerve is a branch of maxillary division of trigeminal nerve. It supplies sensory fibres through its maxillary and alveolar branches to the teeth, alveolar periosteum and gums. Apart from this, it supplies fibres to maxillary and nasal regions and the upper lip. The nerve can be approached for blockage at the infraorbital foramen. This foramen is situated on the lateral surface of maxillary bone at the level of first cheek tooth.

The infraorbital foramen is palpated as a depression in the alveolar mucosa opposite the first cheek tooth just rostral to the facial crest that extends rostroventrally from the facial tuberosity. The facial tuberosity, facial crest and the first cheek tooth are used as landmarks for identifying the location of the infraorbital foramen. The needle is placed rostrocaudally to the entrance of the foramen. This will desensitize all dentition, labial, buccal area and the bone and soft tissue of the maxillary jaw.

Supraorbital nerve block

The supraorbital nerve block is indicated in the cases of operations on upper eyelid, trephining of frontal sinus and management of wounds on the forehead. The supraorbital (frontal) nerve is a branch of ophthalmic nerve. It emerges through the supraorbital foramen which is situated in the supraorbital groove about 2.5 cm medial to the root (base) of the supraorbital (zygomatic) process. The site of the foramen is identified by pressing the forehead and feeling the groove and the depression in the groove by fingertips.

Mandibular alveolar nerve block

The mandibular alveolar nerve block is indicated for surgical conditions of molar and incisor teeth of the lower jaw, body of the mandible and the lower lip. The mandibular nerve is a branch of the mandibular division of the trigeminal nerve. The nerve enters the mandibular canal through the mandibular foramen, passes through the canal and gets exit through the mental foramen after giving out the alveolar branch to pass through the body of the mandible.

The mandibular foramen lies at the middle of the medial surface of the vertical part of the ramus of the mandible. The site for blocking the nerve at the mandibular foramen is approached by inserting the needle from the lower angle of the jaw. The foramen is located at the crossing point of the horizontal line passing along the masticatory (table) surfaces of the mandibular cheek teeth and the perpendicular line passing through the lateral canthus of the eye.

Mental nerve block

The mental nerve block is indicated for surgical interventions on the chin and lower lip. The mental nerve is the branch of the mandibular alveolar nerve. It exits through the mental foramen and supplies to the skin on the chin and the mucous membrane of the lower lip.

The mental foramen is situated on the lateral surface of the ramus of the mandible near its junction with the body of the mandible. The foramen lies in a depression, the mental fossa on the lateral side of inter dental space about 5 cm behind the

4th incisor. The depression (fossa) can be felt as a oval soft area by pressing with the thumb. The needle is inserted rostro-caudally parallel to the surface of the mandible.

Shining of eyes in the dark

The eyeballs of some animals (e.g. cattle) look shining in the dark night. This is due to the presence of variously coloured area, the tapetum lucidum in the dorsal part of the fundus of the choroid of the eyeball. This part is avascular in nature. The tapetum cells consist of crystalline rods arranged in such a way that the light striking them is split into its components resulting in the characteristic iridescence. When the animal looks towards the light, the tapetum makes the eyes to shine.

The tapetum is supposed to be nocturnal in adaptation, so by reflecting the light it stimulates the light sensitive receptor cells in the overlying retina and thus helps into seeing in the dark.

Clinical examination of neck

In the clinical examination of neck in the cattle, buffalo and horse, the cervical part of the **trachea** can be palpated throughout its length starting from the laryngeal mound to the thoracic inlet where it continues further as thoracic part. Throughout its length the ventral surface of the cervical part of trachea is covered by sternocephalicus and sternothyrohyoideus muscles. These muscles of the opposite sides form a thin sheet on the ventral surface of trachea and can be followed to their laryngeal and hyoid insertions. The muscles of the opposite sides diverge from each other at the level of 4th tracheal ring, leaving the trachea to become subcutaneous from first to fourth tracheal ring. This area is the site best suitable for tracheotomy. The **thyroid gland** can be palpated on the lateral surface of trachea just caudal to larynx. It is very soft and flat and is covered by sternocephalicus muscle.

The **oesophagus** lies lateral to trachea in the middle third of the neck. It is viewed by observing the act of swallow or eructation. In case of chocking due to obstruction, the oesophagotomy is preferred to be performed at this site.

For observations on **jugular vein**, it is distended by compressing over the jugular in the lower part of the neck. The jugular when passes through the jugular groove (furrow) which is bounded dorsally by brachiocephalicus, ventrally by sternocephalicus and medially by sternomastoid part of sternocephalicus muscle. It is covered externally by skin and fascia. Venipuncture is usually performed above the middle of the neck, where the jugular vein is separated from the carotid artery by the omohyoideus. Some times carotid pulse is seen in the jugular groove. This can be identified by palpation. It is a resultant of insufficiency of the right atrioventricular valve. It can be obliterated by pressing at the lower cervical part in front of the first rib.

Clinical affections in neck

The most common affections in the neck is the **yoke gall** in cattle and buffalo and the **fistula wither**, **poll evil** and **bursitis** in horses. There is a common factor in all these conditions that it is the acute inflammation of skin and subcutaneous tissue over the dorsum of the neck. In extreme conditions it may lead to damage of the nuchal ligament. The anatomy of nuchal ligament is described under the chapter on the joints of head and neck.

PART-1.3: ANATOMY OF THORAX

SECTION-A
MUSCULO-SKELETAL COMPONENT

40

Skeleton of Thorax

The skeleton of thorax (Fig. 3-1) consists of a bony cage formed by thirteen thoracic vertebrae constituting its dorsal boundary and roof, thirteen pairs of ribs forming its lateral walls, the costal cartilages which assist the ribs to form the lateral walls and the sternum forming its floor.

The general architecture of the vertebrae and the vertebral column is described in the chapter on skeletal system under PART ONE (Systemic anatomy) of this book. Only the deviations from the general characteristics of vertebrae as occur in the thoracic vertebrae are described here in the following account on the thoracic vertebrae.

Thoracic vertebrae

These are thirteen in number in ox (Fig. 3-1 A and B) The characteristic features of these vertebrae are the presence of capitular facets for articulation with the head of the rib and the greater development of dorsal spinous processes (neural spines).for attachment of muscles of the back and the supraspinous ligament that helps in the ligamentum nuchae to extend and suspend the head with the body trunk.

The bodies of the thoracic vertebrae are shorter than those of the other regions of the body. On either sides of the cranial and caudal articular ends of the body, are concave semi lunar capitular facets which with those of the adjacent vertebrae and the intervertebral substance form costal cavities for articulation with the head of the rib. Thus each rib articulates with two adjacent vertebrae by way of these capitular facets. The last thoracic vertebra has no capitular facet. The notches in the pedicles at the cranial edges of the arch of the vertebrae are shallower than those at the caudal edges. Those of the caudal edges in the last few thoracic vertebrae are converted into foramina. The body of the thoracic vertebrae is distinctly constricted in the middle and on its ventral surface it bears a thin edged ventral crest in addition to the usual notches.

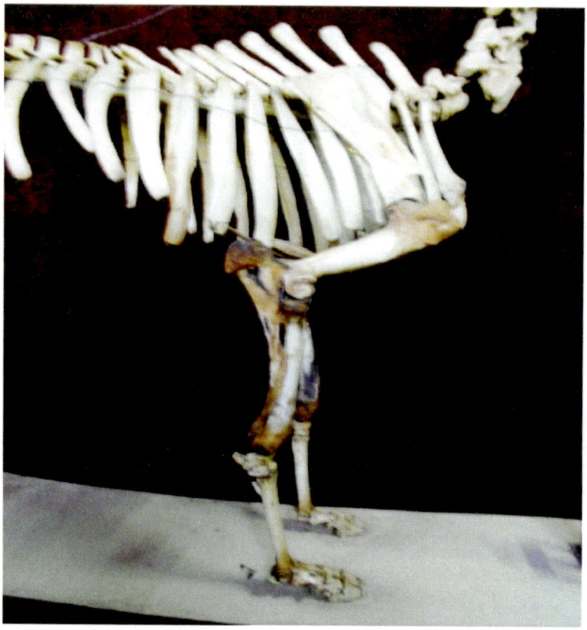

Fig. 3–1: Skeleton (Bony cage) of thorax

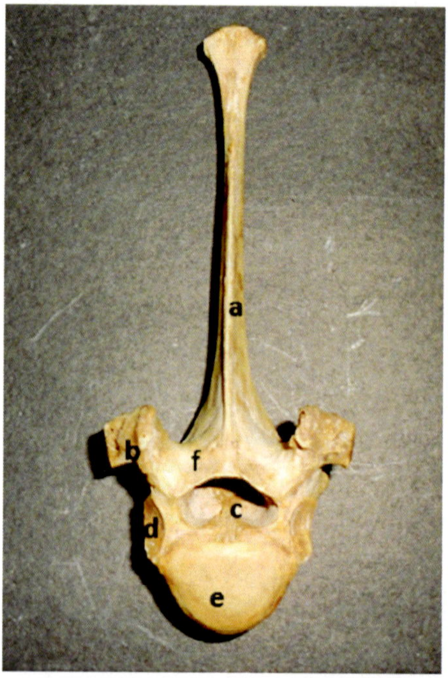

Fig. 3–1 A: Thoracic vertebra of Ox

a. Supraspinous process; b. Transverse process; c. Neural ring; d. Costal facet, e. Body of thoracic vertebra; f. Cranial articular facet.

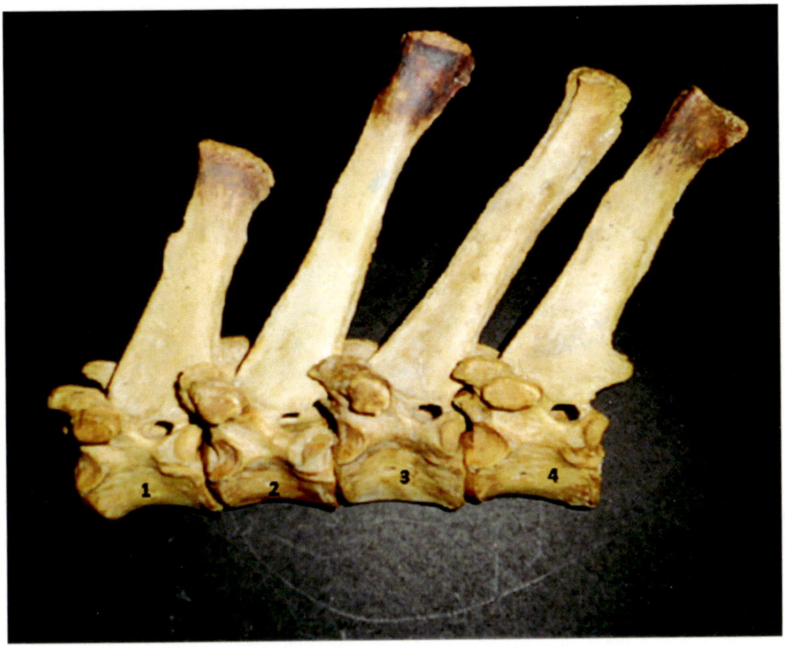

Fig 3–1 B: Thoracic vertebrae of Ox (2nd to 5th)
1.First Thoracic vertebra; 2. Second Thoracic vertebra; 3. Third Thoracic vertebra; 4. Fourth Thoracic vertebra

The spinous processes of thoracic vertebrae are distinctly longer than those in the other regions. The first is shorter than the second, the second and third are prominently high and caudal to this there is a gradual diminution in height. This particular part of the back of the animal forms humph region in bovine animals. The backward slope of the spinous processes is slight initially but it increases gradually up to the tenth thoracic vertebra. The last thoracic vertebra has a straight vertical spine. The transverse processes are thick, short, undivided, strong and tuberous at their free borders. On the ventrolateral aspect, the transverse process presents a tubercular facet for articulation with the tubercle of the corresponding rib. These tubercular facets gradually decrease in size craniocaudally in the series. The articular processes are very small. The cranial ones in the series are represented by small oval facets on the cranial part of the arch.

Ribs

The ribs (Fig. 3-1 C) are elongated, flat curved bony plates which form the skeleton of lateral walls of the thorax. They are arranged in pairs extending obliquely downward from the vertebrae on both side and joining with the sternum at the floor of the thorax. They are serially arranged in pairs and their number corresponds with the number of thoracic vertebrae. In ox there are thirteen pairs of ribs. The first eight of these are termed as sternal ribs or true ribs because they reach to and articulate with the sternum individually by means of their cartilages. Whereas, the remaining five ribs are called as asternal or false ribs because they join each other at their ventral extremity by means of a common cord of cartilage that articulates on either side of the caudal end of the sternum. Each rib has a body and two extremities. The elongated body is, flattened and curved approximately in upper half of its length while its lower half is twisted and inclined inwards. The point at which the rib is most curved is called as angle of the rib and it bears a rough area for attachment of longissimus thoracis muscle. The lateral surface is convex and bears a wide groove close to its cranial border. The medial surface is smooth, concave and bears a distinct groove close to its caudal border. This is termed as subcostal groove. It runs downward up to the middle of the body of the rib and then disappears. This groove is meant for lodging the intercostal vessels and nerves. The cranial border is concave while the caudal border is correspondingly convex. Both the borders are thin and sharp and provide an area for attachment of intercostal muscles. The dorsal or vertebral extremity presents head, neck and tubercle. The head bears an articular area made up of two convex facets, the cranial and caudal costal facets separated by a nonarticular groove. These two facets articulate with the two adjacent thoracic vertebrae, except the first rib which forms articulation with the last cervical and first thoracic vertebra. The nonarticular groove provides attachment to the intraarticular ligament of the head of the rib. Neck is the constriction below the head and is roughened for the attachment of ligaments. Just caudal to the junction of head and neck is tubercle. At its dorsal surface it presents a transversely placed concave facet for articulation with the transverse process of the caudal of the two thoracic vertebrae with which the head of the rib articulates. This facet of the last two ribs is comparatively smaller and almost flat. The ventral extremity of the rib is smooth and articulated with the costal cartilage.

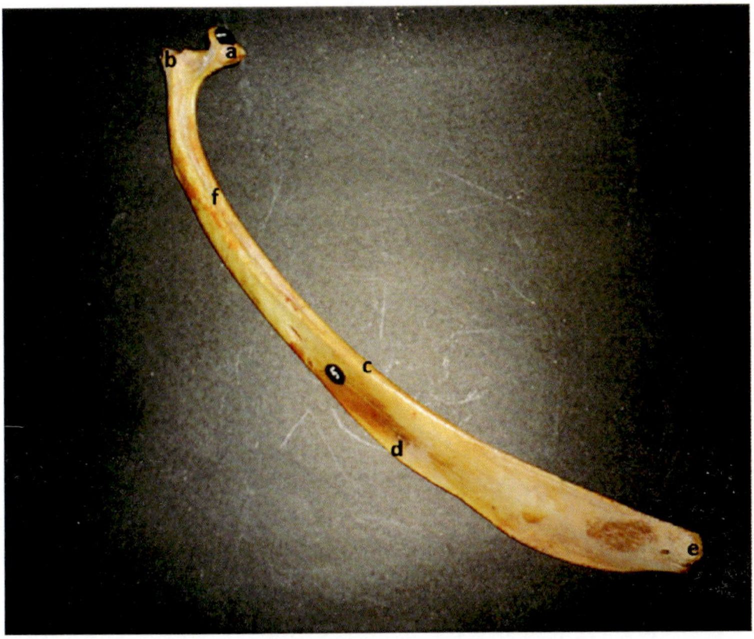

Fig. 3–1 C: Rib of Ox
a.Head of rib; b. Tubercle; c. Cranial border; d. Caudal border; e. Distal extremity; f. Costal groove; 5. Body of rib.

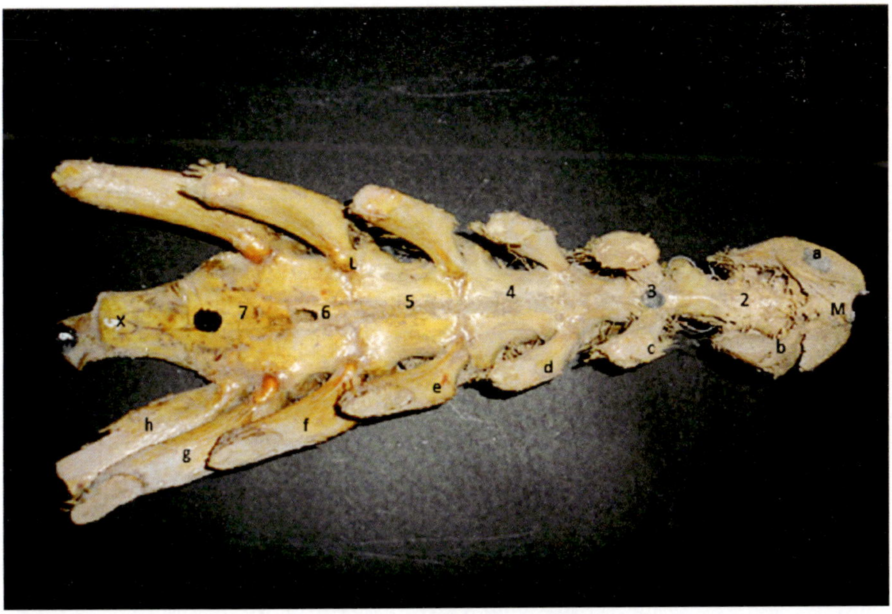

Fig 3–1 D: Sternum of Ox
1-7 Sternabrae; a – h first to eighth costal cartilage; L. Sternochondral junction; M. Manubrium sterni; X . Xiphoid cartilage.

Special characteristics of ribs: The first rib is shortest and least curved. The ventral extremity is greatly widened. The lateral surface presents rough area for attachment of scalenus medius muscle. At the lower part of the cranial border is a smooth impression formed by the axilary vessels. Just dorsal to this is another impression made by dorsal root of brachial plexus. The tubercle of first rib is largest. The eighth, ninth and tenth ribs are longest and widest. Both in front and behind these, the length and width of the ribs diminishes gradually. The head and tubercle diminishes in size from first to last rib.

Costal cartilages

The costal cartilages are elongated cylindrical rods of hyaline cartilage lying between the ribs and the sternum. The upper extremity of the costal cartilage forms an articulation with the rib and continues the corresponding rib to the sternum. While the lower extremity forms a joint with the sternum. The first eight costal cartilages form diorthroidal joints with the sternum and hence are called as costal cartilages of sternal ribs while the rests do not reach to the sternum, hence they are called the costal cartilages of asternal ribs.. They are longer, slender and pointed. They overlap and are attached to each other by elastic tissue to form the costal arch. The first costal cartilage is shortest. Its dorsal (costal) end is wide and thick. The ventral (sternal) end is small. The cartilages of other sternal ribs progressively increase in length and become more rounded.

Sternum

The sternum (Fig. 3-1 D) is medially placed central osseocartilaginous structure forming the floor of the thorax. It consists of seven sternebrae. It is elongated craniocaudally, flattened dorsoventrally and compressed laterally till about its middle. It is directed obliquely downward and backward. It has three parts namely- the cranial presternum or manubrium sterni, the middle mesosternum or body and the caudal xiphi sternum. The dorsal surface is narrow in front and becomes gradually wider behind. It gives attachment to the dorsal sternal ligament running along the central line on this surface. Lateral to the ligament it provides attachment to triangularis sterni muscles. This surface forms the floor of the thorax. The ventral surface is extensive. It is strongly convex at the level of the first sternebra but more or less concave behind the second sternebra. This surface presents attachment to the pectoral muscle and the rectus abdominis muscle. Both the surfaces present transverse marks indicating the lines of fusion of the adjacent sternebrae. The lateral borders are thick in front and thinner behind. Each border has eight concave articular facets for articulating with the corresponding costal cartilages. The first sternebra has two facets while the rests have one each. The cranial extremity of the sternum is formed by the cranial border of the first sternebra and it forms manubrium sterni. Behind this is the body. The caudal extremity is formed by xiphoid cartilage which is attached to the caudal border of the eighth sternebra. The xiphoid cartilage is thin flexible and heart shaped. Its dorsal surface is concave and it presents attachment to diaphragm close to its junction with last sternebra. The part of the xiphoid cartilage behind the line of attachment of diaphragm forms the part of floor of abdomen and it presents on its ventral surface an area for attachment of rectus abdominis muscle and linea alba.

41

Comparative Anatomy of Skeleton of Thorax

Horse

The **bony cage** of thorax is longer but narrower in horse than that in ox. It is compressed laterally

The **thoracic vertebrae** are eighteen in number. Their bodies are shorter. The spinous process of the first one is shorter and it is curved backward. The height of the spinous process increases up to third and fourth and there after it diminishes gradually up to fifteenth beyond which it is almost same. The backward inclination of the spinous process is most pronounced in the second. The spine of the sixth vertebra is straightly vertical and that of the last two vertebrae is directed slightly forward.

The **ribs** are in eighteen pairs. First eight pairs are sternal and the remaining ten pairs are asternal. These are shorter, narrower and more curved. The length of the ribs increases up to sixth and then it diminishes. The cranial borders of the ribs from second to sixth are sharp and from ninth to eighteenth they are rounded and thick. The lower edges of the ribs are excavated for receiving the costal cartilages. The first rib inclines little forwards, the second rib is vertical and the rests slope backwards.

The first pair of **costal cartilages** articulates at their distal ends with each other and with the sternum. The upper ends of the cartilages form synarthroidial joints with the ribs.

The **sternum** of horse is composed of seven sternebrae. It is canoe or boat shaped and presents three faces, three borders and two extremities. It is compressed laterally in front and dorsoventrally behind. The dorsal surface is narrow and triangular. It is concave craniocaudally. The lateral surfaces are convex above and slightly concave below. The lateral borders separate the dorsal surface from the lateral surfaces and they give attachment to two lateral sternal ligaments. The ventral border is the direct continuation of the cariniform cartilage of the cranial extremity of the sternum. It is thin, sharp and convex from before backwards. It is very prominent and can be felt by palpation in live animal. It is also called as sternal crest or keel. The cranial extremity presents a laterally compressed cariniform cartilage which presents a deep notch dorsally for articulation with the first pair of costal cartilages. The first sternebra is fused with second and the manubrium is made up of cariniform cartilage and the first sternebra.

Dog

The **bony cage** of the thorax of dog is barrel shaped.

The **thoracic vertebrae** in dog are thirteen in number. The bodies of the vertebrae are wider. The transverse processes of the vertebrae except the first two or three possess mammillary processes. The last three thoracic vertebrae posses accessory processes projecting backwards from the caudal end of the arch of the vertebrae. In these three vertebrae the caudal facets of the vertebral body are absent. The spinous processes of the thoracic vertebrae mark wide variations. The first three or four and the last three spines are equal in height but these are greater than the middle six or seven spines. The spines in the middle series decrease gradually from fourth to tenth. The spine of the eleventh segment is nearly vertical while those of first ten are directed backwards and the last two are inclined slightly forward.

The **ribs** are thirteen pairs in number. The first nine are sternal and the last four are asternal. The last pair of ribs is usually floating. The shafts of the ribs are cylindrical and very strongly curved. The shaft of first eight or nine ribs increases in width at their distal extremity. The first rib is very long and highly curved.

The **costal cartilages** are long and curved ventrally and cranially. The length and curvature of the first costal cartilage is especially characteristic.

The **sternum** of dog is composed of eight sternebrae and these are usually fused in extreme old ages. It is rod like, constricted in the middle and wide at the extremities. The first segment, manubrium is the longest. Its cranial end is blunt and pointed and it bears a short conical presternal cariniform cartilage. The last segment, xiphoid cartilage is long and narrow.

Sheep and Goat

The bony cage of the thorax is wider than that of horse.

The **thoracic vertebrae** in sheep and goat are usually thirteen in number but in rare cases fourteen or even twelve may occur. The bodies of the vertebrae are relatively wider and less constricted than those in ox. The extremities (convexity and concavity) of the vertebral bodies are not strongly curved. The intervertebral foramina are relatively larger.

The **ribs** are usually thirteen pairs but occurrence of fourteen pairs is not uncommon. The last rib is usually floating and its cartilage is very short. The fourteenth rib if present is necessarily floating. The first eight ribs are sternal and the last five are asternal. The ribs are narrow and are strongly curved in the cranial segments.

The second to eleventh **costal cartilages** form synovial joints with their ribs. The costal cartilages are relatively short.

The **sternum** is wider, flatter and relatively longer than that of the horse and ox. It consists of seven sternebrae. The manubrium is somewhat wedge shaped and laterally compressed. The dorsal part of manubrium sterni has a large notch on each side for articulation with first costal cartilage. The presternal cariniform cartilage of the manubrium is absent. The xiphoid cartilage is similar to that of ox but relatively larger than it.

Pig

The **bony cage** of thorax is long and more barrel shaped in pig than that in ox and horse since ribs in pig are more strongly curved and are of almost equal length.

The **thoracic vertebrae** are fourteen or fifteen in number. The bodies of these vertebrae are relatively long. They are constricted in the middle. The ventral crest of the body is absent. The extremities of the body are elliptical, depressed in the middle and prominent at the periphery. The arch is perforated by a foramen on each side. This foramen communicates with the lateral vertebral foramen which is formed at the root of the transverse processes of the vertebrae. The mammillary processes project from the cranial articular processes of the last five or six vertebrae. The first spinous process is broad, very high and is inclined slightly craniad. The spinous processes of the rest of the vertebrae diminish gradually up to tenth vertebra and behind this they are equal in height. The second to tenth spinous processes are directed slightly caudad, the eleventh is nearly vertical and the rests up to the last one are inclined cranially.

The **ribs** are fourteen or fifteen pairs in number. The first seven are sternal and the last seven or eight are asternal. The fifteenth pair when present is usually floating. All the ribs are strongly curved. The first rib is prismatic and has a large ventral end and a short cartilage. The width of the ribs from third to sixth is greatest and the length of sixth and seventh ribs is greatest.

The **costal cartilages** are wide and plate like. The second to fifth costal cartilages form synovial joints with the ribs.

The **sternum** resembles to that of ox in form. It consists of six sternebrae. The first one, the manubrium sterni is long and is laterally flattened. The cranial end of the manubrium bears a blunt cartilage and its caudal end forms a synovial joint with the body of the sternum. The body of the sternum is flattened dorsoventrally and wide transversely in the middle and it is narrow at either ends. The last sternebra has a narrow long xiphoid process that bears the xiphoid cartilage.

Fowl

The **thoracic vertebrae** are seven in number. The first and sixth are free, second to fifth are fused into a single piece and the seventh is fused with the lumbosacral segment of the vertebral column. Each vertebra presents a complete capitular cavity (instead of capitular facet) for the head of the rib. The dorsal and ventral spines are well developed. The transverse processes are plate like and present tubercular facets.

The **ribs** are seven pairs in number. Each rib is made up of the dorsal portion called the vertebral rib and the ventral portion called the sternal rib. The first, second and usually the seventh rib do not have sternal portion. The dorsal and ventral parts (vertebral and sternal ribs) articulate with each other in a diorthroidal joint. The head of the rib articulates with the capitular cavity of the vertebra. Except the first and seventh, the caudal border of each vertebral rib presents an uncinate process which is directed backwards and upwards to overlie on the lateral surface of the next rib.

The **sternum** of fowl is a large quadrilateral curved plate of bone. It forms the floor of the thoracic cavity and partly of the abdominal cavity. The dorsal surface of the central mass of the bone, the **body** is concave craniocaudally as well as transversely. It continues caudally into a long process called as **metasternum**. The ventral surface of the body presents a prominent median longitudinal sternal crest called as **keel** which presents a large area for attachment of strong breast muscles that help in flying in birds. The cranial end of the body presents a median process projected craniodorsally which is called as **rostrum.** The furculum of the clavicle is attached by a ligament to the rostrum. On either side of the rostrum are elongated saddle shaped areas for articulation with the lower end of the coracoids. The rostrum is pierced at its root by a foramen. The craniolateral and caudolateral processes extend respectively from the craniolateral and caudolateral aspect of the body. The **craniolateral processes** one each on either side project forward and are called as **costal processes**. These costal processes present five double facets for articulation with the sternal ribs. The **caudolateral processes** project backwards as a single plate on each side and divides into dorsal and ventral parts. The short dorsal parts overlap the last two ribs while the longer ventral parts terminate into the **xiphoid process**.

42

Articulations of Thorax

Articulations of thoracic vertebrae

These are (1) **Intercentral articulations** which are amphiarthroses formed between the bodies of the adjacent vertebrae and (2) **Inter neural articulations** which are diarthroses formed between the articular processes of the vertebrae. These articulations are similar to the articulations described for typical vertebrae of the cervical region. The only difference is that the supraspinous ligament in the thoracic part of vertebral column is single as against two parts the funicular and lamellar parts of the cervical part of this ligament. The supra spinous ligament in the thoracic part is the backward continuation of the funicular division of its cervical part which extends medially behind from the occipital eminence , passes through the cervical region as nuchal ligament and continues behind over the summits of the spinous processes of the thoracic and lumbar vertebrae and finally terminates on the sacrum.

Articulations of ribs

Costovertebral articulations

The articulations of the ribs with thoracic vertebrae are called the costovertebral articulations. These are of two types, the costocentral and costotransverse.

The **costocentral articulation** is a trochoid or rotatory joint formed between the head of the rib and the capitular facets of the two adjacent vertebrae and the intervertebral disc between the corresponding vertebrae. The two facets separated by nonarticular groove on the head of the rib correspond to the capitular facets of the two adjacent vertebrae. The joint thus formed is covered by the **capsular ligament** (joint capsule). The joint capsule is supported from outside by the **accessory ligaments**. These are the radiate ligament and the round ligament. The **radiate ligament** extends from the neck of the rib, divides into three filaments which pass one each on the bodies of the corresponding two adjacent vertebrae and the intervertebral disc between them. The **round** (conjugal) intraarticular **ligament** is attached to the groove on the head of the rib, passes transversely into the vertebral canal under the dorsal common vertebral ligament, divides into two branches, one of these gets attached to the body of the vertebra of the cranial segment of the concerned joint and the other reaches across to the head of the rib of the opposite side and gets attached to it. While crossing the side, this ligament is attached to the intervertebral disc of the concerned segment. The joint cavity of the costocentral articulation is divided into two divisions by the round ligament. The round ligament is, however, absent in the first costocentral articulation.

The **costotransverse articulation** is a gliding joint formed between the tubercle of the rib and the tubercular facet on the transverse process of the corresponding thoracic vertebra. The joint has a **capsular ligament** which is reinforced by two other ligaments called the cranial and caudal costotransverse ligaments. The **cranial costotransverse ligament** connects the neck of the rib to the ventromedial part of the transverse process of the concerned vertebra. The **caudal costotransverse ligament** connects the tubercle of the rib to the lateral of the transverse process of the concerned vertebra.

The **movement** performed by these joints is the rotation around an axis connecting the centre of the head and tubercle of the rib.

Costochondral articulations

The costochondral articulations are diarthroses (synovial) with little movements and are formed between the ventral end of the ribs and the cartilages that are interposed between the rib and the sternum (costal cartilages). Each of these joints are covered by the joint capsule that is reinforced externally by the collateral ligaments. These joints are formed by only second to eleventh ribs in ox. The first pair of ribs articulates separately with the first sternebra.

Chondrosternal articulations

The chondrosternal articulations are the diarthroses formed between the cartilages of the sternal ribs (second to eleventh) and the sternum. The first chondrosternal joint is formed between the ventral ends of the first pair of ribs and the first sternal segment. Each of this pair is a separate joint with a separate joint capsule. A strong cruciate ligament keeps the joint capsule of the two sides apart from each other. The chondrosternal articulations from second to eighth sternal ribs are formed between the ventral ends of the respective costal cartilages and the corresponding articular facets which are placed laterally on the junctions of the sternal segments. The ligaments of these joints are the capsular ligament and the dorsal and ventral chondrosternal ligaments. The capsular ligament surrounds the joint. The dorsal chondrosternal ligament connects the ventral end of the cartilage to the dorsal surface of the sternum.

The ventral chondrosternal ligament connects the ventral end of the cartilage to the ventral surface of the sternum. The movement performed at this joint is rotation around the vertical axis except at the first chondrosternal joint.

Interchondral articulations

The asternal cartilages are united at their free ventral extremities to the cartilages of their respective cranial costal cartilages by small elastic interchondral ligament thus forming the costal arch which is attached to the Ziphoid cartilage of the sternum. The eighth and ninth costal cartilages are united with each other by fibrous tissue and are also attached to the Ziphoid cartilage by chondroxiphoid ligament.

Articulations of sternum

The sternal articulations are amphiarthroses. The seven segments (sternebrae) are joined to one other through the discs of cartilages. The first sternebra is articulated to second forming a diarthrosis which permits movements. The rests are the amphiarthroses. The different segments are connected by a common suprasternal ligament. To start with in the first segment this ligament is narrow and as it passes caudally it widens and ends on the last sternebra,

Comparative anatomy of articulations of thorax

There ere no major differences in the articulations of bones of thorax in ox, horse, dog and pig. The articulations of the bones of thorax of fowl have some deviations which have been mentioned with the description of the concerned bones.

43

Muscles of Thorax

Cutaneous muscle

The cutaneous muscle of the thoracic region is a part of the cutaneous muscle of the trunk. It arises from the interbrachial fascia on the medial surface of the arm and elbow and the lateral aspect of the arm and shoulder. It extends as a broad sheet between the shoulder and arm cranially and the stifle and thigh caudally and then upward to the middle of the dorsum and the tuber coxae.

Fascia of thorax

The fascia of the thoracic region is the caudal continuation of cervical fascia. It is in two layers, the superficial and deep. The superficial fascia is continuous with that of the skin and the cutaneous muscle. The deep fascia forms a well developed sheath for aponeurosis with the longissimus muscle. It is attached medially to the supraspinous ligament and the summits of the spinous processes of the thoracic vertebrae while laterally it is attached to the lateral surface of the ribs. From here it continues ventrolaterally and passes medial to the scapula under the rhomboideus thoracis muscle.

Muscles of thorax

The muscles of thorax (Fig. 3-2A) are grouped in two major groups, the muscles of thoracic vertebrae and the muscles of the thoracic wall. The **muscles of vertebrae** in the thoracic region are the erector muscles of the spine. These are also named as muscles of the back region of the trunk. The main function of these muscles is to erect the spine (back) of the trunk. The **muscles of the thoracic wall** are the muscles attached to the lateral and ventral part of the thoracic wall. The main function of these muscles is to assist in the act of expiration.

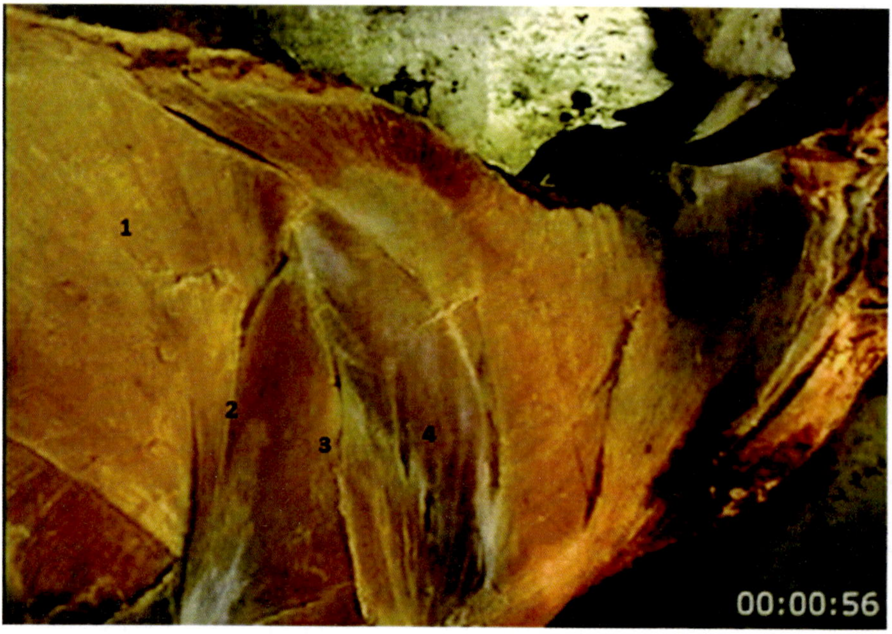

Fig. 3–2 A: Muscles of Thorax

1. Latissimus dorsi; 2. Tensor fascia antebrachii; 3. Long head of triceps brachii; 4. Infraspinatus; 5. Serratus ventralis thoracis; 6. Brachiocephalicus; 7. Teres minor; 8. Trapezius; 9. Omotransversarious.

Muscles of spine (Back)

Iliocostalis thoracis

Is a segmented muscle starting from the transverse process of fourth lumbar vertebra and passing cranially up to fifth rib on the dorsolateral aspect of the thorax. The muscle is composed of series of bundles. Each segment of these bundles originates on the lateral surface of the rib crosses a few ribs and intercostal spaces cranially and ends on the caudal border of the preceding third or fourth rib.

Origin: The cranial border and lateral surface of the ribs, except the first five and the ends of transverse processes of first four lumbar vertebrae.

Insertion: The caudal border of all ribs and transverse process of last cervical vertebra.

Relations: It is related superficially to serratus dorsalis and ventralis, latissimus dorsi and obliquus abdominis externus muscles and deeply to the lateral surface of ribs and external intercostal muscles. It is medially related to longissimus dorsi muscle.

Action: Erection of the spine.

Blood supply: Dorsal intercostal arteries.

Nerve supply: Thoracic spinal nerves.

Longissimus dorsi

The longissimus dorsi is the largest and longest muscle of the body extending from sacrum and ilium to the atlas vertebra covering the pelvic, abdominal, thoracic and cervical parts. It is a prism shaped three sided muscle lying in the angle between spinous processes and the transverse processes of the vertebrae and the dorsal ends of the ribs. The thoracic part of this muscle is named as longissimus thoracis.

Longissimus thoracis (Longissimus costarum)

The thoracic part of the longissimus muscle is quite fleshy and is arranged in to two distinct masses with separate tendons of insertions. Each segment of the muscle originates into a series of fasciculi directed obliquely forward and downward, passes cranially crossing two or three intercostal spaces and then terminates on the caudal border of the rib.

Origin: The thoracic (costal) part of the longissimus (longissimus thoracis) muscle originates on the anterior border and the lateral surface of the dorsal parts of the last eight or nine ribs.

Insertion: The thoracic part of the muscle inserts on the caudal border of ribs from first to tenth ribs and to transverse process of the last cervical vertebra.

Relations: This muscle is related superficially to serratus dorsalis, deeply to the ribs, external intercostal muscle and medially to longissimus dorsi muscle.

Action: This muscle is powerful extensor of the back (dorsal spine). It assists in the act of expiration.

Blood supply: Dorsal intercostal arteries.

Nerve supply: Dorsal branches of thoracic spinal nerves.

Semispinalis thoracis (longissimus thoracis)

This is a thick mass of muscle extending from the transverse process of first lumbar vertebra to the third cervical vertebra.

Origin: From transverse process of first lumbar vertebra and last four thoracic vertebrae.

Insertion: The lateral surface of the dorsal spines and the interspinous ligament from first to tenth thoracic vertebrae.

Action: to assist in erection of spine.

Blood supply: Dorsal intercostal arteries.

Nerve supply: Dorsal branches of thoracic spinal nerves.

Multifidus thoracis

The Multifidus is a long and segmented muscle attached to the spinous processes of the vertebrae from sacrum to neck and is named as Multifidus dorsi. In the thoracic part (Multifidus thoracis), each segment or bundle of the muscle is flattened. It originates on the transverse processes of the thoracic vertebra and passes obliquely upward and forward to insert on the lateral surface and caudal border of the spinous process of the second or third vertebra preceding the vertebra of its origin.

Origin: The transverse processes of the thoracic vertebrae.

Insertion: Summits of the spinous process of the second or third thoracic vertebra preceding the vertebra of origin.

Relations: The Multifidus thoracis is related laterally to the longissimus dorsi, medially to the supraspinous processes of the vertebrae and the interspinous ligaments.

Action: It is extensor of the spine.

Blood supply: Dorsal intercostal arteries.

Nerve supply: Dorsal branches of thoracic spinal nerves.

Blood supply: Dorsal intercostal arteries.

Nerve supply: Dorsal branches of thoracic spinal nerves.

Muscles of thoracic wall

Levatores costarum

This is a segmented muscle having eleven pairs in ox. They constitute a series of small muscles which overlie the vertebral ends of the intercostal spaces. The muscle at each segment is triangular in shape. It arises by tendinous fibres which pass caudally, ventrally and laterally to insert on the cranial border of the succeeding rib. Near its termination, the muscle segment intimately blends with the corresponding external intercostal muscle.

Origin: Transverse processes of the thoracic vertebrae

Insertion: The cranial border of succeeding ribs, second to thirteenth.

Relations: The muscle levatores costarum is related superficially to the longissimus thoracis and Iliocostalis thoracis muscles and deeply to the ribs, internal intercostal muscle and the intercostal vessels and nerves.

Action: To draw the ribs craniad and thus to assist in inspiration.

Blood supply: Dorsal intercostal arteries.

Nerve supply: Intercostal nerves.

External intercostal (Intercostalis externi)

The intercostal muscles fill in the intercostal spaces. Each of these muscles extends from the levatores costarum to the distal extremity of the rib. These muscles do not reach to the interchondral spaces. These muscles contain the fleshy as well as tendinous fibres. The fibres of these muscles pass obliquely downward and backward from the caudal border of one rib to the cranial border of the succeeding rib.

Origin: The caudal border of each rib.

Insertion: the cranial border of the succeeding rib.

Relations: Laterally to latissimus dorsi, serratus thoracis and many more muscles of shoulder girdle. It is medially related to the internal intercostal muscle and the intercostal vessels and nerve.

Action: To assist in inspiration.

Blood supply: Dorsal intercostal arteries.

Nerve supply: Intercostal nerves.

Internal intercostal (Intercostalis interni)

The internal intercostal muscles also lie in the intercostal spaces with the preceding muscle. It lies internal to the preceding muscle feeling the intercostal space from the levatores costarum to the interchondral spaces up to the sternum. The fibres of these muscles extend in opposite direction to that of the preceding muscle. This muscle extends from the cranial border of the rib, pass forward and upward and terminate on the caudal border of the preceding rib.

Origin: The cranial borders of the ribs and their cartilages.

Insertion: The caudal borders of the preceding ribs and their cartilages.

Relations: Laterally it is related to the external intercostal and levatores costarum muscles and the intercostal vessels and nerves. Medially, it is related to the costal pleura, diaphragm and other muscles of the thoracic wall.

Action: The intercostal part of the muscle assists in expiration and the interchondral part assists in inspiration.

Blood supply: Dorsal intercostal arteries.

Nerve supply: Intercostal nerves.

Retractor costae

It is a small, flat, thin triangular muscle located in the angle formed by the last rib and the ends of the lumbar transverse processes.

Origin: Transverse processes of the first three or four lumbar vertebrae.

Insertion: The caudal border of the last rib.

Relations: It is related superficially to the last segment of the serratus dorsalis caudalis, longissimus lumborum and Iliocostalis lumborum muscles and deeply to the aponeurosis of the transversus abdominis muscle.

Action: To retract the last rib and assist in the forced expiration.

Blood supply: Dorsal costoabdominal artery.

Nerve supply: Costoabdominal nerve.

Serratus dorsalis

This muscle has two divisions, the cranial and caudal, which are attached to the corresponding areas of the dorsolateral thoracic wall.

Serratus dorsalis cranialis

Origin: By means of aponeurosis on the thoracolumbar fascia.

Insertion: The cranial border of lateral surface of sixth to ninth ribs.

Relations: It is related superficially to serratus ventralis thoracis and latissimus dorsi and deeply to the ribs, intercostal external, iliocostalis and longissimus thoracis muscles.

Action: It assists in inspiration by drawing the ribs craniad and laterad.

Blood supply: Dorsal intercostal arteries.

Nerve supply: Intercostal nerves.

Serratus dorsalis caudalis

Origin: By means of aponeurosis on the thoracolumbar fascia.

Insertion: On the last lateral surface of the last four ribs.

Relations: This muscle is related superficially to the skin, fascia and latissimus dorsi and deeply to the ribs, external intercostal and retractor thoracis muscles.

Action: Same as cranial division.

Rectus thoracis

The rectus thoracis is a thin and flat muscle lying on the cranioventral aspect of the thorax especially the first three intercostal spaces.

Origin: Ventral half of the caudolateral aspect of the first rib, ventral to the insertion of scalinus muscle.

Insertion: Costal cartilages of third to fifth ribs and the adjacent area of the sternum.

Relations: Superficially, the deep pectoral, deeply to the external intercostal muscles in the first, second and third intercostal spaces and the internal intercostal muscles in the third, fourth and fifth intercostal spaces, the ribs and costal cartilages.

Action: It assists in inspiration by drawing the ribs and cartilages craniad and laterad.

Blood supply: Dorsal intercostal arteries.

Nerve supply: Intercostal nerves.

Transversus thoracis

The transversus thoracis is flat muscle situated on the upper (thoracic) surface of the sternum and the cartilages of the sternal ribs. The muscle thus covers the dorsal surface of the sternum and the medial surfaces of the costal cartilages.

Origin: The sternal (suprasternal) ligament and the adjacent area of the upper (dorsal or thoracic) surface of the sternum.

Insertion: The cartilages and ribs from second to sixth ribs and the seventh and eighth costal cartilages.

Relations: Dorsally (superiorly) the sternal fascia, 'pericardium and pleura. Deeply (inferiorly), the sternum and sternal cartilages, internal intercostal muscles and the internal thoracic vessels.

Action: To assist in expiration.

Blood supply: Perforating branches of internal thoracic artery.

Nerve supply: Second to sixth Intercostal nerves.

Diaphragm

The diaphragm is a large, broad, unpaired muscle which forms a partition between the thoracic and abdominal cavities. It is dome shaped with its convexity towards the thorax and corresponding concavity towards the abdomen. Its thoracic surface which is strongly convex is covered by a serous membrane called the pleura while the abdominal surface which is deeply concave is covered by another serous membrane called the peritoneum. Its peripheral part, the rim is fleshy while the central part is tendinous. The fleshy rim has the sternal and costal and lumbar parts. Its lumbar part has two strong tendinous crura or pillars. On the abdominal side, the diaphragm is connected with the liver and on the thoracic side it is connected with the heart and lungs by double fold of serous membrane.

Attachments of diaphragm: Its costal part is attached in a straight line from about the middle of last rib to the eighth rib. The sternal part is attached to the dorsal face of the xiphoid cartilage. The lumbar part is attached through its crura to the ventral longitudinal ligament of the lumbar vertebrae, first four or five on the right side and first two on left side. The diaphragm presents three foramina, the hiatus aorticus for the passage of aorta, hiatus oesophageus for passage of oesophagus and the foramen venae cavae for caudal vena cava.

Relations: The thoracic surface of the diaphragm is related to the lungs and pericardium, the phrenic vein and the phrenic nerve. The abdominal surface is related to rumen, reticulum, omasum, abomasums, spleen and liver. Its lumbar part has two strong tendinous crura or pillars.

Action: The diaphragm is the chief muscle of inspiration.

Blood supply: Phrenic artery and its branches

Nerve supply: Phrenic nerve..

Muscles of thoracic (shoulder) girdle

In addition to the muscles of spine (back) and the muscles of thoracic wall, there is another set of muscles attached to and located on the dorsolateral as well as ventrolateral aspect of the thorax. This group of muscles is the muscles of thoracic girdle (shoulder girdle) and forms the musculature of the thorax. With the help of these muscles, the thoracic limb or the fore limb is attached to the body trunk especially to the cervical and thoracic regions of the body. The main function of muscles of this group is to support and hold the forelimb against the body trunk and to assist in the movements of the forelimb. These muscles are as under.

Trapezious

This is an extensive, thin, flat and irregularly triangular muscle. Its base extends along the dorsal median line from the level of atlas to about the last thoracic vertebra and the apex reaches ventrally to the lateral aspect of the shoulder. Since it extends from cervical to thoracic region, this muscle is considered to have two parts as trapezious cervicis and trapezious thoracis. The trapezious cervicis has already been described under the dorsal muscles of the neck. The trapezious thoracis is as under.

Origin: The summits of the spinous processes and the supraspinous ligament from first to twelfth thoracic vertebra.

Insertion: The tuberous part of the scapular spine and the fascia of the shoulder and arm.

Relations: Laterally this muscle is related to and is covered by the skin and fascia of the back and the thorax. Medially it is related to rhomboideus, latissimus dorsi, supraspinatus and infraspinatus muscles.

Action: The trapezious thoracis is an elevator of the shoulder. It carries the shoulder dorsad and caudad.

Blood supply: Vertebral artery.

Nerve supply: Dorsal branches of thoracic spinal nerves.

Latissimus dorsi

This is another extensive muscle on the lateral wall of thorax extending from the thoracolumbar spine to the arm. Its upper (dorsal) part is aponeurotic and lies under the skin while the lower (ventral) part is muscular which is covered by cutaneus muscle.

Origin: The origin is by aponeurosis on the fascia of the thoracolumbar spine extending from the level of third thoracic vertebra to the level of the last lumbar vertebra.

Insertion: The cranial part of the insertion blends with the tendon of teres major muscle. The middle part ends on the tendon of triceps muscle and the caudal part terminates on deep pectoral muscle.

Relations: The latissimus dorsi muscle is related laterally to the skin, fascia, cutaneous muscle, trapezious, tensor fasciae antibrachia and the triceps muscles. Medially it is related to rhomboideus, serratus dorsalis, longissimus dorsi and a few more muscles.

Action: It assists in the flexion of the shoulder joint.

Blood supply: Thoracodorsal and dorsal intercostal arteries.

Nerve supply: Thoracodorsal nerve.

Rhomboideus

This is also a large muscle extending from the mid level of the funicular fart of the ligamentum nuchae in the neck to about the ninth or tenth thoracic vertebra in the thoracic region. It consists of two parts, the cervical part as **rhomboideus cervicis** and thoracic part as **rhomboideus thoracis**. The cervical part is already described with the muscles of the dorsolateral group of cervical muscles. The thoracic part is as under.

Rhomboideus thoracis

This is a thin, flat and irregularly quadrilateral.

Origin: Summits of the spinous processes of thoracic first nine or ten thoracic vertebrae.

Insertion: The medial aspect of the scapular cartilage.

Relations: Laterally the upper part of this muscle is related to trapezious muscle and its lower part is related to deep face of the subscapularis muscle along with the scapular cartilage. Medially it is related to the serratus dorsalis cranial and caudal.

Action: Extension of the shoulder. The rhomboideus thoracis draws the shoulder upwards.

Blood supply: Dorsal intercostal arteries.

Nerve supply: Thoracic spinal nerves.

Superficial pectoral (pectoralis superficialis)

This muscle is in two parts, the cranial and caudal. It extends from the ventral and cranial part of the sternum to the medial surface of the arm and forearm.

Cranial superficial pectoral

This is a short, thick and slightly rounded muscle extending from manubrium sterni to the cranioventral aspect of the arm. This muscle forms a prominent brisket in the living animal. The outer (superficial) surface of this muscle is convex and its internal (deep) surface is flat.

Origin: The ventrolateral aspect of the first sternebra along with manubrium of the sternum.

Insertion: In common with the brachiocephalicus on the ventral part of the crest of humerus and fascia of the arm.

Relations: Superficially, fascia and skin; deeply, caudal deep pectoral and biceps brachii.

Action: To adduct the limb and draw it forward.

Blood supply: External thoracic artery.

Nerve supply: Cranial pectoral nerve.

Caudal superficial pectoral

This is a thin flat muscle extending from ventrolateral aspect of the sternum to the medial side of the forearm.

Origin: From the ventrolateral aspect of the sternum in the region of second to sixth sternebra.

Relations: Superficially, The pectoral fascia and skin, cranial superficial pectoral and deeply, the part of the sternocephalicus, deep pectoral and the pectoral vessels and nerve.

Action: To adduct the fore limb.

Deep pectoral

This is a large fleshy muscle extending from sternum at the level of xiphoid cartilage to the shoulder joint.

Origin: The ventral surface of sternum from xiphoid cartilage to the level of second rib and tunica abdominalis.

Insertion: The lesser and greater tubercles of the humerus.

Relations: Superficially the skin, fascia, cutaneous muscle of the trunk, cranial superficial pectoral muscles and the external thoracic vessels and nerves and deeply the tunica abdominalis, obliquus abdominis external, rectus abdominis, and rectus thoracis muscles and the vessels and nerves of the axillary region.

Action: To adduct and retract the fore limb.

Blood supply: External thoracic artery.

Nerve supply: Caudal pectoral nerve.

Serratus ventralis

This is a large fleshy muscle located on the lateral aspect of the neck (serratus cervicis) and the serratus thoracis. The cervical part is already described with the muscles of the neck. The thoracic part is described hereunder.

Serratus ventralis thoracis

This is a flat, thin muscle that covers the cranial half of the lateral surface of the thoracic wall. It overlaps the caudal part of the serratus ventralis cervicis. Its lower (ventral) border is serrated possessing six digitations.

Origin: The lateral surface of fourth to ninth ribs.

Insertion: On the muscular line of the scapula, the caudal angle of the scapula and the **cartilage** by means of aponeurotic attachment with the subscapularis muscle of the scapula.

Relations: It is related superficially to cleido occipitalis, omotransversarius, scalinus, and other muscles of the shoulder girdle and deeply to the ventral border of splenius, serratus, longissimus and intercostal muscles.

Action: Pulls the fore limb caudad. It acts as a muscle of forced inspiration.

Blood supply: Costocervical, supreme intercostal, second to fourth dorsal intercostal and dorsal scapular arteries.

Nerve supply: Fifth to eighth cervical thoracic and long thoracic nerves.

Subclavius

It is a small, round bundle of fleshy muscle that arises from the cartilage and the ventral end of the first rib and ends on the deep face of the brachiocephalicus muscle cranial to the shoulder joint.

Origin: The sternal end of the cartilage of first rib.

Insertion: The medial surface of brachiocephalicus in the area of clavicular intersection.

Relations: Superficially, it is related to a part of brachiocephalicus and deep pectoral muscles and deeply to the sternocephalicus muscle.

Action: Adduction of the limb.

Blood supply: Superficial cervical artery.

Nerve supply: Cranial pectoral nerve.

44

Comparative Anatomy of Muscles of Thorax

Muscles of the back (spine), muscles of thorax and muscles of thoracic girdle of **Horse, Dog, Sheep and Goat, and Pig** almost resemble those of ox except for a few miner differences due to variations in the number of bony segments of the vertebrae, ribs and sternebrae.

Fowl

Muscles of back (spine)

Spinalis thoracis is the thoracic part of the spinales complexus. It originates by aponeurosis on the spinous processes of the thoracic vertebrae including the dorsal median ridge of the synsacrum, dorsal surface of the bases of the transverse processes and the cranial border of the ilium. The muscle inserts by multiple tendinous slips on the spinous processes, vertebral arches, transverse processes of several thoracic vertebrae and the vertebral ribs. This muscle helps in straightening of the head and neck of the fowl.

Iliocostalis et longissimus dorsi is the segmented muscle originating on the transverse processes of the thoracic vertebrae and inserting on the vertebral parts of the ribs. This muscle assists in elevating the thorax.

Muscles of thoracic walls

Levatores costarum is the muscle with several slips originating on the transverse processes of the thoracic vertebrae and inserting on the vertebral ribs. It helps in elevating the rib cage and thereby in inspiration.

Scalinus dorsalis muscle originates on transverse processes of last cervical and first thoracic vertebrae and inserts on the lateral surface of first and second vertebral ribs. It assists in inspiration by elevating the first two vertebral ribs.

External and internal intercostal muscles lie in the intercostal spaces of sternal ribs and have origin and insertion on the opposite borders of the adjacent rib. The external intercostal muscle assists in inspiration and the internal intercostal muscle helps in expiration.

Costosternalis muscle has two divisions, the pars major and pars minor. The **pars major** originates on the caudal surface of sternocoracoidal process and the **pars minor** originates on the dorsocaudal surface of sternocoracoidal process of the sternum. The insertion of pars major is on the second vertebral rib, third sternal rib and its caudal extension on the fourth and fifth ribs. The pars minor inserts on the first and second vertebral ribs. The pars major is inspiratory and pars minor expiratory muscle.

Costopulmonaris muscle is formed by fleshy slips from the medial surface of several vertebral ribs near their articulations with the corresponding sternal parts. These slips insert in series on the pulmonary fascia by aponeurosis.

Muscles of thoracic girdle

Latissimus dorsi thoracis originates on the spinous processes of the thoracic vertebrae and inserts by aponeurosis on the scapular or humeral region of the wing of the bird. It helps to draw the wing caudally and flexing and elevating the humerus in flying.

Rhomboideus thoracis originates on the spinous processes of thoracic vertebrae and inserts on the scapular spine by a tendon to help in elevating the wing for flying.

Serratus superficialis resembles to serratus ventralis of the mammalian species of animals while **serratus profundus** resembles to serratus dorsalis of mammals.

SECTION-B

THORACIC CAVITY AND VISCERA

45

Thoracic Cavity

Boundaries

The cavity of thorax (**thoracic cavity**) is formed like a truncated cone which is compressed laterally in its cranial part and some what wider in its caudal part. The dorsal wall or roof of the thorax is formed by the thoracic vertebrae and the ligaments and muscles connected with them. The lateral walls are formed by the ribs and intercostal muscles and other muscles supporting the walls internally and externally. The floor or the ventral wall is formed by the sternum and costal cartilages along with the ligaments and muscles attached to them. The caudal wall or the base of the thorax is formed by the diaphragm. It slopes craniad and ventrad. It is bound dorsally by the last thoracic vertebra, ventrally by xiphoid cartilage and laterally by the last pair of ribs and the costal arch formed by the union of costal cartilages of asternal ribs. The apex of the cone is narrow, nearly oval or triangular in form and it is directed cranially. The cavity of the apex is bound dorsally by the first thoracic vertebra, laterally by the first pair of ribs and ventrally by the first sternebra along with manubrium sterni. The apex is fully occupied by the longus colli muscle, oesophagus, trachea, vessels, nerves and lymph nodes. The width of the thorax is greatest at the level of ninth ribs. The wall of the thorax is internally lined by the **serous membrane** which is a part of the **pleura.**

Mediastinum

The **mediastinum,** although means a median partition, here in the present case it is a central median space or interval between the two pleural sacs. It extends from the thoracic inlet to the diaphragm and is bound dorsally by the vertebral column, ventrally by the sternum and laterally by the pleural sacs. It divides the thoracic cavity into two lateral chambers. Each of these chambers is lined by the pleura and its cavity is the pleural sac which is occupied by lung. The mediastinum, although is said as median in position, is inclined more to the left side because the main and the major content of the mediastinum, the heart is inclined more on left side than the right side. So also, the right lung which is larger in size than the left lung pushes the mediastinum towards the left side. All the contents of the thoracic cavity, except the lungs with pleural sacs are placed in the mediastinum. The space of the mediastinum occupied by the heart and pericardium is the middle mediastinum and the space cranial and caudal to it is the cranial mediastinum and caudal mediastinum respectively.

46

Viscera of Thorax

The thoracic cavity (Fig. 3-3 A, B and C) contains lungs and pleura, the heart and pericardium, the great vessels connected with the heart (the aortae, azygos veins and venae cavae), the oesophagus, trachea, the lymph nodes, vessels, nerves and lymphatics. All of these contents except the lungs and pleural sacs are located in the mediastinum, while the lungs along with the pleural sacs are situated on either sides of the mediastinum.

Lungs

The right and left lungs (Fig. 3-3 A and B) are paired organs which occupy greater space of the thoracic cavity. Each lung is enclosed in a double layered bag of serous membrane called the pleural sac. The right lung is larger, almost double in size than the left one. The difference in size is mainly due to an additional lobe called the intermediate lobe and the greater size of an apical lobe of the right lung. Each lung is divided into different lobes formed by deep fissures extending from the ventral border to almost the area of the root of the lung. Each lung is soft, light weighted, spongy and elastic. The surface of the lung is smooth and glistening and it is mapped out into irregular areas indicating the lobules of the lungs. In the fresh, unpreserved cadaver the lung collapses to about one third of its original size and looses its normal shape. The colour in fresh state is pink, in bled animals it is pale grey and in unbled animals it is dark red. In embalmed specimens, the outer surface of the lungs is marked by the imprints of other organs and structures that are related to lungs in the thoracic cavity.

Each lung presents two surfaces, two borders, a base and an apex. The **lateral or costal surface** is convex in conformity to the ribs, cartilages and intercostal spaces of the inner surface of the lateral wall of the thorax. In hardened specimens, costal impressions appear on the lateral surface of the lung. The **medial or mediastinal surface** is vertical but irregular and is molded on the organs in contact with it on this side. The cardiac impression is large, concave and prominent area on this surface. It is larger and more extensive on the right

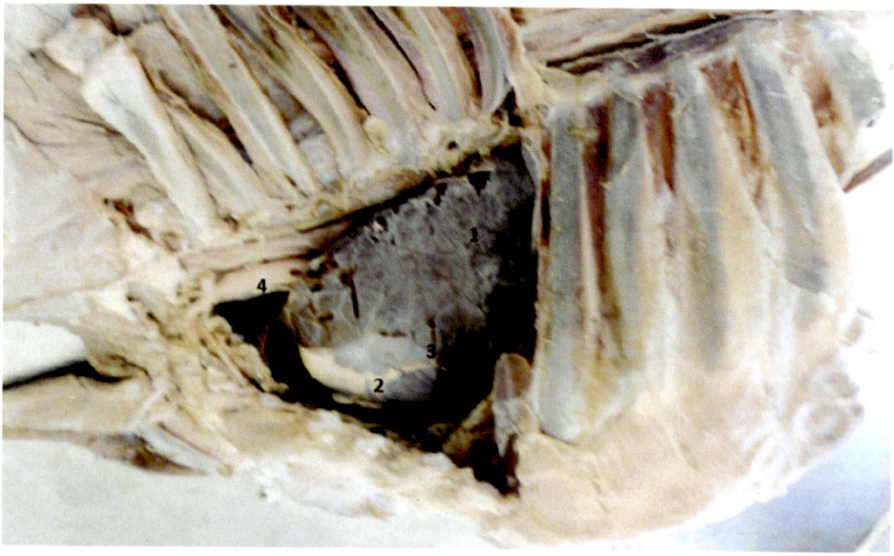

Fig. 3–3 A: Viscera of thorax; Left side. in situ.
1. Left Lung; 2. Heart; 3. Cardiac notch; 4. Cranial aorta.

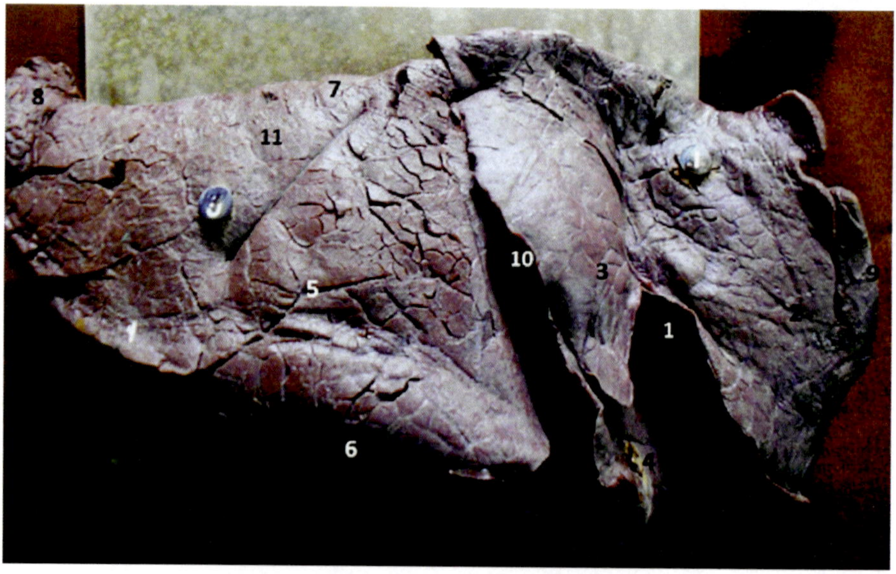

Fig. 3–3 B: Lateral surface of Right lung
1. Cardiac notch 2. Cranial part of apical lobe 3. Caudal part of apical lobe 4. Cardiac lobe 5. Diaphragmatic lobe 6. Ventral border 7. Dorsal border 8. Apex of lung 9. Base of lung 10. Interlobar fissure 11. Costal impression

lung than the left one. It appears mostly on the apical and cardiac lobes of both the lungs. Just above the cardiac impression is the **hilus** of the lung. It contains the bronchus, the pulmonary artery and vein, the bronchial artery, lymph vessels and nerves. Above and behind the hilus is the aortic groove, which is deeper on the left lung. Ventral to the aortic groove is the oesophageal groove. It is deeper on the right lung. On the mediastinal surface of the right lung running between the intermediate and cardiac lobes is groove for caudal venacava. The **basal surface (base)** or the **diaphragmatic surface** of the lung is oval, concave and smooth and it is related and molded to the dome of the diaphragm. The **apex** is conical and it occupies the space within the cupula of the pleural sac. The apex of the right lung is much larger than that of the left lung. In situ it appears to be extended to left side of the thoracic cavity passing ventral to the trachea and great vessels, cranial to the heart. In the young animals, the extension of apex of right lung to left side is limited because of the presence of thymus.

The **dorsal border** of the lung is thick and rounded. It forms the dorsal boundary between the costal surface and the vertebral part of the medial surface. The **ventral border** is thin and sharp. It is irregular and shorter than the dorsal border. It is indented at the level of the heart and forms the **cardiac notch** through which the pericardium along with the apical part of the heart is exposed to the wall of the thorax. This is variable in size in the two lungs. In the left lung, the ventral border is 'L' shaped and the angle of the 'L' forms the cardiac notch. In ox it lies opposite the ventral third of the third intercostal space, fourth rib and the fourth intercostal space. This is much more extensive area than on the right side. Hence the area of left cardiac notch is the preferred site for examination of the heart in animals.

The **right lung** is divided into four lobes formed by deep interlobar fissures. These lobes are the **apical** (cranial), **cardiac** (middle), **accessory** (intermediate) and **diaphragmatic** (caudal) **lobes.** The apical lobe is large and extends to the left of the median plane, ventral to the trachea and great vessels cranial to the heart and pericardium. The medial surface of the apical lobe presents greater part of the cardiac impression. The apical lobe is subdivided into two, the cranial and caudal parts by a fissure that extends from the cardiac notch. The middle lobe is an elongated three sided part of the lung which is separated from apical and diaphragmatic lobes by interlobar fissures. The medial surface of the middle lobe presents a part of the cardiac impression because of its relation with the heart. Its caudal surface is related to diaphragmatic lobe and the diaphragm. The diaphragmatic lobe is the largest lobe and is caudal in position. The cardiac lobe is attached to the medial surface of the diaphragmatic lobe. The accessory lobe is pyramidal in shape and it forms a part of the diaphragmatic surface of the right lung. At the site of its attachment with the diaphragmatic lobe it presents a groove for the passage of caudal venacava,

The **left lung** possesses three lobes, the **apical** (cranial), **cardiac** (middle) and the **diaphragmatic** (caudal). The medial surface of the apical and the cardiac lobes present a cardiac impression. The diaphragmatic lobe is in contact with the diaphragm.

The **root of the lung** which connects the lung with the trachea and the heart lies at the horizontal level of about the junction of dorsal and middle third of the sagittal diameter of thoracic cavity opposite the fifth rib and intercostal space. The root is formed by the structures entering and leaving the lung through its hilus. These structures include the principal bronchus, pulmonary vessels, bronchial vessels, lymphatic vessels and the nerves. All these structures are embedded in the connective tissue mass and the entire bunch of these structures is externally covered by the pleura. The sheath of the pleura that wraps the root of the lung extends caudally to form the pulmonary ligament.

Each lung is composed of the external **serous layer**, the **subserous** layer of areolar connective tissue and the **parenchyma**. The serous coat is the visceral (pulmonary) layer of the pleural sac. It is thin and transparent. Next to this, is the layer of areolar connective tissue which is mixed with the fibres of elastic tissue. It closely adheres to the external surface of the lung and invests deeply into the parenchyma of the lung giving lobular appearance on the surface of the lungs. The parenchyma is composed of numerous distinct lobules. Each lobule (pulmonary lobule) is composed of lobular bronchiole, the air cell in which the pulmonary bronchiole opens, the vessels, lymphatics and the nerves.

The architecture of the lung is based on the framework of **bronchial tree**. The **principal bronchus** after entering the substance of the lung through the hilus, gives rise to relatively large bronchi called the lobar bronchi that ventilate the pulmonary lobes. Each **lobar bronchus** gives rise to smaller bronchi called the **segmental bronchi** that ventilate a large independent area (segment) called the **bronchopulmonary segment** of the pulmonary lobe. The segmental bronchi divide into **subsegmental bronchi** ventilating still smaller segments of the parenchyma. The subsegmental bronchi further continue to divide into smaller and smaller branches till they reach to the diameter of about 0.5 to 1.0 mm. and loose the cartilaginous plates and are called the **bronchioles.** The terminal bronchioles ultimately lead to the **respiratory bronchioles** and join the alveolar ducts. The framework of bronchi and bronchioles thus formed in the lungs is called the **bronchial tree.**

The **blood supply** to lungs is of two types. It has the functional and nutritional blood supply. The functional blood is carried to the lungs through the pulmonary artery from the right ventricle of the heart. This is a large artery with a large primary branch for each lung. It gives out secondary branches to each lobe of the lung. The secondary branches of the pulmonary artery further divide into smaller branches to reach the air cells. In addition to the two primary branches, a separate branch is given out from the right primary branch of the pulmonary artery for the apical lobe of the right lung. These arteries and arterioles carry deoxygenated blood to the air cells of the lungs. The oxygenated blood is carried back to the heart through the pulmonary venules and veins. Within lungs the veins are the satellites of the arteries. The veins of different lobes do not unite but open separately into the left atrium of the heart. The nutritional blood is supplied to the lungs through the bronchial artery which arises from the aorta.

The **nerve supply** to lungs is through the pulmonary nerves which are the branches of the autonomic nervous system. The parasympathetic nerve fibres from the vagus nerve join the sympathetic nerve fibres from the cervical and thoracic sympathetic ganglia and form the pulmonary plexus as an extension of the cardiac plexus at the base of the heart. The autonomic nerve fibres from the pulmonary plexus run along the branches of the bronchial artery to reach the parts of the lungs. The afferent nerve fibres from the lungs pass along with the autonomic nerves to the spinal cord, but they are not the part of autonomic system.

Pleura

The pleura is a thin serous membrane arranged in the form of two closed sacs, the right and left occupied by the lung of the concerned side. The space in the centre between the two, left and right, pleural sacs is the mediastinum. Each pleural sac is double layered. The inner visceral layer is tightly adhered to the external surface of the lung while the outer parietal layer is closely adhered to the inner surface of the wall of the thorax. Between these two layers is a thin space called the pleural cavity which is filled in by a thin film of serous fluid. This fluid helps in the two layers to glide over each other during respiration. The part of the pleura against the lateral wall of the thorax is called the costal pleura, that against the diaphragm is the diaphragmatic pleura and the part against the mediastinum is the mediastinal pleura. Cranially, the pleura extends to the thoracic inlet or in some cases beyond the thoracic inlet into the cervical region and is called the cervical pleura or cupula of the pleura. The reflection of the pleura in the costal region is called the costal reflection, the one on the diaphragm is called the diaphragmatic reflection and that on the mediastinal region is the mediastinal reflection. The lungs invest the pleural sacs from the mediastinal side and the two sheets of the pleura together form the pulmonary ligament.

Heart

Gross Features

The heart (Fig. 3-3 D) is a cone shaped thick walled and four chambered muscular organ. It lies obliquely craniocaudal in the middle mediastinum in between the left and right lungs and covered by pericardium inside the thoracic cavity. The major part of heart (about 60 per cent) lies to the left of the middle mediastinum. The broad upper end is the base of the heart. It lies at the junction of the dorsal and middle third of the dorsoventral diameter of thorax at the level of about third rib and it faces craniodorsally. The narrow lower end is the apex. It lies just dorsal to the sternum at the level of about sixth rib and it faces caudad and ventrad. The surfaces, right and left are convex. They meet cranially at the right ventricular border and caudally at the left ventricular border. The right (cranial) border is strongly convex. It runs ventrally and caudally. The greater part of this border lies parallel to the sternum. The left (caudal) border is much shorter and nearly vertical. The surfaces of the heart are marked by grooves which indicate the division of the heart into four chambers the two atria dorsally and the two ventricles ventrally. The atria are separated internally by the interatrial septum. The ventricles are separated by interventricular septum. The circular coronary groove indicates the division of the heart in to atria dorsally and ventricles ventrally. It encircles the heart in its upper third part except at the level of the origin of pulmonary artery. The coronary groove is quite deep and wide. It provides passage for the coronary artery and vein..Apart from these, it is deeply filled with fat. The right (subsinuosal) interventricular groove and left (paraconal) interventricular groove indicates the line of separation between the two (right and left) ventricles by the interventricular septum. Both of these grooves run downward from the coronary groove towards the apex parallel to the respective borders and terminate just above the apex. The right and left ventricular grooves are occupied by the respective coronary vessels along with fat.

Structure

The wall of the heart is composed of three layers from without inwards the epicardium, myocardium and the endocardium. The **epicardium** is the visceral layer of the serous pericardium and it is firmly adhered to the heart muscle. The **myocardium** is the cardiac muscle that forms the middle and thickest layer of the wall of the heart. The **endocardium** is the smooth glistening endothelial lining of the cavities (chambers) of the heart. The specialty of the myocardial muscle is that the muscle cells are in the form of striated fibres. The muscle fibres are branched and appear 'Y' shaped. The fibres anastomose with the neighbouring fibres by thick plasma membranes called intercalated

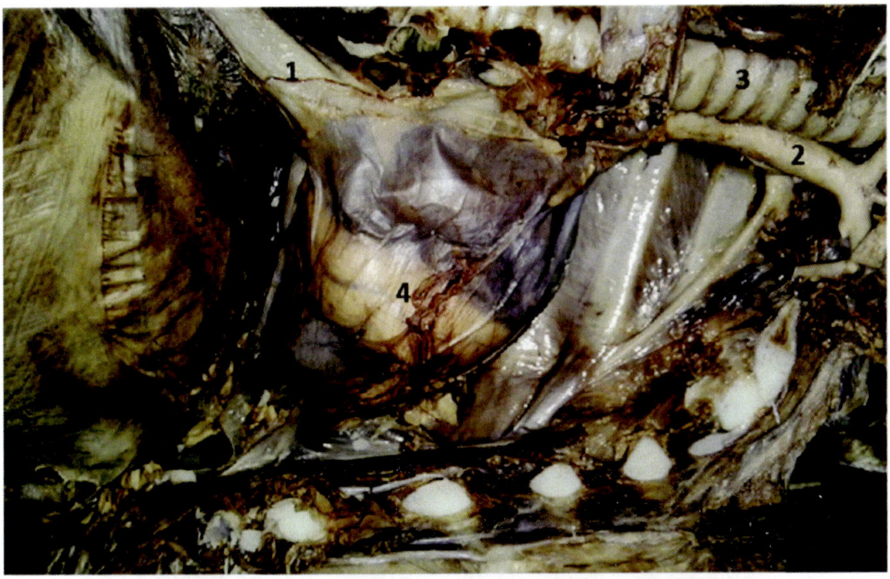

Fig. 3 – 3 C: Viscera of thorax; Right side in situ
1. Caudal aorta 2. Common brachicephalic trunk 3. Trachea 4. Heart 5. Diaphragm

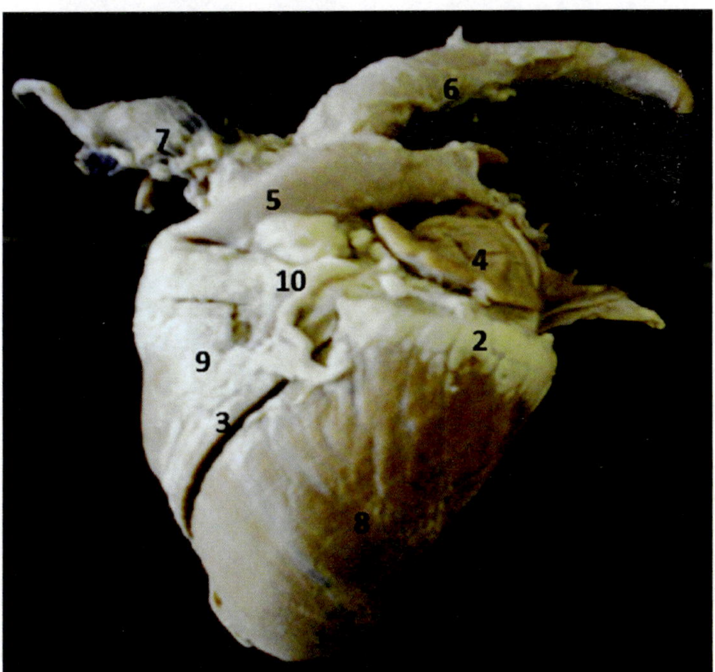

Fig. 3 – 3 D: Heart of Ox (External structure)
1. Apex 2. Coronary groove 3. Left longitudinal groove 4. Left atrium 5. Pulmonary artery 6 Caudal aorta 7. Cranial aorta 8. Left ventricle 9. Right ventricle 10. Base of Heart

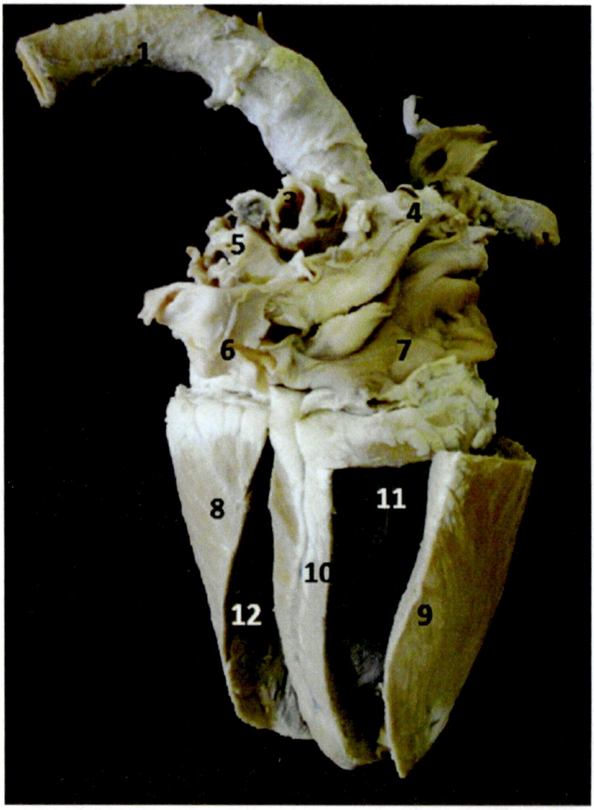

Fig. 3–3 E: Heart of Ox (Internal structure)
1: Descending aorta; 2. Brachiocephalic trunk; 3. Cranial venacava; 4. Caudal venacava; 5. Pulmonary veins; 6. Left atrium; 7. Right atrium; 8. Left ventricle; 9. Right ventricle; 10. Interventricular septum; 11. Chordae tendinae; 12. Papillary muscle.

discs thus forming the complex network which allow the muscle cells to resist high blood pressure and continuous working. The cardiac muscle contracts and relaxes alternately in rhythmic fashion. This contraction and relaxation of the cardiac muscle is involuntary and is regulated for the whole life of the animal. In addition to these specialized cardiac muscles, the wall of the heart contains dense connective tissue that forms the fibrous skeleton of the heart. This fibrous skeleton is composed of dense connective tissue rings that surround the four major orifices of the heart i.e. the right atrioventricular orifice, left atrioventricular orifice, orifice of the pulmonary artery and the orifice of the aorta. This skeleton contains the fibrocartilage in which small nodules of bone (ossa cardis) may develop in certain species like cattle. These rings serve as a point of attachment for the heart valves. It prevents the valves from overstretching as blood passes through them.

Chambers of the Heart

The heart contains four chambers (Fig. 3-3 E). The two upper chambers are the atria and the two lower chambers are the ventricles. Each atrium extends cranially into a pouch like appendage called the auricle which provides additional space and increases the capacity of the atrium.

Right Atrium

The right atrium forms the right cranial part of the base of the heart and lies dorsal to the right ventricle. It consists of a principle cavity the sinus venosus (sinus venarum cavarum) into which the greater veins (the cranial and caudal venae cavae and the pulmonary veins) open and a blind diverticulum- the auricular appendix which is called the auricle. The sinus venosus is the part of the cavity between the openings of the two venae cavae and the atrioventricular opening. The auricle is a conical diverticulum which curves around the right and cranial surfaces of the aorta. The wall of the atria is thinner than that of the ventricles. The inner endocardium is smooth and glistening. It continues into the blood vessels opening into this chamber. However, the wall of the auricle is crossed with bands of muscles called the pectinate muscles. Some of these bands terminate dorsally into a crest called crista terminalis. A intervenous crest projects ventrad and craniad from the dorsal wall of the atrium just cranial to the opening of the cranial vena cava. It directs the flow of blood from the cranial vena cava to the atrioventricular opening. In the interatrial septum there is an oval fossa called the fossa ovalis. This is the remnant of the foramen ovale which is an opening through which the two atria communicate in the foetus. The right atrium presents openings for the following vessels.

1. The opening of the cranial vena cava that brings blood from the cranial parts of the body and opening into this chamber at its craniodorsal part.
2. The opening of the caudal vena cava bringing blood from the caudal parts of the body and opening into this chamber at its caudodorsal part.
3. The right atrioventricular opening is placed in the floor of the sinus.
4. The coronary sinus is the opening of the great coronary vein into the sinus venosus below the opening of the caudal vena cava.
5. Several small orifices of venae cordis parvae are concealed in the depressions between the pectinate muscles. These are the openings of small venules that return blood from the substance of the heart muscle.

Right ventricle

The right ventricle forms the right cranial part of the ventricular mass of the heart. It forms the entire length of the cranial border of the heart but does not reach its apex which is formed entirely by the left ventricle. It is triangular in outline and crescentic in cross section. It communicate above at the base with the right atrium through the right atrioventricular orifice (opening) but its left part projects higher forming the **conus arteriosus** from which the pulmonary artery arises. The atrioventricular orifice and the cavity of the conus arteriosus are separated by a thick ridge the **crista supraventricularis**. The long axis of the cavity extending from the conus arteriosus to the apex forms a spiral curve to right ventrally and caudally. The walls of the ventricle bear the muscular ridges or bands called the **trabeculae carneae**. Some of these are somewhat conical flattened projections called the **musculi papillares**. These are three in numbers in right ventricle. These papillae are continuous at their bases with the wall of the ventricle. Whereas, at their apices they give attachment to the **chordae tendinae** which are fibrous bands attached at the other end to the cusps of the atrioventricular wall. In addition to these, there are moderator bands that extend from the interventricular septum runs transversely across the cavity of the ventricle and terminate into the lateral wall of the ventricle. These are musculotendinous bands and help in preventing over distention of the ventricle.

The atrioventricular orifice (opening) is oval. It is guarded by the right atrioventricular (tricuspid) valve made up of three large cusps. Of these, one is between the right atrioventricular opening and the conus arteriosus, the other one is septal that lies against the interventricular septum, and the third is on the right margin of the orifice. In addition, there are three small intermediate cusps intervening between the large cusps. The peripheral edges of the cusps are attached to the fibrous ring that is embedded in the periphery of the atrioventricular opening. The free edges of the cusps are serrated and ventrally directed. They give attachment to the chordae tendinae which are attached ventrally to the three papillary muscles. Each cusp of the valve receives chordae tendinae from two papillary muscles.

The pulmonary orifice, an opening of the pulmonary artery is circular and is situated at the summit of the conus arteriosus. It is guarded by the pulmonary valve comprised of three semilunar cusps, one medial (right), one lateral (left) and one caudal (intermediate). The peripheral margin of each cusp is convex and is attached to the fibrous ring at the junction of the pulmonary artery and the conus arteriosus. The central margin is free and concave. Each cusp is made of a double fold of endocardium with an intermediate layer of fibrous tissue. The edge of the conus arteriosus forms three arches with intermediate projecting angles or horns, to all of which the cusps are attached and opposite each cusp is a sinus of the pulmonary artery.

Left Atrium

The left atrium forms the caudal part of the base of the heart. It lies behind the pulmonary artery and the aorta and dorsal to the left ventricle. It consists of the sinus (main chamber) and the appendix (diverticulum). The appendix extends laterad and craniad on the left side and its blind end lies behind the origin of the pulmonary artery. The sinus receives about 4 to 7 pulmonary veins. The wall of the sinus is smooth while that of the auricle is crossed with pectinate muscles. The interventricular septum presents the fossa ovalis the remnant of the foramen ovale, the communication between the right and left atria in the foetus. The left atrioventricular opening lies on the caudal side of the floor of the atrium. Openings of small veins the venae cordis parvae from the substance of the heart are present in the spaces of the pectinate muscles of the appendix auriculae.

Left Ventricle

The left ventricle forms the left caudal part of the ventricular mass. It is more regularly conical than the right ventricle and its wall is much thicker except at the apex. It forms all the caudal contour of the ventricular part and the apex of the heart. Its base is continuous with the left atrium and the aorta. The cavity is circular in cross section. The endocardium is smooth. The trabeculae carneae are same as those of the right ventricle. The musculi papillaris are larger and the chordae tendinae are larger and stronger than those of the right ventricle. The moderator bands are more tendinous and branched. The left atrioventricular opening is circular and is guarded by bicuspid or mitral valve consisting of two cusps cranial and caudal. Both the cusps are larger and thicker. The cranial part of the base opens into the aorta. The aortic opening is guarded by aortic valve which is composed of three semilunar cusps. The cusps of the valve are right, left and caudal (septal). They are similar to those of pulmonary valves but are stronger and larger than those of the pulmonary valves. The interventricular septum is convex on the right side and concave on the left side. Hence the right ventricle appears crescentic and the left ventricle appears circular in cross section.

Conduction system of heart

The rhythmic contractions of heart are due to its conduction system. It consists of the Sinuatrial node, Atrioventricular node, atrioventricular bundle, and the conducting fibres (Purkinje fibres).

Sinuatrial Node (SA Node): It is a small mass of modified heart muscle. It is located in the crista terminalis at the junction of the cranial vena cava and right auricular appendix. The fibres of the SA Node merge with the atrial musculature which in its turn conducts the impulses to the atrioventricular node.

Atrioventricular Node (AV Node): It lies cranial to the orifice of the coronary sinus, beneath the endocardium in the septal wall of the right atrium. It is also made of a special type of cardiac muscle fibres and these fibres are connected with the atrioventricular bundle.

Atrioventricular Bundle (AV Bundle): It is a bundle of specialized cardiac muscle fibres which begin at the AV Node and run along the membranous part of interventricular septum beneath the endocardium. The bundle first divide into two divisions the right and left crura. The right crus runs down beneath the endocardium along the right surface of the interventricular septum towards the apex. The fibres of this crus of the bundle later distribute over the papillary muscles and moderator band and finally reach the lateral wall of the right ventricle. The left crus runs down beneath the endocardium along the left surface of the interventricular septum and later break down into number of conducting fibres.

Conducting Fibres (Purkinje Fibres): These are the terminal fibres from the right and left parts of AV Bundle, distributed over the lateral and medial walls of the ventricles, papillary muscles and moderator bands. These fibres are ensheathed by fibrous sheaths to separate them from the myocardium. These fibres merge with the myocardium at their terminal ends.

Blood circulation through the heart

When the heart contracts it pushes the blood out into two measure loops or circulations. These are the systemic circulation and the pulmonary circulation.

Systemic Circulation: In the systemic circulation the oxygen rich blood collected in the left atrium is forced down through the mitral valve in to the left ventricle. From here it is pushed out through the aortic (semilunar) valve into the aorta which by way of arteries, arterioles and capillaries transports this blood to various organs, structures and tissues of the body. The blood circulated by this way is oxygen rich. This oxygen rich blood gets its oxygen exchanged with carbon dioxide at the cellular level and the oxygen poor blood returns back through the venules and veins that join the cranial and caudal vena cava which ultimately open into the right atrium. The systemic circulation is regulated by the left side of the heart.

Pulmonary Circulation: In the pulmonary circulation, the oxygen poor blood received into the right atrium through the cranial and caudal vena cava flows down through the tricuspid valve into the right ventricle. This blood with the contraction of the right ventricle is pushed out through pulmonary (semilunar) valve into the pulmonary artery and reaches into the lungs where in the exchange of gasses. It releases carbon dioxide and gets charged with the oxygen. This oxygen rich blood returns to the left atrium of the heart through the pulmonary veins. The pulmonary circulation is regulated by the right side of the heart.

Blood supply to heart (Coronary Circulation)

The heart muscle like any other tissue in the body needs supply of oxygen rich blood for survival and at the same time it needs to get rid of carbon dioxide through the venous blood. The supply of oxygen rich blood to heart muscle is made through coronary arteries and the draining out of deoxygenated blood from heart muscle is made through coronary veins. The circulation of blood thus effected is called the coronary circulation.

Coronary Arteries

There are two main coronary arteries that branch out from the aorta. These are the left and right coronary arteries.

Left coronary artery: The left main coronary artery arises from the left aortic sinus and turns to left just below the left auricle, divides in to the paraconal (left) interventricular artery and the circumflex artery. The paraconal interventricular artery runs down along the paraconal (cranial) interventricular groove on the cranial (left) surface of the heart towards the apex. From here it turns around, runs to the caudal (right) surface of the heart and terminates giving rise to number of small capillary branches that forms anastomoses with the subsinuosal (right) interventricular artery. This artery supplies blood to the walls of the left and right ventricles and the interventricular septum.

The circumflex artery: The circumflex artery runs along the coronary (atrioventricular) groove, gives rise to the left marginal artery and then continues through interventricular groove around the base of the heart and finally terminates on the caudal surface of the heart. It supplies blood to the wall of both the left and right atria of the heart.

Right coronary artery: The right coronary artery arises from the right aortic sinus at the origin of the aorta, occupies the right part of the coronary groove, gives out a branch called the subsinuosal (right) interventricular artery and continues into the coronary groove to its left side. The subsinuosal interventricular artery runs down the subsinuosal (right) interventricular groove turns round the apical part of the heart and reaches the left surface of the heart and terminates by branching out small capillary branches that anastomose with the similar branches of the paraconal (left) interventricular artery. This artery also supplies blood to the wall of both the left and right ventricles of the heart.

Coronary Veins

The coronary veins return blood from the myocardium back to the right atrium. About 80 per cent of the deoxygenated blood is returned to the right atrium by several prominent veins that run along the surface of the heart.

The great coronary vein: The great cardiac vein collects blood from the areas of heart which are supplied by left coronary artery. It originates at the apex of the heart and runs along the cranial interventricular groove in association with the left interventricular artery. Near the left atrium it turns to left and enters the coronary groove, through which it reaches to caudal side of the heart and merges with the coronary sinus that empties into the right atrium.

Middle coronary vein: The middle cardiac vein collects blood from the areas of heart supplied by right coronary artery. It ascends the cranial interventricular groove and after reaching to the coronary groove gets merged with the great cardiac vein.

Small cranial coronary vein: The small cranial cardiac vein which derives the deoxygenated blood from right atrium and ventricle enter directly into the right atrium.

About 20 per cent of the deoxygenated blood flows directly into the right atrium through numerous **veins of Thibesium** that open into the foramina of Thibesium in the right atrium of heart.

Nerve supply to heart (innervation of heart)

The nerve supply to heart is from two sets of nerves originating in the medulla of the brain. These nerves are part of involuntary (autonomic) nervous system. One of the sets is formed of the sympathetic nerves while the other is formed of parasympathetic nerves.

The sympathetic cardiac nerves arise from the middle cervical, cervicothoracic and thoracic sympathetic ganglia. These are bilateral and the nerves of both the left and right side join and coalesce in the cardiac plexus at the base of the heart.

(1) **Middle cervical sympathetic cardiac nerves**: The left and right middle cervical cardiac nerves after their origin from the middle cervical sympathetic ganglion of the corresponding side, run backward along the

caudal limb of the ansa subclavia up to the origin of subclavian artery and then dissociate from the ansa subclavia and join the cervicothoracic cardiac nerve of the respective side for further course.

(2) **Cervicothoracic sympathetic cardiac nerves**: These are two the cranial and caudal cervicothoracic cardiac nerves on each side. The cranial cervicothoracic cardiac nerve extend from the respective gland and runs toward the ansa subclavia, join the middle cervical cardiac nerve of the respective side. Hereafter, it passes through a groove between the trachea and caudal vena cava, reaches the base of the heart and join the cardiac plexus. The caudal cervicothoracic cardiac nerve after joining the middle cervical cardiac nerve descends along the vena azygos to reach the vascular triangle formed between the pulmonary artery, descending aorta and the base of the heart and join the cardiac plexus.

(3) **The thoracic cardiac nerves**: The origin of these nerves varies from second to fifth thoracic sympathetic ganglia on both sides. The nerve fibres after extending from the ventral border of the respective ganglion run downward and backward and join each other to form one or two nerve trunks. These nerve trunks further course along the vena azygos and reach over the base of the heart where they join the cardiac plexus.

The parasympathetic nerve supply to the heart is through the vagus nerve. The left and the right vagus nerves descend over the carotid artery of the respective side along with the cervical sympathetic nerve trunk through the neck. The left trunk runs along the ventrolateral aspect of the oesophagus and the right trunk along the ventrolateral aspect of the trachea. After entering the thoracic cavity the vagus nerves deviate from the sympathetic trunk, give out the left and right cardiac branches and then continue behind along with the oesophagus to reach the abdominal cavity. The cardiac branches of the vagus nerve run down towards the tracheal bifurcation and reach the cardiac plexus at the base of the heart.

Cardiac plexus

The cardiac plexus is formed by the cardiac (sympathetic) nerves and the vagus (parasympathetic) nerves at the base of the heart. The efferent fibres from this plexus run along the cardiac vessels to reach the myocardium. This plexus is formed in two parts. The superficial cardiac plexus lies beneath the aortic arch in front of the right pulmonary artery. It is formed by the left and right middle cervical and cranial cervicothoracic cardiac nerves and the cervical cardiac branch of the vagus nerve. A small ganglion the superficial cardiac ganglion lies in this plexus. The superficial cardiac ganglion possesses the junctions of the afferent and efferent fibres of the sympathetic cardiac nerves. The parasympathetic nerve fibres of the vagal branches bypass the ganglion and mix with the efferent sympathetic fibres emerging from the superficial cardiac ganglion for their further course to reach the myocardium of the heart. Three principle branches extend from the superficial cardiac plexus. One branch is the cranial coronary branch that supply to the cranial (left) side of the heart. The second branch is the left pulmonary branch that reaches to the pulmonary plexus. The third branch contributes to the deep cardiac plexus. The deep cardiac plexus is situated in front of the tracheal bifurcation above the point of division of the pulmonary artery and behind the aortic arch. It is formed by the caudal cervicothoracic and the thoracic cardiac nerves and the vagal cardiac nerves. The deep cardiac plexus is formed in two parts the right and the left. The nerve fibres from the right part of the deep cardiac plexus are supplied to the right (caudal) surface of the heart and also to the pulmonary plexus. The left part supplies fibres to the left atrium and the pulmonary plexus.

The sympathetic nerves act as cardiac accelerator and they cause the increase in heart rate while the parasympathetic nerves act as cardiac inhibiter and these nerves cause decrease in cardiac rate.

Pericardium

The pericardium is the serous membrane that surrounds and protects the heart. It is composed of two layers the visceral and parietal which are separated by a thin cavity. The visceral layer is firmly attached to the wall of the heart and forms its outermost layer the epicardium. The parietal layer of pericardium is composed of inelastic connective tissue. The cavity between the two layers contains a little volume of fluid the pericardial fluid. It serves as lubricant for minimizing the friction during the possible movement of heart inside the pericardium. The pericardium is fastened with the wall of the thoracic cavity by the sternopericardiac ligament that extends from the parietal layer of pericardium and terminates onto the dorsal (thoracic) surface of the sternum in cattle and horse. Another ligament called the phrenopericadiac ligament extends from the parietal layer of pericardium and terminates on the tendinous part of the diaphragm in dog and swine.

Other contents of mediastinum

Great vessels

The great vessels that are connected to heart and are situated in the mediastinum include, the pulmonary trunk and the pulmonary veins, the ascending and descending aorta, the azygos veins and the cranial and caudal vena cava.

Pulmonary trunk

The pulmonary trunk (pulmonary artery) arises from the right ventricle at the conus arteriosus. It curves dorsad and caudad and divides behind the aortic arch into **right and left pulmonary arteries.** It is related cranially to the right appendix auriculi, caudally to left appendix auriculi and medially to the aorta, with which it is enclosed in a common sheath of the visceral part of the pericardium. Near its termination into left and right branches, it is connected to the aorta by the ligamentum arteriosum. This ligament is the remnant of the ductus arteriosus which connects the pulmonary trunk to the descending aorta as a short cut for conducting oxygenated blood in foetal circulation. The pulmonary trunk is bulbous at its origin and has three pouches called as sinuses of the pulmonary trunk corresponding to the cusps of the pulmonary valve. Beyond this, the trunk diminishes in size.

The **right pulmonary artery** is a little longer than the left one. It passes under the bifurcation of the trachea to the hilus of the lung and inside the organ it accompanies the bronchial tree on its ventral surface. The **left pulmonary artery** is shorter than the right one. It passes caudad and enters the lung ventral to the left bronchus. Its further distribution is similar to that of the right artery.

Pulmonary veins

The pulmonary veins conduct oxygenated blood from lungs to the heart. The tributaries of the pulmonary veins arise from the capillary plexuses of the pulmonary lobules and then converge to form larger and larger trunks (veins) which are the satellites to the pulmonary arteries as well as the branches of the bronchial tree. The larger trunks thus formed finally converge into six or seven large venous trunks called the pulmonary veins at the root of the lungs. These six or seven pulmonary veins open into the left atrium through three sinuses. The right sinus receives three veins, two from the cranial lobe and one from the middle lobe of the right lung. The left sinus receives two or three veins from the cranial lobe of the left lung and the caudal sinus receives two veins from the caudal lobes of both lungs. The pulmonary veins do not have valves at their openings into the sinuses of left atrium.

Aorta

The aorta (Fig. 3-4 A) is the main systemic arterial trunk. It begins as **ascending aorta** at the base of the left ventricle, passes craniad and dorsad between the pulmonary artery on the left and the right atrium on the right and then turns caudad inclining slightly to the left, thus describing a curve called the aortic arch with its convexity directed upward and forward and the concavity facing downward and backward. From here it proceeds caudad on the ventrolateral surface of the thoracic vertebrae and the longus colli muscle as the **descending aorta**. At its origin from the base of left ventricle, the caliber of the aorta is greatest forming the **bulbus aorta** and here it presents three dilatations called the **aortic sinuses.** As the descending aorta reaches the level of the seventh thoracic vertebra it continues behind as **thoracic aorta** running through the middle and caudal mediastinum between the left and right lungs. The ascending aorta gives out the following branches.

Coronary arteries

The right and left coronary arteries arise from the respective aortic sinuses and are distributed almost entirely to the heart. These have been described above under the title 'Blood supply to heart.

Thoracic aorta

The thoracic aorta is the continuation of the descending aorta running caudally beyond the level of the fourth thoracic vertebra. From here it passes caudally between the two pleural sacs. Initially at the level between the fourth and seventh thoracic vertebrae, it is crossed on its right surface by the oesophagus and trachea and on left surface by the left vagus nerve. The left recurrent laryngeal nerve winds round the aorta at its concavity from lateral to medial side. In this course it lies to the left of the median plane. Beyond the level of the seventh thoracic vertebra, it gradually inclines inwards medially and occupies median position when it reaches to the diaphragm. It then passes through the hiatus aorticus of the diaphragm and enter the abdominal cavity as **abdominal aorta**. In its course at the level of seventh or eighth to thirteenth thoracic vertebra, the vena hemiazygos lies along the dorsolateral aspect of the aorta on its left side and thoracic duct on its right side.

From the convexity of the aortic arch extends cranially the **brachiocephalic trunk**. It is very large vessel directed cranially and dorsally in the cranial mediastinum ventral to the trachea. It gives off branches supplying the head, neck, cranial portion of thoracic cavity and the fore limb (pectoral limb).

Relations: At its origin the aorta is related to the pulmonary artery, the thoracic aorta is related on its left to the left lung, left pulmonary artery, left vagus and the left vena azygos and on right it is related to the oesophagus and trachea. In the caudal mediastinum, it is related to the lungs laterally and the bodies of the thoracic vertebrae along with longus colli muscle dorsally. The abdominal aorta is related dorsally to the bodies of the lumbar vertebrae along with the psoas muscles and ventrally to the pancreas and rumen. On its right it is related to the caudal vena cava and on the left to the left adrenal, left kidney and the left ureter.

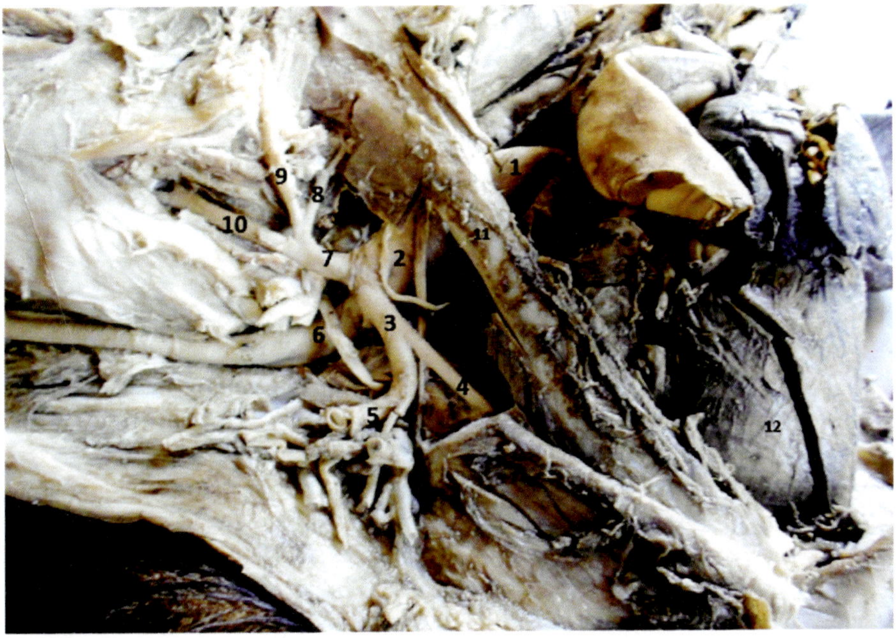

Fig. 3-4 A: Blood vessels of thorax

1. Cranial Aorta; 2. Common Brachiocephalic Trunk; 3. Left Axillary Artery; 4. Internal Thoracic Artery; 5. Brachial Artery 6. Common Carotid Artery; 7. Costo Cervical Trunk; 8. Sub Costal Artery; 9. Dorsal Artery; 10. Superior Cervical or Deep cervical Artery; 11. Second Rib; 12. Heart.

Vena azygos (Vena hemiazygos)

The azygos vein is an unpaired vein that collects venous blood from the wall of the thorax and returns it into the right atrium through the great coronary vein of the heart. In ox, the vena azygos is placed on the left side and is called the vena hemiazygos. The tributaries of the vena hemiazygos are the intercostal veins from fourth to twelfth intercostal spaces.

The vena hemiazygos begins at the left ventrolateral aspect of the last thoracic vertebra collecting the venous blood from the muscles of the back (spine) in this region through the dorsal costoabdominal vein. From here it passes cranially along the bodies of the thoracic vertebrae and the left dorsolateral surface of the thoracic aorta up to the fourth thoracic vertebra. Here it turns downward across the aorta and the pulmonary artery and reaches the left atrium at the base of the heart. Here, it turns backward and to the right side and joins the great coronary vein on the caudal surface of the heart. The coronary vein in its turn opens into the coronary sinus of the right atrium of the heart. During its course from the level of the last thoracic aorta, the vena hemiazygos receives dorsal intercostal veins at each intercostal level from twelfth to fourth intercostal space. These dorsal intercostal veins collect the venous blood from the roof (back), floor (sternal part) and the lateral walls of the thoracic cavity. The first to third dorsal intercostal veins join the costocervical or the supreme intercostal (subcostal) vein. The dorsal intercostal veins from the right side cross the median plane ventral to the bodies of the thoracic vertebrae to join the vena hemiazygos on the left side. Occasionally, the right vena hemiazygos also occurs and it is joined by tributaries from fifth and sixth intercostal veins and it joins the right supreme intercostal vein.

Cranial vena cava

The cranial vena cava is a large, short vessel extending from the cranial border of the first rib to the right atrium of the heart. It is formed by the union of the right and left common jugular veins, and the right and left subclavian veins at the lower part of the thoracic inlet. It passes caudally in the cranial mediastinum lying ventral to trachea on the right side of the aorta and after reaching at the level of the fourth rib it opens into the sinus venosus of the right atrium of the heart. At the beginning of its course, it is median in position but as it passes caudally it gradually inclines towards right side and occupies a position to the right of the aorta. In this course, it is related dorsally to trachea, cranial mediastinal lymph node, laterally on the left side to the aorta, on the right to the vagus and sympathetic cardiac nerves and the phrenic nerve.. Its tributaries include the right and left internal thoracic veins, the vertebral, costocervical, and caudal cervical veins and the subcostal veins. Venous blood is received into the cranial vena cava from head, neck, thoracic limbs, withers (back), cranial part of the thoracic walls, the floor of the thorax and the cranial part of the abdominal wall and its floor.

Caudal vena cava

The caudal vena cava is the largest and longest venous trunk in the animal body. It is formed by the union of the left and right common iliac veins in the sublumbar region ventral to the sixth lumbar vertebra in the abdominal cavity. From here it passes cranially in the sublumbar region, follows the abdominal surface of the diaphragm to the foramen vena cava, and enters the thoracic cavity through this foramen of the diaphragm.

In the thoracic cavity, the caudal vena cava runs cranially and slightly ventrad in the groove formed between the cardiac and mediastinal lobes of the right lung enclosed in the fold of right pleural sac in company with the right phrenic nerve and opens into the sinus venosus of the right atrium of the heart. The right and left phrenic veins are the only tributaries of the caudal vena cava in its thoracic part.

Thoracic part of trachea

The thoracic part of the trachea (Fig. 3-4 A) is the caudal continuation of its cervical part. It enters the thorax through the thoracic inlet. Within the thorax, the trachea lies in the cranial and middle parts of mediastinum. At the beginning of its thoracic course from thoracic inlet to about the level of third rib or intercostal space, the trachea lies on the right side of the oesophagus and thereafter it sleeps down ventral to the oesophagus at the level of fifth rib or intercostal space where it terminates by bifurcating into the right and left bronchi. The thoracic part of the trachea is related dorsally to the longus colli muscle except at its bifurcation where it is related dorsally to the oesophagus. Its ventral relations include the brachiocephalic vein, the cranial vena cava, the brachiocephalic trunk, the right common carotid artery, the right pulmonary artery, the left recurrent laryngeal nerve, the right sympathetic cardiac nerves and the cranial mediastinal lymph nodes. On the left lateral side it is related dorsolaterally to the oesophagus except in the region of its termination, laterally to vagus nerve, the left sympathetic cardiac nerves, the aortic arch, the left tracheobronchial lymph node. in young animals it is related to thymus gland. On the right lateral side, the trachea is related to the common trunk of the costocervical, deep cervical and vertebral arteries, the satellite veins of these arteries, the right azygos vein, the ansa subclavia, vagus verve, right sympathetic cardiac nerves and the tracheobronchial lymph nodes.

Thoracic part of oesophagus

The thoracic part of oesophagus begins at the level of first rib in continuation of its cervical part. At the junction of the neck and thorax, the oesophagus undergoes a slight curvature with its convexity directed ventrally and then it continues caudally into the cranial mediastinum. After reaching at the level of the third or fourth rib dorsal to the base of the heart and bifurcation of the trachea it forms second curvature which is convex dorsally. Here it crosses the right face of the aortic arch and then passes straight back in the caudal mediastinum ventral to the thoracic aorta up to the level of eighth or ninth intercostal space where it passes through the hiatus oesophageus of the diaphragm, enters the abdomen and opens into the rumen immediately behind the diaphragm.

Relations: At its entrance into the thorax, the oesophagus is related medially to trachea, and laterally to the first rib, and a common trunk of the vertebral, costocervical and caudal cervical veins.As it passes through the cranial middle mediastinum, it is related to the thoracic duct and aortic arch on the left side and the right and left longus colli muscles, common trunk of right costocervical and sub costal veins and the right vagus nerve on the right side. In its course through the caudal mediastinum, the oesophagus is related to the right and left lungs, the vagus nerve and the bronchial and oesophageal arteries on its left.

Phrenic nerve

The phrenic nerves are the motor nerves of the diaphragm. The origin of these nerves is the ventral roots of fifth, sixth and seventh cervical nerves. The major course of these nerves is through the mediastinum of the thorax. The right and left phrenic nerves cross the lateral surface of the scalenus ventralis muscle, enter the thorax ventral to subclavian artery and continue backward in the mediastinal space.

The sixth and seventh cervical roots of **right phrenic nerve** on entering the thoracic cavity runs backwards along the right face of the cranial vena cava in the cranial mediastinum and then crosses the upper part of the pericardium in the middle mediastinum. Behind the base of the heart, it runs backward in company with the caudal vena cava enclosed within a special fold of pleura in the caudal mediastinum, crosses the right face of caudal vena cava and terminates into the right side of the tendinous centre of the diaphragm.

The **left phrenic nerve**, on entering the thoracic cavity unite with the fifth cervical root at the level of first intercostal space and passes backwards along with the vagus nerve in the cranial mediastinum. It then gradually gets separated from the vagus, crosses the upper part of the pericardium in the middle mediastinum and then passes through the caudal mediastinum to reach the diaphragm.

47

Comparative Anatomy of Viscera of Thorax

Lungs and pleura

Horse

The lungs of horse are comparatively larger and longer than those of ox. These are not divided into lobes by deep fissures. The surface markings of lobules of lungs are indistinct due to reduced amount of interlobular connective tissue. The upper part of the medial surface of left lung has two grooves which are the markings of the aorta and oesophagus. These markings are comparatively faint and less marked. The ventral border of both lungs presents cardiac notch. The left cardiac notch is quadrilateral and more extensive than the right one. It extends from third to sixth ribs. The right cardiac notch is smaller and triangular. It extends from third to fifth ribs.

Dog

The lungs of dog are short and wide in order to be accommodated in the correspondingly similar shape and size of the thoracic cavity of dog. The fissures in the ventral border of the lungs are deeper and extend up to the hilus of the lung giving it an appearance of independent lobes. The right lung has four lobes and the left lung has two lobes. The intermediate (accessory) lobe of the right lung presents on its lateral surface a groove for caudal vena cava and right phrenic nerve. The cardiac impression on the mediastinal surface of the cardiac lobe is deeper in the right lung than that in the left lung. The right cardiac notch is triangular and it lies at the level of fourth and fifth interchondral spaces. The left cardiac notch is more ventral in position at the level of fifth and sixth interchondral space. The lobules are small and the surface lobulation is not distinct because of less amount of interlobular connective tissue.

Sheep and Goat

The lungs of sheep and goat are relatively longer than those of ox. The cardiac notch lies opposite the ventral part of fifth rib and fifth intercostal space. The basal border of the lungs follows a slightly curved line from the sixth costochondral junction to the vertebral end of the eleventh intercostal space. The lobes of the right and left lungs in sheep and goat are similar to those in ox. The lobules, however, are not clearly demarcated in all except the apical and middle lobes of the right lung due to incomplete interlobular connective tissue.

Pig

The lungs in pig are more or less similar to those in ox. The right lung has four lobes, the apical, cardiac, diaphragmatic and accessory. The left lung, however, has only two lobes the apical and the diaphragmatic. The cardiac notch is narrow and deep in the right lung. It lies opposite the ventral end of the third rib and third intercostal space. In the left lung, the cardiac notch is wide and shallow. It lies opposite the ventral end of the second and third intercostal space. The cardiac notch in pig is bounded cranially by the apical lobe of the right lung and dorsally and caudally by the ventral border of the left lung similar to that in ox.

Fowl

The lungs in fowl are relatively small. These are flattened and nearly rectangular structures lying in the roof of the cranial end of the celom. They are closely applied against the ventrolateral surfaces of the vertebrae and the ribs to which they are attached by cellular tissue. The left and right lungs occupy only a small space of the thoracic cavity. The base of the lung is covered by the pleura and is in contact with a rudimentary diaphragm as the diaphragm is absent in birds. The dorsal edge of the vertebral surface of the lungs is marked by five deep furrows caused by second to sixth vertebral ribs. The visceral surface is broad and flat. On this surface, the parabronchi and parts of four great medioventral secondary bronchi are visible.

Heart and pericardium

Horse

The heart of the horse is completely conical in shape and it is slightly flattened on each side. Its long axis from middle of the base to the apex is much more oblique ventrally and caudally. The base of the heart of horse is larger than that of the ox. It lies at about the junction of the dorsal and middle third of the dorsoventral diameter of the thorax. It is opposite the lateral wall of the thorax at the level of second to sixth intercostal space or from second to sixth rib. The apex is completely conical and it lies centrally dorsal to the last sternebra about one centimeter dorsal to the sternum and about two to three centimeter away from the sternal part of the diaphragm. The cranial (right ventricular) border is strongly convex and more so than that in ox. Its greater part lies parallel to the sternum. The caudal (left ventricular) border is shorter and is nearly vertical and is opposite the sixth rib or sixth intercostal space. The intermediate or caudal groove is absent. The ossa cordis, the bones of the aortic fibrous rings are absent. The right atrium is larger than the left one.

The ventral part of the pericardium is in partial contact with the thoracic wall. On the left side, the area of contact is from third rib to sixth rib. On right side, it is opposite to the ventral part of third and fourth intercostal spaces.

Dog

The heart of the dog greatly differs in form and position from that of other domestic animals. It is usually ovoid in form and its apex is blunt and rounded. The long axis of the heart is more oblique in dog than in other species. The base of the heart faces towards the cranial thoracic aperture and the thoracic vertebrae and it is opposite the ventral part of third rib. The apex is on the left side at the sixth interchondral space or seventh costal cartilage. It is in close relation to the sternal part of the diaphragm. The right and left interventricular grooves unite at the right side of the apex.

The pericardium in dog has no attachment with the sternum The apical part of the pericardium is, however, attached to the sternal part of the diaphragm by tendinous band called as phrenico-pericardial ligament.

Sheep and Goat

The heart in sheep and goat is elongated and conical in shape and it lies at the level of second to fifth intercostal space. It lies obliquely across the median plane with the base in the mediastinum and the apex to the left side of the cavity towards the diaphragm. The main portion of heart lies to the left of the median plane. The cranial border of the heart corresponds to second intercostal space and the caudal border lies opposite the fifth intercostal space. The left ventricular border is convex. The right ventricular border in sheep is convex in the dorsal part and concave in the ventral part. In goat it is nearly straight except its apical portion which is slightly concave. The os cordis is single in sheep but paired in goat.

The pericardium is attached to the sternum by two fibrous sternopericardiac ligaments at the paired notches of sixth costal cartilages.

Pig

The heart in pig is small in proportion to the body weight. It is broad, short and blunt. In hardened specimens, it appears as compressed dorsoventrally. The auricular surface is ventral in position and it is moderately convex. It overlies the sternum extending from second to seventh sternebra. The dorsal or atrial surface is more convex. The intermediate groove is present. The apex is blunt and is almost median in position overlying the seventh sternebra.

The pericardium is attached to the sternum by sterno pericardiac ligament and with the diaphragm by phrenico- pericardial ligament. It is in contact with the lateral thoracic wall from second intercostal space to fifth rib.

Fowl

The heart of chicken is placed in the cranial part of the thoracic (thoracoabdominal) cavity. It lies exactly on the midline of the cavity and is directed caudoventrally. It has the form of an acute cone. It has three surfaces, the sternal (cranioventral), hepatic (caudodorsal) and pulmonary (dorsal). The base of the heart is formed by left atrium and part of right atrium and it lies at the thoracic inlet. The apex lies between the left and right lobes of the liver. It is separated from the sternum by pulmonary air sac.

The right atrium is larger than the left atrium. The venous blood returns to right atrium by two cranial and one caudal venae cavae. The right atrioventricular opening is a slit like. It is guarded by a leaf like strong muscular fold in place of tricuspid valve of the mammalian animals. The right ventricle is more crescentic than that of mammals. The pulmonary opening is guarded by pulmonary valve consisting of three small semilunar cusps.

The two pulmonary veins instead of opening separately in the left atrium, join each other on the dorsal wall of the left atrium before entering the left atrium and open by a common opening. The left atrioventricular opening is guarded by membranous cusps like those of bicuspid valve of the mammals. The aortic opening has three semilunar valves.

The pericardium of fowl is thin and membranous. It gives attachment to the falciform ligament of the liver. It is related to the lobes of liver laterally, sternum ventrally and trachea and oesophagus dorsally.

Other contents of mediastinum

Horse

The **thoracic part of trachea** is almost circular with its transverse and vertical diameter nearly equal. However, at the site of its crossing the aortic arch at the level of third rib, the trachea is slightly compressed from side to side. As a result, the vertical diameter at this level becomes greater than the transverse diameter. The tracheal rings in horse are larger than those in ox. In the thoracic part of trachea, the tracheal rings do not meet dorsally. The tracheal muscle made of smooth muscle fibres extends transversely across the incomplete ends of tracheal rings closing the gaps between the two ends. The rest of the features about the course and relations of thoracic part of thorax in horse are more or less similar to those of ox.

The gross anatomical features of the **thoracic part of the oesophagus** in horse are almost similar to those in ox. The oesophagus in horse enters the thorax through the thoracic inlet passing dorsally and caudally between the left face of the trachea and first rib. It passes caudally lying dorsal to trachea and reaches the third thoracic vertebra where it crosses the aortic arch and gains the position on the right of the median plane. From here it passes caudally between the lungs inclining gradually to the left and reaches the hiatus oesophageus passing through which it enters the abdomen and terminates at the cardiac orifice of the stomach in the abdomen. The musculature of the wall of the oesophagus at the level of the base of the heart is of striped type while in rest of its length it is unstripped.

The **thoracic aorta** and the thoracic part of **caudal vena** cava in horse resembles to that of ox. The **vena azygos** is however is on the right side. The right vena azygos runs cranially along the right side of the ventral surfaces of the thoracic vertebrae to about sixth or seventh thoracic vertebra, passes ventrally and cranially across the right side of the thoracic duct, trachea and oesophagus and either into the cranial vena cava or the coronary sinus. Some times the left vena azygos (vena hemiazygos) occurs in horse.

Dog

The **thoracic part of trachea** in dog lies in the cranial and middle mediastinum similar to that in other species. The gross features including the course and relations with other contents of the mediastinum are also similar to those of ox and horse. The tracheal rings in dog, however, are bent because of which the trachea in cross section appears like an ellipse with its shortest diameter in the sagittal plane. The outline of thoracic trachea is almost cylindrical. The tracheal rings are incomplete dorsally, the gaps between the two ends being filled by the tracheal muscle.

The **thoracic part of oesophagus** in dog is relatively wide and dilatable. It enters the thorax lying dorsal to trachea and ventral to left longus colli muscle. After reaching the base of the heart, it inclines medially with aortic arch on its left and passes back over the bifurcation of the trachea. From here it continues to pass caudally between the lungs inclining slightly to the left and then passes through the hiatus oesophageus to terminate into the cardiac opening of the stomach in the abdominal cavity.

The **thoracic aorta** has the same course as in ox. The bronchial and oesophageal arteries arise in a common trunk as broncho-oesophageal artery from the convexity of the aortic arch. The intercostal arteries are eighteen pairs in dog instead of twelve in ox. The first pair comes from the superior cervical artery and the next three from the subcostal artery, and the remaining fourteen arise from the aorta. Two or three phrenic arteries arise from the aorta during its passage through the hiatus aorticus.

The **thoracic part of caudal vena cava** resembles to that of ox. The right **vena azygos** also resembles to that of ox. The left vena azygos is inconsistent in appearance in dog, if present, it resembles to that of horse.

Sheep and Goat

The **thoracic part of trachea** passes through the cranial mediastinum and terminates in middle mediastinum similar to that in ox. The course and relations with other contents of the mediastinum are also similar to those of ox. However, a slight deviation occurs in the morphology of the tracheal rings in sheep and goat. In the goat, the cartilaginous plates of trachea are bent in a form of 'U' with open end dorsal and the wall of the trachea between the open ends of the plate is flat and entirely membranous. In the sheep, the left end of the plate overlaps the right end in the fixed material but in the fresh material the dorsal crest is formed by the elevation of the left ends of the plates. The two free ends are joined by the tracheal muscle in both, sheep and goat like that in ox.

The **thoracic part of oesophagus** in sheep and goat resembles that of ox. The course and relations of **thoracic aorta** in sheep and goat are similar to those in ox. However, little differences occur in regard to the arterial branches arising from the aorta. The broncho-oesophageal artery arises in a common trunk from the aorta in sheep and goat as against a separate origin of bronchial and oesophageal arteries in ox. The dorsal intercostal arteries correspond to the intercostal spaces both in sheep and goat as well as in ox. The **caudal vena cava** and the **left azygos vein** resemble that of ox.

Pig

The course and relations of the **thoracic part of trachea** in pig are similar to those in ox. The tracheal rings are incomplete dorsally. The free ends of the plates overhang a little dorsally with the right side overlying the left. The tracheal muscle fills in the gaps between the ends of the tracheal rings. Under the action of the tracheal muscle, the lumen of the trachea becomes smaller than that of the larynx.

The **thoracic part of oesophagus** resembles that of ox. However the remarkable feature of the porcine oesophagus is that it becomes transversely flattened while passing through the hiatus oesophagus of the diaphragm owing to vertically elongated slit like contour of the oesophageal hiatus in pig.

The course and distribution of **thoracic aorta**, **caudal vena cava** and **vena azygos** in pig is more or less similar to that of ox.

Fowl

The **trachea** in fowl which is on the right side of the neck in its cervical course becomes almost median in position as it enters the thorax. At its entry in the thorax the crop lies to its right side. After its entry into the celom, it is ventral to oesophagus. The tracheal rings are like signet rings and they are complete dorsally.

The **pulmonary trunk** is very short and lies slightly left and ventral to the root of the aorta. It bifurcates just dorsal to the brachiocephalic artery and to the left of the medial plane. The right pulmonary artery is longer than the left artery because, after its origin to the left of the midline, it has to cross over the midline and then to undertake intrapericardial course before piercing the pericardial sac to reach the right lung. The left pulmonary artery leaves the pericardial sac between the left brachiocephalic artery and the left cranial vena cava. After entering the lung through its hilus, each pulmonary artery gives out the cranial ramus which distributes blood to the cranial third of the lung substance. Thereafter, the main trunk of each artery divides into two, the caudomedial and caudolateral ramus to supply the remaining two thirds of the lung.

The **oesophagus** in birds gets enlarged and forms a saccular diverticulum called as crop just cranial to thoracic inlet. While entering the thorax it returns to its tubular form similar to that of the cervical part. The thoracic part of oesophagus is shorter than the cervical part. It extends caudally dorsal to the trachea and the base of the heart. It is covered dorsally by the cervical air sac and ventrolaterally by the clavicular air sac. Caudal to fifth rib it passes caudally between the cranial thoracic air sacs to the medial surface of left lobe of the liver. In its most caudal part it is considerably reduced in diameter. The internal surface of the wall of the oesophagus presents numerous longitudinal folds which are lined by stratified squamous epithelium. At its junction with proventriculus, the oesophagus presents oesophageal tonsil.

The left and right **pulmonary veins** unite and form a common venous trunk that opens into the left atrium.

There are two **cranial venae cavae** in fowl, the right and left. Each of these is formed by the union of jugular vein that brings from head and neck and the subclavian vein that collects blood from the cranial part of thorax and the wings.

The **caudal vena cava** is short and collects blood from the viscera and the wall of the thoracoabdominal cavity and the limbs.

The **aorta,** ascending and descending aorta dose not have any remarkable deviations in fowl.

SECTION-C

BLOOD VESSELS AND LYMPHATICS

48

Arteries of Thorax

The wall of the thorax and its contents (the viscera) are supplied by the following branches of the thoracic aorta.

Brachiocephalic trunk

The brachiocephalic trunk (Fig. 3-4 A) is a large vessel distributing arterial branches to the head, neck, thoracic limbs (fore limbs) and the cranial part of thorax especially to the region of the withers, thoracic floor and parts of the cranial third of the lateral thoracic wall. It arises from the convexity of the aortic arch between the right auricle and pulmonary artery within the pericardium. It is directed cranially and dorsally in the cranial mediastinum ventral to the trachea. It is partly covered on the right side by the cranial vena cava and on the left it is crossed by the vagus nerve. The recurrent laryngeal nerve runs between it and the trachea. It gives off the left subclavian artery opposite the second intercostal space or the third rib and the right subclavian artery opposite the first rib and then continues cranially as the common bicarotid trunk.

The **subclavian arteries** entirely furnish blood supply to the thoracic limbs. Except for different (separate) origins and the left artery being longer than the right artery, the **right and left** subclavian arteries are identical in their course and distribution. A short portion of each artery is within the thoracic cavity and is called as intrathoracic course. Each of these arteries leave the thorax by encircling and crossing the cranial border of the first rib below the insertion of the scalinus ventralis muscle and above the brachial vein. The intrathoracic branches of the subclavian arteries are the costocervical, caudal cervical and internal thoracic arteries.

The **costocervical** and **caudal cervical** arteries have been described with the arteries of the neck.

The **internal thoracic artery** is large and arises from the ventral surface of the subclavian artery at the level of the first rib. It passes downward and backward to the dorsal surface of the sternum. It then continues behind covered by the transverse thoracis muscle to the seventh interchondral space where it divides into the musculophrenic and cranial abdominal branches. During this course, each internal thoracic artery gives off two, the dorsal and ventral, collateral branches at each interchondral space. The dorsal branch is called the ascending intercostal artery. It passes upward and anastomoses with the intercostal artery of the respective intercostal space. The ventral branches supply the pleura, transverse thoracis muscle and the pericardium. The thymic branches are given out from the cranial part of the internal thoracic artery in young animal.

Bicarotid trunk

The bicarotid trunk is the continuation of the brachiocephalic trunk after the right subclavian artery is given off. It is very short and lies on the ventral surface of the trachea at the thoracic inlet and divides into **right and left common carotid arteries.**

Other collateral branches of thoracic aorta

The thoracic aorta gives off **visceral branches** to the thoracic viscera and **parietal branches** to thoracic walls and the thoracic part of the spinal cord and its meninges. The visceral branches are the bronchial and the oesophageal arteries. The parietal branches include the dorsal intercostal, dorsal costoabdominal and the cranial phrenic arteries.

Bronchial artery

The bronchial artery is a single (unpaired) slender branch that arises from the right ventral face of the thoracic aorta at the level of sixth thoracic vertebra. It is the artery for nutritional blood supply to the lungs. After its origin from the aorta, it descends across the left face of the oesophagus and on reaching the tracheal bifurcation, divides into the left and right branches. The right branch is slightly larger than the left one. Each of these further proceeds to the root of the lung and enters the hilus of the lung of the corresponding side. At the hilus of the lung, each artery splits into two to three branches which accompany the branches of the bronchial tree. At the hilus of the lung, each of the bronchial arteries detaches small branches to the bronchial lymph nodes, pulmonary pleura and the mediastinum.

Oesophageal artery

The oesophageal artery is a small branch that arises from the ventral face of the thoracic aorta just behind the origin of the bronchial artery. Immediately after its origin, it divides into several branches that supply blood to the wall of the middle and caudal thoracic part of the oesophagus. A few of these branches are supplied to the caudal mediastinum and the caudal mediastinal lymph nodes.

Dorsal intercostal arteries

The intercostal arteries, except the first three, are parietal branches of the aorta and supply the lateral thoracic wall. There are twelve pairs of intercostal arteries in ox. Of these, the first three pairs arise from the costocervical trunk or the supreme intercostal artery (a branch of costocervical) and the rests arise directly from the thoracic aorta. The last one (thirteenth intercostal) is called the dorsal costoabdominal artery as it arises from the aorta caudal to the last rib and do not run in the intercostal space. The dorsal intercostal arteries arise in pairs from the dorsal surface of the thoracic aorta and cross the vertebral bodies to reach the caudal border of the corresponding rib where they divide into dorsal and ventral branches. The dorsal branch passes upward to supply the dorsal muscles of the back (spine). It gives off the spinal branch which passes through the intervertebral foramen and is distributed to the vertebrae and meninges and joins the ventral spinal artery. The ventral branch passes outward in the intercostal space where it lies first between the external and internal intercostal muscles but soon becomes subpleural. They anastomose with the intercostal branches of the internal thoracic arteries and supply the intercostal muscles, pleura and the ribs. The branches from these intercostal arteries are also supplied to the latissimus dorsi, serratus thoracis and the cutaneous muscles and the skin. The last intercostal artery supplies the oblique abdominal muscles.

Dorsal costoabdominal artery

The dorsal costoabdominal artery resembles the dorsal intercostal arteries in its origin and distribution. It descends caudal to the last rib and supplies the obliquus abdominis externus and internus muscles.

Cranial phrenic artery

The cranial phrenic arteries are usually two or three small branches arising from the ventral surface of the thoracic aorta at the hiatus aorticus either separately or in a common trunk. These branches are distributed to the crura of the diaphragm, usually one branch for each crus. In some cases this artery may arise from the abdominal part of the aorta or from the celiac or mesenteric branches of the abdominal aorta.

49

Veins of Thorax

The venous drainage from the wall of the thorax is performed by the **dorsal intercostal veins**. These veins are distributed as below.

The **dorsal intercostal veins** are twelve pairs in number. Of these, the fourth to twelfth intercostal veins from right side and fifth to twelfth intercostal veins from the left side join the **vena azygos**.

The **costocervical vein** arises at the second intercostal space. It passes dorsocranially towards the thoracic inlet and join a common trunk of the supreme intercostal, dorsal scapular and vertebral veins to finally join the cranial vena cava.

The **supreme intercostal vein** is formed by the union of first three dorsal intercostal veins, runs towards the thoracic inlet to join the common trunk with the vertebral vein which finally join the cranial vena cava.

The **internal thoracic vein** lies on the dorsal surface of the sternum under cover of the transversus thoracis muscle except at the first rib where it is covered by the pleura. It is formed by the union of epigastric (cranial abdominal) and musculophrenic veins at the xyphoid cartilage of the sternum and terminates on the ventral surface of the cranial vena cava at the level of first rib. Along its course it receives ventral intercostal, mediastinal and thymic veins. The ventral intercostal veins form anastomoses with the dorsal intercostal veins of the corresponding intercostal space.

Musculophrenic vein lies in a groove between the seventh and eighth costal cartilages and behind this between the attachment of diaphragm and transversus abdominis muscle. Its tributaries are from the lateral part of the abdominal floor and the lower part of the thoracic wall.

The **oesophageal veins,** about four or five small branches extend from the dorsolateral face of the oesophagus in the middle and caudal thoracic part and open into the vena azygos.

The right and left **bronchial veins** emerge through the hilus of the corresponding lung, pass through the root of the lung and runs craniodorsally to join either in a common trunk or separately to the vena azygos.

50

Lymphatics of Thorax

The lymphatics of the thoracic region are comprised of large number of lymph nodes which are arranged in different groups like the aortic, sternal, mediastinal and bronchial. The efferent ducts from these lymph nodes ultimately join the thoracic duct which carries lymph from all over the body except the head neck and fore limb to open in the cranial venacava.

Thoracic aortic and sternal lymph nodes

The lymphatics of the thoracic and sternal region is comprised of thoracic aortic, intercostal, cranial and caudal sternal, and the xiphoid lymph nodes and the thoracic duct which conducts the lymph collected from most of the parts of the body except the head, neck and fore limbs.

The **thoracic aortic lymph nodes** are located along the dorsolateral border of the aorta, ventral to the sympathetic trunk. The afferents for these lymph nodes are received from the muscles of thoracic wall, diaphragm, pleural and pericardial sacs and the intercostal lymph nodes. The efferents from the thoracic aortic lymph nodes are connected to the thoracic duct either directly or through other lymph nodes of the thoracic cavity.

The **intercostal lymph nodes** are situated dorsal to the sympathetic trunk in the intercostal spaces along the course of the intercostal vessels. The afferents for these lymph nodes come from intercostal muscles, the muscles of the back (spine), the costal (parietal) pleura, and ribs. The efferents of these lymph nodes open into the thoracic aortic lymph nodes or directly into the thoracic duct.

The **cranial sternal lymph nodes** are situated along the internal thoracic vessels on the floor of the thoracic cavity. This is usually a large lymph node located in the first intercostal space cranial to the transversus thoracis muscle. The afferents of this lymph node are received from the muscles of ventral and lateral thoracic wall, abdominal muscles, diaphragm, and the ventral aspect of the pleural and pericardial sacs. The efferents from this lymph node are connected to the thoracic duct or tracheal trunk either directly or through the mediastinal lymph nodes.

The **caudal sternal lymph nodes** vary in size, number and arrangement. Some of these are located on the transversus thoracis muscle along the internal thoracic vessels and one of these is present at the angle between the eighth and ninth costal cartilages and the sternum. The afferents of these lymph nodes are received from the muscles of the ventrolateral aspect of the thorax, and abdomen, the ribs and the sternum. The efferents usually connect these lymph nodes to the cranial sternal lymph node.

The **xiphoid lymph node** is a medium sized single lymph node located on the xiphoid cartilage of the sternum. The afferents for this lyph node comes from diaphragm, costal pleura, pericardium and the caudal mediastinum. The efferent of this lymph node are connected to the caudal sternal lymph nodes.

The **phrenic lymph nodes** are small and are located at the foramen vena cava of the diaphragm and at the termination of phrenic nerves. One of these is located mostly at the angle of the caudal vena cava with the diaphragm. The afferents come from diaphragm and the mediastinum and the efferents join the caudal mediastinal lymph nodes.

Mediastinal lymph nodes

The mediastinal lymphocentre has three lymph nodes in this group. These are the cranial, middle and caudal mediastinal lymph nodes.

The **cranial mediastinal lymph nodes** are a group of variable number of small lymph nodes located on the great vessels, trachea and oesophagus. The afferents from these lymph nodes come from the thoracic portion of oesophagus, trachea, thymus, lungs, pericardium, heart, costal and mediastinal pleura and the intercostal and thoracic aortic lymph nodes. The efferents from these lymph nodes connect them directly with the thoracic duct.

The **middle mediastinal lymph nodes** are about four to five small lymph nodes situated on the right or dorsal aspect of the aortic arch and in some cases extends to right face of the oesophagus. Their afferents arrive from the oesophagus, trachea, lungs, pericardium, mediastinum and the intercostal and tracheobronchial lymph nodes. The efferents from these lymph nodes open into the thoracic duct.

The **caudal mediastinal lymph nodes** are usually one large lymph node accompanied by three to four small lymph nodes situated in the caudal mediastinum, ventral to the aorta along the dorsal and lateral faces of the oesophagus. The afferents for these lymph nodes are received from oesophagus, lungs, pericardial sacs, diaphragm, mediastinum and some organs of the abdominal cavity. The efferents unite to form a common trunk that joins the thoracic duct.

Bronchial lymph nodes

The bronchial lymph nodes include the left tracheobronchial, right tracheobronchial, cranial and middle tracheobronchial and pulmonary lymph nodes.

The **left tracheobronchial lymph node** is relatively larger in size and it is situated at the angle between the aortic arch and the left branch of pulmonary artery. The afferents for this lymph node are received from the oesophagus, heart, and the pulmonary and thoracic aortic lymph nodes. Its efferent vessel joins the thoracic duct either directly or through the caudal mediastinal lymph nodes.

The **right tracheobronchial lymph node** is located on the right side of the bifurcation of trachea, near the dorsal border of the right branch of pulmonary artery. The afferents for this node come from the lungs and the pulmonary and middle tracheobronchial lymph nodes. The efferent vessel of this node joins the middle mediastinal lymph node.

The **cranial tracheobronchial lymph node** is situated at the origin of the bronchus of the apical lobe of the lung. Its afferents come from lungs and the pulmonary lymph nodes. The efferent vessel from this node joins the cranial mediastinal lymph node.

The **middle tracheobronchial lymph node** is situated at the bifurcation of the trachea. Its afferent vessels are from the lungs and the efferent vessel is connected to middle mediastinal lymph node.

The lymph from these lymph nodes of thoracic cavity is collected into the thoracic duct which conducts this lymph to the cranial vena cava.

Thoracic duct

The thoracic duct arises from the cisterna chyli at the hiatus aorticus. In most cases this duct divides into two divisions, the right and the left, which lie on the respective sides of the dorsal face of the thoracic aorta. During their course, the right and the left ducts are intermittently united by anastomotic lymph vessels. The two ducts finally join each other at the level of the fifth thoracic vertebra and form a common trunk. This trunk turns from right to left side in an 'S' shaped curve at the cranial mediastinum from where it courses cranioventrally on the left side of the trachea and oesophagus and terminates in the cranial vena cava in front of the first rib. At its opening into the cranial vena cava, the thoracic duct ampulates.

51

Comparative Anatomy of Blood Vessels and Lymphatics of Thorax

Arteries of thorax

Horse

The **bronchial** and **oesophageal arteries** in horse have a common trunk of origin as broncho-oesophageal artery. It arises from the convexity of aortic arch, passes ventrally and caudally on the right side of the aorta and divides into bronchial and oesophageal arteries. The oesophageal artery passes caudally in the caudal mediastinum along the dorsal face of oesophagus and supplies branches to oesophagus, caudal mediastinal lymph nodes and pleura and anastomoses with the pleuro-oesophageal branch of the gastric artery.

The **intercostal arteries** are eighteen pairs in number. The first pair arises from the superior artery, the next three pairs come from subcostal artery and the remaining four arise from the thoracic aorta.

The **phrenic arteries** are not variable in origin as in the ox. They are small and are two to three in number. They arise on the ventral face of the aorta while it passes through the hiatus aorticus and enter the crura of the diaphragm.

The rest of the arterial branches of thorax in horse are similar to those in ox.

Dog

The **bronchial arteries** do not arise from the aorta. Some of the oesophageal arteries supply bronchial branches to reach the hilus of the lungs. About four to five oesophageal arteries arise from different parts of thoracic aorta, pass ventrally into the mediastinum and supply the oesophagus.

The **phrenic arteries** do not originate from the thoracic part of the aorta. Instead, the phrenico-abdominal artery arises from the abdominal part of the aorta to supply the diaphragm.

The **intercostal arteries** are thirteen pairs in number. Their distribution is similar to that in ox.

The rest of the arterial branches of thorax in horse are similar to those in ox.

Sheep and Goat

The broncho-oesophageal artery arises by a common trunk from the thoracic aorta at the level of fifth intercostal space. This artery divides into bronchial and oesophageal arteries.

The dorsal intercostal arteries correspond with the number of thoracic vertebrae. The last of these arteries is called the costoabdominal artery. The first and second intercostal arteries arise from the supreme intercostal artery.

Pig

A common trunk of the **bronchial and oesophageal arteries** frequently arises separately from the thoracic aorta. The bronchial artery passes ventral to the tracheal bifurcation and divides into four branches together with the bronchial veins. The oesophageal arteries are usually two branches supplying the cranial and middle mediastinal segments of the oesophagus. In addition, there are some branches directly arising from the thoracic aorta to supply the caudal thoracic segment of the oesophagus.

The **cranial phrenic arteries**, usually two, arise from the thoracic aorta in the region of hiatus aorticus.

The **dorsal intercostal arteries** are thirteen or fourteen pairs. Of these, eight or nine pairs arise from thoracic aorta. The first dorsal intercostal artery arises from vertebral artery on the right side and from the deep cervical artery on the left side. The second dorsal intercostal arteries originate from the dorsal scapular artery. The third, fourth and fifth dorsal intercostal arteries arise from the supreme intercostal artery.

The rest of the arterial branches of thorax in horse are similar to those in ox.

Fowl

The dorsal intercostal arteries of the first two or three intercostal spaces arise from the vertebral artery. The remaining three intercostal spaces are supplied by the dorsal intercostal arteries arising from the descending aorta. The dorsal rami of the dorsal intercostal arteries supply the spinal cord, vertebral column, dorsal axial musculature and the overlying skin. The ventral rami supply the musculature of the body wall.

Veins of thorax

The veins of thorax in horse, dog, sheep and goat and pig almost resemble those of ox. In the fowl, the sterno-clavicularis, thoracic and axillary veins drain out the venous blood from the thorax.

Lymphatics of thorax

The **lymph nodes and lymph vessels** of thorax in **horse, dog, sheep and goat and pig** resemble those of ox.

However, **in fowl** the lymphatics are thymus dependent wherein the lymphoid tissue is in two groups, the central and peripheral. The central group of lymphoid tissue consists of thymus and bursa as against that of thymus in mammalian species.

The peripheral **lymph nodes** in fowl are very few and very small in the form of nodules in the cranial part of thorax and in the walls of the alimentary canal.

The **lymphatic vessels** are very thin and narrow lymphatic ducts running along the large blood vessels.

SECTION-D

NERVES

52

Nerves of Thorax

Spinal nerves

The thoracic spinal nerves are thirteen pairs in ox. These are named and numbered according to the vertebra caudal to which they emerge from the vertebral canal. They emerge from the vertebral canal through the respective lateral vertebral (intervertebral) foramina. Each nerve, after its emergence, divides into dorsal and ventral branches. Each dorsal branch passes up dorsally between the transverse processes of the vertebrae and divides in to medial and lateral branches. The medial branch passes upward and supplies the dorsal muscles of the back. The lateral branch passes laterally on the deep surface of the longissimus dorsi muscle. At the lateral border of this muscle it passes between this and longissimus costarum muscles and becomes a cutaneous nerve which divides into ascending and descending branches supplying the muscles and the skin of this region.. Before its division, the lateral branch supplies muscular branches to the longissimus dorsi and longissimus costarum muscles.

The ventral branches continue ventrally as intercostal nerves. The first and second thoracic nerves, before their continuation as intercostal nerves, give out a branch to the brachial plexus. At a short distance from the spinal nerve, the ventral branch of each of these nerves is connected to sympathetic trunk by a ramus communicans containing preganglionic and postganglionic sympathetic fibres. The intercostal nerves run down ventrally through the intercostal spaces, lying between the external and internal intercostal muscles close to the caudal border of the respective rib and in company with the intercostal vessels. Along this course they supply these muscles. After a variable distance, the intercostal nerves and vessels traverse through the internal intercostal muscles and become subpleural in position. The second to eighth nerves end in the transversus thoracis muscle. The rests behind these end in the rectus abdominis and other abdominal muscles and the skin in this region.

Autonomic nerves

The sympathetic division of autonomic nervous system in thoracic cavity is represented by thoracic sympathetic trunk and the parasympathetic division is provided by the branches of the vagus nerve.

Sympathetic nerves

The thoracic sympathetic trunk (Fig. 3-5 A) lies bilaterally ventral to the costovertebral articulations along the lateral border of the longus colli muscle. This trunk is the continuation of the cervical sympathetic trunk and it extends caudally from the cervicothoracic ganglion ventral to the head of the first rib or the costovertebral articulation on the ventrolateral surface of the longus colli muscle to the crura of the diaphragm and continues between the crura of diaphragm and the psoas muscle as the lumbar sympathetic trunk. The thoracic sympathetic trunk bears thirteen sympathetic ganglia, one each at the respective intercostal space. The first thoracic ganglion is fused with the caudal cervical ganglion and is called as cervicothoracic (stellate) ganglion. Cranially the thoracic sympathetic trunk is connected to the cervical sympathetic trunk by the ansa subclavia. Each ganglion is connected with the ventral branch of respective thoracic spinal nerve by a ramus communicans. These are of two types, the white and grey rami communicantes.

Cervicothoracic ganglion

The cervicothoracic ganglion is bilaterally situated medial to the first rib or first intercostal space ventral to first thoracic costovertebral articulation. The left ganglion lies obliquely dorsoventral on the lateral face of longus colli muscle and the oesophagus while the right ganglion lies dorsoventral on the lateral face of longus colli muscle and the trachea. Its dorsal end is narrow and the ventral end is wide. The ganglion is compressed mediolaterally. It is related medially in its dorsal third to the longus colli muscle on either side. The ventral third of the medial surface of the right ganglion is related to trachea while that of the left ganglion is related to oesophagus. Laterally this ganglion is related to vertebral artery and vein. The cervicothoracic ganglion is connected to first thoracic spinal nerve through the **first thoracic ramus communicans**. When second thoracic ganglion is fused with the cervicothoracic ganglion is connected to second thoracic spinal nerve through **second thoracic ramus communicans**. In addition to these, the cervicothoracic ganglion is connected to second to seventh cervical spinal nerves through the nervous transversarius.

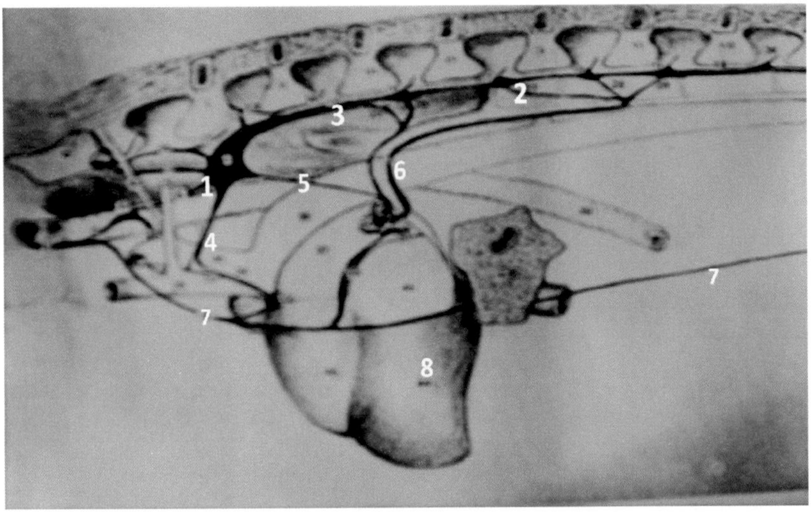

Fig. 3 – 5 A: Thoracic Sympathetic cardiac nerves
1. Cervicothoracic ganglion; 2.Thoracic Sympathetic ganglion 3. Thoracic Sympathetic trunk 4. Cranial cervicothoracic cardiac nerve 5. Caudal cervicothoracic cardiac nerve 6. Thoracic sympathetic cardiac nerve 7. Vagus nerve 8. Heart

The **nervous transversarius** extends from the cranioventral part of the cervicothoracic ganglion, passes upward and forward over the lateral face of the longus colli muscle parallel to the vertebral artery up to the seventh cervical spinal nerve. Here it detaches a ramus to seventh cervical spinal nerve and then enters the transverse canal along with the vertebral artery. During its course forward through this canal it furnishes ramus communicans to each of the sixth to second cervical nerve.

The **ramus communicans to eighth cervical spinal nerve** extends from the craniodorsal aspect of the cervicothoracic ganglion. It courses caudal and parallel to the nervous transversarius along the lateral face of the longus colli muscle and join the ventral branch of the eighth cervical spinal nerve.

The **visceral nerves** extending **from cervicothoracic ganglion** include the left and right cervicothoracic cardiac nerves, nerve fibres to oesophagus from left ganglion and to trachea from the right gland and the fibres to major blood vessels and lymph nodes in the middle mediastinum.

Cervicothoracic cardiac nerves: Usually one or sometimes two cardiac nerves extend from the cervicothoracic ganglion. These are named as **caudoventral** and **caudodorsal** cervicothoracic cardiac nerves since these arise from the ventral and dorsal part of the caudal border of the ganglion respectively. The left caudoventral cervicothoracic cardiac nerve arises from the caudal border of the ganglion and passes ventrally over the left surface of the aorta and reaches at the intervascular triangle where it enters the cardiac plexus and joins the cardiac sympathetic ganglion in this plexus. The left caudodorsal cervicothoracic cardiac nerve passes down following the brachiocephalic trunk, then passes caudally to the right of the aortic arch and enters the cardiac plexus. The right cervicothoracic cardiac nerves, after arising from the caudal border of the cervicothoracic ganglion or from the cranial or caudal limbs of the ansa subclavia, pass caudoventrally on the right face of the cranial vena cava and then between the cranial vena cava and aorta to reach the pretracheal portion of the cardiac plexus. Here these nerves enter the cardiac plexus and join the cardiac ganglion.

Sympathetic nerves to oesophagus, trachea and mediastinal lymph nodes are supplied to the respective organs through the fibres separated from the cardiac nerves during their course from cervicothoracic ganglion to cardiac plexus.

Sympathetic fibres to great vessels are supplied from the cardiac plexus as an extension of cardiac plexus or as its sub plexuses on these vessels.

Thoracic sympathetic ganglia

The thoracic sympathetic trunk bears 13 ganglia on each side. The first and occasionally the second ganglion is included in the cervicothoracic ganglion. It lies ventral to the first costovertebral articulation. The second or third to thirteenth thoracic sympathetic ganglia are situated medial to the vertebral end of the corresponding intercostal spaces. These ganglia are mostly oval or triangular in shape. The third to sixth ganglia are slightly larger than the succeeding ganglia. All the thirteen ganglia are connected with the corresponding thoracic spinal nerves by rami communicantes. Third to sixth ganglia gives out thoracic cardiac nerves. Other visceral nerves extending from these ganglia include the nerve fibres supplied to the great vessels, oesophagus lungs and lymph nodes. Seventh to thirteenth ganglia mainly contribute fibres to the major splanchnic nerve which distributes sympathetic fibres to the viscera of the abdomen.

Thoracic cardiac nerves arise from the lateral border of the thoracic ganglia. These nerves on the left side arise from second to fifth thoracic ganglion and on right side from third to sixth thoracic ganglion. The left thoracic cardiac nerves pass ventrally over the lateral surface of the aorta and then continue along the vena hemiazygos to the cardiac ganglion of the cardiac plexus at the left intervascular triangle. The right thoracic cardiac nerves pass ventrally between the thoracic aorta and oesophagus and then along the right face of the cranial vena cava to reach the pretracheal portion of the cardiac plexus.

Sympathetic nerves to lungs, great vessels, oesophagus and trachea are supplied to these organ through the small extensions of the cardiac plexuses or the sub plexuses formed by the nerve fibres extending from cardiac plexuses.

The **major splanchnic nerve** is a major nerve formed by the nerve fibres furnished by the sixth to thirteenth thoracic sympathetic ganglia in the thoracic cavity. The nerve fibres from each of the sixth to thirteenth thoracic sympathetic ganglia pass caudally and join this nerve along the ventral aspect of the thoracic sympathetic trunk and gets exit from the thorax along with the sympathetic trunk passing between the crus of the diaphragm and the psoas minor. After entering the abdomen the major splanchnic nerve gets separated from the sympathetic trunk and joins the celiac plexus on the celiac artery.

Parasympathetic nerves

The parasympathetic part of autonomic nerve supply to the viscera of thorax is through the branches of thoracic part of the vagus nerve.

Vagus nerve

The vagus nerve (Fig.3-5A) which accompanies the sympathetic trunk in the vagosympathetic trunk passes down the neck and reaches the thoracic inlet. In its further course before entering the thoracic cavity, it separates from the sympathetic trunk and then enters the thorax. After entering the thorax, the right and left vagus nerve follows somewhat different course. The right vagus nerve passes backward under the right subclavian artery and between the subclavian artery and the bicarotid trunk. It then passes caudally and slightly dorsally crossing obliquely the lateral surface of the brachiocephalic artery and the right face of the trachea and after reaching near the bifurcation of trachea it divides into dorsal and ventral branches. The left vagus nerve enters the thorax along the ventrolateral face of the oesophagus, crosses it obliquely under the left subclavian artery and then passes caudally on the lateral surface of that artery. Behind this, it courses caudally over the left face of the aorta and reaches at the root of the left lung and the dorsal face of the oesophagus where it divides into dorsal and ventral branches. At this place, the dorsal and ventral branches of the left vagus unite with the dorsal and ventral branches of right vagus and form the combined dorsal and ventral vagal trunks that pass caudally on the corresponding surfaces of the oesophagus in the caudal mediastinum and then pass through the hiatus oesophageus along with the oesophagus and enter the abdominal cavity. During its thoracic course, the vagus nerve contributes parasympathetic nerve fibres to the autonomic plexuses in the thorax for the viscera of the thorax. In addition, it gives out a branch named as recurrent laryngeal nerve on either side which ascends through the neck and terminates on the larynx. The right and left recurrent laryngeal nerve s differ in their origin from vagus nerve in the thorax.

The **right recurrent laryngeal nerve** originates from right vagus opposite the second rib, passes from medial to lateral side dorsal to subclavian artery and caudal to costocervical trunk and then ascends in the neck on the right ventral surface of the trachea to reach the larynx.

The **left recurrent laryngeal nerve** arises from the left vagus nerve at the aortic arch, passes caudal to ligamentum arteriosus and reaches to the right surface of the aorta. From here, the left recurrent laryngeal nerve ascends the neck along the left ventral part of trachea to reach the larynx.

The **vagal cardiac nerves** arise from the right and left vagus nerves caudal to the origin of recurrent laryngeal nerves. The left vagal cardiac nerve passes caudally into the pretracheal portion of the cardiac plexus. About one to three right vagal cardiac nerves pass cranially and reach cranial to the ventromedial aspect of the tracheal bronchus to join the cardiac plexus.

The **bronchial nerves** arise from each vagus nerve near the dorsal surface of the bronchi. In addition some fibres of vagus nerve extend from the ventral vagal trunk in the caudal mediastinum and some fibres extend from the cardiac plexus. All these nerves pass to the bronchial tree.

The **oesophageal branches** originate directly from the right and left vagal nerves and also from the dorsal and ventral vagal trunks.

The other structures in the thorax including the vessels and lymphatics receive parasympathetic fibres through the cardiac, pulmonary and bronchial autonomic plexuses.

53

Comparative Anatomy of Thoracic Nerves

The thoracic spinal nerves of the horse, dog, sheep and goat, pig and fowl almost resemble to those of ox in origin, disposition and distribution. The number of pairs of thoracic spinal nerves, however, vary and it corresponds to the number of thoracic vertebrae present in those particular species of animal.

The thoracic sympathetic trunk, ganglia and the visceral nerve branches extending from the thoracic sympathetic ganglia in different species also resemble to those of ox with some minor variations.

The parasympathetic nerve supply to thoracic viscera in these animals is also through the vagus nerve and its branches similar to that in ox.

SECTION-E

APPLIED ANATOMY

54

Applied Anatomy of Thorax

Surface locations for clinical examination on the wall of thorax

Lymph nodes

Prescapular lymph node is palpable as a cylindrical object just cranial to the point of shoulder. Palpation can be performed by putting the base of the hand on the cranial edge of the scapula and pressing forward with fingers. This enables to roll the skin and feel the lymph node flicking underneath the fingers.

Heart

The clinical examination of heart is performed by percussion and auscultation on the thoracic wall.

For **percussion** of heart, usually the fifth rib is identified opposite the olecranon of a straight vertical limb. Two fields are identified for percussion of heart. (1) The area of absolute cardiac dullness corresponds to the area of contact of the pericardium with the thoracic wall. It gives a flat sound on light percussion. (2) The area of relative cardiac dullness indicates the outline of heart which is covered by the thin margin of lung. It needs somewhat stronger percussion to define this area which is usually difficult in animals. The absolute dullness is used to test the hypertrophy, displacement and pericardial effusion. In ox, the normal area of absolute dullness is explored in the fourth and fifth intercostal spaces. Traumatic pericarditis may result in absolute dullness in these spaces extending above a horizontal line through the shoulder joint. In horse this area is a triangle bounded by the triceps in front, the sternum below and the lung along the line joining these two. On left side of the normal horse, the dullness extends about 7 cm above the olecranon in the fourth intercostal space and about 3 cm above the olecranon in the fifth space. On the right side, the dullness extends about 3 cm above the olecranon in the fifth space only. In dog, the area of absolute dullness extends about 1 to 2 cm above the sternum in the fourth and fifth intercostal spaces in the line with the corresponding costochondral junction.

The **auscultation** of heart is performed usually on the left side of thorax to obtain heart rate as well as to listening abnormalities in the rhythm or the heart murmurs. The auscultation of heart in ox and horse is performed at the fourth and fifth intercostal space near the olecranon and in dog it is at fifth intercostal space.

Lungs

A thorough auscultation and percussion of lung field is a critical part of clinical examination in mild respiratory disease or consolidated lung fields. The **area of auscultation of lungs** in all animals is almost same. Its cranial limit is the caudal border of triceps brachii from the caudal angle of scapula to the olecranon. The dorsal border is on the line running from the caudal angle of scapula to the tuber coxae. The basal border is a line joining the olecranon to the dorsal end of the last intercostal space. The basal border of the **area of percussion of lungs** in ox is almost straight but in horse and dog it is concave. The exact variations are as below.

In **cattle**, the basal border is almost straight. It intersects the cranial border at the olecranon. In the seventh intercostal space the basal border intersects the line through shoulder joint. At the eleventh space it meets the dorsal border. This is the smallest area as compared to other animals.

In **horse**, the basal border intersects the horizontal line through shoulder joint at the tenth intercostal space. At the fourteenth intercostal space it intersects a horizontal line through the tuber ischii. In the sixteenth space it reaches a line through the ventral part of tuber coxae where the basal border meets the dorsal border.

In **dog,** the basal border of the percussion area passes from the level of the olecranon at the sixth rib through the middle of the eighth rib to intersect the dorsal border at the eleventh intercostal space.

Site for Thoracocentesis

The thoracocentesis is a technique used for removing the fluid or air from the pleural space. It can be used as a diagnostic tool as well as for therapeutic intervention. In this technique, the catheter or a needle is passed inside the pleural cavity through the 7th or 8th intercostal space on either side but usually the right side is preferred. This site is common for both, the cattle and horse. However, in dog the site for thoracocentesis is seventh to ninth intercostal space. For removal of air the needle or catheter is passed in the dorsal half of the space and for removal of fluid, the ventral half of the space is used. The procedure is performed under the guidance of sonography and under local anaesthesia.

PART-2.1: ANATOMY OF ABDOMEN AND PELVIS

SECTION-A

MUSCULO-SKELETAL COMPONENT

55

Skeleton of Abdomen and Pelvis

The skeleton of abdomen and pelvis (Fig. 4-1) consists of the lumbar vertebrae that form the dorsal boundary or roof of the abdomen, sacral vertebrae or the sacrum that forms the dorsal boundary or the roof of the pelvic cavity, the xiphoid cartilage of the sternum that provides attachment to the strong ligaments of the abdominal floor and the pelvic bone (pelvis) that forms the floor and lateral wall of the pelvic cavity.

Lumbar vertebrae

The lumbar vertebrae (Fig. 4-1 A) in ox are six in number. These are characterized by great size and form of their transverse processes. The other characteristic features of lumbar vertebrae are as below.

The body of the vertebra is much compressed dorsoventrally. The convexity of the cranial extremity and concavity of the caudal extremity of the body of the vertebra is moderate. The arch of the first lumbar vertebra is similar in size to that of the last thoracic vertebra but behind this the arches of the second to sixth lumbar vertebra gradually increase in height and width. The caudal notches are deeper than the cranial one. The intervertebral foramina of the first few lumbar segments are often double.

The articular (oblique) processes are large. They are placed a little further apart and are strongly curved. The cranial articular processes are concave and are directed inwards and they present mammillary processes on their external aspect. The caudal articular processes are convex and they are directed inwards. These processes project from the arch at the base of the spinous process.

The transverse processes are elongated plates flattened dorsoventrally and they project outwards at right angles to the body of the vertebra. Each transverse process is slightly curved downwards. Its dorsal surface is slightly concave and ventral surface is slightly convex. All the transverse processes of lumbar vertebrae are directed little forwards. The transverse processes of first lumbar vertebra are shorter than the second ones and the length gradually increases up

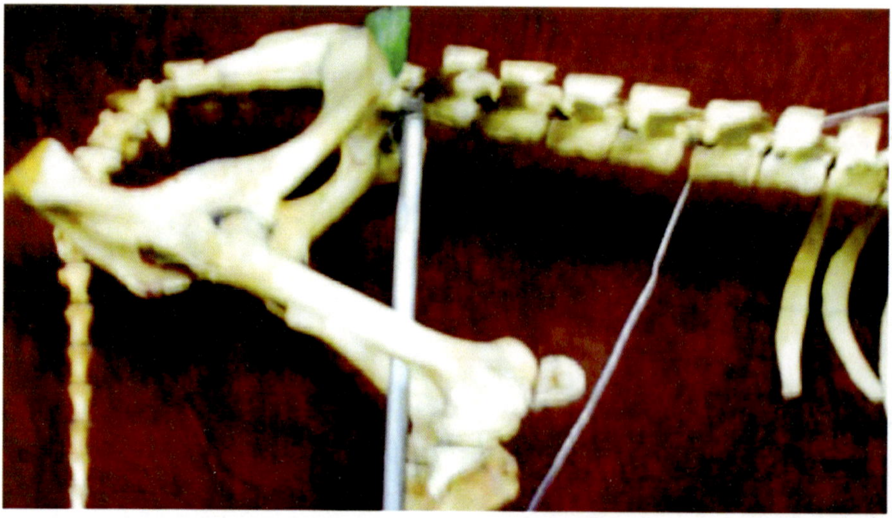

Fig. 4 – 1: Skeleton of Abdomen and Pelvis of Ox

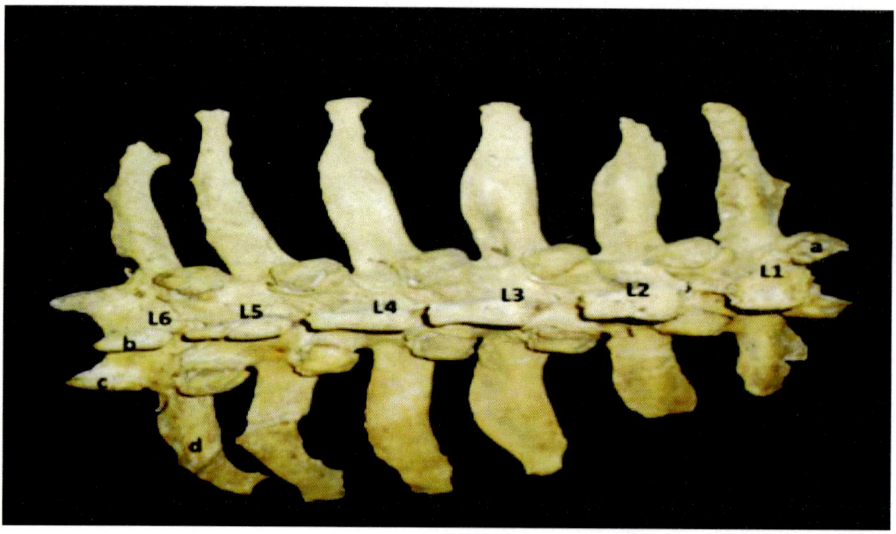

Fig. 4 – 1 A: Lumbar Vertebrae of Ox

a. Cranial articular process b. Superior spine c. Caudal articular process d. Transverse process of lumbar vertebra; L1. First lumbar L2. Second lumbar, L3. Third lumbar, L4. Fourth lumbar, L5. Fifth lumbar, L6. Sixth lumbar vertebra

to fifth lumbar vertebra so that the transverse processes of fifth lumbar vertebra are longest and those of the sixth are shorter than the fifth one. The intertransverse spaces are quite large gaps which are filled by the intertransversalis lumborum muscles.

The supraspinous processes of lumbar vertebrae are broad, flattened plates and are of the same height as that of the last thoracic vertebra. The spinous process of the last lumbar vertebra is the narrowest of all the six lumbar vertebrae. The ventral spinous processes are rudimentary and they present attachment to the ventral common ligament of the bodies of the vertebrae.

Sacral vertebrae (Sacrum)

The sacral vertebrae which are five in number in ox are fused to form a large single piece of bone called the sacrum (Fig. 4-1 B). It forms the roof of the pelvic cavity. It is triangular in form and is wedged between the left and right iliac bones of the pelvic girdle to form the roof of the pelvic cavity. The sacrum has two surfaces, two borders, a base and an apex.

The dorsal surface (Fig. 4-1 B) presents a median sacral crest that extends craniocaudally from the base to the apex of the sacrum. This median sacral crest is formed by fusion of the spinous processes of the five sacral vertebrae. The summit of the crest is rough and tuberous. On either side of this crest is another crest running parallel to the median sacral crest. These are the lateral sacral crests which are formed by fusion of the articular processes of five sacral vertebrae. Just above the lateral sacral crests and on either side of the median sacral crest are four dorsal sacral foramina placed at the site of the junction of the adjacent segments of the sacrum. These foramina present the passage for the dorsal division of the sacral spinal nerves.

The ventral surface (Fig. 4-1 C) is flat, smooth and arched forming concavity facing craniocaudally. This surface forms the roof of the pelvic cavity. It presents a median longitudinal groove for the passage of middle sacral artery. The ventral surface is also marked by four transverse lines which indicate the lines of fusion of the bodies of the five sacral vertebrae. On either ends of these transverse lines are ventral sacral foramina which present the passage for ventral divisions of the sacral spinal nerves.

The lateral borders are thin, concave and provide attachment to the sacrosciatic ligament.

The base or cranial extremity of the sacrum is formed by the cranial extremity of the first sacral vertebra. Centrally it bears head which is wide, transversely elongated and dorsoventrally flattened. Its cranial surface is convex and articulates with the caudal extremity of the last lumbar vertebra. The edges of the pedicles of the cranial extremity present the cranial notches which with the caudal notches of the sixth lumbar vertebra form the intervertebral foramina through which passes the sixth lumbar spinal nerves. The neural ring is triangular in form but its angles are rounded off. On either side of the arch and above the

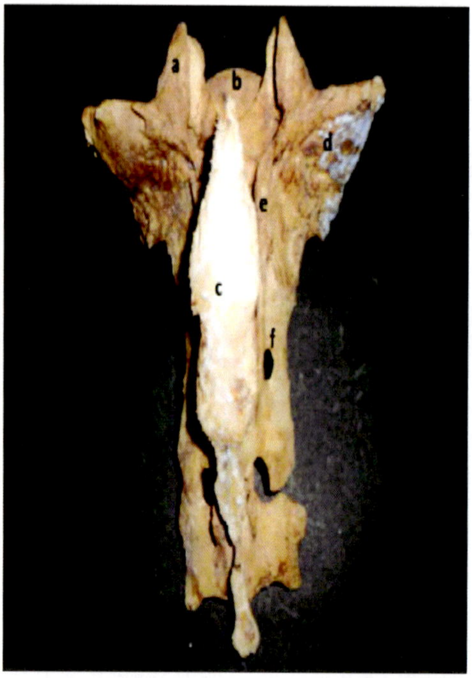

Fig. 4 – 1 B: Sacrum of Ox; Dorsal view
a. Anterior articular process b. Body c. Median sacral crest d. Wing e. Lateral sacral crest f. Dorsal sacral foramen

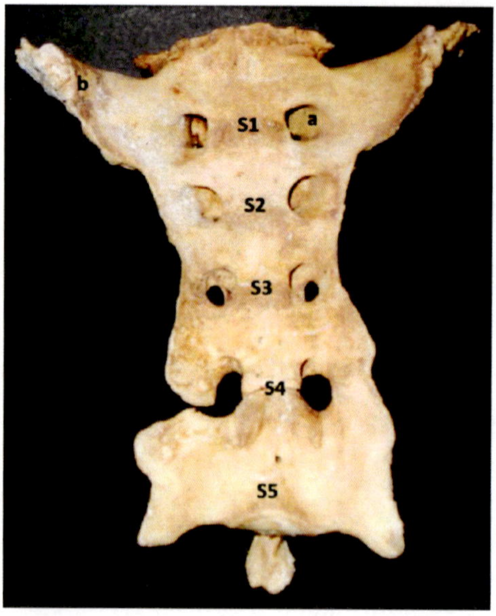

Fig. 4 – 1 C: Sacrum of Ox; Ventral view
a. Ventral sacral foramen; b. Wing of sacrum; S1- S5 sacral vertebrae

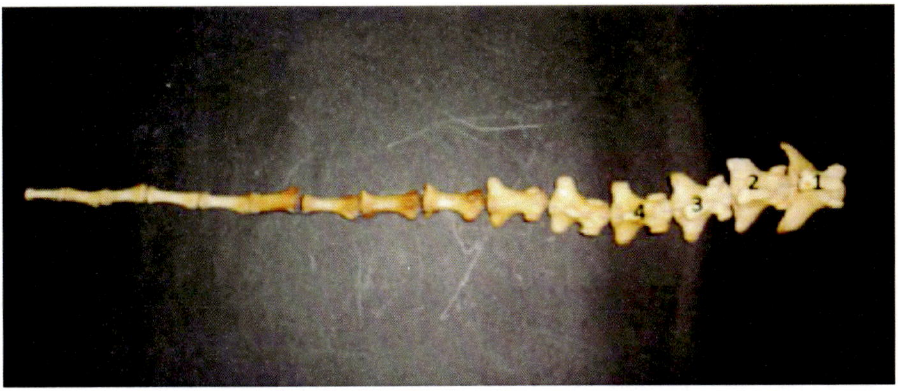

Fig. 4 – 1 D: Coccygeal Vertebrae
1 – 4 First to fourth coccygeal vertebrae with vertebral canal

notches are the cranial articular processes which are very large and widely separated. The lateral parts of the base are the alae or wings of sacrum. Each wing is a thick and compressed quadrilateral plate which is directed downwards and forwards. Its cranial surface is extensive and concave mediolaterally. The caudal surface is rough in its lower part and presents a triangular area called the auricular facet for articulation with the ilium of the pelvic bone.

The apex or the caudal extremity of the sacrum is the caudal extremity of the last (fifth) sacral vertebra. Centrally it presents a small triangular neural ring. Above the neural ring is a pointed projection of caudal end of the median sacral crest. On either side of the body of the last segment (vertebra) of the sacrum are caudally directed projections indicating the transverse processes of the last (fifth) sacral vertebra.

Coccygeal vertebrae

The coccygeal (caudal) vertebrae (Fig. 4-1 D) mainly constitute the region of the tail and partly contribute to complete the roof of the pelvic cavity. In ox they vary in number from fifteen to twenty. They gradually diminish in size from first to last. The first five or six coccygeal vertebrae are typical vertebrae. Beyond these, they are gradually suppressed of arches and processes so that the caudal ones are made up of bodies only. The first coccygeal vertebra may be fused with the sacrum. The first two or three are almost horizontal in position and they partly rest over the ischial arch forming the roof of the caudal limit of pelvic cavity. The third or fourth to seventh or eighth vertebrae gradually incline to become oblique in position and the rest of them are straightly vertical. The first twelve coccygeal vertebrae present small craniocaudally elongated processes called the haemal processes one each on either side of the median line on the ventral surface of the body of these vertebrae. These processes enclose a groove or a sulcus called the sulcus vasculosus through which passes the middle coccygeal artery.

Pelvic girdle

The pelvic girdle (Fig. 4-1 E and F) is formed by the union of two (left and right) os coxae (pelvic bones) which are fused ventrally at the pelvic symphysis and are articulated firmly with the sacrum dorsally. The two os coxae together with the sacrum and first two or three coccygeal vertebrae constitute the bony pelvis. The sacrum and first two or three coccygeal vertebrae form the roof or dorsal wall and the parts of the pelvic bones form the floor and lateral walls of the bony pelvis. Each pelvic bone consists of three parts, the ilium, ischium and the pubis. These three bony segments of the pelvic bone meet each other at the cotyloid cavity called the acetabulum.

The **ilium** is the largest of the three parts. It is irregularly triangular with a wide dorsal part, prismatic middle part and expanded lower part. The narrow prismatic middle part is the shaft and the wide proximal part is the wing of the ilium. It has two surfaces, three borders and three angles.

The lateral or gluteal surface faces ventrad and caudad. The ventral third of this surface presents rough lines for the attachment (origin) of deep gluteus muscle. A prominent oblique ridge, the gluteal line running parallel to the lateral border traverses the most of the length of this surface. It becomes continuous dorsally with the superior ischiatic spine and provides attachment to the middle and deep gluteus muscle. The medial or pelvic surface has two parts, the proximal rough articular facet for articulation with the sacrum and the lower comparatively smooth area for attachment of iliacus muscle. A rough iliopectineal line separates these two areas on the medial surface of the ilium. It begins at the lower margin of the sacral articular facet, joins the cranial border of the pubis and forms the lateral boundary of the pelvic inlet. It bears at about its middle, the psoas tubercle which provides attachment to the psoas minor muscle.

The lateral or cotyloid border is concave and rough. It separates the gluteal and iliac surfaces and reaches the cotyloid cavity. The caudal or ischiatic border is deeply concave and forms at about its middle the cranial boundary of greater sciatic foramen (greater ischiatic foramen) through which pass the sciatic and gluteal nerves and the gluteal vessels. In its lower part it is convex, rough and continuous with the superior ischiatic spine which gives attachment to the sacrosciatic ligament (sacrotuberal ligament) at its free edge and to the deep gluteus muscle at its lateral aspect. The dorsal border is thick and irregular and forms the iliac crest on either ends of which are angles.

The **ischium** is smaller than ilium. It is irregularly quadrilateral and placed behind the ilium and pubis. It has two surfaces and two borders. The dorsal (pelvic) surface is slightly concave transversely and forms the caudal two thirds of the floor of the pelvic cavity. The ventral surface is nearly flat and presents about its middle a rough ridge for the attachment of origin of the adductor muscle of the thigh. The cranial border is concave and forms the caudal boundary of the obturator foramen. The caudal border slopes downward and forward and together with the same border of the ischium of opposite side forms the ischial arch which forms the ventral boundary of the pelvic outlet. The medial border meets with that of the bone of opposite side and forms the ischial symphysis (symphysis ischii). The ventral edge of the ischial symphysis is roughened in the form of a ridge. The lateral border is thick, smooth and concave and forms the lesser sciatic notch (lesser ischiatic notch) which forms the lower boundary of the lesser sciatic foramen (lesser ischiatic foramen) that provides passage for the caudal gluteal vessels. The craniolateral angle of the ischium joins the ilium and pubis at the acetabulum. The caudolateral angle is rough and thick and forms trifid process called the tuber ischii which can be felt on palpation in the living animal. It provides origin to the biceps femoris, semitendinosus and semimembranosus muscles. The craniomedial angle meet the pubis and forms the medial boundary of the obturator foramen while the caudomedial angle meet the same angle of the opposite bone at the ischial arch.

The **pubis** is the smallest of the three parts of the pelvic bone. It is placed between the ischium and pubis. It is irregularly triangular and has two surfaces, three borders and three angles. The dorsal or pelvic surface is smooth and rounded. It forms the cranial third of the floor of the pelvic cavity. The urinary bladder rests on this surface. The ventral surface is slightly convex and roughened for the attachment of muscles of hip and thigh. The cranial border is smooth, thick and rounded. It presents an oblique sub pubic groove. Lateral to this groove is an iliopectineal eminence which provides attachment to the common prepubic tendon of the abdominal muscles. The medial border meets the same border of the opposite bone and forms the pubic symphysis. The caudal border is smooth and concave and it forms the cranial boundary of the obturator foramen. The craniomedial angle meets the same angle of the opposite bone at the pubic symphysis. The craniolateral or acetabular angle joins the ilium and ischium at the acetabulum. The caudal angle meets the craniomedial angle of the ischium.

The **acetabulum** is a cotyloid cavity formed on the ventrolateral aspect of the pelvic bone by joining its three components. It faces laterad and caudad and has an articular and nonarticular part. The articular part is nearly circular and articulates with the head of the femur. The nonarticular part is deep and is

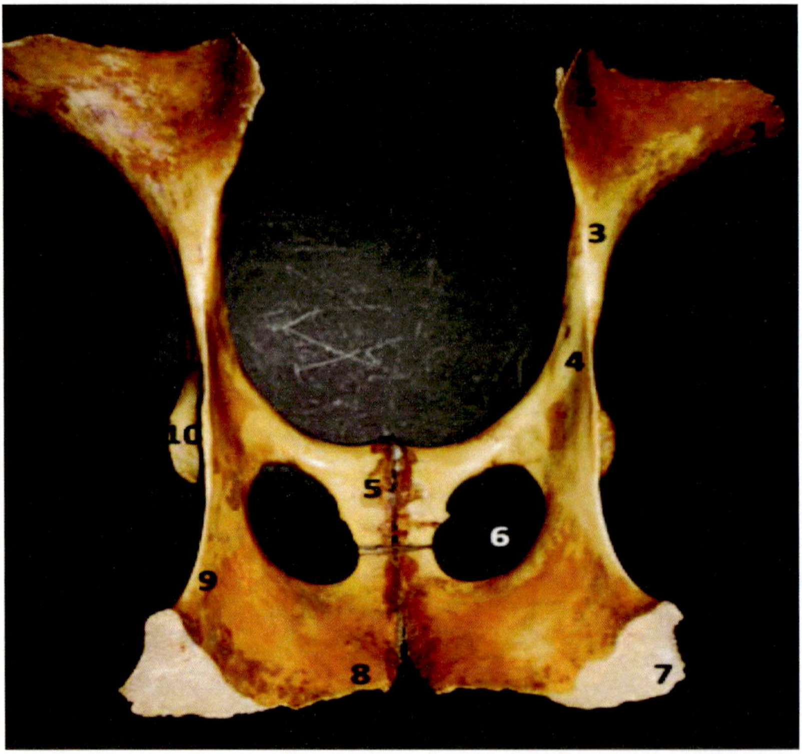

Fig. 4 – 1 E: Pelvic bone of Ox (dorsal view)

1. Tuber coxae 2. Tuber sacrale 3. Gluteal line 4. Psoas tubercle 5. Pelvic floor 6. Obturator foramen 7. Tuber ischii 8. Ischial arch 9. Lesser ischiatic notch 10. Superior ischiatic spine

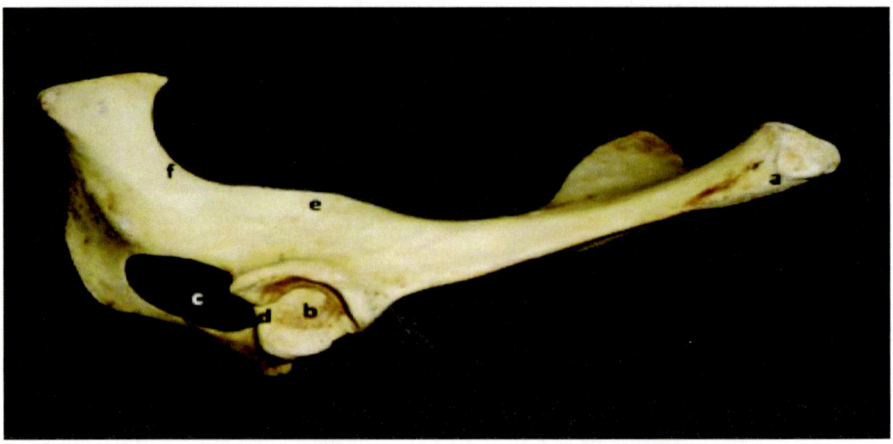

Fig. 4 – 1 F: Pelvic bone of cow; Lateral view

a. Tuber coxae b. Acetabulum c. Obturator foramen d. Acetabular notch e. Superior ischiatic spine f. Lesser ischiatic notch

called the acetabular fossa. The bottom of this fossa is rough for attachment of round ligament of the hip joint. The rim of the acetabulum on its caudomedial aspect is cut into a deep notch called the acetabular notch which leads into the acetabular fossa. In addition, there are two more notches, the lateral and mediolateral notch but these are small and shallow and do not reach the acetabular fossa.

The **obturator foramen** is a large, oval or elliptical opening on the floor of the pelvis and is circumscribed by the ischium and the pubis. Its margin is thin and sharp except at its lateral part. It is covered dorsally by obturator internus and ventrally by obturator externus muscles. The obturator ligament is also attached to the dorsal surface of this foramen in such a way as to leave a narrow space for the passage of obturator nerve.

In female animals the ischial arch is wider and the pelvic outlet is larger than that in male animals. The conjugate and transverse diameters of the pelvic girdle in females are also greater than those in males. The pubis and the ischia of the opposite side meet at a wider angle in female animals than that in the male animals. Because of these differential characteristics, the pelvic girdle of female animals become more roomy which is required for accommodating the growing foetus in females.

56

Comparative Anatomy of Skeleton of Abdomen and Pelvis

Horse

The **lumbar vertebrae** in horse are six in number. The bodies of these vertebrae are shorter. The first three of them have a distinct ventral spine which subsides thereafter. The transverse processes increase in length from first to third or fourth and then diminish. The first one or two slightly curve caudad and the last two or three curve craniad and the third is at right angles. The caudal border of the transverse process of the fifth vertebra at its base has an oval concave facet which articulates with a convex facet on the cranial border of sixth vertebra. The sixth transverse process is thick at the base and thin, narrow at its free end. It is curved forward. It has a large concave facet on its caudal border by which it articulates with the corresponding facet on sacrum.

The **sacrum** of horse is formed by the fusion of five sacral vertebrae similar to that in ox. However, the fusion of the spinous processes is incomplete. On either side of the base of the each spinous process is a groove which presents the dorsal sacral foramen. There are four foramina on each side of the dorsum of the sacrum of horse. The ventral surface of sacrum of horse is not so deeply arched as that of ox. The wings of sacrum are prismatic. Each wing has a large oval convex facet for articulation with similar facet on the caudal border of the transverse process of last lumbar vertebra.

The **coccygeal vertebrae** are eighteen to twenty in number in horse. The laminae of the neural arch of the coccygeal vertebrae beyond fourth vertebra fail to meet dorsally.

The **pelvic bone** (os coxae) of horse is in general similar to that of ox. The gluteal line on the gluteal surface of the ilium is faint. The ilium is placed more obliquely. The articular surface of ilium is rough and large and extends nearly to the external angle. The internal angles of the ilium of opposite sides are more close to each other. The external angles are formed of four tuberosities each.

The ischium of the two sides meets at a greater angle because of which the pelvic floor is bowl like. The ischial arch is wide and shallow. The ridge on the ventral surface of ischium is absent. The tuber ischii is not trifid. The lower border of tuber ischii forms the ventral ischiatic spine. The ventral surface of pubis is crossed by pubic groove which leads to acetabular notch that transmits the pubic femoral ligament.

Dog

The **lumbar** vertebrae in dog are seven in number. The bodies of the vertebrae increase in width from first to last. The transverse processes are plate like and they are directed craniad and ventrad. The length of the transverse processes increases from first to fifth or sixth. The extremities of the transverse process, except the last are expanded. The cranial articular (oblique) processes are surmounted by mammillary processes. The accessory processes project caudad. The supraspinous processes are equal in height to that of the last thoracic vertebra.

The **sacrum** of dog is comparatively and relatively smaller. It is formed by fusion of three sacral vertebrae. The vertebral segments are short, wide and quadrangular. The median sacral crest is notched. The articular processes are vestigial and are represented by a pair of tubercles placed on either side of the median crest. External to these tubercles are dorsal sacral foramina. The ventral (pelvic) surface of the sacrum is arched deeply concave and presents a pair of ventral sacral foramina. The wings of the sacrum are prismatic.

The **coccygeal vertebrae** in dog are eighteen to twenty three in number. The first five or six are fully developed with all the processes like those in a true (typical) vertebra. The neural rings are present in first six. The articular processes of first four or five coccygeal vertebrae form synovial joints.

The **pelvic bone** of dog is in general similar in constitution to that of ox. The ilium is nearly vertical and its gluteal surface is more concave and is directed laterad. Its pelvic surface is nearly flat. The crest of the ilium is strongly convex. The ischium has a twisted appearance and the ischial arch is very wide. The greater sciatic notch is very shallow. The lesser sciatic notch is absent. The acetabulum and the acetabular fossa are deep. The obturator foramen is triangular in outline and its angles are rounded off.

Sheep and Goat

The **lumbar vertebrae** in sheep and goat are six or seven in number. Some times the number reduces to five. The bodies of the vertebrae are more flattened dorsoventrally than those of ox. Their cranial ends are little concave transversely and the caudal ends are almost flat. The cranial articular processes are strongly curved and they overlap the caudal ones. The transverse processes curve cranially and their free ends are expanded.

The **sacrum** of sheep and goat is normally formed by fusion of four sacral vertebrae. However, the fourth vertebra in some cases remains separate or incompletely fused. The vascular groove on the ventral (pelvic) surface is absent. The spinous processes of the first and second sacral segment remain separate and the rest of them are fused. The transverse processes of the last segment are distinct and outstanding.

The **coccygeal vertebrae** in sheep and goat vary in number from three to twenty four or more. The bodies of the vertebrae have no haemal processes on their ventral surface. The transverse processes are long and thin and they project caudally.

The **pelvic bone** of the sheep and goat differs greatly from that of the ox. The long axis of the ilium is almost in a line with that of ischium. The gluteal line on the gluteal surface of the ilium is in the form of a ridge that is nearly parallel to the lateral border of the shaft of the bone. The lateral angle of the ilium (tuber coxae) is thickened and the medial angle (tuber sacrale) is pointed. The crest (cranial border) of ilium is concave medially and convex laterally. The ischiatic spine is low. The pubis is similar to that of ox but its cranial border is thin and sharp. The ischium slopes ventrad and caudad and it meets the bone of the opposite side at a larger angle. The tuber ischii is flattened, The lesser sciatic notch is shallow. The acetabulum is more laterad than that in ox. The floor of the pelvic cavity is wide and shallow.

Pig

The **lumbar vertebrae** in pig are six or seven in number. The bodies of the lumbar vertebrae are longer than those of thoracic vertebrae of the same species. In caudal part of the series, the bodies become wider and flattened dorsoventrally. The neural arches are deeply notched and are separated dorsally. The mammillary processes project laterad and caudad. The transverse processes are bent ventrad and they are inclined slightly craniad.

Their length gradually increases up to fourth and thereafter reduces so that the transverse processes of last lumbar vertebra are shortest. The transverse processes form no articulations with each other or with the sacrum. These processes at the caudal part of their roots present a notch in the cranial segments of the series and foramen in the caudal segments of the series. The supraspinous processes are broad and inclined cranially except the last one which is narrow and vertical.

The **sacrum of pig** consists of four vertebrae which in the initial part of the life are separated and later on gets fused in the later part with the advancement of age. The fusion is, however, slightly incomplete. It is less curved than in ox. The supra spinous processes are less developed and even absent in some part of the bone. The dorsal surface of the arch is flattened and smooth in the middle and presents openings in to the sacral canal. On either side of these openings are the dorsal sacral foramina and the dorsal tubercles which represent the dorsal lateral crest. The cranial articular processes are very large. The wings of the sacrum in pig are similar to those of ox. The pelvic surface of the sacrum is less curved and the transverse lines of fusion of the vertebrae are distinct.

The **coccygeal vertebrae** of pig are twenty to twenty three in number. The first four of these are characterized by the presence of functional articular processes. Beyond these, the articular processes of the rest of the vertebrae are nonarticular and smaller. The neural arch of the first five or six vertebrae is complete while in the rests it is incomplete or totally absent. The transverse processes are broad and plate like in the cranial segments of the series and behind these they gradually become diminished and finally completely absent. The first coccygeal vertebra most often unites with the sacrum.

The **pelvic bones** of the opposite sides unite and fuse with each other by synostosis along the median line (pelvic symphysis). The ilium and ischium are almost in line with each other and are nearly sagittal in direction. The wing of the ilium bends laterally much less than in ox. The gluteal surface of the ilium is divided into two fossae by a ridge which is continuous with the ischiatic spine caudally. The pelvic surface of ilium presents extensive rough area caudally The rest of this surface is smooth and is bounded dorsally by a ridge. The iliac crest is convex and thick. It is rough and prominent in the middle forming the highest point of the bone. The medial angle (tuber sacrale) is smooth and is at lower level than the crest. It is directed caudally and is articulated with the sacrum. The lateral angle (tuber coxae) is still lower and is comparatively thinner. The ischium is flattened and diverge at a greater angle in females than in males. The ischiatic spine is slightly curved inwards. The muscular ridges on the lateral surface of the ischium are pronounced. The pubic bones of two sides meet each other in a horizontal plane. The iliopubic eminence is prominent and the psoas tubercle is well marked.

Fowl

In fowl, the **lumbar and sacral vertebrae** are fused into a single piece of bone called as **synsacrum**. It is often fused laterally with the ilium. Caudal to synsacrum are four to nine **coccygeal vertebrae**. The varying numbers of these vertebrae (four to eight) are often fused to form a single triangular piece of bone called the **pygostyle** which is the characteristic feature of birds. The two preen glands are separated by the pygostyle. It provides attachment to the feathers of the tail in birds.

The **pelvic bone** is formed by the union of three bones, the ilium, ischium and pubis similar to that in mammalian species. The ilium is fused with the synsacrum. The pelvic bones of two sides do not meet with each other at the symphysis. The pelvic symphysis is absent. The two pelvic bones are widely separated ventrally. The ilium is the longest and largest segment of the pelvic bone. It is elongated and firmly attached to the transverse processes of the fused lumbar and sacral vertebrae. The cranial half of the lateral surface of the ilium is concave while the caudal half is convex. The medial surface presents two deep cavities into which the kidneys are lodged. The ischium is smaller than ilium and is continuous with it except at the obturator foramen. The sciatic notch is converted into sciatic foramen. The pubis is thin, narrow and elongated in the form of a thin strip of bone which runs caudad along the ventral border of the ischium. Its cranial part is fused with ilium while caudal part is curved inwards and is free. The acetabulum is relatively large and deep and its bottom is pierced by a large opening.

57

Articulations of Abdomen and Pelvis

Sacroiliac articulation

The sacroiliac articulation (Fig. 4-2 A) is a synovial (diorthroidal) joint formed between the articular surface on the wing of the sacrum and pelvic surface of the proximal extremity of the ilium. The articular area of the wing of the sacrum has a rough eminence while that of the ilium has a reciprocal rough depression. Both the articular areas are covered by a thin layer of cartilage. The joint cavity is a thin like a cleft and is crossed by fibrous bands.

The joint capsule is closely fitting around the margins of the articular surfaces. The joint capsule is reinforced by the ventral sacroiliac ligament which surrounds the joint. The dorsal part of this ligament is quite strong and it occupies the angle between the ilium and wing of the sacrum. The movements are inappreciable at this joint.

Ligaments of pelvic girdle

There are four ligaments of pelvic girdle.

(1) Dorsal sacroiliac ligament

(2) Lateral sacroiliac ligament

(3) Ilio lumbar ligament and

(4) Sacrosciatic ligament.

Although these ligaments are not involved directly in the formation of sacroiliac articulation, they reinforce the girdle muscles and contribute for completing the pelvic cavity and hence are regarded as accessory ligaments of the sacroiliac joint.

The **dorsal sacroiliac ligament** is a strong band which is attached to the summits of the sacral spines and the sacral tuberosity. The spinal attachment of this ligament blends with the supraspinous ligament.

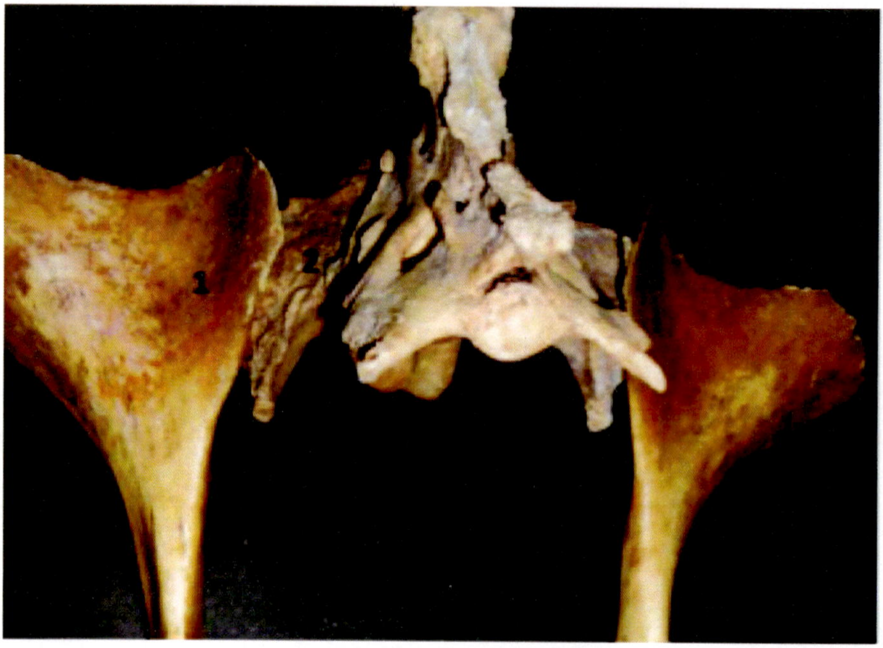

Fig. 4 – 2 A: Sacroiliac articulation
1. Ilium 2. Wings of sacrum

The **lateral sacroiliac ligament** is triangular thick sheet which is attached cranially to the sacral tuberosity and adjacent part of the medial border of ilium dorsal to the greater ischiatic notch and ventrally to the lateral border of sacrum. It blends ventrally with the broad sacrosciatic (sacrotuberal) ligament.

The **ilio lumbar ligament** is a triangular sheet which connects the ends of lumbar transverse processes to the ventral surface of ilium, ventral to the attachment of longissimus muscle.

The **sacrosciatic ligament** (sacrotuberal ligament) is an extensively broad quadrilateral sheet which completes the lateral wall of the pelvic cavity. The dorsal border of this ligament is attached to the lateral border of sacrum and transverse processes of first and second coccygeal (caudal) vertebrae. The ventral border is attached to the ischiatic spine and the tuber ischii. Between these two ventral attachments over the lateral border of ischium, the ligament forms the lesser sciatic (ischiatic) foramen through which passes the caudal gluteal vessels. The cranial border of the ligament is concave and with the greater sciatic (ischiatic) notch over the middle of the caudal border of the ilium it completes the formation of the greater sciatic (ischiatic) foramen through which passes the sciatic nerve and cranial gluteal vessels. The caudal border of the ligament forms the lateral boundary of the pelvic outlet. A large broad sciatic nerve after passing through the greater sciatic foramen runs down along the lateral surface of this ligament which is covered laterally by the middle and deep gluteal and the biceps femoris muscles. The cranial part of the medial (pelvic) surface of the ligament is covered by the peritoneum and the caudal part is connected to the ischiococcygeus and retractor ani muscles.

Obturator ligament (membrane) is a sheet of thin membrane made of fibrous tissue which covers the obturator foramen and which is traversed by obturator vessels and nerve.

Pelvic symphysis

The pelvic symphysis (ischio-pubic symphysis) is formed by the union of medial borders of pubis and ischium of the os coxae of the opposite sides. In young animals the articular surfaces are covered by a layer of cartilage but as the age advances the cartilage is gradually replaced by the bone. A transverse band called the cranial pubic ligament covers the cranial border of pubis and the fibrous band called the arcuate ischiatic ligament extends across the ischial arch.

58

Comparative Anatomy of Joints and Ligaments of Abdomen and Pelvis

Horse

In addition to the common articulations of vertebrae, the lumbar region of horse has two special articulations, the inter-transverse articulations and lumbosacral articulations.

The **intertransverse articulations** are bilateral joints formed between the transverse processes of the fourth and fifth and between the fifth and sixth lumbar vertebrae. The articular surfaces of these joints are the oval facets on the transverse processes of these vertebrae, the cranial ones being concave while the caudal ones the convex. These are synovial joints (diarthrodial). The capsule of the joint is reinforced ventrally.

The **lumbosacral articulations** are diarthrodial joints formed between the transverse processes of the sixth lumbar vertebra and the wings of the sacrum. These joints are similar to the intertransverse articulations.

The **sacroiliac articulation** of the pelvis is similar to that of ox. However, the **sacrosciatic ligament** is broader. Its lateral surface is related to middle gluteus, biceps femoris and semitendinosus muscles.

Dog

The joints and ligaments of the lumbar, sacral and coccygeal regions of the dog are more or less similar to those of ox.

The joints of the pelvic bone also do not present any striking differences except that the sacrotuberal ligament is a narrow but strong band which extends from the caudal part of the lateral margin of the sacrum to the tuber ischii.

Sheep and Goat

The joints and ligaments of abdomen and pelvis in sheep and goat have no differences from those in ox.

Pig

The joints and ligaments of abdomen and pelvis have no differences in pig from those in ox.

Fowl

Most of the vertebrae of the lumbar and sacral regions in fowl are fused forming a single piece of bone the synsacrum and those of coccygeal region are fused forming the pygostyle. The ilium is also fused with the sacrum. Thus, there are no joints of the bones in this region in fowl.

59

Muscles of Abdomen and Pelvis

Cutaneous muscle

The cutaneous muscle of abdomen and pelvis is the continuation of cutaneous muscle of thorax. This has been described under the muscles of thorax.

Abdominal fascia

Beneath the skin in the abdominal region, there are two layers of fascia, the superficial and deep, similar to those of the fascia of thoracic region.

The **superficial fascia** is next to skin. It is fused dorsally with the thoracolumbar fascia. Cranially it is continuous with the superficial fascia of shoulder and arm and caudally with that of the gluteal region. In the inguinal region it forms part of fascia of penis in male and of mammary glands in female animals. At the flank, it continues as fascia of thigh region.

The **deep fascia** forms the **abdominal tunic**. It is especially well developed as a thick sheet of tunic in the ventral and the adjacent lateral parts of the abdominal floor. It extends cranially over the ribs and external intercostal and the caudal digitations of the serratus thoracis muscles. Caudally it is attached to the external angle of the ilium and thoracolumbar fascia. The suspensory ligament of prepuce in males and that of the mammary glands (udder) in females is an extension of this tunic. It strongly supports the abdominal muscles to bear the weight of abdominal viscera.

Abdominal muscles

The muscles of the abdomen are in three groups. These are the muscles of spine (lumbar spine), the sublumbar muscles and the muscles of the wall of the abdomen.

Muscles of lumbar spine (Back and loins)

The muscles of lumbar spine (Fig. 4-3 A) are part of the muscles of back and loins. Most of these muscles begin on the wing of the sacrum or the ilium, run cranially over the spinous processes or the transverse processes of the lumbar vertebrae and then continue on the thoracic part of the spine as muscles of the back which have already been described. The lumbar parts of these muscles are described below.

Longissimus

The longissimus muscle is the longest and largest muscle of the body. It consists of four parts, the atlantis, cervicis, thoracis and the lumborum. It extends from sacrum and ilium to the neck. It has a three sided form like a prism and it fills in the space between the spinous processes and the transverse processes of the vertebrae. The lumbar part, **longissimus lumborum**, is distinct from the other parts.

Longissimus lumborum

Origin: The longissimus lumborum originates on the iliac crest and the lateral surface of the ilium and the spinous processes of the sacrum and lumbar vertebrae along with the supraspinous ligament.

Insertion: The lumbar part of the muscle inserts on the transverse processes of the lumbar vertebrae.

Action: The longissimus lumborum assists the spine to erect. Acting together the longissimus muscle is a strong erecter of the spine and acting singly it causes lateral flexion on the side of contraction.

Iliocostalis lumborum

The iliocostalis is also long but a segmented muscle that lies medial to the longissimus muscle.

Origin: It originates by tendinous fibres from iliac crest and by aponeurosis from the longissimus lumborum muscle and lumbar fascia.

Insertion: The muscle, lumbar part of iliocostalis, inserts on the caudal border of the last rib.

Action: It assists the preceding muscle in erection of spine.

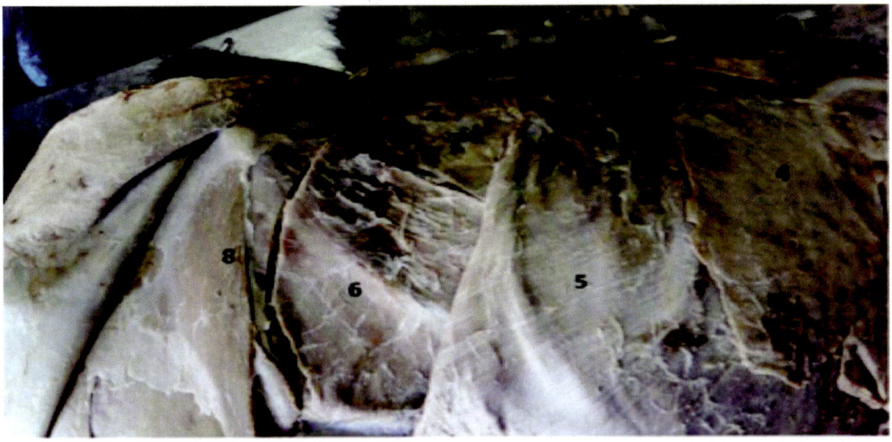

Fig. 4 – 3 A: Muscles of abdomen (back & loin)
1. Longissimus dorsi 2. Longissimus costarum 3. Serratus dorsalis 4. Latissimus dorsi 5. Obliquus abdominis externus 6. Obliquus abdominis internus 7.Rertractor costarum 8. Tensor facia lata

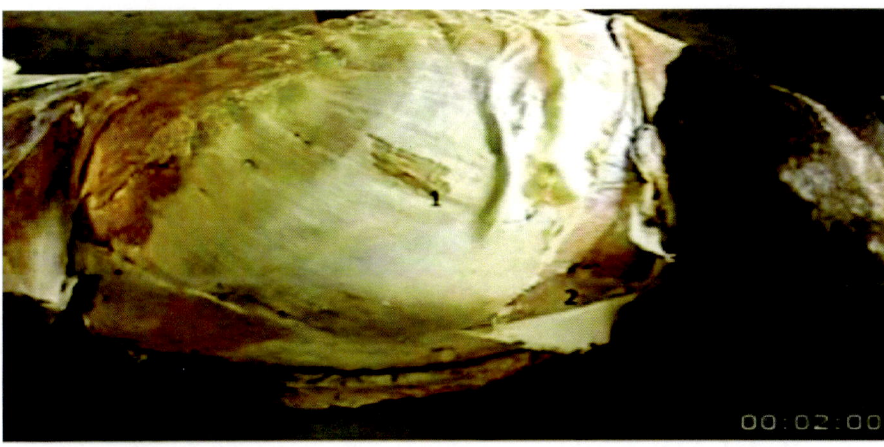

Fig. 4 – 3 B: Muscles of wall of abdomen (superficial dissection)
1. Obliquus abdominis externus 2. Rectus abdominis

Multifidus lumborum

The Multifidus muscle is composed of a series of small segmented muscles extending from third cervical vertebra to sacrum. Each of the segments of this muscle extends from articular, mammillary or transverse process of one vertebra to the spine of the adjacent cranial vertebra. The fibres of this muscle may pass craniodorsally and medially over one or more vertebrae before their insertion on the preceding vertebra.

Origin: The segments of the lumbar part of the muscle originate on the mammillary and articular processes of lumbar vertebrae.

Insertion: The segments insert on the caudal border and lateral surface of the spines of first four lumbar vertebrae.

Action: Same as the preceding muscle

Intertransversarii lumborum

The intertransversarii lumborum are small paired muscles lying on either sides of the lumbar vertebrae and occupying the spaces between the transverse processes of the lumbar vertebrae.

Origin: Caudal borders of the transverse processes of lumbar vertebrae.

Insertion: Cranial borders of the transverse processes of adjacent succeeding lumbar vertebrae.

Action: To assist in lateral flexion of lumbar region and stabilizing the lumbar processes.

Blood supply to all the muscles of lumbar spine is through the lumbar arteries.

Nerve supply to these muscles is through the dorsal divisions of the lumbar spinal nerves.

Sublumbar muscles

The muscles of sub lumbar region are mainly placed on the ventral surface of the lumbar vertebrae and their transverse processes. But these are not confined to sublumbar region and extend beyond this region both cranially and caudally. These muscles form the roof of the abdominal cavity. This group of muscles consists of four muscles on each side of the vertebral column.

Psoas minor

The psoas minor is most medial of the four sublumbar muscles. It is a long muscle arising on the ventrolateral aspect of the last thoracic vertebra and passing caudally gradually diverging in its course to ilium.

Origin: The ventrolateral aspect of the bodies of vertebrae from last thoracic to fifth lumbar.

Insertion: Psoas tubercle on the shaft of the ilium.

Action: To flex and arch the lumbar spine (loin).

Psoas major

The psoas major is the largest and most lateral of the four sublumbar muscles. Because of its closeness with the iliacus, the two muscles are jointly considered as a single muscle named as iliopsoas muscle.

Origin: The muscle originates by filaments on the vertebral ends of last two ribs and the ventrolateral surfaces of the bodies and ventral surfaces of transverse processes of the lumbar vertebrae.

Insertion: It inserts on the lesser trochanter and the neck of the femur in common with the insertion of iliacus muscle.

Action: To flex the hip joint and to rotate the thigh laterad.

Iliacus

The iliacus is a short, thick and rounded muscle. It is situated on the ilium lateral to the sacroiliac articulation. It occupies the ventrolateral part of the shaft of ilium. The iliacus muscle is longitudinally grooved to accommodate in it the belly of the psoas major muscle and the two muscles are so intimated that they are jointly termed as iliopsoas muscle.

Origin: The body of the sixth lumbar vertebra, the ventrolateral surface of the shaft of the ilium, the iliopectineal line, the ventral sacroiliac ligament and the sacrum.

Insertion: The lesser trochanter of the femur in common with the psoas major muscle.

Action: To flex the hip joint and to rotate the femur laterad.

Quadratus lumborum

The quadratus lumborum is a thin and flat bundle of muscle lying on the ventral surfaces of the lumbar transverse processes deep to the psoas major muscle.

Origin: The ventrolateral surface of the bodies of last four thoracic vertebrae, the caudal border of the last rib and the ventral surface of the lumbar transverse processes.

Insertion: The ventral surface of the wing of sacrum, the sacroiliac ligament and the cranial border of the transverse process of the succeeding lumbar vertebra.

Action: Acting jointly to flex the lumbar region and acting singly to flex it laterally.

The **blood supply** to all the four muscles is through the lumbar arteries and **nerve supply** through the lumbar nerves.

Muscles of abdominal wall

The abdominal muscles form the entire ventral and most of the lateral parts of the abdominal wall (Fig. 4-3 B and C). These are four muscles and are named according to the direction of their fibres. Thus, these are oblique (external and internal), transversus and rectus abdominis muscles. The oblique muscles form the major part of the lateral walls, the rectus lies along the floor and the transversus mainly form the flank region. The contraction of these muscles causes pressure on the visceral organs and thus assists in different acts like micturition, defecation, parturition, forced expiration, coughing etc.

Obliquus abdominis externus

The obliquus abdominis externus is the largest of the abdominal muscles. It is irregularly triangular in shape with narrow part in front and wide part behind. Its fibres pass ventrad and caudad.

Origin: This muscle originates on the lateral surfaces of ribs from lower part of the fifth intercostal space to just above the middle of the last rib and the thoracolumbar fascia. The fibres of this muscle pass ventrad and caudad before their termination by aponeurosis at linea alba on the floor of the abdomen.

Insertion: It inserts on linea alba and prepubic tendon by aponeurosis along with other abdominal muscles.

Obliquus abdominis internus

The obliquus abdominis internus lies underneath the obliquus abdominis externus. Its fibres pass ventrad and craniad. It has muscular and aponeurotic parts. The aponeurotic part blends with that of the externus muscle and then it gets attached to the rectus abdominis muscle and finally terminates on the linea alba. The muscular part occupies mostly the dorsolateral aspect (flank region) and a part of inguinal region of the abdominal wall.

Origin: It originates by aponeurosis on the external angle of ilium and the adjacent thoracolumbar fascia.

Insertion: This muscle inserts on linea alba, prepubic tendon and the lateral surface of the last two or three ribs and their cartilages.

Rectus abdominis

The rectus abdominis muscle is mainly the muscle of the floor of the abdomen. It is a wide band of muscle that extends from sternum to pubis. It lies between the obliquus abdominis laterally and transversus abdominis medially.

Origin: It originates from the lateral border and the ventral surface of sternum and third to ninth costal cartilages.

Insertion: It inserts on linea alba and the pubis by prepubic tendon.

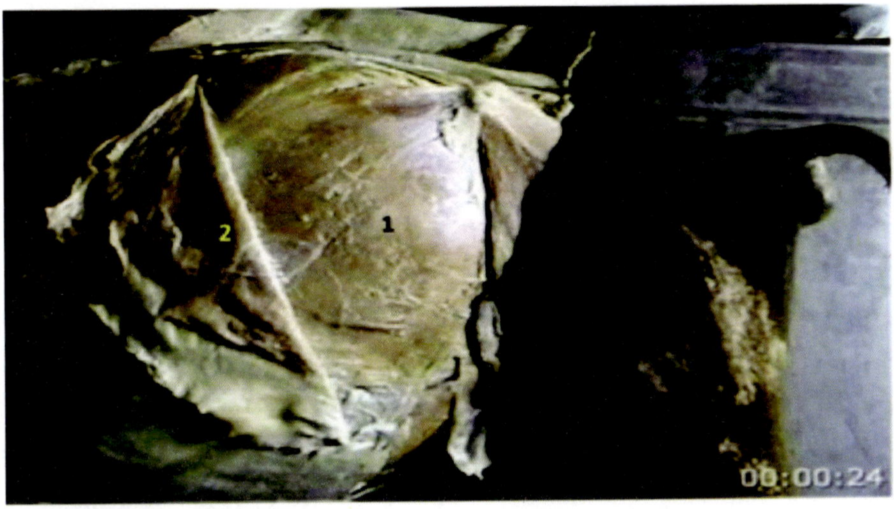

Fig. 4 – 3 C: Muscles of wall of abdomen ; (Deep dissection, Dorsal side)
1. Obliquus abdominis internus 2. Obliquus abdominis externus

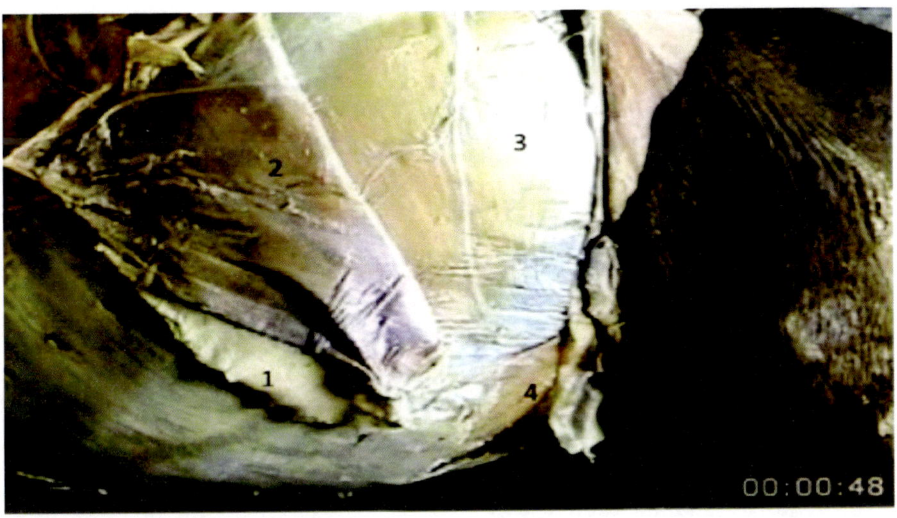

Fig. 4 – 3 D: Muscles of wall of abdomen ; (Deep dissection, Ventral side)
1. Obliquus abdominis externus; 2. Obliquus abdominis internus 3. Transversus abdominis 4. Rectus abdominis

Transversus abdominis

The transversus abdominis muscle forms the innermost muscular layer of the abdominal wall and is lined internally by the peritoneum. Laterally it is covered by the obliquus abdominis internus muscle. Like other abdominal muscles, this muscle also has muscular and aponeurotic parts. The muscular part forms the layer of lateral wall of the abdomen and the aponeurotic part forms its ventral part. The fibres of this muscle run transversely from above downwards.

Origin: It originates on the medial surface of the cartilages of asternal ribs and the transverse processes of lumbar vertebrae through thoracolumbar fascia.

Insertion: It inserts by aponeurosis on linea alba and prepubic tendon along with the external and internal oblique muscles.

Action: All these four abdominal muscles jointly act and exert pressure and compress the abdominal viscera in the act of micturition, defecation, parturition, forced expiration and coughing.

Linea alba

The linea alba is a white fibrous raphe that is formed by union of aponeurotic parts of the oblique and transverse abdominis muscles in the ventral part (floor) of the abdomen. It extends from xiphoid cartilage of the sternum to the prepubic tendon that is attached to the pubis.

Prepubic tendon

The prepubic tendon is a common tendon of insertion formed by all abdominal muscles in the midline of the abdominal floor and ventral to the abdominal tunic extending from xiphoid cartilage to the iliopectineal eminence on the cranial border of the pubis.

Inguinal canal

The inguinal canal is a slit like oblique passage through the caudal part of the abdominal floor. This is a paired canal which lies on either side of the prepubic tendon. The canal begins at the deep inguinal ring and extends obliquely ventromedially to the superficial inguinal ring. It passes through the muscles and fascia of the abdominal wall. The deep inguinal ring is the abdominal opening of the inguinal canal. It is bounded cranially by the margin of obliquus abdominis internus, caudally by inguinal ligament, medially by the lateral border of prepubic tendon and laterally by the attachment of obliquus abdominis internus to the inguinal ligament. This canal in males serves for the passage of spermatic cord, tunica vaginalis, cremaster externus muscle, pudendal artery and the artery and vein of the cord. The canal in female is rudimentary and provides passage for mammary vessels and nerve.

Cremaster externus muscle

The cremaster externus muscle is a narrow flat band of muscle detached from the internal oblique muscle of the abdomen. It passes into the inguinal canal along with the spermatic cord, encloses the vaginal tunic into which it inserts at the level of the head end of the testicle.

Origin: Obliquus abdominis internus muscle and iliac fascia.

Insertion: Tunica vaginalis

Action: To raise the tunica vaginalis and with it the testicle.

Preputialis

These are two short muscles, the preputialis cranialis and preputialis caudalis which are modified cutaneous muscles.

The **preputialis cranialis** arises in the form of numerous fascicles from the fascia slightly caudal to xiphoid cartilage, pass caudally and converge to insert about the preputial orifice. It assists in protracting the prepuce and protecting the penis.

The **preputialis caudalis** arises in the form of five or six cutaneous fascicles in the caudal portion of the inguinal canal. The fibres course cranially and ventrally to unite on the abdominal wall slightly cranial to the scrotum. The fibres then converge around preputial orifice. This muscle acts as retractor of the prepuce.

Muscles of tail

The muscles of tail (coccygeal muscles) are placed around the tail. These are enclosed in a strong coccygeal fascia which blends with the ventral iliosacral and sacrosciatic ligaments and the cranial gluteal fascia. Strong septa extending from the deep face of this fascia pass between the coccygeal muscles and then get attached to the coccygeal vertebrae. This fascia is loosely attached to the root of the tail but behind that it gets closely adhered to the coccygeal muscles and vertebrae. There are five pairs of coccygeal muscles. These are the dorsal, lateral and ventral sacrococcygeal, the coccygeus and the intertransversarii caudalis.

Sacrococcygeus dorsalis

The sacrococcygeus (sacrocaudalis) dorsalis muscles of the opposite sides lie parallel and close to each other on the dorsal aspect of the caudal half of the sacrum and coccygeal vertebrae in the cranial third of the tail. This muscle is erector of the tail.

Origin: On the summits and sides of the last three or four sacral spines and the spines of first five or six coccygeal vertebrae.

Insertion: On the dorsal and lateral aspect of the coccygeal vertebrae.

Action: The muscles of two sides acting together elevate and extend the tail. Contraction of the muscle of one side flexes the tail laterally on the side of the acting muscle.

Sacrococcygeus lateralis

The sacrococcygeus (sacrocaudalis) lateralis muscle is situated lateral to the preceding muscle. At its cranial end it meets with the multifidus dorsi.

Origin: The spinous process of the last lumbar vertebra jointly with multifidus dorsi and the transverse processes of the coccygeal vertebrae.

Insertion: The lateral surface of the bodies of coccygeal vertebrae starting from second to the rests in caudal direction.

Action: Acting together it acts to elevate the tail and acting singly it flexes the tail on the corresponding side.

Sacrococcygeus ventralis

The sacrococcygeus (sacrocaudalis) ventralis muscle is thicker than the preceding two muscles. It lies along the ventral aspect of the sacrum and coccyx. It has two separate divisions, the lateral and medial, which lie parallel to each other.

Origin: The lateral division of this muscle originates from the lateral aspect of the ventral surface of the sacrum and the medial division arises from the medial aspect of the ventral surface of the sacrum.

Insertion: The lateral division of the muscle inserts on ventral surface of the transverse processes of the coccygeal vertebrae while the medial division is inserted on the ventral surface of the bodies of the coccygeal vertebrae.

Action: Acting together it acts to depress the tail while acting singly it causes lateral flexion of the tail on the corresponding side.

Coccygeus

The coccygeus is a thin, flat and triangular muscle situated against the lateral wall of the pelvis between the sacrosciatic ligament and the rectum. In that context, this muscle in reality forms the lateral wall of the pelvic cavity in association with the sacrosciatic ligament.

Origin: It originates on the medial surface of the sacrosciatic ligament and the dorsal border of the ischiatic spine.

Insertion: It inserts on the ventral surface of the transverse processes and the bodies of the first two or three coccygeal vertebrae and the coccygeal fascia.

Action: Same as the preceding muscle.

Intertransversarii caudalis

The intertransversarii caudalis is a segmented muscle that lies in fascicles as independent muscles running from one vertebra to another occupying the intertransverse spaces of the coccygeal part of the vertebral column.

Origin: The first segment of this muscle arises from the caudal part of the lateral border of the sacrum and each of the succeeding segments arise from the caudal border of the transverse process of preceding coccygeal vertebra.

Insertion: The segmental fascicles of this muscle inserts on the cranial border and the dorsal surface of the transverse process of the succeeding coccygeal vertebra.

Action: Same as the preceding muscle.

Blood supply to these muscles is through the middle and lateral coccygeal arteries

Nerve supply through the coccygeal spinal nerves.

Perineum

The perineum is the region of the pelvic outlet. In ox, it is greatly elongated and very much extensive. It is bounded dorsally by the base of the tail and ventrally by the caudal attachment of the scrotum in male and udder in female. The lateral boundaries are formed by the sacrosciatic (sacrotuberal) ligament, the dorsal and ventromedial processes of the tuber ischi. The perineal region is divided into the urogenital and anal regions by a line connecting the ventromedial processes of the tuber ischi.

The urogenital group of muscles in male includes the ischiourethralis, bulboglanduralis, bulbospongiosus, ischiocavernosus and retractor penis muscles.

The urogenital group of muscles in female includes the sphincter urethrae, constrictor vulvae, bulboglanduralis, ischiourethralis, retractor clitoridis and sphincter ani externus muscles.

The anal region consists of the levator ani (retractor ani) and the coccygeus muscles.

60

Comparative Anatomy of Muscles of Abdomen and Pelvis

Horse

The **muscles of lumbar spine** in horse are more or less similar to those of ox. Of the **sublumbar muscles,** the **psoas minor** lies under the bodies of the lumbar and last three thoracic vertebrae. It arises from dorsal ends of sixteenth and seventeenth ribs and eighteenth thoracic vertebra and the first five lumbar vertebrae.

The **psoas major** arises from dorsal ends of last two ribs and the ventral faces of the transverse processes of the lumbar vertebrae. It is much wider than that of ox and covers the quadratus lumborum entirely.

The origin of **iliacus muscle** is limited to sacrum and ilium only. It has no lumbar origin and it is not so intimately united with psoas major muscle.

The **quadratus lumborum** is less developed.

The **intertransversarii lumborum** is absent between the fifth and sixth lumbar transverse processes.

The **muscles of abdominal wall** in horse do not have any striking differences, except that the **obliquus abdominis externus** is thicker and more extensive. The muscular portion of this muscle reaches the external angle of ilium and as high as lumbar transverse processes.

The **obliquus abdominis internus** is less developed. The additional origin from thoracolumbar fascia that occurs in ox is absent in horse.

The **rectus abdominis** has its origin from the cartilages of fourth or fifth to ninth ribs. The muscle is widest in the middle. It has eleven transverse linea.

The **transversus abdominis** arises from medial faces of the distal ends of cartilages of the asternal ribs at the place of the costal attachment of the diaphragm.

The **muscles of the tail** of the horse resemble in general to those of ox except that the coccygeus muscle is less developed. The lateral part of this muscle is inserted to the first four or five coccygeal vertebrae.

Dog

The **muscles of lumbar spine** in dog are more or less similar to those of ox. Of the **sublumbar muscles**, the **psoas minor** is relatively larger than the psoas major. Its cranial part blends with the quadratus lumborum but does not extend into the thoracic cavity.

The **psoas major** is short and it begins at third or fourth lumbar vertebra.

The **iliacus** is very small in its outer portion and large in the inner portion. The inner part fuses with the psoas major.

The **quadratus lumborum** is better developed in dog as compared to other animals. It extends outwards beyond the iliacus and psoas major. It arises in common with psoas minor from the last three or four thoracic vertebrae and terminates on the dorsal aspect of the pelvic surface of the ilium.

The **intertransversarii lumborum** is similar to that in ox.

The **muscles of the abdominal wall** in dog have a few differences as below. The **abdominal tunic** is absent.

The **obliquus abdominis externus** is well developed and its aponeurotic end has a clear border. It arises from the thoracolumbar fascia and the caudal eight or nine ribs.

The **obliquus abdominis internus**, though an oblique muscle, has vertical fibres. It arises from the thoracolumbar fascia and the lateral angle of the ilium.

The **rectus abdominis** has five transverse linea.

The **inguinal canal** in bitch lodges the round ligament of the uterus enclosed in a tubular process of peritoneum.

The **muscles of tail** in dog are more or less similar to those in ox. The **sacrococcygeal** muscles originate on lumbar vertebrae also. An **accessory sacrococcygeus** muscle arises on the lateral border of the sacrum, the transverse process of first coccygeal vertebra and the caudal border of ilium. It is inserted to the dorsal and lateral coccygeus muscle.

Sheep and Goat

The general disposition including the origin, insertion, relations and action of the abdominal and pelvic muscles in sheep and goat is more or less similar to that in ox.

Pig

The **iliocostalis lumborum** continues cranially as iliocostalis thoracis, and through cervical region extends to the wing of the atlas.

The **longissimus lumborum** can be separated from the rest of the common muscle mass on the loins that begins on the first lumbar vertebra.

The **multifidus lumborum** is similar to that of horse.

The **interspinales and the intertransversarii** are same as those of ox.

The **psoas minor** is intimately adhered to psoas major. It begins at the first lumbar vertebra and inserts by long small tendon on the psoas tubercle.

The **psoas major** is large and rounded. It begins at the last rib.

The **quadratus lumborum** is well developed and extends to the last two or three thoracic vertebrae.

The **abdominal tunic** is developed but not so strong.

The **obliquus abdominis externus** has an extensive fleshy portion while its aponeurotic part is narrow and is reflected to form the inguinal ligament.

The **obliquus abdominis internus** resembles to that of ox. A small slip detached from this muscle crosses the inguinal canal obliquely and gets attached to the abdominal surface of the inguinal ligament.

The **rectus abdominis** is extensive and thick and it has about seven to ten transverse linea. Its tendon of insertion fuses with the common tendon of the gracilis.

The **transversus abdominis** has a well developed fleshy part and it blends cranially with the transversus thoracis.

The **cremaster externus** is present in both, males and females.

The **sacrococcygeus dorsalis medialis** is considered to be the caudal continuation of multifidus muscle.

The **sacrococcygeus dorsalis lateralis** represents the longissimus muscle in the caudal region.

The **sacrococcygeus ventralis lateralis** is better developed as compared to the sacrococcygeus ventralis medialis. It is a strong bilateral muscle that arises on second and third coccygeal vertebrae and extends to first eleven coccygeal vertebrae.

The **sacrococcygeus ventralis medius** is poorly developed. It lies medial to the preceding muscle and is located on the ventral surface of the tail.

Fowl

The **subcutaneous abdominalis** is the cutaneus muscle of the abdominal region in fowl. It extends in common with the thoracic part of this muscle beneath the skin over the lateral surface of the breast and abdomen in close association with the ventral feather tract. It passes caudally to the subcutaneous fascia where it overlies the muscles of the abdominal wall and pelvis.

The muscles of the wall of the abdomen include the **obliquus abdominis externus** and **internus, rectus abdominis** and the **transversus abdominis**. The general disposition of these muscles in fowl is similar to that in mammalian species.

SECTION-B

VISCERA

Visceral cavities

There are three major cavities known as visceral cavities. These are the **thoracic, abdominal** and **pelvic** cavities. The **thoracic cavity** accommodates most of the organs of respiration and heart. The **abdominal cavity** contains within it the majority of organs of the digestion, excretion and reproduction. Some of the organs forming the terminal part of these systems are contained in the **pelvic cavity**. The thoracic cavity and its contents have been described under the Anatomy of Thorax. The remaining two cavities and their contents are as below.

Abdominal cavity

The abdominal cavity is the largest of the three cavities. Cranially it is separated from the thoracic cavity by diaphragm while caudally it continues with pelvic cavity. The line of demarcation between the abdominal and pelvic cavities is the pelvic brim or pelvic inlet. The abdominal cavity is ovoid in form and somewhat compressed laterally. Its long axis extends obliquely from the centre of the pelvic inlet to the sternal part of diaphragm. Its greatest dorsoventral diameter is at the level of the first lumbar vertebra and the transverse diameter is near the pelvis. It presents a roof, the floor, the two lateral walls and the cranial wall. The **roof** is formed by the lumbar vertebrae, the lumbar part of diaphragm and the sublumbar muscles. The **lateral walls** are formed by the external and internal obliquus and the transversus abdominis muscles, the abdominal fascia, the central part of the ilia with their muscles, the cartilages of the sternal ribs and the parts of the caudal ribs below the attachment of diaphragm. **The floor** or the ventral wall is formed by the two rectus abdominis muscles, the aponeuroses of the external and internal obliquus abdominis and the transversus abdominis muscles, the abdominal fascia and the xiphoid cartilage. The **cranial wall** is formed by the diaphragm which is deeply concave resulting into greatly increasing the size of the abdomen at the cost of the thorax. The abdominal walls are pierced by **five foramina (apertures)**. Three of these are in the diaphragm and are named as hiatus oesophageus, hiatus aorticus and the foramen vena cava. The **hiatus oesophageus** transmits through it the oesophagus and along it the dorsal and ventral oesophageal trunks of the vagus nerves. The **hiatus aorticus** provides passage for the caudal aorta and the **foramen vena cava** for the caudal vena cava. The other two apertures are in the floor of the abdominal cavity and these are the **left** and **right inguinal apertures** (openings) through which pass the spermatic cord in the male and the external pudendal vessels and nerves in the female. In foetus, there is an additional opening called the umbilical opening in the floor of the abdominal cavity.

Pelvic cavity

The pelvic cavity is the smallest of the three visceral cavities. It is continuous in front with the abdominal cavity. The line of demarcation between the abdominal and pelvic cavities is the pelvic inlet. The dorsal wall or roof of the cavity is formed by the sacrum and first three coccygeal vertebrae. The ventral wall or floor is formed by the pubic and ischial bones of the pelvis and the lateral walls are formed by parts of ilia and the sacrosciatic ligaments. The pelvic inlet is bounded by base of the sacrum dorsally, the iliopectineal lines laterally and the cranial borders of the pubic bones ventrally. The pelvic outlet is formed by the third coccygeal vertebra dorsally, the ischial arch ventrally and the caudal edges of the sacrotuberal ligament and the semimembranosus muscles laterally. The outlet is closed by the perineal fascia consisting of the superficial and deep layers attached to the margin of the pelvic outlet, the anus and its muscles and the vulva in female and root of penis in male. The organs contained in the pelvic cavity include rectum, parts of urinary and genital organs, muscles vessels and nerves.

Peritoneum

The peritoneum is a serous membrane which lines the abdominal cavity and to some extent the pelvic cavity and covers the organs contained in them. In the male it is a completely closed sac but in female it has two small openings the abdominal openings of the oviduct or the fallopian tubes. The peritoneal cavity is a potential space formed between two layers, parietal and visceral which are normally in contact with each other. It contains a thin film of serous membrane. The parietal layer lines the boundaries of the wall of the cavity and then reflects over the organs contained in it forming the visceral layer. The double folds of peritoneum thus passing from the walls of the visceral cavity to the organs contained in it constitutes a pathway for the vessels and nerves supplying to the concerned organs. The folds that connect the stomach to other viscera is called omentum, the one that passes from the dorsal wall to the intestine is called the mesentery while the folds which are attached to the organs other than those of the gastro-intestinal tract (gut tube) are called as ligaments. However, these folds i.e. ligaments except the broad ligament of uterus does not transmit vessels and nerves.

Topographic regions of the abdominal cavity

For topographic purposes the abdomen is divided into nine regions by imaginary planes. Two transverse planes divide the cavity into three regions, the cranial abdominal, middle abdominal and the caudal abdominal region. The first (cranial) of these two planes passes through the caudal border of the costal arch while the second (caudal) passes through the level of the tuber coxae. These three regions are further divided by two sagittal planes into left, central and right divisions with three sub regions each as below.

Abdominal regions	Abdominal regions created by sagittal planes		
Created by transverse planes	Left	Central	Right
Cranial abdominal region:	Left hypochondriac	Xiphoid	Right hypochondriac
Middle abdominal region:	Left lumbar	Left inguinal	Umbilical
Caudal abdominal region:	Prepubic	Right lumbar	Right inguinal

In addition to these, there are some more regions referred in relation to abdominal cavity. These are named as sublumbar, diaphragmatic, lumbar and the flank regions.

The **sublumbar region** is the part of the abdominal cavity that is below the lumbar vertebrae and their transverse processes. This is the dorsal part of the abdominal cavity.

The **diaphragmatic region** is the portion of the abdominal cavity that is in the vicinity of the diaphragm towards the cranial part of the cavity.

The **inguinal region** is the part in front of the inguinal ligament and the parts of the abdominal cavity in the vicinity of the left and right inguinal canal.

The **flank region** is the part of the abdominal cavity that is formed by the soft part of the abdominal wall. On the dorsal part of this region is a triangular part which is called as **paralumbar fossa**. It is bounded dorsally by the longissimus muscle, ventrally by the dorsal border of obliquus abdominis internus muscle and cranially by the last rib.

Viscera

Viscera are the organs contained inside the visceral cavities of the body. Most of these organs have a linear or circular or irregular cavity within them. There are some organs which do not have cavity within them and are solid organs with parenchyma within them. The hollow organs or the organs with cavity or lumen are covered from outside and lined internally by a layer of thin, translucent, moist membrane. These membranes are serous, muscular or mucous in nature. The wall of the hollow visceral organs is made of different layers which are called as tunics. The outer tunic is a serous layer and is differentially called as tunica serosa, tunica adventitia and tunica albuginea or tunica fibrosa in different organs. The serous fluid secreted by the cells of these membranes reduces the chances of friction of the organs. The middle layer is the tunica muscularis. It is formed by smooth or striated muscle fibres. The muscle fibres may be arranged differently in different organs. This layer is responsible for movements of the wall of the organs. The inner layer is called tunica mucosa. It lines the internal surface of the wall of the organs. The submucous layer of this tunic produces a viscus coating for surface facing the lumen of the organ.

In ruminants, the major part of the abdominal cavity is occupied by the stomach. It occupies nearly three fourths of the abdominal cavity. It fills in the entire left half except a small space at the dorsum occupied by spleen, and extends well into the right half of the cavity. The rest of the organs contained in the abdominal cavity are the small and large intestines, the accessory organs of digestion like the liver, pancreas, and spleen, the organs of urinary system like kidneys, ureters, urinary bladder and the urethra, the internal genital organs and their accessory glands, adrenal glands, lymph glands, vessels and nerves.

61

Digestive Organs

Stomach

The stomach of ruminants (Fig. 4-4 A) is compound stomach with four parts; the rumen, reticulum, omasum and abomasum. The first three compartments comprise the forestomach or proventriculus. These parts have a nonglandular mucous membrane lined by a stratified squamous epithelium and are concerned with maceration, fermentation and cellulose digestion while the last part, the abomasum has a glandular mucous membrane which is concerned with digestion of the food material with the help of gastric juices. The relative sizes of the four compartments change with the age of the animal. In new bourn calf the rumen and reticulum together have about half the capacity of abomasum. But, as the diet of the animal is restricted to milk during this period, these two compartments remain collapsed and functionless. At eight weeks of age, the total capacity of rumen and reticulum equals to that of the abomasum and at twelve weeks of age the combined capacity of rumen and reticulum doubles to that of the abomasum. During this period the growth of the omasum is slow and steady. At about one and half years of age the omasum and abomasum equals in their capacity. At this age the four parts reach to their definitive size, shape and capacity. The relative capacity of the four compartments at this stage is rumen eighty per cent, reticulum five per cent, omasum seven per cent and abomasum eight per cent. The total capacity of average sized cattle varies between hundred fifteen to hundred fifty litre.

Rumen

The rumen (Fig. 4-4 A) is the largest and voluminous part of the bovine stomach. It occupies most of the left half of the abdomen and extends considerably over the median plane to the right side of the abdominal cavity. In the abdominal cavity, the rumen extends from the level of the seventh or eighth intercostal space to the pelvic inlet. It is somewhat compressed from side to side and presents two surfaces, two borders and two extremities. The **parietal surface** is convex and is related to diaphragm, the left wall of the abdomen and the

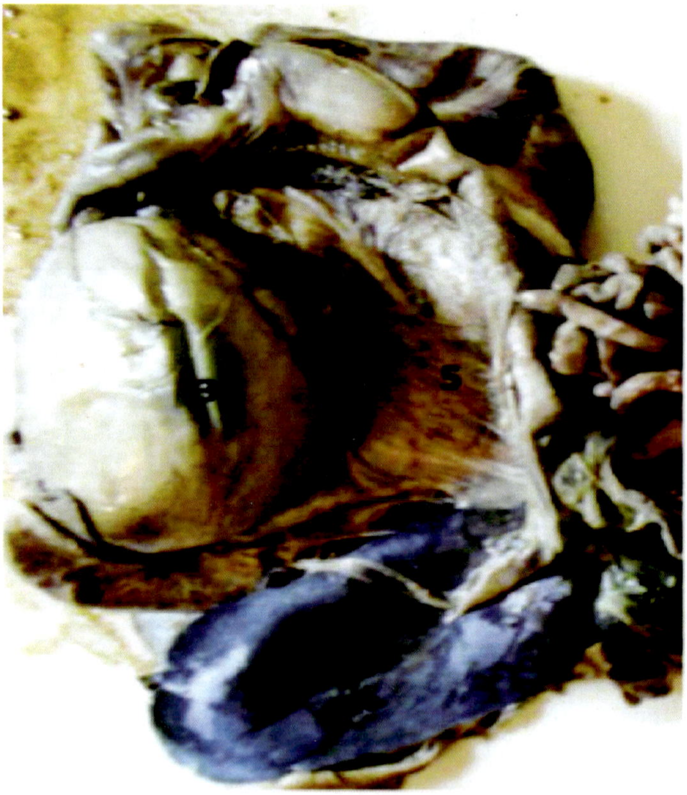

4 – 4 A: Stomach of Ox; External features (Right side)
1. Rumen; 2. Reticulum; 3. Omasum; 4. Abomasum; 5.Omentum 6. Liver 7. Gall bladder (Liver and Gall Bladder have been dissected and pulled away from their original location)

spleen. The **visceral surface** is irregular and is related to the omasum, abomasum, intestine, liver and pancreas, left kidney and adrenal, aorta and the caudal vena cava. The **dorsal border** (curvature) is convex and is in contact with the dorsal wall of the abdomen through peritoneum and connective tissue as far back as to the level of fourth lumbar vertebra. The **ventral border** (curvature) is also convex and is for most part in contact with the floor of the abdomen.

The two surfaces are marked by **right and left longitudinal grooves** indicating externally the division of the cavity of rumen into **dorsal and ventral sacs**. The **cranial extremity** is divided ventrally by a **cranial transverse groove** into two sacs. The dorsal sac is called **atrium ruminis** and it is continuous caudally with the dorsal sac of the rumen and cranially with the reticulum. It curves over the ventral sac which is rounded and blind. Externally the junction of atrium ruminis and reticulum is marked by a groove which is called the

ruminoreticular groove. It is distinct ventrally but dorsally the two compartments form a sort of dome named as **atrium ventriculi** on which the oesophagus terminates. The **caudal extremity** of the rumen extends to the pubis and is related to the intestine and urinary bladder. It is divided by a **caudal transverse groove** into dorsal and ventral sacs both of which are blind. All the grooves on the external surface of the rumen are lodged by vessels and nerves of the rumen.

Reticulum

The reticulum is the most cranial and the smallest of the four compartments of bovine stomach. It extends from level of sixth to seventh or eighth ribs and its greater part lies to the left of the median line. It is somewhat piriform in shape and is compressed craniocaudally. The **parietal** (diaphragmatic) **surface** faces craniad. It is convex and lies against the diaphragm and liver. The **visceral surface** faces caudad and is flattened by the pressure from atrium ruminis. It ends dorsally by joining the rumen. The concave line of junction of the rumen and reticulum corresponds to a ridge in the interior which forms the lower margin of the ruminoreticular orifice. The **lesser curvature** of rumen faces to the right and dorsally and is connected to the omasum. The **greater curvature** faces to the left and ventrally. It lies against the diaphragm opposite the sixth and seventh ribs. The **right extremity** (fundus) of the reticulum forms a rounded cul-de-sac which is in contact with the sternal part of the diaphragm, the liver, omasum and abomasum. It is opposite the ventral end of sixth intercostal space.

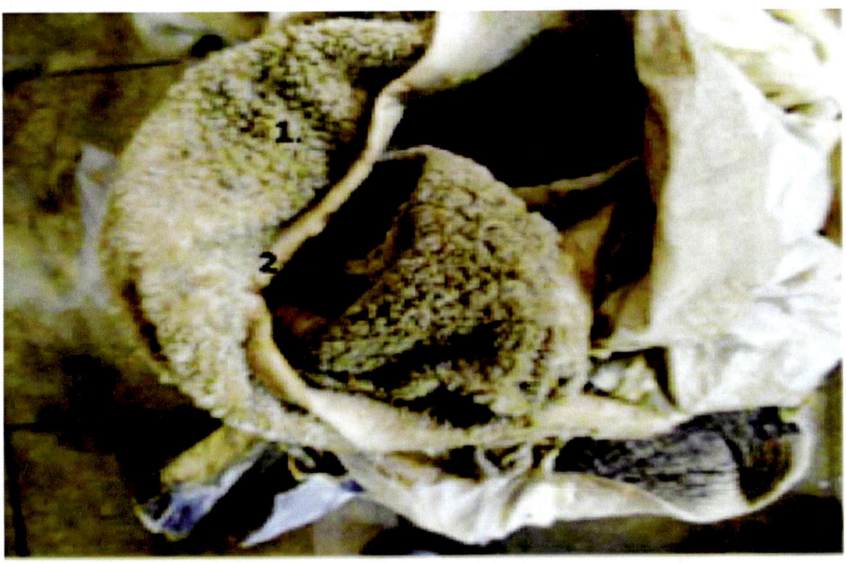

Fig. 4 – 4 B: Internal surface of rumen
1. Papillae; 2. Pillar

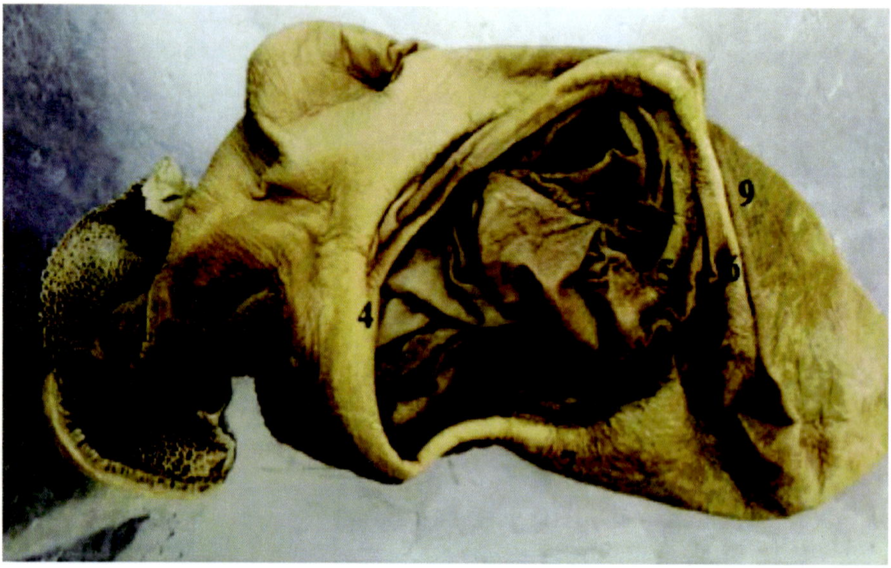

Fig. 4 -4 C: Internal structure of rumen and reticulum of Ox
1: Chambers of reticulum; 2. Rumino-reticular groove; 3. Cranial end of dorsal sac; 4: Cranial pillar of rumen; 5. Coronary pillars; 6. caudal pillar of rumen; 7. right ventral sac of rumen; 8.Caudo ventral pillars; 9. Caudo dorsal bind sac

Omasum

The omasum is ellipsoidal in form and is somewhat compressed between its parietal and visceral surfaces. Its long axis is nearly vertical. It is clearly marked off from the other compartments of the stomach. It lies to the right of the median line from the level of seventh to eleventh ribs. The **parietal surface** faces to the right and craniad and is related to the diaphragm and liver. The **visceral surface** faces to the left and caudad and is in contact with the right surface of the rumen, the reticulum and the abomasum. The **dorsal** (greater) **curvature** faces caudad and to the right. The **lesser curvature** (base) is very short and faces cranially, ventrally and to the left. It is connected at its upper part with the reticulum by a very short narrow neck of omasum. Below it joins the abomasum. The junction with abomasum is much more extensive externally than the omasoabomasal orifice.

Abomasum

The abomasum is an elongated sac which lies chiefly on the abdominal floor extending caudad from the xiphoid region. Its cranial blind end, the **fundus,** is at the xiphoid region in relation to the reticulum, the atrium ruminis and the ventral sac of rumen. The **body** extends back between the ventral sac of rumen and the omasum and turns to the right behind the omasum. It is constricted in the middle forming the cranial larger part and the caudal pear shaped smaller part. The **pyloric part** inclines dorsally and joins the duodenum at the ventral part of the tenth rib. The **parietal surface** is in contact with the abdominal floor. The **visceral surface** is related to the rumen and omasum. The **greater curvature** gives attachment to the superficial part of the greater omentum. The **lesser curvature** is related to the greater curvature of omasum.

Attachments of ruminant stomach

The dorsal curvature of the rumen is attached to the crura of diaphragm and sublumbar muscles by connective tissue at the dorsal wall of the abdomen. This attachment extends from the hiatus oesophageus to the fourth lumbar vertebra. The sheet of peritoneum extending from the abdominal wall to the rumen and spleen converts into **gastrophrenic and splenicophrenic ligaments.** In addition to these, there are two larger extensive sheets of peritoneum which connects the rumen and other parts of the stomach to the parietal layer of peritoneum. These are called the lesser omentum and greater omentum.

The **lesser omentum** connects the portal fissure of the liver to the lesser curvature of rumen. It is attached to the visceral surface of liver along the line from the oesophageal impression to the portal fissure. The line of attachment to the stomach passes from the ventral side of oesophagus, along the reticular groove, the parietal surface of the base of omasum and the lesser curvature of the abomasum. The terminal part of lesser omentum attached to the cranial part of duodenum is the hepatoduodenal ligament.

The **greater omentum** consists of two layers. The **superficial layer** extends from the left groove of rumen, curves ventrally around this organ, ascends to the right and ends on the second part of duodenum and greater curvature of abomasum. The **deep layer** is attached ventral to the right groove of rumen, curves to the right side and blends with the mesoduodenum enclosing the intestinal mass, extends as far as the first bend of colon and gets attached to the liver and pancreas. The superficial and deep parts blend with each other at the duodenum. The **epiploic foramen** which is the communication between the peritoneal sacs of lesser and greater omentum is a sagittal slit between the caudate process of liver laterally, the vena cava dorsally and the hepatoduodenal ligament ventrally.

Interior of ruminant stomach

The **cavity of rumen** (Fig. 4-4 B) is divided into two sacs by the **pillars** of rumen which are muscular folds and correspond to the grooves on the exterior. They project like shelves into the cavity of the organ. The **cranial pillar** has a thick concave free edge. The **caudal pillar** is horizontal and also presents a thick free edge. Between these free edges the two sacs of rumen communicate with each other. The **right and left pillars** connect the cranial and caudal pillars and are less prominent.

The **ruminoreticular fold** on the interior corresponds to the ruminoreticular groove on the exterior. Its free edge is concave and forms the ventral and lateral margins of the large oval ruminoreticular aperture. The **cardia** which marks the entry of the oesophagus into the rumen is about four to five inches ventral to the vertebral end of the eighth or ninth rib. This opening is slit like. The mucous membrane of rumen is brown in colour and is thickly studded with **large conical papillae** except on the pillars where the mucous membrane is pale and is without papillae.

The **interior of** the **reticulum** (Fig. 4-4 C)is raised into folds about half inch high enclosing four to six sided spaces or cells. These spaces are subdivided by smaller folds and their bottoms are studded with pointed horny papillae. This peculiar arrangement of the mucous membrane of the reticulum gives it **honey comb like appearance**. The round **reticulo-omasal** orifice is situated at the lesser curvature of reticulum five or six inches above its bottom. The **oesophageal groove** begins at the cardia of the rumen and passes ventrally on the internal face of the right wall of atrium ruminis and the reticulum to end at the reticulo-omasal orifice. It is about seven or eight inches in length. It is directed dorsoventrally. The groove is twisted in a spiral fashion so that its thickened edges project at first caudad, then to the left and finally craniad. The twist mainly concerns with the left lip of the groove.

The **cavity of omasum** (Fig. 4-4 D) is occupied by about a hundred **longitudinal muscular folds** which spring from its greater curvature and are called as **laminae omasi**. The largest of these, which are about ten to twelve in number, have a superior convex attached edge and a thick concave free edge. A groove, the **sulcus omasi** extends from the reticulo-omasal opening to the omasoabomasal opening and is about four inches long. It is free from laminae. The omasoabomasal orifice is oval and is about four inches long.

The cavity of **abomasum** (Fig. 4-4 E) is divided into two parts by a constriction. The first part (**fundus**) is lined with glandular epithelium forming about twelve or more oblique folds. The folds extend from the sides of the abomasal groove towards the greater curvature and pyloric part. The second (**pyloric**) part is narrower and pear shaped and presents a brownish coloured mucous membrane. It contains pyloric glands. This part is without any folds. The **pylorus** is small and round.

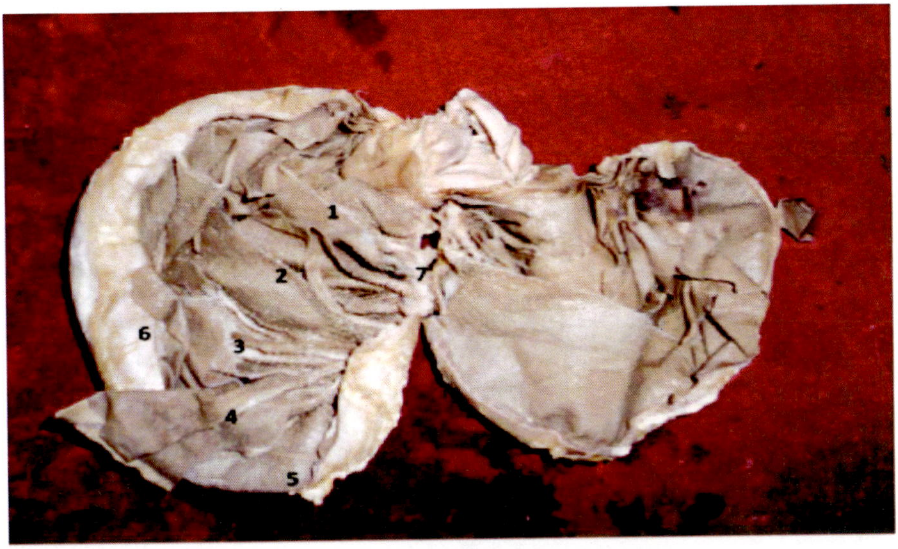

Fig. 4 – 4 D: Internal structure of Omasum of Ox
1. Abomasal folds; 2. Fundus; 3. Pylorus; 4. Pyloric sphincter

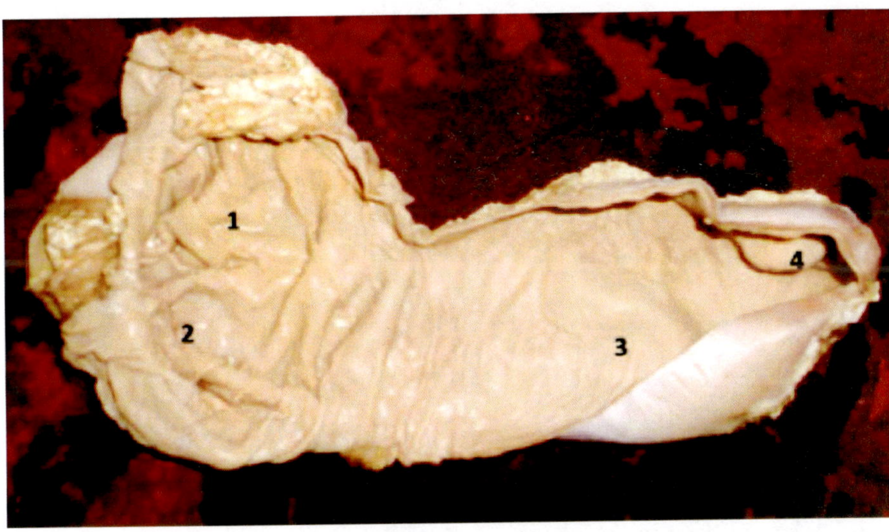

Fig. 4 – 4 E: Internal structure of Abomasum of Ox
1. Abomasal folds; 2. Fundus; 3. Pylorus; 4. Pyloric sphincter

Intestines

The intestine (Fig. 4-4 F) is about twenty times in length of the body. It is situated almost entirely to the right side of the median plane in contact with the visceral surface of the rumen and is attached to the sublumbar region by the mesentery. The intestine has two major parts, the small intestine and large intestine.

Small intestine

The small intestine continues the gastrointestinal tract caudally from the pylorus of the abomasum. It measures about 40 m (130 feet) in average sized Indian cattle and has a diameter of about 5 to 6 cm (2 inches). It consists of three parts in succession. The first part is a fixed part and is called duodenum. The second and third part is mesenteric and is called as jejunum and ileum.

Duodenum

The duodenum is about 1m (3 to 4 feet) long. It begins at the pylorus of the abomasum at the level of ventral end of tenth rib. It first passes dorsally and cranially to the visceral surface of liver where it forms an S-shaped curve, the **ansa sigmoidea** (sigmoid flexure) and turns back and then continues as **descending part** running dorsally to the tuber coxae. Here it forms the **caudal (iliac) flexure** passing from right to left side around the caudal mesenteric

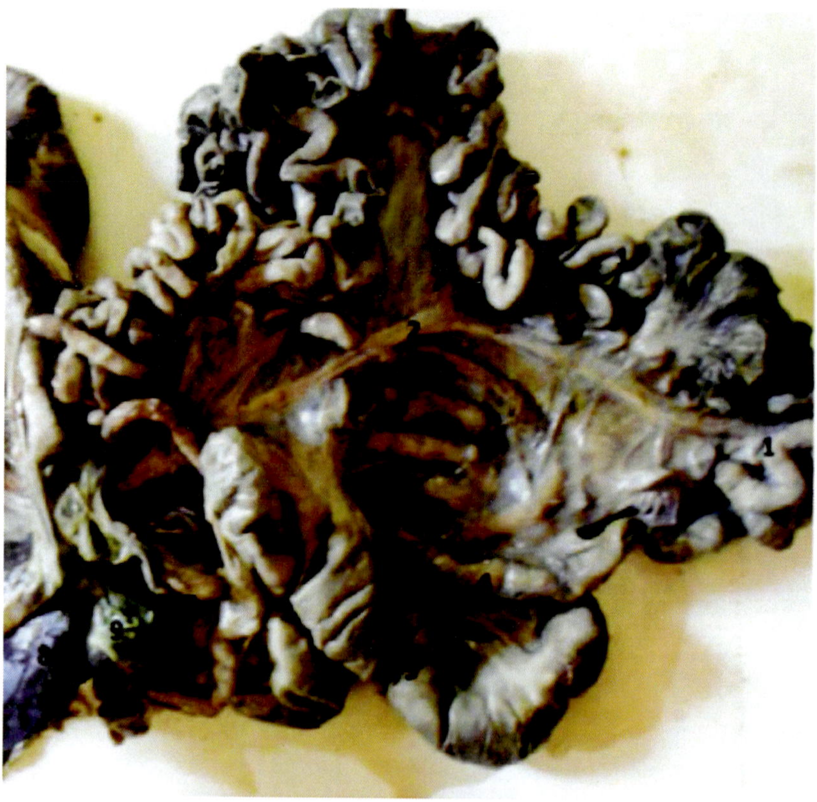

Fig. 4 – 4 F: Intestines of ox
1. Jejunum 2. Mesenteric blood vessels 3. Ansa spiralis 4. Eleum 5. Caecum 6. Duodenum 7. Mesentery 8. Visceral surface of liver 9. Gall Bladder

artery and then continues as ascending part running cranially to its termination at the **duodeno-jejunal flexure** on the left side of the cranial mesenteric artery. The **cranial part** of the duodenum is attached to the liver by the lesser omentum. The descending part and the caudal flexure are attached dorsally to the mesoduodenum and ventrally to the superficial wall of omental bursa. The **ascending part** of the duodenum is attached to the descending colon caudally by the **duodenocolic ligament**. The **bile duct** opens into the second bend of the S-shaped curve about 60 cm from the pylorus. The **pancreatic duct** opens into the descending part of duodenum about 30 cm caudal to the bile duct.

Jejunum

The jejunum is the continuation of small intestine from duodenum. It is arranged in the form of several close coils like festoon attached to the edge of the mesentery. Caudally just before joining the ileum it prolongs into a U-shaped series of loops on the extended part of the mesentery and then continues into a straight part as ileum without any distinct mark of division. The jejunum chiefly lies on the right side of the rumen in the supraomental recess bounded medially by the right (visceral) surface of the rumen, laterally by the abdominal wall, dorsally by large intestine and cranially by omasum and abomasum. It can be easily exposed by drawing the caudal fold of omentum cranially.

Ileum

The ileum is the terminal part of the small intestine is a straight tube about 1 m in length. It leaves the edge of the mesentery, runs cranially between the caecum and colon and opens on the medial face of the caecum.

Mesentery

The mesentery is a fan shaped double walled fold of peritoneum which attaches the jejunum and ileum to the dorsal wall of the abdomen. Between the walls of the mesentery run the vessels and nerves supplying the intestine. The **visceral border** of the mesentery is attached to the intestines and contains the mesenteric lymph glands while its **parietal border** or root is attached to a small area around the cranial mesenteric artery under the first and second lumbar vertebrae. The mesentery is short at first but soon it extends and reaches to a length of about 50 to 60 cm, sufficient to allow the intestine to reach the abdominal floor.

Structure: The **wall** of the **small intestine** has the outer **serous coat**, medial to it is the **muscular coat** and then the **submucous coat** and the innermost **mucous membrane**. The submucous coat contains **Brunner's glands** in the first twelve to fifteen feet. The free surface of the mucous membrane presents numerous finger like projections, the **villi** between which are the intestinal glands.

The intestinal glands are present throughout the intestine. The lymphoid tissue occurs in the form of distinct nodules which are either scattered solitary glands or in groups, the **Payer's patches**. These patches are large and are about eighteen to forty in number in the adult cattle and about twenty five to fifty in calves. Usually there is a very long patch close to the ileo-caecal valve.

Large intestine

The large intestine extends from the termination of ileum into caecum to the anus. It measures about thirty five to forty feet in length. Its diameter is almost similar to that of the small intestine or slightly greater than it. It is situated into the supraomental recess, between the layers of the mesentery in the right dorsal part of the abdominal cavity and is related to the rumen on its left side. It consists of three parts, the caecum, colon and rectum.

Caecum

The caecum is a great cul-de-sac intercalated between the small intestine and the colon. It measures about 75 cm in length and 12 cm in diameter in the average sized cattle. It is directly continuous cranially with the colon. The line of demarcation between the two is the junction of ileum with large intestine. From this junction, on the medial surface of the caecum at the ventral end of the last rib, the caecum extends caudodorsally along the right flank. Its rounded blind end commonly lies at the right side of the pelvic inlet. The cranial two thirds of the caecum is adhered to the right side of the mesentery. It is dorsally attached by a short caecocolic fold to the proximal loop of colon and ventrally by ileo-caecal fold to the ileum.

Colon

The colon is about 10 m long and its diameter is at first the same as that of the caecum but diminishes to about 5 cm in the course of the proximal loop. The greater part of caecum is arranged in double elliptical coils between the two layers of the mesentery. It begins as a direct continuation of caecum at the ileo-caecal orifice, runs cranially for a short distance to a point opposite the ventral part of last two ribs and then turns dorsad and caudad. From here it continues caudad in relation to the right flank laterally and caecum ventrally to the caudal part of the sublumbar region. Here it again turns forwards and runs parallel to the second part of duodenum as far as second lumbar, turns backwards and is continued by the spiral part. In this part there are usually two full centripetal turns, the central flexure and two centrifugal turns. The terminal part, the distal loop proceeds from the last centrifugal gyrus dorsally and caudally on the proximal loop, turns around the caudal border of the mesentery from left to right side and runs cranially medial to the proximal loop. It then continues as a short transverse colon which passes from right to left around the cranial mesenteric artery and is continued by the descending colon. The descending colon runs caudally dorsal to the ascending duodenum, inclines to the right under the right kidney, forms a sigmoid flexure near the pelvic inlet and joins the rectum. This part is attached by a short mesocolon to the sublumbar region.

Rectum

The rectum is the terminal part of the gastrointestinal tube. It extends from the pelvic inlet to the anus. It measures about 30 cm in length. The cranial part of the rectum till the level of first coccygeal vertebra is covered by peritoneum and is attached by the mesorectum to the roof of the pelvis. The caudal part which is not covered by the peritoneum (retroperitoneal part) presents a dilatation called the ampullae recti.

The rectum runs almost straight or obliquely through the pelvic cavity. It is related dorsally to the roof of the pelvic cavity, ventrally to the bladder, seminal vesicles, prostrate, vasa differentia, Cowper 's glands and urethra in the male and the uterus and vagina in female animals.

Structure: The **serous coat** covers the **large intestine** except at the portion of the adherent surfaces. And the retroperitoneal part of the rectum. The later part is covered by connective tissue. The **muscular coat** has longitudinal and circular layers. The **submucous coat** has ramifications of vessels. The mucous membrane does not present any villi as in the small intestine but it has **intestinal glands**. The **ileo-caecal orifice** is located on an elevation formed by mucous membrane and the ileal musculature and this structure is called the **papilla ilealis** which protrudes slightly into the lumen of the large intestine.

Anus

The anus is the terminal part of alimentary canal and is placed below the root of the tail forming a rounded projection with a central depression when contracted. It is covered externally by thin skin which is devoid of hairs but provided with numerous sweat and sebaceous glands. Its lumen, the anal canal is about 5 cm long and is always closed by the contraction of sphincter muscles and folds of the mucous membrane except during defecation. The mucous membrane is pale, glandless and covered with thick squamous stratified epithelium.

Muscles of anus

The **sphincter ani internus** is the terminal thickening of the circular coat of bowel and the **sphincter ani externus** is a broad ring of striped muscle outside the preceding muscle. The action of both the muscles is to close the anus. The **retractor ani** is a flat striped muscle which lies between the rectum and the sacrosciatic ligament ending below the sphincter ani externus. It reduces the partial prolapse, the anus undergoes during defecation.

The **suspensory ligament** of anus is a band of plain muscle that arises from the first coccygeal vertebra, passes down under the retractor ani and unites with its fellow of the opposite side below the anus. In the male, it is continued as retractor penis muscle. In the female, it blends with the constrictor vulvae.

Glands

Liver

The liver (Fig. 4-4 G) is the largest compound tubular gland in the body. It lies almost entirely to the right of the median plane. It is red brown in colour and its weight in cattle ranges from 4.5 to 5.5 kg. It extends obliquely cranioventral from the lumbocostal angle to the level of the eighth rib. It is strongly curved and is accurately adapted to the abdominal face of the diaphragm. It presents two surfaces and four borders.

The **parietal or diaphragmatic surface** (Fig. 4-4 G) is convex and for the most of its part is applied against the right part of the diaphragm and a small part of it is in direct contact with the last two ribs and flank at the lumbocostal angle. This surface is marked by an oblique ridge which divides it in to two areas. The falciform ligament is attached to this surface along a line from the oesophageal impression to the notch for the round ligament. A small area at the dorsomedial part of this surface has no parietal covering as it is adhered to the diaphragm.

The **visceral surface** (Fig. 4-4 H) is concave and very irregular. It presents impressions of organs with which it is in contact. The most important and a prominent structure on the visceral surface of liver is the **portal fissure (porta hepatitis)**. The portal vein and hepatic artery enter and common hepatic duct leaves the liver at this portal fissure. Several hepatic lymph nodes are also present in this fissure. It is bounded by the papillary process, caudate process and the area of adhesion of pancreas. Below the portal fissure, a large central and dipper impression is caused by omasum and hence is named as **omasal impression.** It extends from below the portal fissure and produces most of the concavity of the liver. Below the omasal impression is the **reticular impression**. It is narrower and shallower than the preceding one. The **cystic impression** is formed by the gall bladder. This impression is formed on the lateral part of the portal fissure and is in the form of a deep furrow. A part of the pancreas is also in contact with the visceral surface of the liver slightly dorsal and lateral to the portal fissure. The **duodenal impression** is in the form of a faint groove by the sides of the portal fissure. In the right ventral area is the **abomasal impression.**

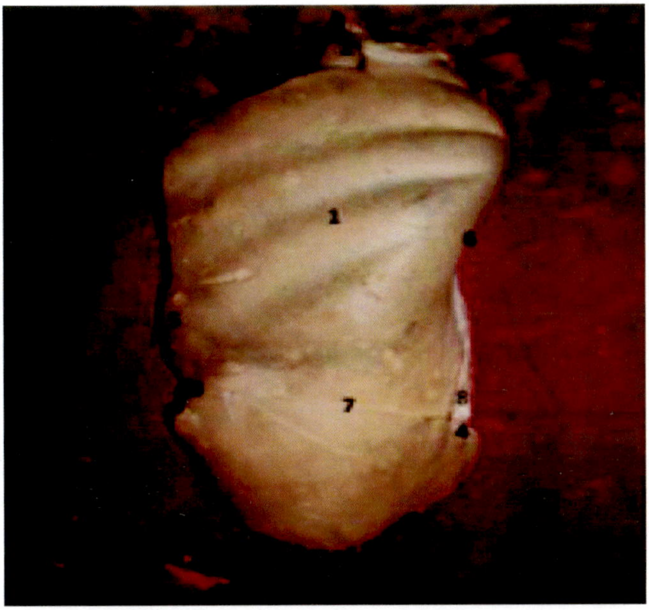

Fig. 4 – 4 G: Liver of Ox; Parietal surface

1. Costal impression 2. Caudate lobe 3. Umbilical fissure 4. Oesophageal notch 5. Lateral (right) border 6. Medial (left) border 7. Falciform ligament 8. Caudal Vena cava

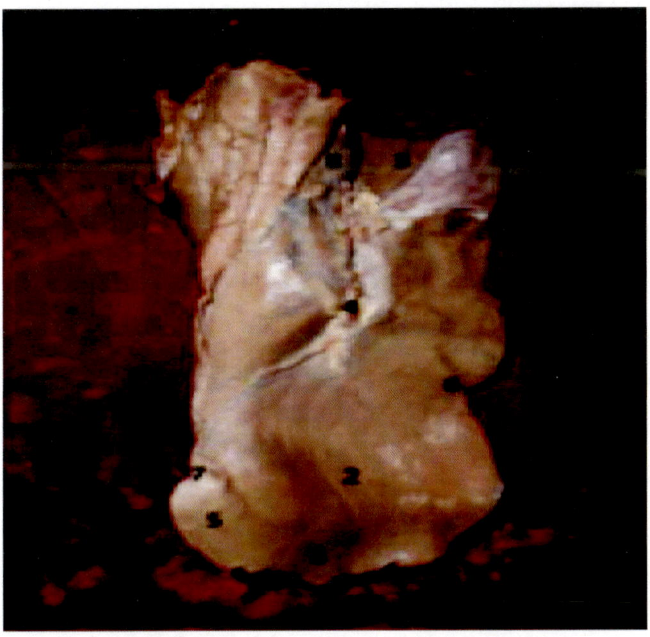

Fig. 4 – 4 H: Liver of Ox; Visceral surface

1. Abomasal impression 2. Omasal impressiion 3. Renal fossa 4. Portal fissure 5. Reticular impression 6. Umbilical fissure 7. Oesophageal notch 8. Caudate lobe

The **dorsal border** is short and thick. It presents towards its right a **caudate lobe** and towards its left, a deep **renal impression** in which the right kidney is lodged and a notch or deep **sulcus for the vena cava**. The **ventral border** is short, thin and convex. It presents a **gall bladder fossa** and the notch for the round ligament. The **lateral or the right border** presents the **umbilical fissure** to which the round ligament is attached. The **medial or the left border** is smoothly curved and is continuous with the dorsal and ventral borders.

Ligaments: The liver is hold in its position with the help of several ligaments. The **right lateral ligament** attaches the dorsal border to the sublumbar region. The **caudate ligament** attaches the caudate lobe to the ventral face of the right kidney. The **falciform ligament** is a crescentic fold which attaches the sternal part of the diaphragm to the parietal surface of the liver. The **round ligament** which is in the free border of the falciform ligament extends from the umbilical fissure of the liver to the umbilicus. The **lesser omentum** attaches the liver from the oesophageal notch to the portal fissure with the parietal surface of the omasum. The parietal surface is adhered to the diaphragm. The caudal vena cava embedded in its left dorsal border holds it in position.

Structure: A fold of serous membrane extending from the peritoneum forms the outer **serous coat** of the liver. Internal to this is a **fibrous coat** that adheres to the serous coat and invests the organ. After investing the organ, it enters the liver through the portal fissure, forms a sheath around the structures entering and leaving this organ, pierces the gland substance and divides it into numerous minute lobules. Thus it constitutes the interlobular connective tissue and forms lining to the various **portal canals**. The gland substance of liver thus consists of minute **lobules** which are separated from each other by interlobular connective tissue. Each lobule consists of numerous **hepatic cells** between which are the blood and bile capillaries. The hepatic cells are either round or polygonal and resemble the cells of squamous epithelium. The cells are without enveloping membrane and contains adepose granules along with one or two nuclei and the nucleolus with coloured biliary matter.

The **portal vein** and the **hepatic artery** enter the liver through the portal fissure and are enclosed together with the **hepatic duct** in a connective tissue sheath, the **hepatobiliary capsule** and ramify in the connective tissue capsule throughout the substance of the liver accompanied by nerves and the lymph vessels. The **portal vein** is the functional vessel of the liver. The **hepatic vein** and **artery** are vessels for supply of blood to the liver tissue. The **hepatic duct** leaves the liver through the portal fissure and unites with the **cystic duct** to form the **bile duct** that opens into the duodenum.

Gallbladder

The gallbladder is considered as a diverticulum of the bile duct enlarged to form the reservoir for bile. It is pear shaped musculomembranous sac measuring about 10 to 15 cm long. It is partly in contact with and attached to the visceral surface of the liver and most of its part lies in contact with the abdominal wall at the ventral part of the tenth or eleventh rib. It has a large part called the fundus or the body and a narrow constricted part the neck. The neck is continued by the **cystic duct** which is joined by the **hepatic duct** emerging from the liver and these two unite to form the **bile duct**. The bile duct thus formed opens into the second curve of the duodenum 80 cm from the pylorus and terminates on the summit of a papilla. Before opening into the lumen of the duodenum, the bile duct penetrates the duodenal wall obliquely because of which the valve like arrangement is formed to prevent the regurgitation from the intestine.

Structure: The **wall** of the gallbladder and the cystic and bile duct consists of **serous, muscular and mucous coats.** The **serous coat** is the reflection of visceral peritoneum. The **muscular coat** consists of muscle fibres running in different directions. The fibres in the neck of the gallbladder are circular. The **mucous membrane** is covered by columnar epithelium and contains numerous groups of branched tubular glands.

Pancreas

The pancreas is a racemose gland situated transversely across the dorsal part of the abdominal cavity and lies almost to the right of the median line. When fresh, it is reddish cream in colour and resembles salivary glands in appearance. It weighs about 500 gm in ox and is irregularly quadrilateral in outline. The part of the gland on the right side of the portal vein is considered to be its right lobe and that on the left side as left lobe, the right lobe being larger than the left one. However, there is no clear demarcation between the two. The gland as a whole presents two surfaces, four borders and four angles.

The **dorsolateral surface** faces cranially and dorsally and is covered by peritoneum. It is attached to the liver at and lateral to the portal fissure and crura of diaphragm. Between these attachments it is free and forms the ventral wall of the epiploic foramen. On the right side it extends beyond the caudate lobe of liver between the layers of the mesoduodenum. This part of the pancreas is in contact with the right flank of the abdominal wall at lumbocostal angle. This surface is related to the liver, ventral face of the right kidney and adrenal, caudal vena cava and portal vein. The **ventromedial surface** faces ventrally and caudally and is in contact with the dorsal curvature of rumen and the intestine. It presents a deep notch for the portal vein, hepatic artery and hepatic lymph nodes.

The **right border** is nearly straight and is related to the second part of duodenum. The **left border** is concave and is related to the rumen and splenic vessels. The **caudal border** is irregular and presents a deep notch through which the portal vein passes obliquely to reach the portal fissure of the liver. The **cranial border** is also straight, and is situated across the liver at the level of portal fissure.

The **craniolateral or duodenal angle** is at the level where the duodenum forms a bend and where it receives the bile duct. The **caudolateral angle** is placed at the site where the pancreatic duct leaves the gland and opens into the duodenum. The **craniomedial angle** is at the level where the splenic vessels pass between it and the liver. The **caudomedial angle** forms the left extremity of the gland and is related to the rumen.

The pancreas is attached by connective tissue to the kidneys, the suspensory ligament of the spleen and the caudal vena cava.

Structure: The pancreas is made up of small **lobes** separated by small amount of interstitial tissue. Each lobe is made up of a number of **lobules**. Each lobe has its own duct which is the tributary of the pancreatic duct. The interstitial tissue is so meager that the gland is easily torn. The colour is dark in embalmed specimens and light pinkish in fresh specimens. Pancreas is both endocrine as well as exocrine gland. The exocrine part of the gland is a compound tubulo-alveolar type of gland with serous acini. The endocrine part of the gland is known as islets of Langerhans. It is composed of alpha, beta and delta cells. The alpha cells secrete glucagon, beta cells secrete insulin and delta cells secrete somatostatin.

Spleen

The spleen (Fig. 4-4 I and J) is the largest of the ductless glands and is situated on the left side of the abdominal cavity. It is elongated, flat and elliptical in outline. Its both extremities are thin and rounded. It is bluish red or purple in colour. It measures about 50 cm in length and 15 cm in width. It presents two surfaces, two borders and two extremities. The **dorsal** or **parietal** surface (Fig. 4-4 I) is convex and is related to diaphragm. A small narrow area on this surface at its upper part near the cranial border is uncovered by the serous coat and is adhered to the diaphragm. The **ventral** or **visceral surface** (Fig. 4-4 J) is concave and is related chiefly to the parietal surface of rumen and a narrow adjacent area of reticulum. About cranial half of the visceral surface of the gland is adhered to the rumen and is devoid of the serous coat. The **cranial border** is concave and the **caudal border** is convex. The **hilus** of the spleen is situated on the dorsal third of the visceral surface near the cranial border. The **dorsal extremity** lies under the dorsal ends of the last two ribs. The **ventral extremity** lies opposite the eighth and ninth ribs about hands breadth above their sternal ends.

Structure: The **serous coat** is incomplete. A thick **capsule** containing **fibrous** and **elastic** connective tissue and **unstripped muscle** covers the external surface next to serous coat. Numerous **trabeculae** from the deep surface of the capsule pass into the substance of the spleen. They join each other forming irregular spaces and constitute the interstitial tissue. The **spleen pulp** is a soft, dark red tissue occupying the spaces founded by the trabeculae.

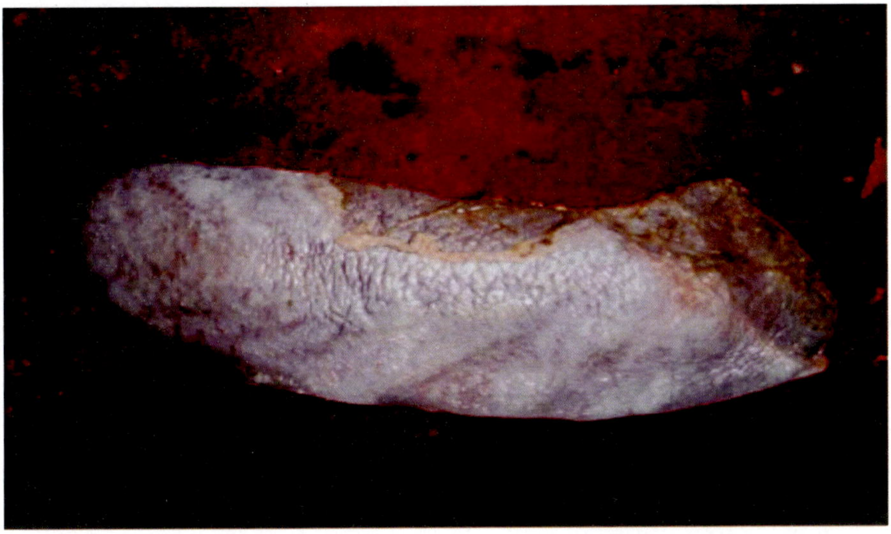

Fig. 4 – 4 I: Spleen of Ox; Parietal surface

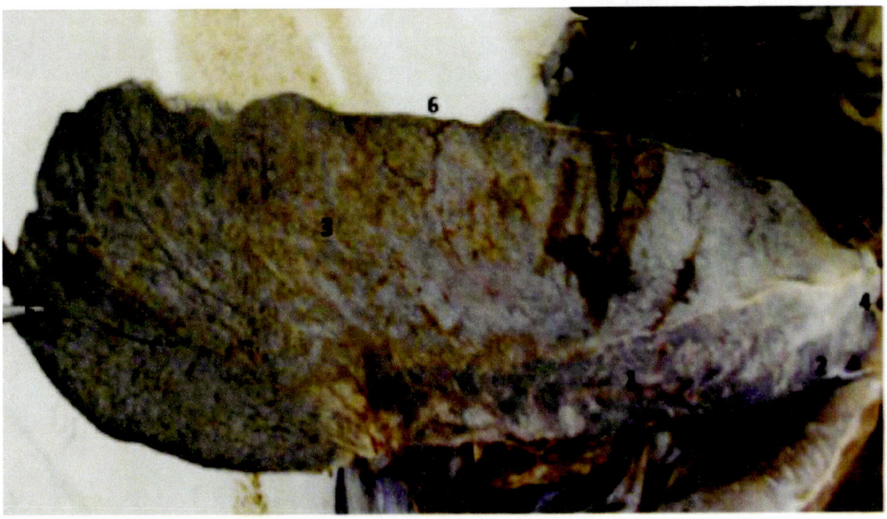

Fig. 4 – 4 J: Spleen of Ox; Visceral surface

1. Area of attachment with rumen; 2. Hilus; 3. Area o in contact with diaphragm; 4. Proximal extremity; 5. Distal extremity; 6. Caudal border; 7. Cranial border

62

Comparative Anatomy of Digestive Organs

Stomach

Horse

The stomach of horse is a **simple stomach**. It is **'J' shaped** sac with its right part very much shorter than the left part. It is situated in the dorsal part of the abdominal cavity behind the diaphragm and liver mainly to the left of the median line. The **parietal surface** faces craniad and dorsad and to the left. It is related to the diaphragm and liver. The **visceral surface** faces caudad and ventrad and to the right. It is related to the small intestine and colon. Its **lesser curvature** is short and the **greater curvature** is extensive. The **left extremity** is called the **saccus caecus**. It lies ventral to the sixteenth or seventeenth rib. It is related to pancreas and terminal part of greater colon caudally and to the base of the spleen laterally. The **right extremity** is the **pylorus**. It is smaller and is continued by duodenum. The stomach is fastened by several **ligaments** which include the **gastro-phrenic ligament**, the **gastro- pancreatic ligament**, the **greater omentum**, the **lesser omentum** and the **gastro-splenic ligament**. The capacity of the equine stomach is about 8 to 15 liters.

The wall of the stomach consists of four coats, the **serous, muscular**, **submucous** and the **mucous**. The mucous membrane is clearly divided into two parts by sinuous ridge called the **margo plicatus**. The part which is towards the left extremity is **nonglandular** while that towards the right extremity is **glandular.**

Dog

The stomach of dog is simple stomach. When full, it is **piriform** in shape. Its **capacity** is about 2.4 liters. Its **left part** is large and rounded while the **right part** is small and cylindrical. The **parietal surface** is extensive and convex. It faces craniad and ventrad towards the left side. It is related to the liver, diaphragm and the left ventral abdominal wall as far caudally as a transverse plane through the second or third lumbar vertebra. The **visceral surface** is less extensive and is related to the intestine, pancreas and left kidney. The **lesser curvature** is nearly straight and vertical but its lower part forms a deep narrow angle as a result of pyloric part directed craniad and dorsad. The **greater curvature** is nearly four times longer than the lesser curvature. In the full stomach it extends considerably caudal to the left costal arch. Ventrally it lies on the abdominal floor.

Sheep and Goat

The stomach of the sheep and goat is a **ruminant (compound) stomach**. In general, it resembles to that of ox having four compartments, the rumen, reticulum, omasum and abomasum. The total capacity of the stomach of sheep and goat is about 15 to 18 liters. The rumen and omasum are relatively smaller. The rumen constitutes about 71 percent, the reticulum 8 percent, omasum 2 percent and the abomasum 19 percent.

In sheep and goat, the **ventral sac of the rumen** is relatively larger and extends more to the right of the median plane than in the ox. Its blind sac extends farther caudally than that of the dorsal sac. The **parietal attachment of the dorsal sac** extends caudally to the second lumbar vertebra. The **left longitudinal groove** extends dorsally and caudally for a short distance only and therefore does not connect with the caudal groove. The **right ventral coronary groove** is distinct and extends to the ventral curvature, but the left one does not. The **dorsal coronary grooves** are very short or absent. **The reticulum** in sheep and goat is relatively larger than in the ox. Its ventral part curves more caudally and less to the right than in the ox. The **omasum** is much smaller than the reticulum, its capacity being only about 300 ml. It is oval and compressed laterally, It is situated almost entirely to the right of the median plane, opposite the ninth and tenth ribs in the middle third of the dorsoventral diameter of the trunk and has no contact with the abdominal wall. The **abomasum** in sheep and goat runs obliquely caudally and to the right along the costal arch.

The **cardia** is at the level of eighth intercostal space and about 5 cm ventral to the vertebrae. The left longitudinal pillar of the rumen is short and extends caudodorsally in the direction of the accessory pillar of the bovine rumen. The **oesophageal groove** is about 10 cm in length. It is inclined caudally and the reticulo-omasal orifice is about 2 to 3 cm caudal to the plane of the cardia.

Pig

The stomach of the pig is a simple stomach similar to that of the horse and dog. Its average **capacity** is about 5.7 to 8.0 liters. When full, its **long axis** is transverse and its **greater curvature** extends caudally on the floor of the abdomen midway between xiphoid cartilage and the umbilicus. The **left part** is large and rounded while the right part is small and bends sharply dorsally to join the duodenum. The **parietal surface** faces craniad and is related to the diaphragm and the liver. The **visceral surface** faces caudad and is related to the intestine, greater omentum, mesentery and pancreas. Its greater curvature is related to diaphragm, spleen, liver and abdominal floor. The left extremity is ventral to the dorsal part of thirteenth rib and presents a conical blind pouch called the diverticulum. The oesophagus joins the stomach obliquely just to the left of the median plane and about 10 cm ventral to the thirteenth thoracic vertebra. The pyloric end lies against the right lateral lobe of the liver. The mucous membrane is similar to that of the horse and dog.

Fowl

The stomach of the fowl has two parts, the glandular stomach or proventriculus and the muscular stomach or gizzard. The **proventriculus is** an elongated fusiform thick walled tubular organ which lies to the left of the median plane of the thoracoabdominal cavity. It is related laterally and ventrally to the liver and spleen. It is connected cranially to the oesophagus and caudally to the gizzard.

The **gizzard** is a dense, thick walled muscular rounded disc with two **orifices** placed close together on the craniodorsal aspect of its circumference. It is situated caudal to and between the two lobes of the liver. The mucous membrane lining the gizzard is thrown into ridges and is covered by a dense horny substance.

Small intestine

Horse

The small intestine of horse is about 22 meters in length and its diameter varies from 7.5 to 10.0 cm. Its capacity is about 40 to 50 liters.

The **duodenum** is about one meter long. Its shape is somewhat like a horse shoe with the convexity facing to the right side of the abdominal cavity. The first part of the 'S' shaped curve is in contact with the middle (quadrate) and right lobes of the liver. The **pancreatic duct** and the **bile duct** pierce the wall of the duodenum and open into its lumen at this place which is at a distance of about 12 to 15 cm from the pylorus of the stomach. The second (descending) part passes dorsad and caudad on the right dorsal part of the colon and ventral to the right lobe of the liver to the right kidney and caecum and curves mediad to the median line to continue as third part. Here the third part turns to the left, caudal to the base of the caecum, crosses caudal to the root of the great mesentery to continue as the **jejuno -ileac (mesenteric) part.** The **jejunum** lies in numerous coils mingled with those of the small colon in the dorsal part of the left of the abdomen from the visceral surface of stomach to the pelvis and continues as the ileum. The **ileum** is a straight terminal part of the small intestine. It passes to the medial face of the caecum and joins the same at the lesser curvature of its base. The mesenteric lymph glands are present at the root of the mesentery.

The **mucous membrane** of the duodenum forms a pouch called the **hepatopancreatic ampulla** in which the pancreatic and hepatic (bile) ducts open on a small papilla opposite this level is the opening of additional **accessory pancreatic duct**. The **Payer's patches** are formed on the surface opposite to the mesenteric attachment. The **intestinal** and **solitary glands** are present in the mucous membrane throughout the length of the small intestine. The **Brunner's glands (duodenal glands)** are found in the first six to seven meters of its length.

Dog

The small intestine of dog is about 4 meter long. It occupies most of the abdominal cavity caudal to the stomach and liver. The duodenum and jejunum are clearly demarcated while the division into jejunum and ileum is arbitrary.

The **duodenum** begins at the pylorus and passes caudally and somewhat dorsally, at first on the visceral surface of the liver and then in contact with the right flank to the pelvic inlet. Here it turns medially and passes cranially along the medial aspect of the left part of the colon and the left kidney. Here it bends ventrally and joins the jejunum to the left of the root of the mesentery. The remainder of the small intestine (mostly the **jejunum**) forms numerous coils and is attached by wide mesentery to the sublumbar region. The terminal part (**ileum**) passes cranially along the medial face of the caecum and opens into the colon at the ileo-colic orifice. The **bile** and the **small** (minor) **pancreatic** ducts open into the duodenum about 5.0 to 7.5 cm from the pylorus. The **larger** (major) **pancreatic duct** opens about 2.5 to 5.0 cm further caudad.

The **duodenal glands** (Brunner's glands) occur only close to the pylorus. The **Payer's patches** are numerous (about 20 in young dogs). These begin in the duodenum and are elliptical in outline but the last one is band like and reaches to the end of the ileum. It is about 10 to 40 cm in length in young dogs.

Sheep and Goat

The small intestine in sheep and goat has an average length of 25 m and its diameter is about 2 to 3 cm. It is more or less similar to that of ox. The **common bile duct** opens in the second curve of sigmoid flexure of **duodenum** at a distance of about 25 to 40 cm from the pylorus of the stomach. The **pancreatic**

duct joins the bile duct for its opening into the duodenum. The **jejunum** usually lies in the supraomental recess on the right side of the rumen. The **ileum** enters the junction of caecum and colon obliquely on the medial surface. The collateral branch of the **cranial mesenteric artery** supplying blood to the small intestine that appears in ox is absent in sheep and goat.

Pig

The small intestine of pig is about 15 to 20 meter long. It lies mostly to the right of the median plane extending from the visceral surface of the stomach and liver to about the level of the pelvic inlet.

The **duodenum** arises on the right side from the pylorus at about the level of tenth to twelfth intercostal space. Its cranial part turns sharply medially on the visceral surface of the liver to the right of the portal fissure. The descending part passes caudally in relation to the medial part of the right kidney dorsally and the right colon ventrally. At about the middle of the sublumbar region it turns across the median plane and runs cranially to be continued as mesenteric part (**jejuno-ileum**). The **mesenteric part** of small intestine is arranged in close coils and lies mainly dorsal to the colon and caecum. It extends caudally from stomach to the pelvis. In this course many of the coils of small intestine lie against the right flank and on the caudal part of the floor of the abdomen. The **common bile duct** opens into duodenum at a distance of about 2.5 to 5.0 cm from the pylorus. The **pancreatic duct** opens into duodenum at about 10 to 12 cm caudal to the opening of the common bile duct.

The **Payer's patches** and the solitary glands are numerous and very distinct. The Payer's patches are usually band like and prominent. Their number varies from 16 to 38. They begin at about 20 to 50 cm from the pylorus and the last one continues into the caecum but its height is just about a millimeter. The **Brunner's** (duodenal) **glands** occur at about 3 to 5 cm caudal to the pylorus.

Fowl

The small intestine of the fowl is made up of the duodenum, jejunum and the ileum. The **duodenum** is in the form of a loop with a proximal descending and distal ascending parts. The total length of the duodenum is 22 to 35 cm and its diameter is about 0.8 to 1.2 cm. The **descending part** extends caudoventrally from the cranial part of the right surface of the gizzard and then caudal to gizzard it crosses to left side and bends dorsally to join the ascending part. The **ascending part** extends cranially and ventrally, immediately dorsal to the descending part and opposite the cranial part of gizzard it bents dorsally, crosses the cranial mesenteric artery and joins the jejunum ventral to the right kidney. Between the descending and ascending parts of the duodenum lies the pancreas.

The **jejunum** is arranged in the form of close coils at the edge of the long dorsal mesentery. The loops are close to the right abdominal air sac on the right side, to the ovary caeca, ileum, ascending duodenum and pancreas on left side and to the liver on the ventral side. The distal part of jejunum is continuous with the **ileum** in the midline ventral to the rectum and dorsal to the duodenum. The ileum extends from the jejunum cranially dorsal to the ascending duodenum. and opposite the spleen it bends dorsally and caudally and near the seventh lumbosacral vertebra continues as rectum. The junction of these two is joined by the caeca on either side.

The **Meckel's diverticulum** is a short, blind remnant of yolk sac and yolk stalk present on the coil of the jejunum, opposite the distal parts of cranial mesenteric artery and vein. It is usually at the beginning of the distal half of the jejunum. Its length is about 1.25 cm and diameter is about 0.5 cm.

Large intestine

Horse

The large intestine in horse is about 7.5 to 8.0 m in length. It extends from the termination of ileum to anus. The **characteristic features** of the large intestine of horse are its **greater size**, being **sacculated** in most of its part, possessing **longitudinal bands** and having a more **fixed position**.

The **caecum** is about 1.25 m in length and its capacity is about 25 to 30 liters. It is comma shaped and extends from right ileac region through the right lumbar region to the abdominal floor caudal to the xiphoid cartilage. Its both extremities are blind and the ileo-caecal and caeco-colic orifices are placed closed together on the lesser curvature of the base of the caecum. It presents a base, an apex and a body. The **base** is strongly curved. The **body** is related on the right to the abdominal wall, diaphragm, duodenum and liver and on the left to the left and terminal parts of colon and small intestine. The caecum has four **longitudinal bands** situated on the **dorsal, ventral, left and right lateral** surfaces which cause the four rows of sacculations.

The **great colon** begins at the caeco-colic orifice and ends by joining the transverse colon. It is about 3.0 to 3.7 m long and its average diameter is about 20 to 25 cm. Its capacity is more than double that of caecum. It consists of two parallel parts attached by peritoneum and partially by areolar and muscular tissue. In situ, it is kept folded in the abdominal cavity so that it presents **four parts** which are designated according to their position or numerically. Three bent connecting parts are called the flexures.

The **first part** or the **right ventral part** begins at the lesser curvature of the base of the caecum, passes ventrad and craniad along the right costal arch and then along the floor of the abdomen. At the xiphoid cartilage, it bents sharply to the left and caudally and forms the sternal flexure. The **second or** the **left ventral part** passes caudad on the abdominal floor to the left of the first part and caecum, reaches the pelvic inlet and bends to the right and craniad forming the pelvic flexure. The **third** part or **left dorsal part** passes craniad, dorsal to the second part, reaches to the diaphragm and left lobe of the liver, turns to the right and caudad forming the diaphragmatic flexure. The **fourth** or **right dorsal part** passes caudad, dorsal to the first part, reaches the medial face of the base of the caecum, turns to the left and dorsad behind the saccus caecus of the stomach where it becomes short, narrow transverse colon which joins the small colon below the left kidney. The **diameter** of the great colon varies greatly at ite different parts. At the right and right ventral parts it is 5.0 to 7.5 cm, at the right dorsal part it becomes 20 to 25 cm and at left dorsal part it is 7.5 to 10.0 cm. The bands of the colon vary in differently. The ventral parts have four bands, the right dorsa part has three bands and the left dorsal part first has one band and two more bands are added to it later on.

The **transverse colon** is a constricted part of the colon between the great and small colon. It begins opposite the head of the seventeenth or eighteenth thoracic vertebra where it passes from right to left cranial to the root of the mesentery.

The **small colon** begins at the termination of the transverse colon caudal to the saccus caecus of the stomach and ventral to the left kidney and lies in the form of coils in the space between the stomach and pelvic inlet dorsal to the left part of great colon. They are mingled with those of the small intestine from which they can be identified by means of sacculations and the two muscular bands. It is attached to the sublumbar region by the colic mesentery.

The **rectum** is similar to that of the ox but is slightly larger than that of the ox.

Dog

The large intestine of dog is about 60 to 75 cm in length. Its calibre is about the same as that of the small intestine and has neither sacculations nor longitudinal bands.

The **caecum** is about 12.5 to 15.0 cm in length and is flexuous. It opens cranially into the colon. The other end is pointed and blind. It is situated midway between the right flank and median plane below the duodenum.

The **colon** is attached to the sublumbar region by the mesocolon. It has three parts corresponding to the ascending, transverse and descending parts of the colon of man. The **first, right part (ascending)** is very short, passing cranially medial to the first part of duodenum and reaches to the pyloric part of the stomach. Here it turns to the left crossing the median plane and forming the **second, (transverse) part.** The **third, left (descending) part** passes back in the sublumbar region ventral to the left kidney and inclines to the median plane to be continued as rectum.

The **rectum** is completely covered with peritoneum. At the junction of the rectum and anus, the mucous membrane has stratified squamous epithelium and contains the anal glands. A small opening on either side leads into two lateral anal sacs of the size of hazel nut containing a dirty grey fatty substance having a peculiar unpleasant odour.

Sheep and Goat

The large intestine in sheep and goat is more or less uniform in diameter and it measures similar to that of the small intestine. It lies in the supraomental recess with the small intestine. In its gross disposition it is similar to that of ox. The **caecum** in sheep and goat has an average length of about 30 cm and its diameter is about 8 cm. The **colon** has a length of about 4 to 5 m and the diameter is about 2 cm. The **spiral loop of colon** is somewhat hemispherical. It has usually three centripetal and three centrifugal turns. The last gyrus differs from that of ox being more closely related to the jejunum. The **rectum** and **anus** in sheep and goat has no differences in comparison with the ox.

Pig

The large intestine in pig is about 4.0 to 4.5 m in length and is for the most part wider than the small intestine. It is connected by a mesentery with the dorsal abdominal wall between the kidneys.

The **caecum** is cylindrical, about 20 to30 cm long and 8 to 10 cm wide. It lies against the dorsal and cranial part of the left flank and extends ventrally, caudally and medially caudal to the coiled part of the colon. Its ventral blind end lies on the floor of the abdomen near the median plane and at a variable point between the umbilicus and the pelvic inlet. Its dorsal end continues with the colon and the line of demarcation between the two is indicated by the termination of small intestine. It has three muscular bands and three rows of sacculations.

The **colon** has initially the same diameter as that of the caecum but gradually becomes smaller than the caecum. It lies chiefly to the left of the median plane caudal to the stomach. The ascending colon is arranged in three close double spiral coils in the mesentery. It is related ventrally to the abdominal floor, cranially to the stomach and liver, caudally to caecum and small intestine and medially on right side to the small intestine. On emerging from the spiral, it passes first cranially in the sublumbar region to the right of the median plane and on reaching to the stomach and pancreas, turns to the left as transverse colon. It then passes caudally to the pelvic inlet and is continued as the rectum. The ascending colon has two bands and two rows of sacculations.

The **rectum** is the continuation of the descending colon. It is usually surrounded by large amount of fat. The **anus** is short.

Fowl

The large intestine of fowl consists of a pair of caeca, a colon and a cloaca. The line of demarcation between the ileum and colon is at the opening of the caeca. The **colon** is short and straight, leading from ileum to the cloaca. The short villi project into the lumen of colon. The **caeca** are two blind sacs about seven inches long. They empty into the intestine at the junction of ileum and colon, Its mucosal surface is covered by villi.

The **cloaca** is a tubular structure. It is the terminal part of the gut and it opens to the exterior. It is a common opening for the digestive, urinary and genital systems. It has three parts, the coprodeum, urodeum and proctodeum. The **coprodeum** is the cranial part in which the colon empties. The **urodeum** is the middle part into which the urinary and genital ducts open. The **proctodeum** is the caudal most part which opens to the exterior. The dorsal wall of this part presents an opening for the duct of the **bursa of fabricius** which is a blind sac like lymphoid nodule situated dorsal to the cloaca. It is best developed in the birds of about four months of age and usually disappears at the age of about one year.

Liver

Horse

The liver of horse is larger than that of ox. It extends from the right hypochondriac through epigastric to the left hypochondriac region in a sloping direction from right to left side of the median plane. Its **dorsal border** presents from right to the left side the attachment of right lateral ligament, renal impression, fossa vena cava, oesophageal notch and the attachment of left lateral ligament. The **ventral border** presents two fissures dividing the liver into three main lobes, the **right, middle** and the **left lobe**. The middle lobe is divided by secondary fissure into two small divisions. The **right lobe** is larger and it presents at its dorsal part the caudate lobe and the caudate process. The **middle lobe** is smallest and presents the umbilical fissure and the round ligament. The **left lobe** is smaller than the right and larger than the right lobe, especially in young subjects. The right border is thin and the left border is convex. The latter begins at the oesophageal notch.

The **parietal surface** is convex and presents a median vertical fissure, the fossa vena cava. The **visceral surface** is concave and presents the portal fissure above its middle. The extensive concave area in front of the portal fissure is the gastric impression and that behind it is the colic impression formed by the diaphragmatic flexure of the great colon. The **gall bladder** is absent in horse. The **hepatic duct** opens into the duodenum at a distance of about 12.5 to 15 cm from the pylorus.

In addition to the ligaments of liver in ox, there are two more ligaments in horse. These are the left lateral ligament that attaches the left lobe to the tendinous centre of the diaphragm and the coronary ligaments on either side of the caudal vena cava which unite below to form the falciform ligament.

Dog

The liver in dog has five chief lobes. The **left lateral lobe** is the largest and oval. The **left central lobe** is prismatic, the **right central lobe** is second in size and it presents a tongue shaped quadrate lobe which is separated from the chief lobe by a fissure that lodges gallbladder in it. The **right lateral lobe** is third in size and is oval. On its visceral surface is the **caudate lobe** made by the caudate process on the right and the papillary process on the left.

The **parietal surface** of liver is convex and is related to the diaphragm and the adjacent part of the ventral wall of the abdomen. The **visceral surface** is concave and presents the larger gastric impression on the left lateral lobe. The **portal fissure** is between the caudate and papillary lobes. The **dorsal border** presents a deep renal impression for the right kidney. The caudal vena cava passes in a deep groove on the caudate lobe and then on the parietal surface of the right lateral lobe. The oesophageal notch is large. The **ventral border** lies on the floor of the abdomen at variable distance from the xiphoid cartilage. The gallbladder lies between the two parts of the right central lobe.

Sheep and Goat

The liver in sheep and goat is almost similar to that in ox. It weighs about 550 to 700 gm. The gallbladder fossa extending from portal fissure to the ventral border of the liver is more distinct in sheep and goat than that in the ox. The fissure for the round ligament extending transversely across the visceral surface is well distinct as compared to that in ox. The omasal impression on the visceral surface is smaller in sheep and goat than that in ox. The lobation is more distinct in sheep and goat than that in ox.

Pig

The liver in pig is relatively large. Its average weight is 1.5 to 2.0 kg. It is thick in the centre and thin at the periphery. It is divided into four lobes by three fissures. The **lobes** are **right lateral**, **right central, left central** and **the left lateral**. The **caudate lobe** is at the dorsal part of the right lateral lobe and it is distinctly marked off by a fissure and often subdivided by secondary fissure. The **papillary process** is absent. The **quadrate lobe** lies ventral to the portal fissure and to the left of the gallbladder and cystic duct. The **parietal surface** is convex and is related to diaphragm. The **visceral surface** has a prominent impression of the stomach. A small part of this surface is related to abdominal floor in xiphoid region. The **coronary** and **round ligaments** are similar to those in other species and the falciform ligament is usually absent and if present is very short. The gallbladder is present. The **hepatic** and **cystic ducts** join to form the **bile duct.**

Fowl

The liver in fowl lies in the ventral part of the body cavity. It is suspended by peritoneum in the right and left dorsal and ventral hepatic and coelomic cavities. It has the left and right lobes which join cranially in the midline. The **left lobe** is prism shaped and it is smaller than the right lobe. It is divided by a fissure into caudodorsal and caudoventral parts. It extends from third thoracic to fourth lumbosacral level. The **right lobe** is heart shaped and it extends from third thoracic and fifth lumbosacral level.

The **parietal surface** is smooth and convex. It is close to the ventral and lateral body walls and the thoracic air sacs. The **visceral surface** is irregularly concave and is in contact with oesophagus, glandular stomach, spleen, jejunum and duodenum. The caudal vena cava passes through the cranial part of right lobe close to the dorsal border. The **gallbladder** lies on the visceral surface of the right lobe.

The **hepato-cystic duct** extends from the right lobe to the gallbladder from where the **cystic duct** passes to the termination of the duodenum. The left lobe is drained by the **hepato-enteric duct** which opens directly into the duodenum close to the opening of the cystic duct.

Pancreas

Horse

The pancreas in horse is situated transversely in the dorsal aspect of the abdominal cavity. Its greater part lies to the right of the median plane and the central part is ventral to the seventeenth thoracic vertebra. The gland is triangular in outline. The **dorsal surface** faces dorsally and cranially. It is related to the liver, right kidney, caudal vena cava, portal vein, celiac artery, gastrophrenic ligament and the saccus caecus of the stomach, right and caudate lobe of the liver and the gastropancreatic fold of the peritoneum. The **ventral surface** faces ventrally and caudally. It is related to the caecum, great colon and small colon. The right border is nearly straight and is related to the descending part of the duodenum. The **left border** is slightly concave and is related to the cranial part of the duodenum, the left sac of the stomach and the splenic vessels. The **caudal border** is related to the caudal vena cava. The **duodenal angle** is attached to the concavity of the second curve of the duodenum. The pancreatic duct leaves the gland at this angle. The **left** or the **splenic angle** fits into the space between the saccus caecus of stomach cranially, the left kidney caudally, the spleen dorsally and great colon ventrally. **The right angle** is rounded and lies at the central face of the right kidney. There are two ducts, the larger one is the major duct and is named as pancreatic duct while the smaller one is a minor duct and is named as accessory duct. The **pancreatic duct** opens along with the bile duct in the diverticulum of the duodenal mucous membrane about 15 cm from the pylorus while the **accessory duct** opens into the duodenum on a papilla opposite to the opening of the pancreatic duct.

Dog

The pancreas in dog is 'V' shaped consisting of two lobes meeting at an acute angle caudal to the pylorus. The **right lobe** extends caudad above the first part of the duodenum and ends at a short distance caudal to the right kidney. The **left lobe** passes to the left and caudally between the visceral surface of stomach and the transverse colon and ends at the cranial pole of the left kidney. There are two ducts. The **smaller duct** opens into the duodenum with the common bile duct or close to it. The **larger duct** opens into the duodenum about 3 to 5 cm caudal to the opening of the smaller duct.

Sheep and Goat

The pancreas in sheep and goat is almost similar to that in ox. It weighs about 50 to 70 gm. In sheep and goat there is only one pancreatic duct as against the occurrence of two ducts (including accessory duct) in ox.

Pig

The pancreas in pig extends across the dorsal wall of the abdominal cavity caudal to the stomach. It is triangular in shape. The **right lobe** is attached to the first curve of the duodenum. The **left lobe** is related to the left extremity of the stomach, the dorsal end of the spleen and the cranial pole of the left kidney.

The **middle portion** is related to the portal vein and root of the mesentery. The **pancreatic duct** passes from the right lobe and opens into the first curve of the duodenum at about a distance of 10 to 12 cm from the pylorus.

Fowl

The pancreas in fowl is a long narrow lobulated gland which is situated in a space between the two (ascending and descending) parts of the duodenum. The **lobes** are **dorsal, ventral and splenic.** The splenic lobe is shorter than the other two lobes. The gland has two or three **ducts** that extend from the dorsal and ventral lobes. The splenic lobe has no separate duct. The pancreatic duct opens into the ascending part of the duodenum close to the opening of the hepatic duct.

Spleen

Horse

The spleen in horse is bluish red in colour. It is situated in the left hypochondriac region in close relation with the left part of the greater curvature of the stomach. It is scythe shaped and weighs about 1 kg. Its length is about 50 cm and width about 20 to 25 cm. Its **parietal surface** is convex and is related to diaphragm. The **visceral surface** is concave and presents a **ridge** which divides this surface into two unequal areas. The **hilus** is on a groove situated on the ridge. The area cranial to the ridge is **gastric impression** and that caudal to the ridge is the **colic impression** caused by the left part of the colon. The **caudal border** is convex. The **base** is beveled and presents the renal impression.

Dog

The spleen in dog is bright red in colour. It is somewhat falciform, long and narrow and its ventral part is widest. It weighs about 50 gm in a medium sized dog. Its **dorsal end** is narrow and is ventral to the vertebral end of last rib and first lumbar transverse process. The **ventral end** is wider and variable in position. The **parietal surface** is convex and lies largely against the left flank. The **visceral surface** is concave in its length and is marked by a longitudinal ridge to which the greater omentum is attached.

Sheep and Goat

The spleen in sheep and goat is triangular in shape with the angles rounded off. It weighs about 100 gm. Its length is about 12 to 15 cm and width about 7.5 to 10.0 cm. Its long axis is oblique and corresponds to a line drawn from the vertebral end of the last rib to about the middle of the tenth intercostal space. The **parietal surface** is convex and is related to diaphragm. In hardened specimens it shows the impressions of the last three ribs. The **visceral surface** is concave and its cranial half is attached to the dorsal curvature of the rumen. The borders are thin. The **dorsal end** or **base** is attached to the left crus of diaphragm under the last two ribs. The **hilus** is on the visceral surface close to the cranial angle. The **ventral end** is narrower and thinner than the base. It is situated opposite the tenth intercostal space.

Pig

The spleen of the pig is long and narrow. Its long axis is nearly dorsoventral in direction and corresponds to the left part of the greater curvature of the stomach. The **dorsal end** lies under the vertebral end of last three ribs. It is related cranially to the stomach, caudally to left kidney and medially to the left extremity of the pancreas. The **visceral surface** has the longitudinal ridge which divides the surface into two nearly equal areas. The cranial one is the gastric area and the caudal one is the intestinal (colic) area. The **hilus** is situated on the ridge on the visceral surface. The **parietal surface** is convex and is related to the left lateral and ventral wall of the abdomen. The **ventral end** is smaller than the dorsal end. It lies in the umbilical region on the abdominal floor. The spleen is attached very loosely to the stomach.

Fowl

The spleen in fowl is reddish brown in colour. It is a rounded body situated dorsally and to the right of the junction of proventriculus and gizzard. It weighs about 3.0 gm in female and about 4.5 gm in males. Its diameter is about 1.5 cm.

63

Urinary Organs

The urinary organs include the kidneys, ureters, bladder and urethra (Fig. 4-5 A).

Kidneys

The kidneys are two compound tubular glands situated retroperitoneally in the sublumbar region. They are elongated, the right kidney being elliptical in outline and the left one slightly oval. They are red brown in colour. The weight of each kidney varies from 500 to 700 gm, the left kidney being about 25 gm heavier than the right kidney. The outer surface of the bovine kidneys is marked by polygonal lobes which are about twenty in number and are separated from each other by deep grooves (fissures). The grooves are filled in by fat. Both the kidneys are embedded in a large amount of perirenal fat termed as adipose capsule.

The **right kidney** is flattened dorsoventrally. It is 15 to 17 cm long, 8.5 to 10 cm wide and 5 cm thick. It lies ventral to the last rib and first two or three lumbar transverse processes. The dorsal surface is rounded and nearly convex. It is related to sublumbar muscles. The ventral surface is less convex and is related to the liver, pancreas, duodenum and colon. The hilus is situated at the cranial part of this surface near the medial border. The medial border is nearly straight and lies parallel to the caudal vena cava. The lateral border is convex. The cranial extremity is thick. It lies in the renal impression of the liver and is capped by the adrenal. The caudal extremity is narrow and pointed.

The **left kidney** is three sided. It is about 13 to17 cm long, 7.5 to 8.5 cm wide and 5.5 to 7.5 cm thick. It is variable in position. The position of the left kidney of ox depends on the state of fullness of the rumen. When the rumen is full, it pushes the left kidney caudally and across the median plane, so that it is situated on the right side, caudal and a little ventral to the right kidney. It then lies ventral to the third, fourth and fifth lumbar vertebrae. When the rumen is not so full, the left kidney may lie partly to the left of the median plane. The left kidney has three surfaces. The dorsal surface is convex and presents on its craniolateral

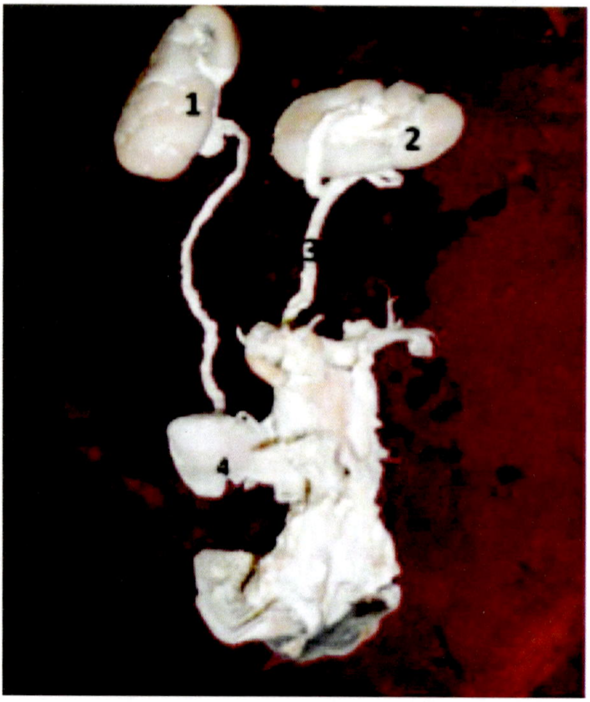

Fig. 4 – 5 A: Urinary organs of cow
1. Left kidney 2. Right kidney 3. Ureter 4. Urinary bladder

part the hilus, which opens laterally. The ventral surface is nearly flat and is related to the intestine. The third face, the ruminal surface, is more or less flattened and lies in contact with the rumen. The cranial extremity is small and narrow and the caudal extremity is large and rounded. At the hilus, the renal artery is dorsal, the renal vein in the middle and the ureter is ventral to it. A thick layer of fat surrounds these structures in the hilus.

Structure: The kidneys are covered by a strong capsule of fibrous tissue. A circumferential section of the kidney revels that it is made up of a reddish brown layer, the **cortex** and an internal paler part, the **medulla**. The cortex presents a granular appearance and is studded with numerous minute dark structures, the renal or **Malpighian corpuscles,** which are the dilated origins of renal tubules containing the tuft of capillaries called the **glomerulus.** The medulla is pale and presents at its junction with the cortex an intermediate vascular zone. It is in the form of pyramids which are called as **renal pyramids**, about twenty in number, with their bases directed towards the cortex. Between the pyramids, a part of the cortex deeps inwards forming the renal columns named as **columns of Bertini**. Each renal pyramid present radially striated appearance, the medullary rays and presents at its apex the renal papilla. Each

renal papilla is enclosed or embraced by the funnel shaped end of a tube, the **calyx major**. Two such calyces major from the two extremities unite at the hilus to form the excretory duct, the **ureter.**

Ureters

The ureters are the excretory ducts of the kidneys. Each ureter begins at the junction of the calyces majores and terminates at the bladder. It is about 25 mm in diameter. The right ureter emerges out of the hilus of the right kidney on its ventral surface, runs mediad, gains the medial border of the kidney and runs along it. The left ureter emerges out of the hilus of the left kidney on the craniolateral aspect of the dorsal surface of the left kidney, crosses over this face medially gains its medial border and runs caudally.

Each ureter consists of abdominal and pelvic parts. The abdominal part runs caudad and mediad, the right ureter being related to the medial face of the caudal vena cava and the left one to the aorta, passes back in the sub-peritoneal tissue on the ventral surface of the psoas major and psoas minor muscles, crosses the internal iliac artery and enters the pelvic cavity. The pelvic part passes caudad and ventrad on the lateral wall of the pelvic cavity, turns mediad and pierces the dorsal wall of the bladder near its neck. In the male, the pelvic part of the ureter enters the genital fold and crosses vas deferens and in the female, it is situated in the dorsal part of the broad ligament.

Urinary bladder

The urinary bladder is a musculomembranous sac which differs in form, size and position according to the amount (volume) of its contents, the urine. When contracted and empty, it is a dense piriform mass of about the size of a fist and lies on the floor of the pelvic cavity. When moderately full, it is oval in shape and extends a variable distance on the floor of the abdominal cavity. Its capacity ranges from 2.8 to 3.8 liters. It has three parts. The cranial rounded blind end is termed as the **apex** or **vertex**. On the middle of the vertex is a mass of cicatricial tissue, a vestige of the urachus which in foetus forms a tubular connection between the bladder and the allantois. The middle part or **body** is rounded and somewhat flattened dorsoventrally except when distended. It presents two surfaces, the dorsal and ventral which are convex when full, the dorsal surface being more strongly convex than the ventral surface especially in its caudal part cranial to the entrance of the ureters. The caudal narrow part is the **neck** and it joins the urethra.

The relations of the bladder vary according to the degree of fullness of the organ and the sex of the animal. The **ventral surface** lies on the ventral wall of the pelvis and extends over the ventral wall of the abdomen when the bladder distends due to fullness. The **dorsal surface** in the male is related to the rectum, the genital fold, the terminal parts of ductus deferens, the seminal vesicles and the prostate. In the female, it is related to the body of the uterus and the vagina. When bladder is full the vertex reaches to the rumen and the small intestine.

Ligaments: The bladder is fixed or held in position with the help of three peritoneal folds which are called the middle and lateral ligaments of the bladder. The **middle ligament** is the median ventral triangular fold of peritoneum that extends from the ventral surface of the bladder to the ventral wall (floor) of the pelvis and abdomen. The **lateral ligaments** extend transversely from the lateral aspect of the bladder to the lateral wall of the pelvis. Each contains in it a round cord named as **round ligament**, the remnant of the foetal umbilical artery. The caudal part of the bladder is devoid of peritoneal covering and is called the **retroperitoneal part**. It is attached to the surrounding parts by fat and connective tissue.

Structure: The wall of the uterus has the outer **serous coat** (in the cranial part only), the middle **muscular coat** and the inner coat of **mucous membrane**. The mucous membrane is pale and thin and is loosely attached to the submucous tissue. It is modified over a triangular area on its caudodorsal aspect which is called the **trigonum vesicae** where the mucous membrane is firmly attached without any folds. The two cranial angles of this space present the openings of the two ureters and the caudal central angle presents the opening of the bladder into the urethra. This opening is termed as **internal urethral orifice.**

Urethra

The urethra is a mucous tube that extends caudally from the internal urethral orifice at the neck of the bladder. In its further course it shows distinct sex differences.

In the **female**, it begins at the internal urethral orifice at the neck of the urinary bladder and terminates by opening into the external urethral orifice situated in the cranial part of the floor of the vaginal vestibule. The urethra is situated centrally on the pelvic floor. It is about 10 cm long and the diameter of its lumen is about 25 mm and is remarkably dilatable. The striated urethral muscle surrounds almost the full length of the tube. It is related ventrally to the pelvic floor and dorsally to the wall of the vagina with which it appears to be fused.

In the **male,** the urethra has the pelvic part and the extra pelvic part. The **pelvic part** is about 10 cm long and its diameter is almost equal to that of the female urethra. It is surrounded by **pars disseminata** of the prostate gland. Outside this gland, the urethra is enclosed by thick **urethral muscle** and the aponeurosis. **The aponeurosis** is dorsal and the muscle is lateral and ventral to the urethra. It is related dorsally to the rectum and prostate, ventrally to the obturator muscle and laterally to the seminal vesicles or the Cowper's glands. The internal surface of the cranial half of the pelvic part of the urethra presents on its dorsal wall a rounded and elongated prominence, the **colliculus seminalis**. About 5 cm behind the internal urethral orifice and on either side of it are the two openings of the vasa deferentia and vesiculae seminalis. A little lateral and caudal to the colliculus are the openings of the ducts of the prostate and behind these the ducts of Cowper's glands. Behind this, the pelvic part of urethra continues as extra pelvic part.

The **extra pelvic (penile) part** of the male urethra passes between the two crura penis turns cranially around the ischial arch and is included in the body of the penis. Its further course is described with the course and structure of penis as male genital organ.

Adrenal glands

The adrenal glands are the **endocrine glands** related to kidneys. The right and left adrenals differ in shape, location and relations.

The **right adrenal** is located between the cranial extremity of the right kidney and the caudal vena cava and partly it lies into the renal fossa of the liver. It is roughly 'V' shaped or pyramidal in shape with its **base** cranial in position and in contact with the liver. The **apex** is pointed and it lies in the angle between the caudal vena cava and the dorsal border of the liver. Its flat, triangular **medial surface** is adhered to the caudal vena cava and it lies in close opposition with the right crus of the diaphragm. In the area of adhesion, the adrenal vein opens into the vena cava. The **lateral surface** is also triangular but concave in shape and is in contact with the right kidney. The **ventral surface** is triangular and uneven and is in contact with the pancreas. It presents a groove for the passage of caudal vena cava. The right adrenal in cattle measures about 8 cm in length, 3 cm in breadth and 2 cm in thickness. It weighs about 12 to 13 gm in adult cattle.

The **left adrenal** is located approximately on the midline cranial to left kidney and caudal to the cranial mesenteric artery on the medial face of the caudal vena cava. It is flat, triangular and roughly 'C' shaped with a deep notch in the caudal border. Its **lateral surface** is slightly convex and is related to the visceral surface of the dorsal sac of the rumen. The **medial surface** is flat and it is related to the caudal vena cava. The left adrenal in adult cattle measures about 8 cm in length, 6 cm in breadth and 3 cm in thickness. The gland weighs about 14.5 gm.

Structure: The **fibrous capsule** of the gland is closely fitted and adhered to it. The **parenchyma** of the gland has the outer part, the cortex and the inner one, the medulla. The **cortex** forms a peripheral layer and sends trabeculae into medullary portion. The **medulla** forms the central part of the gland and has yellowish colour.

The **adrenal arteries** two for each gland arise from the renal artery and the aorta. The short **vein** leaves the deep notch of the gland in the area of adhesion and immediately enters the renal vein on the left and caudal vena cava on the right. Rich **nerve supply** to the adrenals is from the **splanchnic nerves** and the **coeliacomesenteric plexus**.

64

Comparative Anatomy of Urinary Organs

Horse

The kidneys of horse slightly differ in form and size than those of ox. The outer surfaces of kidneys of horse are smooth and plane as against lobulated kidneys of ox. The right **kidney** is like the heart of the plying cards while left kidney is bean shaped. The **right kidney** is placed under the vertebral ends of the last two ribs and first lumbar transverse process. The **left kidney** is situated under the last rib and the first two or three lumbar transverse processes. The hilus of both the kidneys is at about the middle of the medial border of the respective kidneys. The cranial extremity of the right kidney is thicker while the caudal extremity of the left kidney is wider and thicker. The **hilus** of the kidneys lead into the renal sinus in the interior for the lodgment of the renal pelvis which is the dilated origin of the ureter. The inner central part of the medulla forms a concave ridge called the renal crest. It presents numerous openings through which the large ducts open into the renal pelvis. This part is called the area cribrosa.

The ureter of the horse kidney begins at the renal pelvis and is about 70 cm in length and 6 to 8 mm in diameter.

The **urinary bladder** of horse is shorter but wider than that of the ox. Its capacity is about 2.8 to 3.8 liters. The rest of the features are same as those of ox.

The **female urethra** is about 5.0 to 7.5 cm long and about 1.5 cm in diameter. It is remarkably dilatable. The **pelvic part of the male urethra** is about 10 to 12 cm long and 1.5 to 2.0 cm in diameter. The **extrapelvic or penile part** of male urethra is almost of the same diameter as that of the pelvic part. The **colliculus seminalis** presents on either side a common ejaculatory orifice. Behind this are the openings of the prostate and further back are the openings of the ducts of Cowper's glands.

Dog

The **kidneys** of the dog are smooth and bean shaped. In a medium sized dog the weight of each kidney is about 50 to 60 gm. The left kidney is usually heavier than the right kidney. The right kidney is situated under the bodies of the first three lumbar vertebrae. The left kidney is under the second, third and fourth lumbar vertebrae. When the stomach is full, the left kidney is pushed to the level of third to fifth lumbar vertebra, so that the cranial pole of left kidney lies behind the caudal pole of the right kidney. The hilus is at the middle of the medial border of each kidney. The medulla of the kidney presents the renal crest.

The **ureters** are about 12 to 16 cm long, the right ureter being slightly longer than the left one because of the more cranial position of the right kidney.

The **urinary bladder** when full is abdominal in position and in this situation, its neck lies at the cranial border of the pubic bones. In the distended condition of the bladder, its vertex reaches to the umbilicus and when empty it is entirely in the pelvic cavity. It is not covered by the greater omentum. It is about 3.5 to 4.0 cm in length and its diameter is about 2.5 to 3.0 cm. It has a capacity of about 150 to 180 ml in average sized dog.

The **female urethra** is, about 2.5 to 3.0 cm in length. It is marked on the floor of the vagina as longitudinal swelling reaching to the vestibule. The **pelvic part of the male urethra** is relatively long.

Sheep and Goat

The **kidneys** of sheep and goat are bean shaped and smooth and the lobation on the external surface is shallow and superficial. Both the kidneys are elliptical in shape. The dorsal and ventral surfaces are convex and the cranial and caudal extremities are rounded. The length of each kidney is about 7.5 cm, width about 5 cm and thickness about 3 cm. Its average weight is about 100 to 125 gm. The kidneys of goat are, however, narrower than those of the sheep. The right kidney lies ventral to the first three lumbar transverse processes. The position of the left kidney varies with the fullness of the rumen and is similar to that in ox. The hilus of each kidney is in the middle of the medial border and it is deeper in sheep than in goat.

The ureters and the **urinary bladder** in sheep and goat have no differences from those of ox.

The **female urethra** in ewe is about 4 to 5 cm long and in goat it is about 5 to 6 cm. It is narrower and much more dilatable than in cow. The rest of the features of **female** and **male urethra** in sheep and goat are almost similar to those in ox.

Pig

The **kidneys** of pig are smooth and bean shaped. They are more flattened dorsally, more elongated and smaller at the extremities than those of dog. Both, the right and left, kidneys are symmetrical in position and are placed ventral to the first four lumbar transverse processes. The left kidney, in some cases, may be a little cranial in position. The right kidney is usually separated from the visceral surface of the liver by a space of about 2.5 cm. Each kidney is about 12.5 cm long and about 6.0 to 6.5 cm wide. Its weight is about 200 to 250 gm.

The **ureters** of the pig have a special feature with regards to its course and calibre. It is relatively wide in the initial course and then gradually diminishes in calibre in the rest of the course so that at its termination (opening) into the bladder it is quite narrow. In its initial course, the ureter is slightly flexuous and it leaves the kidney in a sharp caudal curve.

The **urinary bladder** in pig is relatively very large when full. It lies chiefly in the abdominal cavity. Its dorsal surface is almost completely covered with peritoneum but ventrally it is little short of its length.

The **female urethra** is about 7 to 8 cm long. Its caudal part is fused with the vagina and produces a corresponding elevation on the floor of the vaginal vestibule. The **male urethra** has a very long pelvic part, about 15 to 20 cm long in adult animals. The penile part is of small calibre and is surrounded by erectile tissue similar to that in other species. However, in pig it does not reach to the extremity of the penis.

Fowl

The **kidneys** of fowl are long, elongated and lobed. Each kidney has four lobes on its external surface and is dark red in colour. The right and left kidneys in fowl are symmetrical in poison. These are placed on either side of the vertebral column in contact with the pelvis and synsacrum dorsally. The cranial extremity reaches to the lungs and the caudal extremity nearly to the caudal end of the synsacrum. The length of each kidney is about 7 cm and width is about 2 cm. Each kidney is divided into three divisions by deep grooves which are occupied by the vessels and nerves.

The **ureter** in fowl arises on the cranial part of the ventral surface of the kidney. It runs caudally in relation to the vas deferens or oviduct and opens into the cloaca medial to the opening of the vas deferens or oviduct. The length of the ureter is about 5 cm and its diameter is about 2 mm.

The **urinary bladder** is absent in the fowl. The ureters open immediately dorsal to the genital opening into the dorsal region of the urodeum of the cloaca. Hence the **urethra** is absent.

65

Female Genital Organs

The female genital organs (Fig. 4-6 A) comprise the ovaries where the female gametes (ova) are produced, the uterine (fallopian) tubes which convey the ova to the uterus and where the fertilization takes place, the uterus in which the ovum and the embryo develops, the dilatable passage formed by the vagina and vulva through which the foetus is expelled to the exterior and the mammary glands (udder) which is functionally associated with the female genital organs. All of these except the mammary glands are located in the abdominal and pelvic cavity while the mammary glands are located outside the cavity in the perineal region.

Ovaries

The ovaries are two small oval glands measuring about 3.5 to 4.0 cm in length, 2.5 cm in width and about 1.5 cm in thickness and they weigh about 15 to 20 gm. They are oval in form and are situated a little above the middle of the pelvic inlet and approximately 40 to 45 cm cranial to vulvar opening in a middle sized cow. They are attached to the sublumbar region by the cranial part of the broad ligament of uterus, the **mesovarium.** Each ovary presents for description two surfaces, two borders and two extremities. The **medial** and the **lateral surfaces** of the ovary are smooth and rounded. The **attached** or **mesovarial border** is convex. It is enclosed in a part of the broad ligament termed as mesovarium. The vessels and nerves reach the ovary by way of mesovarium to this border and enter the gland through the hilus. The **free border** which is also convex presents a notch in its middle. The ovarian vessels and nerves enter the gland through this notch. The **cranial or tubal extremity** is rounded and is related to the fimbriated end of the uterine tube. The **caudal or uterine extremity** is also round but narrower and is connected to the horn of the uterus by the ovarian ligament.

Structure: The peritoneal covering is absent except at a narrow zone along the attached border. The greater part of the surface of the ovary is covered with **germinal epithelium**. The substance of the gland is divided into an outer **cortex**

and the inner **medulla**. The stroma of the cortex is a network of connective tissue. In the meshes of the stroma there are numerous **ovisacs** containing **oocytes.** The immature oocytes are surrounded by follicle cells, those in the advanced stage of development are enclosed by several layers of follicle cells forming the stratum granulosum. The **follicles** of various sizes project on the surface of the ovary.

In the process of development, some of the follicles become **thica folliculi** by the condensation of the stroma. Within the thica folliculi is the fluid called **liquor folliculi**. In the most advanced stage, a few oocytes are covered by a hip of follicle cells and become the **Graafian follicles**. As the Graafian follicles mature, they enlarge and become visible as vesicles of a diameter of about a centimeter or more on the surface of the ovary. At a definite interval the matured Graafian follicles rupture and their contents escape in the process of **ovulation.** After rupture, the cavity of the Graafian follicle is partly filled in by a blood clot. As a result of fatty changes, proliferation and enlargement, the follicle cells are transformed into **lutin cells** and a yellow mass called the **corpus luteum** is formed. During this period, if impregnation of the fertilized ovum takes place, the corpus luteum reaches to its maximum size and it projects on the surface of the ovary. If the impregnation does not occur the site of the ruptured follicle transforms into a **scar tissue** forming the **corpus albicans**.

Uterine tubes

The **uterine tubes**, **oviducts** or **fallopian tubes** are two long flexuous ducts of the ovary. They are not in direct continuity with the gland but are partly attached to them. Each of these is about 30 cm long. It begins as a funnel shaped dilatation called the **infundibulum** adjacent to the ovary and follows a course over a pouch formed by a folding called the **mesosalpinx** over the free edge of the broad ligament which envelopes the ovary. The free border of the infundibulum bears a number of small projections which are called the **fimbriae.** The fimbriae are attached to the free margin of the pouch formed by the mesosalpinx. The portion of the tube leading from the infundibulum is the ampullae and has a diameter larger than that of the rest of the tube. The other end of the tube joins the uterine horn without visible demarcation.

Structure: The uterine tube is covered externally by a **serous coat** formed by the mesosalpinx. The serous membrane is continued on the fimbriae and meets the mucous membrane lining them internally. The **tunica adventitia**, a **fibrous tunic**, continues with the fibrous lamina of the broad ligament. The **muscular coat** contains the outer longitudinal and inner circular strands of the muscle. The **mucous coat** is thin and consists of a single layer of ciliated columnar epithelium.

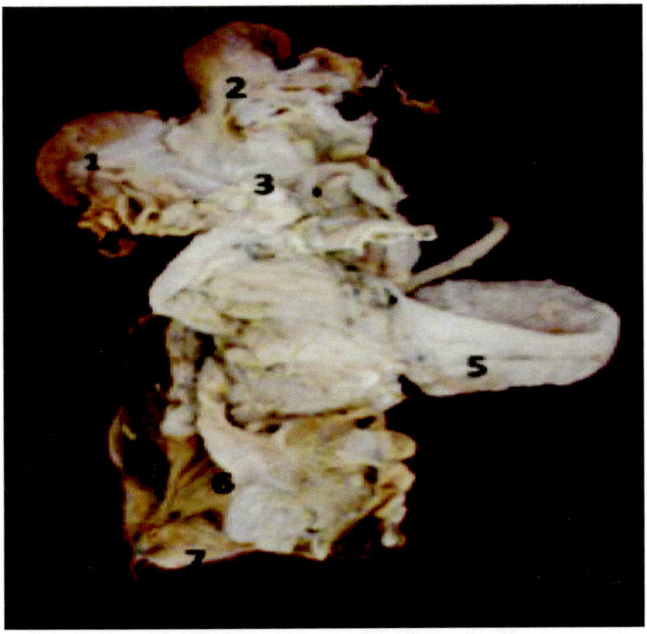

Fig. 4 – 6 A: Genital organs of cow
1. Left horn of uterus 2. Right horn of uterus3. Body of uterus 4. Ovary 5. Urinary bladder 6. Vagina 7. Vulval lip.

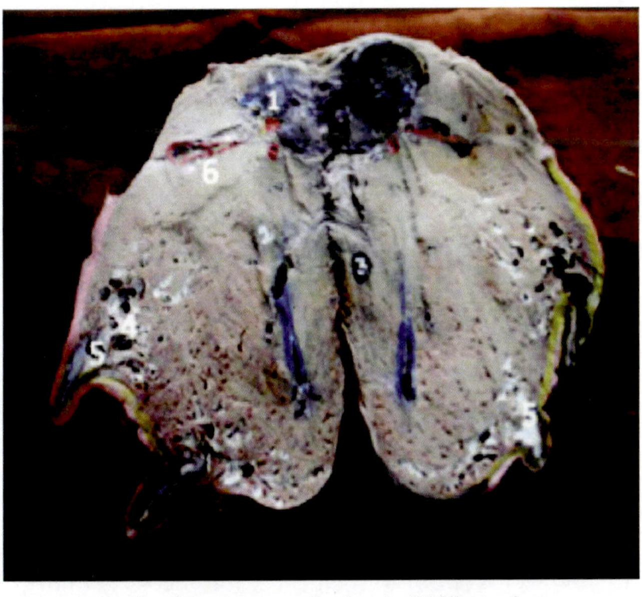

Fig.4 – 6 B: Mammary glands (Udder) of cow
1. Supramammary fat 2. Body 3. Interglandular septum 4. Lactiferous sinus 5. Teat cistern 6. Mammary vessels

The **blood supply** is through the ovarian arteries and the veins are the satellites of these arteries. The lymph vessels from the uterine duct join the lumbar lymph nodes. The **nerve supply** is through the ovarian plexus.

Uterus

The uterus is a hollow musculomembranous organ which is continuous with the uterine tubes cranially and opens into the vagina caudally. It is located entirely into the caudal part of the abdomen. It is attached to the sublumbar region and the lateral walls of the pelvic cavity by two folds of peritoneum which are called as broad ligaments. It consists of a body, the paired horns or cornua and a cervix.

The **body** of the uterus is about 3 to 4 cm long but externally it appears to be about 12 to 15 cm long i.e. longer than its actual length. This is because the two horns of the uterus which extend craniolaterally from the body are united for a short distance from it by connective and muscular tissue and this part of the horns is covered by a common peritoneal covering with the body of the uterus. The body of the uterus is cylindrical and is related to the rectum dorsally and urinary bladder ventrally. The **horns** are about 35 to 40 cm in length but appear to be shorter than this for the reasons stated above. They have uniform diameter through most of their length but the terminal 8 to 10 cm part tappers to the junction with the uterine tube. From the body, the horns are directed craniad and laterad, then they turn ventrad and mediad forming a close spiral which is maintained by the broad ligament. The bases of the horns are closely united as they leave the body and they diverge from each other. The divergence is dorsally marked by **intercornual groove** which increases in depth cranially. The dorsal and ventral short peritoneal folds between the horns are the **intercornual ligaments**. The **cervix** or the neck of the uterus is between the uterine body and the vagina. It lies on the cranial part of the pelvic floor. It measures about 10 cm in length and is remarkably firm and dense. Its external diameter is equal to that of the body but the lumen is considerably smaller than that of the body of the uterus. This is as a result of its excessively thick and firm wall. The thickness of the wall is about 3 cm. The part of the muscle of the wall forms four annular folds or rings which are arranged eccentrically. The **lumen** of the cervix is called the **cervical canal**. It is a passage through the cervix. The direction of this passage is spiral due to the eccentric arrangement of the rings. The vaginal end of the cervix is so fused externally with the vagina that about 2 to 3 cm or more deep recess, the **fornix** is formed dorsally between the cervix and the vaginal wall. However, ventral to the cervix the recess is quite shallow. The opening of the cervical canal into the cavity of the body of the uterus is called the **ostium uteri internus** or the internal os. The **ostium uteri externus** is the vaginal opening of the canal and is commonly called the **os uteri**. The canal is narrow and is very difficult to dilate. At the estrum there is a physiological dilatation sufficient to permit the passage of a small canula and at the time of parturition for the expulsion of foetus.

Structure: The wall of the uterus consists of a **serous covering** (visceral peritoneum), **longitudinal and circular muscle** layers, the **submucosa** and the **mucous membrane**. The mucous membrane of the body of the uterus presents about more than hundred oval elevations called **caruncles.** These extend in the horns also where these are arranged in four rows. During pregnancy, the caruncles undergo remarkable enlargement. The uterine glands are present in the intercaruncular spaces. The mucosa of the cervix forms longitudinal folds. It does not have special glands but the mucous glands are well developed. They are especially active at estrum and during pregnancy.

Attachments (ligaments): The body and horns are attached to the abdominal and pelvic walls by two extensive peritoneal folds, the **broad ligaments of the uterus**. They contain unstripped muscles and uterine vessels. The parietal attachments of the broad ligament are to the lateral pelvic wall and the caudal part of the abdominal walls about four or five inches below the tuber coxae. The uterine attachment is to the lateral surface of the body and to the concavity of the horns of the uterus. The lateral layer of each broad ligament gives off a fold, the **round ligament of uterus** which blends with the parietal peritoneum over the deep inguinal ring. Its cranial end forms an appendix which is attached to the cranial extremity of the horns of the uterus.

The **blood supply** to the uterus is through the cranial, middle and caudal uterine arteries. The **cranial uterine artery** is a branch of utero- ovarian artery. It is distributed to the cranial part of the uterine horn and anastomoses with the middle uterine artery. The **middle uterine artery** is the main source of blood supply of uterus. It reaches the concave border of the horn through the broad ligament and divides into several branches. Increase in size of this artery during gestation is of importance in the diagnosis of pregnancy. The **caudal uterine artery** is the cranial branch of urogenital artery. It passes cranially on the ventrolateral surface of the vagina and then inclines ventromedially to the ventral surface of the cervix and body of the uterus to which it is distributed. It often forms anastomosis with the artery of the opposite side and with the middle uterine artery.

Vagina

The vagina is a tubular passage between the uterus and vulva. It is located in the pelvic cavity. It is about 25 to 30 cm long and about 8 to 10 cm in diameter.

Due to elasticity of the wall its dilatability is limited only by the pelvic wall. There is no line of demarcation between it and the vulva. However, sometimes a slight constriction internally marks the junction of the vagina and vulva. It is related **dorsally** to the rectum, **ventrally** to the bladder and urethra and **laterally** to the pelvic wall. The cervix uteri projects into the cranial end of the cavity of the vagina usually on its floor. The **fornix vaginei** is a space in the cranial part of the vaginal cavity lateral and dorsal to the caudal part of the cervix.

Most of the vagina is **retroperitoneal**. However, its cranial part has peritoneal covering. The **rectogenital pouch** of peritoneum extends caudally to a length of about 12 cm on its dorsal surface, while ventrally the serous coat extends to about 5 cm only. The thin **muscular coat** consists of two layers, the outer longitudinal and the inner circular muscle and contains elastic tissue. In the ventral wall of the vagina, between the muscular and mucous coats there are two longitudinal **ducts of epoophori** (**Canals of Gartner**). These ducts open caudally near the external urethral orifice. The **mucous membrane** is pale, except during estrum and has longitudinal and transverse folds. The **blood supply** is from urogenital artery.

Vulva

The vulva or urogenital sinus is a terminal segment of the genital tract and also that of the urinary tract. It is continuous with the vagina cranially and opens at the vulvar cleft to the exterior caudally. It is short about 10 cm long measured along the floor but only about 5 cm in length on dorsal wall. It is related dorsally to the rectum, ventrally to the floor of the pelvis and laterally to the sacrosciatic ligaments. The **vulvar cleft** is a vertical slit about 10 to 12 cm high and is bounded by the **labia vulvae**. The labia or lips of the vulva are muscular structures covered by a sparsely haired integument. The upper part of the labia blend with the surrounding area. Distally they become increasingly prominent and end in a point which carries several long hairs. They are thick, wrinkled and unite dorsally and ventrally forming the dorsal and ventral **labial commissures**. The dorsal commissure is acute and is about 5 cm below the anus, while the ventral commissure is not so acute and is about 5 cm below the ischial arch.

The cavity of the vulva is called the **vestibule.** In the cranial part of the floor of the vestibule is a **suburethral diverticulum**. The opening of this diverticulum is a longitudinal slit about 2.5 cm long. The urethra opens into the upper part of the cranial wall of this suburethral diverticulum. The **canals of Gartner** are variable tubular structures in the floor of the vagina and vulva. The openings of these canals are on either sides of the opening of the suburethral diverticulum. When the lips of vulva are drawn apart, a fossa is noticed at the ventral commissure. This is the **fossa clitoridis** which lodges the pointed free end of the **glans clitoridis**. Below and in continuation of the glans clitoridis is the **corpus clitoridis** which are attached to the symphysis ischii by suspensory ligament. The **clitoris** is a cylindrical nodule located on the floor of the vulva. It is composed of erectile tissue and is the homologue of the penis.

Structure: The wall of the vulva is retroperitoneal and is composed of muscular and mucous coats. The **muscles** of the vulva are the constrictor vulvae and the constrictor vestibulae. The muscle vestibulae constrictor is a striated muscle in the labia. Most of the fibres of this muscle are parallel to the vulvar cleft and are continuous with the dorsal and ventral commissures. A band of this muscle passes upwards across the sphincter ani externus and attaches to the second or third coccygeal vertebra. Many of the fibres of this band of muscle end in the skin and the perineal fascia. This muscle acts to close the vulvar cleft. The muscle constrictor vestibulae is a thin layer arranged in a circular manner around the vestibule. It constricts the vestibule and empties the diverticulum. The **mucosa** of the vulva is smooth and in life it is pink. Two pairs of glands are situated between the mucosa and the muscle of the vulva. The **major vestibular glands** are in the lateral wall of the vulva and their ducts open lateral to and behind the opening of the diverticulum. The small **minor vestibular glands** are median in position in the vulvar floor caudal to the opening of the diverticulum. The **hymen** is a membranous partition located at the junction of the vulva and vagina. It is present for several months after birth.

The **blood supply** is through the internal pudendal artery and the **nerve supply** through the pudendal nerves.

Mammary glands (Udder)

The mammary glands (Fig. 4-6 B) are modified cutaneous glands associated functionally with the genital organs and are considered as accessory genital organs in cow. These are popularly known as udder and are extra pelvic in position.

The udder of a cow comprises four mammary glands placed two on each side of the median plane in the inguinal region. Each of the four glands is somewhat ellipsoidal in form but flattened transversely. Each presents a base, an apex and two surfaces. The **lateral surface** is convex and the **medial surface** is flattened. The **base** is slightly concave and slopes obliquely ventrally and cranially in adaptation to the abdominal wall to which it is attached by means of a well developed suspensory apparatus (ligament) that is derived from the abdominal tunic. The **apex** of each gland leads ventrally to a teat.

The **suspensory apparatus** extends caudally and is attached to the pelvic symphysis. It consists of four sheets of tissues, two of which are well developed and pass medially forming a septum between the glands of the two sides. The lateral sheets arise from the prepubic tendon. These pass ventrally over the lateral faces of the glands and each divides into two branches, the superficial and deep. The superficial branch is attached to the skin of the udder and the deep branch passes into the substance of the glands. The caudal part of the base has the **supra mammary lymph gland** in relation to it.

It is customary to consider the udder as consisting of **four quarters**. There is no septum or visible division between the two quarters of the same side but at the same time, there is no communication between these two. Each quarter is independent of each other as each is a compound saccular gland. The apex of each quarter is continued by a **teat** which is about 7 to 8 cm in length. Between the bases of teats is **intermammary groove**. At the apex of each teat is an opening of the **lactiferous duct** which widens out dorsally into a **lactiferous sinus** or **milk cistern**. The lower part of the duct, the **outlet,** is narrow and is closed by a **sphincter** of smooth muscle and elastic tissue. The wall of the teat is composed of five distinct layers from without inwards, the **skin, outer fibrous layer, intermediate layer, inner fibrous layer and the mucosa.**

The **blood supply** to the udder is through mammary arteries and perineal arteries and the **nerve supply** is through the inguinal nerve and the caudal mesenteric plexus.

66

Comparative Anatomy of Female Genital Organs

Horse

The **ovaries** in mare are bean shaped and much larger than those of cow. Each is about 7 to 8 cm long and about 3 to 4 cm thick. It weighs about 70 to 80 gm. These are situated in the sublumbar region under the fourth or fifth lumbar vertebra. They are usually in contact with the roof of the abdomen. The average distance of ovaries from the vulvar orifice is about 50 to 55 cm in the average sized mare. The notch on the free border leads to a depression, the ovulation fossa where ovulation occurs.

The **uterine tubes** are shorter and more flexuous in mare than those in cow. Each is about 20 to 30 cm long. At its ovarian end it is wider with a diameter of about 4 to 8 mm and becomes narrower at its uterine end with a diameter of about 2 to 3 mm.

The **uterus** in mare is situated partly in abdomen and partly in pelvis. The horns of the uterus are usually pressed against the sublumbar muscles by the intestine. When moderately distended they are about 25 cm long. The junction of the uterine horns with the body of the uterus is abrupt. The average length of the body is about 18 to 20 cm and its diameter is about 10 cm when moderately distended. The cervix is about 5.0 to 7.5 cm in length and 3.5 to 4.0 cm in diameter. The cervical canal is straight. The mucous membrane of the uterus has no cotyledons.

The **vagina** in mare is shorter than that in cow. It measures about 15 to 20 cm in length and 10 to 12 cm in diameter when slightly distended. Most of the vagina is retroperitoneal.

The **vulva** in mare is about 10 to 12 cm in length. The vulvar cleft lies about 5 to 7 cm ventral to the anus. Its ventral commissure is rounded and thick. The suburethral diverticulum is absent.

The **mammary glands** of the mare have only two glands which are not divided into quarters. These are smaller than those in cow. Each gland has a single teat and the apex of each teat has two openings placed close to each other. Two lactiferous ducts from the teat lead to the sinus of each gland.

Dog

The **ovaries** in bitch are small, elongated, oval and flattened. The average length of the ovary in bitch is about 2 cm These are situated a little caudal to the caudal pole of the corresponding kidney. Thus it lies opposite to the third or fourth lumbar vertebra. Each ovary is enclosed in a peritoneal pouch called the ovarian bursa. The two layers of the pouch constitute the ovarian ligament as they pass to the horn of the uterus. There is no distinct hilus to the ovary.

The **uterine tubes** are small and measure about 5 to 8 cm in length. Each passes at first cranially in the lateral part of the ovarian bursa and then runs caudally in the medial part of the pouch. Each uterine tube is slightly flexuous. Its abdominal opening is large and uterine opening is small.

The **uterus** of a bitch has a small body and very long narrow horns. The body is about 2 to 3 cm and the horns about 12 to 15 cm long. The horns are uniform in diameter throughout their length and they lie entirely within the abdomen. They diverge from the body in the form of 'V' facing towards each kidney. Their caudal parts are united by peritoneum. The neck or cervix is very short and has a thick muscular coat. Dorsally there is no demarcation between the uterus and vagina but the cervix is much thicker than vagina. The mucous membrane has short tubular crypts and the long uterine glands. The broad ligaments are extended in the inguinal canal forming the round ligament. The gravid uterus is entirely abdominal and extends to the stomach and liver.

The **vagina** is relatively long and narrow and the fornix is indistinct. The **vulva** has thick lips which form pointed ventral commissure. The corpus clitoridis is not erectile.

The **mammary glands** are 10 in number and are arranged in two rows, extending from the caudal part of the pectoral region to the inguinal region. They are designated according to their location as thoracic 4 glands, abdominal 4 glands and inguinal 2 glands. The teats are short and the apex of each teat has 6 to 10 openings or orifices of excretory ducts.

Sheep and Goat

The genital organs of sheep and goat resemble, in general, to those of cow except a few special features in these small ruminants.

The **ovaries** of sheep and goat are almond shaped and are about 1.5 cm long. The **uterine tubes** are long and tortuous. They are very flexuous near the infundibulum. There is no demarcation between the uterine tubes and the horns of the uterus.

The **uterus** resembles that of the cow. The horns are 10 to 12 cm long and they tapper towards their junction with the uterine tubes. They join the uterine tubes without any demarcation. They are coiled in close spiral. About 2.5 cm of their caudal parts are united. The body of the uterus is about 2 cm long. The caruncles on the mucosal layer are much smaller than those of cow and they have a depression on their free surface. The cervix is about 4 cm long.

The **vagina** is about 8 cm long and its ventral part contains numerous lymph follicles.

The **vulva** is about 2.5 to 3.0 cm long. Ventral to the urethral orifice is a small diverticulum. The vestibular glands are smaller in size in sheep and are absent in goat. The lips of the vulva are thick and the ventral commissure is pointed and projects ventrally.

The **clitoris** is short and the glans is concealed in clitoral fossa.

The **mammary glands** are two in number. They are globular in form but are flattened on the septal side. They are relatively large in size.

Pig

The **ovaries** in sow are concealed in ovarian bursa. They are more rounded than those in bitch and have a distinct hilus. Their position is variable. Usually they are situated near the lateral margin of the pelvic inlet as that in cow. But in some animals they may lie about 2.5 to 5.0 cm caudal to the kidney. The outer surface of the ovaries appears lobulated due to projection of follicles. The mature follicles measure about 7 to 8 mm and corpora lutea about 12 to 15 mm.

The **uterine tubes** are about 15 to 30 cm long and less flexuous than in the mare. The fimbriated extremity of uterine tube forms an ampulla and has a large abdominal opening.

The **uterus** of pig has many striking features. The body of the uterus is about 5cm long. The horns are extremely long and flexuous. In the non-gravid uterus, the horns are arranged in numerous coils which appear like those of the small intestine. The extremities of the horns taper to about the diameter of the uterine tubes. The cervix is very long, about 10 cm and it is directly continued by the vagina without any intravaginal projection.

The **vagina** is about 10 to 12 cm long in a sow of medium size. It is small in calibre and has a thicker muscular coat which consists of circular fibres between the two layers of longitudinal fibres. The mucous membrane is plicated and united with the muscular coat.

The **vaginal vestibule** is about 7.5 cm long. The urethra opens into the vulva. On either side of the cranial part of the floor of the vulva there is a cul-de-sac bounded medially by a longitudinal fold.

The **vulva** has thick lips which are covered by wrinkled skin. The dorsal commissure of the vulva is rounded and the ventral commissure forms a long pointed projection. About 2 cm cranial to the ventral commissure is the clitoral fossa. About halfway between the clitoral fossa and the external urethral fossa on the floor of the vulva is the deep central depression which is bounded on either side by a thick fold and lateral to these thick folds are the openings of the ducts of vestibular glands.

The **mammary glands** are about 10 to 12 in number and these are arranged in two rows similar to those in bitch. Each teat has two ducts opening at the apex of the teat.

Fowl

The genital organs in the hen are only two and they include the ovary and the oviduct.

In birds, although the ovaries and oviducts of both sides are formed, the left ovary and oviduct exceeds over the right ovary and oviduct in their development. As a result, in the adult life of a bird, only the left ovary and oviduct is fully developed and becomes functional while the right ovary and oviduct remains undeveloped and their rudiments only persist.

The **left ovary** is situated in the dorsal part of the coelomic cavity and it is attached to the dorsal wall of the cavity opposite the last two ribs. It has the left lung and the cranial lobe of the kidney to its dorsal side, proventriculus and spleen to its ventral side and caudal vena cava to its medial side. It appears like bunch of grapes and is formed as a cluster of ova. About tens of thousands of ova in different stages of follicular development are contained in the ovary. Numerous rounded follicles of varying sizes project from the ventral surface of the ovary. The ovary of a matured hen measures about 5 cm or more in craniocaudal or transverse directions and it weighs about 50 gm. After the end of the phase of sexual maturity, the ovary reduces in size as well as the weight.

The **left oviduct** (fallopian tube) is a thick walled convoluted tube extending from the vicinity of the ovary to the cloaca. It completely occupies the left dorsal quadrant of the coelomic cavity and also to some extent the left ventral quadrant also. Occasionally the coils of the oviduct cross the midline and reach to the right side of the cavity and displace the intestinal coils. The topographical relations of the coils of the oviduct include the ventral surface of left kidney, some times right kidney and the dorsal body wall dorsally; the left lateral body wall laterally; the intestine in general and caeca in particular ventrolaterally on the right side and the gizzard and spleen ventrally. The total length of the oviduct is about 65 to 70 cm.

The left oviduct of the fowl consists of five major parts which are sequentially continued with each other. These are the infundibulum, magnum, isthmus, shell gland (uterus) and the vagina.

The **infundibulum** is the first part. It begins with a thin wall, wide, funnel shaped part which tapers ventrally to a narrow tube. It measures about 4 to 10 cm long and its diameter is about 7 to 9 cm. The wall of the tubular part of the infundibulum is thicker than its funnel part but thinner than other parts of the oviduct. Internally the wall forms tall folds.

The **magnum** is the second part. It is the longest and most coiled part of the oviduct. It measures about 20 to 48 cm in length and its diameter is about 2 cm. The wall of this part is much thicker than that of the infundibulum. It is because of massive tubular glands packed into the ridge like longitudinal muscular folds in the wall of the tube.

The **isthmus** is the third part. It is short and its diameter is smaller than that of the preceding part. Its length in a laying hen ranges from about 4 to 12 cm with the average of about 8 cm. Its diameter is about 1 cm. The junction of the isthmus and magnum is sharply marked by a narrow band of tissue (about 1 to 3 mm wide) which appears translucent in fresh specimens. The height of the longitudinal folds in this region is reduced to about 1.5 mm.

The **shell gland part (uterus)** is the fourth part. It is about 4 to 12 cm with a mean of about 8 cm in length and about 3 cm in diameter. It is a sac like expanded region of the oviduct. It is considered to have two regions, the cranial short and relatively narrow region through the egg passes quickly and the caudal pouch region which retains the egg during most of the period of shell formation. The tall muscular folds of the wall of this part are intersected by many transverse and oblique furrows.

The **vagina** is the last (fifth) part. It is a narrow muscular tube sharply curved into a 'S' shaped form of this tube, Its length ranges from 4 to 12 cm with a mean of about 8 cm and is about 1 cm in diameter. The circular layer of the muscle of the wall of this part is much thicker than that in any other parts of the oviduct.

The vagina springs from the uterus at a reverse angle causing to appear its initial part as double walled structure and it acts as a vaginal sphincter and here the lumen of the oviduct is constricted. The mucous membrane is thrown into longitudinal folds. Caudally the vagina opens into the coprodeum of the cloaca.

The **ligaments of the oviduct** consist of the dorsal and ventral ligaments. The oviduct is suspended from the roof of the coelomic cavity by a double layered sheet of peritoneum. This sheet is divided into the dorsal and ventral ligaments of the oviduct.

67

Male Genital Organs

The male genital organs (Fig. 4-6 C) comprise the two testicles (where the male gametes are produced) with their coverings and appendages; the epididymis (which stores and transports the gametes); the ductus deferens (the ducts of the testicles); the seminal vesicles, prostate and bulbourethral glands (accessory sex glands); the urethra and the penis (the organ of copulation).

Testicles (Testes)

The testicles are the essential male gonads. They produce male gametes, the spermatozoa and the endocrine secretion which influences the development and maintainance of masculine characteristics. The testicles are paired compound tubular glands situated in the scrotum below the inguinal canals suspended by spermatic cords. Each testicle is about 15 cm long and about 6.5 to 7.5 cm in diameter. Their long axis is vertical. The left testicle is more often slightly larger and lower in position than the right testicle. In such conditions the scrotum appears asymmetrical. Each testicle is slightly compressed from side to side and presents two surfaces, two borders and two extremities. The **lateral surface** is convex and smooth and is covered by the tunica vaginalis propria. The **medial surface** is slightly flattened due to its contact with the septum scroti. The **cranial border** is convex and it is free and hence is called the free border. The **caudal border** is nearly straight and is attached to the epididymis and hence is called the attached border or the epididymal border. The **dorsal and ventral extremities** are blunt and rounded.

Structure: The gland is compound tubular in structure. It is covered externally by peritoneum, the **tunica vaginalis propria** which is very closely attached to the underlined tissue. Underneath the peritoneum is the capsule of the testicle called the **tunica albuginea** because of its white colour. Numerous trabeculae extend from the capsule into the organ forming the supporting tissue for the **seminiferous tubules** and providing a pathway for vessels. The axial strand of connective tissue extending almost the entire length of the gland is the **mediastinum testes**. Radiating from the mediastinum are the lobes of yellowish

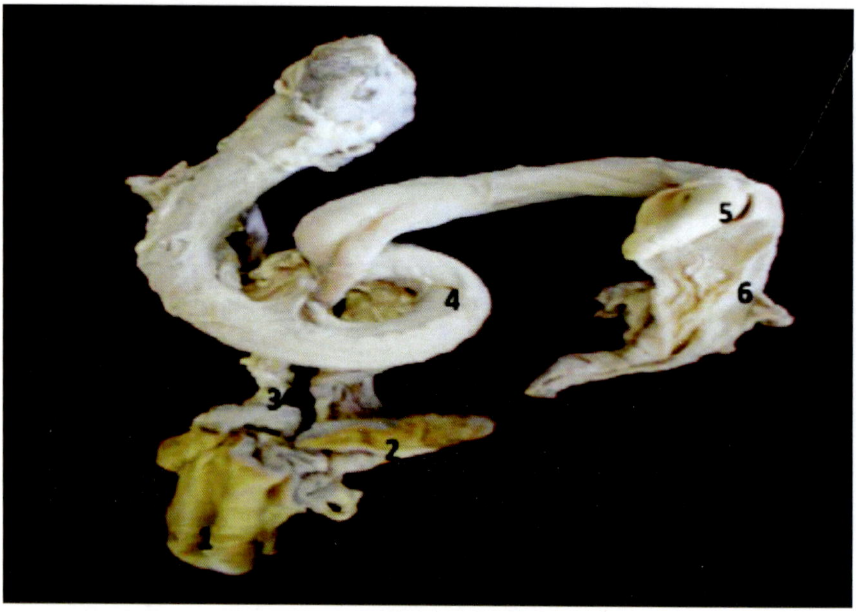

Fig. 4 – 6 C: Genital organs of Ox
1. Scrotum 2. Testicles 3. Spermatic cord 4. Sigmoid flexure 5. Glans penis 6. Prepuce

colour containing the seminiferous tubules. The coiled seminiferous tubules of each lobe unite to form **straight tubules** which enter the mediastinum forming the **rete testes**. The efferent ducts of the rete, about twelve in number, leave the dorsal extremity of the testicle and enter the head of the epididymis.

The **blood supply** is through the internal spermatic artery and the **nerve supply** is through the pelvic plexus.

Epididymis

The epididymis is a tubular structure between the testicle and the ductus deferens. It is attached on the caudal border of the testicle and slightly overlaps its lateral surface. It is comprised of three parts, the dorsal part called the head, the middle part called the body and the ventral part called the tail. The **head** forms a cap like structure on the dorsal extremity of the testicle to which it is closely attached. It extends down the cranial border about one fourth of the length of the testicle. The **body** is in the middle third of the narrow tubular part of the epididymis and it extends down to the ventral extremity of the testicle. It is cylindrical in shape and is attached to the testicle by a fold of peritoneum. The **tail** is spherical and at the ventral extremity of the testicle to which it is attached by **epididymal ligament**. This ligament is formed of connective tissue and unstripped muscle covered by peritoneum. The tail is continued by the vas deferens.

Structure: The epididymis is a compound tubular organ. It is externally covered by peritoneal covering, the **tunica vaginalis**. Beneath this, is a connective tissue capsule containing smooth muscle the **tunica albuginea**. The **interior** of the epididymis is a much **folded tube** formed by the union of efferent ducts in the head and continuing as the ductus deferens at the tail. The epididymis has a considerable storage capacity and an environment favourable to the development of the sperms.

The **blood and nerve supply** is same as that of the testicles.

Vas deferens (Ductus deferens)

The vas deferens or **ductus deferens** is the excretory duct of the testicle. It extends from the tail of the epididymis to the pelvic part of the urethra. At first it pursues a very tortuous course upwards along the caudal border of the testicle. It then becomes straight and becomes part of the spermatic cord with which it enters the abdominal cavity through the inguinal canal. On reaching the internal inguinal ring on the floor of the abdominal cavity it deviates from other structures of the spermatic cord, runs caudally into the pelvic cavity, gains the free edge of the genital fold of the peritoneum by which it is kept attached to the lateral walls of the pelvis. The two ducts are close together here and in their further course caudally on the dorsal surface of the bladder. At this point they leave the genital fold, incline medially and continue to run caudally to reach the caudal part of the bladder. Here the two ducts are in opposition with each other for a distance of about 10 cm bounded and overlapped by the seminal vesicles. Thereafter, they disappear under the prostate and end on the slit like openings on either side of the colliculus seminalis of the urethra, medial to the openings of the seminal vesicles. From its origin to level of the dorsal surface of the bladder, the ductus deferens has a uniform diameter of about 6 mm. It then forms an enlargement, the bulbous part called the **ampulla** which is about 15 to 20 cm long and about 2 cm in diameter. The wall of the ampulla is thicker than the rest of the duct but its lumen remains almost unchanged in its size.

Structure: The wall of the vas deferens is thick and its lumen is very small so that the tube has a firm and cord like character. Its **outer coat** is of **peritoneum**. The **tunica adventitia** is loose and contains numerous vessels and nerves. The **muscular coat** is thick with outer **longitudinal** and inner **circular layer** of smooth muscle. The **mucous membrane** has an epithelium of short and columnar cells. The wall of the **ampulla** is thicker and has numerous **glands.**

The **blood supply** is by the branches of testicular, umbilical and pudendal arteries and the nerve supply is through the nerve fibres from **pelvic plexus**.

Spermatic cord

The spermatic cord is a group of structures that suspend the testicles in the scrotum. It begins at the internal abdominal ring where all structures come together, pass through the inguinal canal and then over the side of the penis and terminates at the attached border of the testicles. Its length varies from 20 to 25 cm depending on the length of the scrotum. The structures forming the spermatic cord are the (1) testicular artery (2) testicular vein (3) lymph vessels (4) autonomic nerve fibres from pelvic plexus to the testicles that run along the artery (5) cremaster internus muscle (6)ductus deferens and (7) visceral layer of the vaginal tunic. These contents of the spermatic cord are grouped into two bundles. The structures 1 to 5 (vessels, nerves and muscle) form the cranial bundle which is the vascular part of the cord while the structure no.6 singularly forms the caudal bundle of the spermatic cord and it is enveloped by structure no. 7 the tunica vaginalis. This caudal part is the nonvascular part of the spermatic cord.

Urethra

The urethra is a Musculo-membranous tube, about 40 to 45 inches long extending from the neck of the bladder to the tip of the glans penis. It has two parts, the pelvic part and the extra pelvic (penile) part. The pelvic part has been described with the urinary organs. The extra pelvic part continues the pelvic part caudally, turns round the ischial arch, passes between the two crura penis , turns forward and is included in the body of the penis. Thus in its further course it becomes a part of the penis.

Scrotum

The scrotum is a cutaneous sac containing testicles and associated structures. It is formed as a diverticulum of the abdomen in front of the inguinal region. It is oval in form and slightly compressed from side to side. It is long and pendulous with a constriction, the **neck** at its junction with the abdominal floor. However, the constriction of the scrotum disappears when it is contracted. The scrotum varies in its form under the influence of cold and heat. The skin is wrinkled and the length of the scrotum is reduced by cold. The heat, debility and fatigue causes the skin to relax and the length of the scrotum to increase. A little cranial to the scrotum is a pair of **rudimentary teat**.

The wall of the scrotum is composed of following four layers.

1. The **outermost layer** is of the **skin** which is thin, elastic and oily. It is haired but less densely than that of the general body skin. It is flesh coloured but usually the colour depends on the breed and the distribution pattern. The outer surface of the scrotum is marked centrally by a raphe called the **raphe scroti**. This is a shallow groove marking the surface longitudinally and indicating the position of the septum scroti.

2. Closely attached to the skin is the **second** layer called the **dartos.** This is an incomplete layer of elastic tissue and unstripped muscle closely attached to the skin. It is dark red in colour and is especially noticeable at the bottom of the scrotum. Temperature changes is the stimulus which causes this layer to contract and relax, thereby influencing the length and surface appearance of the scrotum. The **dartos scroti** forms **septum scroti** dividing the cavity of the scrotum into two unequal parts with the left one larger than the right to accommodate the testicles of the corresponding sides. This septum divides dorsally and becomes continuous with the abdominal tunic.
3. The **third layer** is of the **scrotal fascia.** It is made of a small amount of loose connective tissue between the dartos and the tunica vaginalis. It consists of three layers of visceral fascia derived from the oblique and transverse muscles of the abdomen. These are named as the (a) intercolumnar fascia from the aponeurosis of the external oblique muscle (b) cremasteric fascia from internal oblique muscle and (c) infundibuliform fascia from transverse abdominis muscle.
4. The **innermost layer** is the parietal layer of **tunica vaginalis** which lines the scrotum and is considerably thickened by the addition of connective tissue. It is continuous with the parietal peritoneum of the abdominal cavity at the inguinal ring.

The **blood supply** is by internal testicular artery and **nerve supply** by testicular nerve.

Tunica vaginalis

The tunica vaginalis is a flask shaped serous membrane which extends through the inguinal canal to the bottom of the scrotum. It is an invagination of the parietal peritoneum of the abdomen and consists of two layers, the parietal and visceral. The parietal layer lines the inguinal canal and scrotum. It is reflected from the caudal wall of the inguinal canal around the structures of the cord forming the mesorchium. The visceral layer lines the cord, testicles and the epididymis. The capillary space between the two layers is the cavity of the tunica vaginalis, and it is a diverticulum of the general peritoneal cavity with which it communicates at the vaginal ring.

Cremaster externus muscle

The cremaster externus is a long and narrow voluntary muscle that lies on the caudal and lateral part of the tunic in the inguinal canal. It forms a part of the spermatic cord in the inguinal canal. It acts to raise the tunica vaginalis and the testicle.

Accessory genital glands

The accessory genital glands comprise the seminal vesicles, the prostate and the bulbourethral glands. The secretion of these glands is added to the sperms passing through the vas deferens and the urethra. The semen is a combined secretion of the testicular and the accessory genital glands along with the sperms.

Seminal vesicles

The seminal vesicles are paired compact tubular organs having a thick glandular wall and a small lumen. Their external surface is lobulated. They lie in the genital fold on the caudo-dorsal part of the bladder. It measures about 10 to 12 cm in length, 5 cm in width and 3 cm in thickness in the adult animal. Each gland consists of a thick walled tube folded on itself in a tortuous manner. The dorsal surface of the gland faces dorsally and medially and is partially covered with peritoneum. The ventral surface faces ventrally and is in contact with the bladder. It is not covered with the peritoneum. The duct of this gland opens at the seminal colliculus just lateral to the openings of the ductus deferens.

Prostate gland

The prostate is a musculo glandular organ situated transversely on the neck of the bladder. It is pale yellow in colour. It consists of a **body** and a **disseminate** part. The body is a small transverse mass that stretches across dorsal surface of the neck of the bladder and the origin of the urethra. It measures about 3.5 to 4.0 cm transversely and about 1.0 to 1.5 cm in width and thickness. The disseminate part surrounds the pelvic urethra and in turn is surrounded by the urethral muscle and its aponeurosis. The **prostatic ducts** are about 15 to 20 and these open into the urethra behind the colliculus seminalis in rows.

Bulbourethral glands

The bulbourethral glands are paired, piriform glandular structures located on either side of the pelvic part of the urethra at the ischial arch. These are covered by a dense layer of the fibrous tissue and the bulbo-cavernous muscle. Each gland has a single duct which opens into the urethra behind the ducts of the prostate.

Penis

The penis is a male organ of copulation. It is composed of the erectile tissue and encloses the extra pelvic part of the urethra. It is cylindrical in form and measures about three feet (thirty six to forty inches) in length with the diameter of about 3.5 to 4.0 cm in the adult bull. About twelve inches of its length forms the sigmoid flexure. It extends cranially and ventrally from the ischial arch between the thighs to the umbilical region. The penis consists of three parts, the root, body and the glans.

The **root** of the penis is attached to the lateral parts of the ischial arch by two **crura** which converge and unite below the arch. Ventrally where the two crura unite, it forms a groove which is converted into a tapering **urethral canal** by extension of the tunica albuginea. Through this canal passes the **urethra.** The **body** begins at the junction of the crura and forms the bulk of the organ. At its beginning it is attached to the symphysis ischi by two strong bands, the **suspensory ligaments** of the penis. It forms behind the scrotum an **'S'** shaped curve, the **sigmoid flexure** in which about twelve inches of penis is folded. The body, although cylindrical, is flattened dorsoventrally and presents dorsal, ventral and two lateral surfaces. The **dorsal surface** is narrow and rounded. On this surface are the dorsal arteries and nerves of the penis and a rich venous plexus. The **ventral surface** presents the urethral orifice. It is rounded and along it runs the urethra embedded in the deep urethral groove of the **corpus cavernosum**. The **lateral surfaces** are high and flattened and are covered by the **plexus of veins**. The **glans** is a tapering cranial free end of the penis. It is about three inches long, is not clearly marked off from the body and lies in the cavity of the prepuce. It is pointed and twisted. The twist has a groove and the **external urethral orifice** is at the end of this groove. The prescrotal part of the penis is in a cutaneous pouch, the prepuce.

Structure: The penis consists basically of two bodies, the corpus cavernosum and the corpus spongiosum. The **corpus cavernosum** forms the greater part of the bulk of the penis except at its free extremity. It arises from each side of the ischial arch by a crus penis which is embedded in a ischiocavernous muscle. The **crura** of the two sides unite ventral to the ischial arch to form the body of the corpus cavernosum which presents ventrally the urethral groove. This groove contains the urethra and the corpus spongiosum. Externally, the corpus cavernosum is covered by **tunica albuginea**, which is a thick capsule of white fibrous tissue with some elastic fibres in it. Numerous trabeculae extending from this tunic pass into the substance of the corpus cavernosum and form its framework. Within the framework of these trabeculae is a soft and reddish grey erectile tissue which comprises numerous cavernous spaces. These spaces are regarded as greatly enlarged capillaries which are directly continuous with the veins of the penis. The erection of penis is a result of distention of these spaces with blood. The **corpus spongiosum** forms a tube around the urethra and is continuous cranially with the glans penis. It forms small enlargement at the root of the penis which is termed as bulbus urethrae.

The **blood supply** to penis is by the external pudendal, internal pudendal and obturator arteries. The **nerve supply** is by the sympathetic nerves extending from pelvic plexus.

Muscles of penis

The **ischiocavernous muscle** is a short but strong muscle originating on the medial surface of tuber ischii and inserting on the crura and adjacent part of the body of the penis. Its action is to pull the root and the adjacent part of the body of the penis against the ischial arch.

The **retractor penis** are two bands of unstripped muscle originating on the transverse processes of the first coccygeal vertebra and inserting to the cranial and ventral bend of the sigmoid flexure of the penis. Its action is to retract the penis after protrusion and to maintain the penis in quiescent state.

Prepuce

The prepuce often called as sheath is a tubular structure covering the cranial especially the prescrotal part of the penis. It is about twelve to fifteen inches long and consists of the internal and external layers. The preputial orifice is the opening of the prepuce. It is about 5 cm caudal to the umbilicus. It measures about 35 to 40 cm long and 2.5 to 3.0 cm in diameter but is capable of dilation. It is surrounded by long hairs. The external layer, starting from the base of the scrotum, passes cranially for about 40 cm and reaches to the apex of the glance surrounding the preputial orifice. Here it reflects inwards and continues as the internal or penile layer to run back to the base of the scrotum and again reflects to join the external layer. It thus forms within the cavity of the sheath a secondary tubular invagination. The external layer is continuous with the skin at the orifice and is attached to the adjacent structures by a large amount of loose connective tissue. The free surface has number of longitudinal folds. The internal layer is loosely attached to the body of the penis and is closely attached to the glans.

68

Comparative Anatomy of Male Genital Organs

Horse

The **testicles** in horse are oval in form and they are comparatively smaller in size than those in ox. The long axis of the testicles is parallel to the body of the animal and hence the attached border of the testicle is dorsal while its free border is ventral in position inside the scrotum. The testicle of the stallion is about 10 to 12 cm long, 5 cm wide and about 6 to 7 cm thick. It weighs about 225 to 300 gm. The size of the left and right testicle varies and the left testicle is often larger than the right one.

The **epididymis** is adhered to the attached (dorsal) border of the testicle. The rest of the features of epididymis in horse are similar to those of ox.

The **vas deferens** of horse right from its origin from the tail of epididymis to its course up to the dorsal surface of the bladder it has a uniform diameter of about 6 mm. Thereafter, it forms a fusiform enlargement, the ampulla of the vas deferens and beyond the ampulla the duct abruptly reduces in size. The ampulla is about 15 to 20 cm long and its diameter is about 2 cm. The genital fold is wider and hence the two ducts apart from each other. The vas deferens and the duct of seminal vesicle open in a common ejaculatory orifice on each side of the colliculus seminalis.

The **scrotum** in horse lies under the inguinal canals in the inguinal region. The skin around the scrotum is dark coloured and the rudimentary teats are absent.

The **masculine uterus** is a special feature in the horse. It is the homologue of the female uterus and is situated centrally on the caudal part of the dorsal surface of the bladder. It is a flattened tube of about 7.5 to 10.0 cm length. Its cranial part is narrow and lies in the genital fold and gives off two slender blind cornua. The caudal end of the tube passes under the isthmus of the prostate and opens into the urethra on the summit of the colliculus seminalis or joins the duct of the seminal vesicle or is blind.

The **seminal vesicles** in horse are two elongated and pyriform sacs presenting a fundus, body and the neck. Each is about 15 to 20 cm long. The duct joins the vas deferens.

The **prostate gland** in horse is large and consists of two lobes connected by isthmus. The dorsal surface of the lobes is related to the rectum and the ventral surface is concave and is related to the seminal vesicle. The isthmus is related ventrally to the masculine uterus, vasa deferens and seminal vesicles.

The **bulbourethral glands** are larger, about 5 cm long and are covered by urethral muscle. Each gland has about six to eight ducts which open into the urethra behind the opening of the prostatic ducts.

The **penis** of horse is shorter but has a larger diameter. In the quiescent state it is about 50 cm long and in erected state the length increases to about fifty per cent reaching to about 75 cm. The erectile tissue is very rich in elastic and muscular tissues and hence is very soft. The **glans** is enlarged and its base forms a prominent margin, the **corona glandis**. Its lower part presents a depression, the **fossa glandis** in which the urethra protrudes as a free tube the **urethral process**. The fossa surrounding the urethra opens dorsally into a diverticulum, the **urethral sinus**.

The **prepuce** is shorter and wider. The preputial cavity is only about 15 to 20 cm long.

Dog

The **testicles** in dog are relatively smaller and are oval in form. They are suspended in the scrotum obliquely with their long axis directed dorsally and caudally.

The **epididymis** is large, extremely convoluted and closely attached along the dorsal part of the lateral surface of the testicle.

The **vas deferens** has narrow ampullae which enter the craniodorsal surface of the prostate.

The **scrotum** in dog is situated behind the inguinal region, about halfway between the inguinal region and the anus. The raphe scroti is not very distinct.

The **seminal vesicles** are absent. The **prostate gland** is relatively large and globular. It surrounds the neck of the bladder at or near the cranial border of the pubis. A median furrow indicates the division of the gland into two lobes. The **bulbourethral glands** are absent.

The **penis** of dog presents several special features. In its cranial part, there is a bone, the **os penis** which in large dogs reaches a length of about 10 cm or more. It is considered as ossified part of the corpus cavernosum. Ventrally it is grooved for the urethra, dorsally it is convex and cranially it becomes smaller and has a fibrous curved prolongation. The glans is very long extending over the entire length of os penis. Its cranial part is cylindrical with a pointed free end and caudal to this is a rounded enlargement, the **bulb of the glans**.

The **prepuce** forms a complete sheath around the cranial part of the penis similar to that in ox. The penile layer of the prepuce is closely attached to the cranial part of the glans and more loosely to the bulb of the glans.

Sheep and Goat

The male genital organs in sheep and goat resemble in general to those of the bull (ox). However, the testicles are relatively much larger. The testicle of an adult ram measures about 10 cm long and weighs about 250 to 300 gm. They are broader in proportion to their length. The prostate is entirely disseminate. The bulbourethral glands are relatively very large. In the penis, the urethra lies in a groove on the ventral surface of the corpus cavernosum. Its terminal part projects commonly about 3 to 4 cm beyond the glans penis, forming a twisted urethral process.

Pig

The **testicles** of pig are relatively very large and they are elliptical in form. They are placed in the scrotum in such way that their long axis is directed dorsally and caudally, the free border faces dorsally and the tail of the epididymis is highest. They are comparatively soft in texture. The tunica albuginea contains much elastic tissue but no muscular fibres. From the rete testis, about six to seven efferent ducts proceed to the epididymis.

The **epididymis** is closely attached to the testicle. Its tail is very large and forms a blunt conical projection at the caudal extremity of the testicle.

The **vas deferens** in its testicular part is flexuous and closely attached to the by the vaginal tunic. It does not form a distinct ampulla. The cremaster muscle is very well developed and extends to about the middle of the scrotal part of the tunic.

The **scrotum** is situated at a short distance from the anus and is not so sharply defined from the surrounding parts as in the other animals.

The **seminal vesicles** are exceedingly large and extend into the abdominal cavity. They are three sided pyramidal masses in opposition with each other medially and cover the caudal part of the bladder and ureters, vas deferens, body of the prostate and the cranial part of the urethra and the bulbourethral glands. They are distinctly lobed and glandular in structure. The **prostate gland** is similar to that of ox. Its body is about 2.5 cm wide. It is concealed by seminal vesicles. The **bulbourethral glands** are relatively very large and dense. They are somewhat cylindrical and lie on either side of the pelvic urethra. In a large sized boar, the bulbourethral gland measures about 12 cm in length and 2.5 to 3.0 cm in width. The duct of the gland opens in a cul-de-sac formed by the fold of mucous membrane at the dorsal part of the lumen of the urethra.

The **penis** of a boar resembles in general to that of ox. The sigmoid flexure is, however formed at the prescrotal part. The cranial part of the penis has no glans and it is spirally twisted especially in erection. The external urethral orifice is slit like and is situated ventrolaterally close to the pointed extremity. The penis of adult bore measures about 45 to 50 cm in length.

The **prepuce** has a narrow orifice with stiff hairs around it. The cavity of the prepuce is very long and is partially divided by a circular fold into the cranial wider part and a narrow caudal part. In the dorsal wall of the wide cranial part there is a circular opening that leads to a cul-de-sac, the **preputial diverticulum**.

Fowl

The **testicles** in fowl lie ventral to the cranial lobe of kidneys. The right testicle is against the dorsal part of the right lobe of the liver. The left testicle is related to the glandular stomach. Both the testicles are bean shaped and bear on their concave border, a flattened projection the rudimentary epididymis.

The **vasa deferentia** are extremely tortuous ducts which arise from the so called epididymal projection pass caudally and open into the urodeum on the summit of a papilla lateral to the opening of the ureter.

The **accessory genital glands** are absent in fowl.

The **penis** is not in the regular form as is in the mammalian animals. In fowl, a special type of **copulatory apparatus** exists. It lies in the ventral part of the caudal end of the cloaca and is visible only in the sexually active state of the bird. The copulatory apparatus consists of the paired papillae of the vasa deferentia, the paired vascular bodies, the phallus and the paired lymphatic folds. Each **papilla of the vas deferens** is a conical projection from the wall of the urodeum. Its base is about 5 to 8 mm ventral to the opening of the ureter. This papilla in the sexually matured bird is about 2.5 mm long and 2 to 3 mm in diameter. Its opening is pointed caudomedially. The **vascular body** is a spindle shaped body measuring about 7 mm long and 1 mm wide. It lies in the ventrolateral wall of the urodeum and proctodeum between the dilated end of vas deferens and the phallus in the cloaca. The **phallus** lies in the ventral midline of the proctodeum immediately caudomedial to the papilla of the vas deferens. The **lymphatic fold** lies between the lateral phallus and the papilla of the vas deferens. Out of all these components of the copulatory apparatus, the phallus is nearest to the out side of the body. In the excited state it is visible lying along the crest of the ventral lip or the fold of the **vent.**

SECTION-C

BLOOD VESSELS AND LYMPHATICS

69

Abdominal Aorta and Arteries of Abdomen and Pelvis

The **abdominal aorta** is the continuation of thoracic part of the descending aorta which enters the abdominal cavity through hiatus aorticus of the diaphragm. After entering the abdominal cavity it passes caudally below the bodies of the lumbar vertebrae and psoas minor muscle in contact with the left crus of the diaphragm and the ventral common vertebral ligament. After reaching at the fifth or sixth lumbar vertebra, it terminates into iliac quadrification by dividing into two common iliac arteries. Each of the common iliac arteries further divides into internal and external iliac artery. The internal iliac artery supplies arterial branches to the wall and the viscera of the pelvic cavity while the external iliac artery supplies arterial branches to the pelvic limb of the corresponding side. The abdominal aorta is related dorsally to the bodies of lumbar vertebrae, ventral common ligament, tendon of left crus of diaphragm and psoas minor muscle, ventrally to the pancreas and rumen, on its right to the caudal vena cava and on its left to the left adrenal, left kidney and left ureter. The abdominal aorta gives out parietal and visceral branches that supply the walls and the viscera of abdominal cavity.

Parietal branches

The parietal branches of the abdominal aorta are the six pairs of the lumbar arteries. Out of these, four or five pairs arise from the dorsal surface of the aorta while the fifth or sixth pair depending on where the aorta terminates (fifth or sixth lumbar vertebral level) arises from the internal iliac arteries.

The lumbar arteries, after arising from the dorsal surface of the aorta, pass upward across the bodies of the lumbar vertebrae, reach the intertransverse spaces between the lumbar transverse processes and divide into dorsal and ventral branches. The dorsal branches are larger. They supply spinal branches to reinforce the ventral spinal artery and the muscular branches to supply the muscles and skin over the back (loin) region of the body trunk. The ventral branches run ventrally through the fascia and muscles of the abdominal walls and supply the muscles and skin of the walls of the abdomen.

Visceral branches

The major visceral branches of the abdominal aorta include the phrenic, celiac, cranial mesenteric, renal, testicular or ovarian and caudal mesenteric arteries. Of these, the celiac, cranial mesenteric and caudal mesenteric arteries are single (unpaired) and the phrenic renal and testicular or ovarian arteries are paired.

Phrenic artery

The phrenic artery has a variable origin. Usually two or three small arterial branches of this artery extend from the visceral surface of the abdominal aorta at the level of hiatus aorticus and after a short course along the right crus of diaphragm these are distributed all over the diaphragm. In many cases these arteries arise from the visceral surface of thoracic part of the aorta. Origin of these arteries as a branch of coeliac or coeliaco-mesenteric artery is also not uncommon

Coeliac artery

The coeliac artery originates from the ventral face of the aorta, immediately after the entry of the latter in to the abdominal cavity opposite the first lumbar vertebra. It is about 10 to 12 cm long and passes ventrally on the left face of the rumen turns cranially between the rumen and pancreas on left and the right crus of diaphragm and caudal vena cava on the right and is continued as the left gastric artery. The coeliac artery is often seen originating in a common trunk with the cranial mesenteric artery and in that case is named as the coeliaco-mesenteric trunk. The branches of the coeliac artery given off during its course are as below.

1. The **hepatic artery** arises from the convex side of the coeliac artery as it crosses the caudal vena cava. It passes to the right and somewhat ventrally and cranially with the portal vein to the portal fissure and gives off the following branches.

- The **pancreatic branches** to the pancreas.
- The **right (dorsal) hepatic branch** to the right lobe and caudate process of the liver and the left hepatic branch to the caudate, quadrate and left lobe of the liver.
- The **cystic branch** to the gallbladder

- The **right gastric artery** arises from the hepatic or from its left branch. It passes in the lesser omentum along the duodenum to the lesser curvature of the abomasum, where it anastomoses with the left gastric artery.
- The **gastro-duodenal artery** divides into **cranial pancreatico-duodenal** and the **right gastro-epiploic** arteries. The former supplies the pancreas and second part of the duodenum. The latter supplies the pylorus and anastomoses with the left gastro-epiploic artery (continuation of left gastric artery). It supplies the right face and the caudal one third of the left face of the rumen.

2. The **right ruminal artery** originates either in a common trunk with the splenic artery or separately from the coeliac artery. It forms a sharp curve and runs ventrally and caudally in the right ruminal groove of the rumen, gives off numerous branches to it, reaches the caudal transverse groove, passes into it, reaches the left face of the rumen into the left ruminal groove and anastomoses with the left ruminal artery. It supplies the whole of the right face and a part of the left face of the rumen.

3. The **left ruminal artery** arises from the coeliac artery, descends at first on the cranial part of the right face of the rumen, enters the cranial transverse groove, passes to the left face of the rumen, runs caudally in the left ruminal groove to its caudal end and anastomoses with the right ruminal artery. It supplies the cranial two thirds of the left face of the rumen.

The **reticular artery** is given off from the left ruminal artery immediately after its origin from the coeliac artery, passes along the dorsal (greater) curvature of the rumen, turns ventrally in the rumino-reticular groove and passes to the right where it furnishes branches to the reticulum.

4. The **splenic artery** arising independently from the coeliac artery or in a common trunk with the right ruminal artery, passes cranially, crosses the dorsal curvature of the rumen, reaches the hilus of the spleen and enters through it into the gland.

1. The **left gastric artery** (omaso-abomasal) is the continuation of the coeliac artery. It is about 10 to 15 cm long, passes ventrally and cranially to the greater curvature of the omasum and divides into dorsal and ventral branches.

- The **dorsal branch** passes caudally over the greater curvature of the omasum, then along the lesser curvature of the abomasum supplying branches to these compartments and beyond the pylorus it anastomoses with the right gastric artery.
- The **ventral branch** (left gastro epiploic artery) passes ventrally and cranially to the lesser curvature of omasum, then along the greater

curvature of abomasum giving branches to these compartments and anastomoses with the right gastro-epiploic artery.

Cranial mesenteric artery

The cranial mesenteric artery arises from the ventral surface of the aorta immediately caudal to the coeliac artery and is of the same size as that of the coeliac artery. The coeliac and the cranial mesenteric arteries some times originate from the aorta in a short common trunk that run for few cm down and then gets separated from each other. The cranial mesenteric artery passes ventrally, inclining to the right and somewhat cranially and passes between the pancreas and the caudal vena cava in the concavity of the loop of the terminal part of the colon, leaves the spiral mass, runs along the mesentery and divides into several branches supplying the intestines. It gives off the following branches.

- **Pancreatic branches** supply the pancreas.
- The **caudal pancreatico-duodenal** artery arises from the right side of the cranial mesenteric artery and bifurcates into several branches that supply the descending duodenum.
- The **middle colic artery** runs caudally on the dorsal surface of the colon and anastomoses with the short colic branch of the caudal mesenteric artery.
- The **ileo-caeco-colic artery** ramifies on the right face of the spiral part of the colon. It gives off the ileo-caecal artery which divides into ileac and caecal branches to supply the ileum and caecum.
- The **ramus collateralis** runs in the mesentery along the ventral border of the coils of the colon and unites with terminal branches of the cranial mesenteric trunk.
- The **jejunal arteries** arise from the convex surface of the whole length of the cranial mesenteric artery, pass across the mesenteric lymph nodes and join the arches that supply short, straight arteries to the intestine.
- The **ileal arteries** arise from the terminal branches of the cranial mesenteric artery.

Renal arteries

The renal arteries are the paired arteries. The right and the left artery arise close to each other from the ventral surface of the abdominal aorta about 8 cm caudal to the opening of the cranial mesenteric artery opposite the second lumbar vertebra. The **right renal artery** is shorter than the left while the left renal artery is longer but narrower than the right. The right renal artery passes craniad, laterad and ventrad over the caudal vena cava and enters the hilus of the right kidney. The **left renal artery** passes craniad and ventrad to the hilus of the left kidney. Each renal artery, in its course, gives off branches to the ureter, renal lymph gland and the adrenal gland of the corresponding side.

Testicular artery (in male)

The testicular (spermatic) artery is the longest of the branches of the abdominal aorta. It is a paired artery and the arteries of the opposite side arise in close opposition from the ventral surface of the abdominal aorta close (just cranial) to the origin of caudal mesenteric artery. Each artery passes caudally in the sublumbar region and then ventrally somewhat lateral to the pelvic inlet and reaches to the internal inguinal (deep inguinal) ring. From here it descends through the inguinal canal as a part of the cranial part of the spermatic cord. In its course through the inguinal canal it exhibits remarkably tortuous disposition. It passes out of the external inguinal (superficial inguinal) ring, reaches the head of the epididymis, passes ventrally along the epididymis to the ventral extremity of the testicle, turns upward and runs dorsally along the attached border of the testicle with the other constituents of the cranial part of the spermatic cord. It supplies branches to the vaginal tunic, ductus deferens, epididymis and testicle.

Ovarian artery (in female)

The ovarian (utero-ovarian) artery in female is the homologue of the testicular artery of male. It is a slender vessel which passes caudally in the cranial part of the broad ligament of uterus and divides into **ovarian** and **cranial uterine** branches that supply the ovary and the horns of the uterus respectively. The cranial uterine artery anastomoses with the middle uterine artery.

Caudal mesenteric artery

The caudal mesenteric artery is single (unpaired) artery and it arises from the ventral surface of the abdominal aorta just before its termination. Following its origin, it divides into cranial and caudal branches. The cranial branch is a **colic branch**. It passes cranially in the colic mesentery above the terminal part of the colon which it supplies and anastomoses with the middle colic artery. The caudal branch is the **rectal branch**. It passes caudally into the pelvic cavity along the mesorectum. It terminates near the anus and supplies the rectum and the part of anus.

Median (middle) sacral artery

The median sacral artery is the continuation of the abdominal aorta in the form of a median long but small artery of about 5 mm diameter running through the sacrococcygeal region. It arises as an unpaired vessel from the dorsal aspect of the abdominal aorta before its termination into iliac quadrification. It passes caudally on the ventral face of the sacrum. It gives off in its course spinal branches to the spinal cord and meninges, branches to the epaxial muscles of the sacrococcygeal region and two lateral coccygeal arteries. The **lateral sacral arteries** are transversely connected with the median sacral artery at regular intervals. The median sacral artery, after reaching at the level of first coccygeal vertebra, continues caudally as the **median** (middle) **coccygeal artery** which runs through the haemal arches of the coccygeal vertebrae and supplies the coccygeal muscles.

Internal iliac artery

The internal iliac artery is the main arterial trunk which supplies the pelvic wall and the pelvic viscera. The two internal iliac arteries are the internal branches of the iliac quadrification. Each internal iliac artery passes obliquely caudally and somewhat laterally ventral to the wing of sacrum towards the pelvic cavity on the broad sacrosciatic (sacrotuberal) ligament and terminates about the level of the lesser sciatic (ischiatic) foramen by dividing into caudal gluteal and internal pudendal arteries. During its course the internal iliac artery gives off the following collateral branches.

1. The **umbilical artery** arises from the ventral surface of the internal iliac artery. It is a very large vessel in the foetus and runs in the free border of the lateral ligament of the bladder, passes through the umbilicus and ramifies in the placenta. As this artery is not required after birth it is greatly reduced and is completely obliterated. The part of the obliterated artery beyond the vertex of the urinary bladder to the umbilicus becomes round ligament of the bladder. The umbilical artery from the ventral surface of the internal iliac artery to the vertex of the bladder, however, persists after the birth. This part of the artery gives off following collateral branches.

- The deferential artery supplies the vas deferens in the male.
- The uterine artery (middle uterine) is of a considerable size and is a main artery of uterus in females. It supplies the horns and the body of the uterus. Its branches anastomose with those of the cranial uterine artery (a branch of ovarian artery) cranially and caudal uterine artery caudally.
- The ureteric branch is a slender branch that supplies the wall of the ureter.

- The cranial vesicular artery is a small branch that passes along the lateral ligament of the bladder and supplies the cranial aspect of the urinary bladder.

2. The **ilio-lumbar artery** is a common trunk arising from the internal iliac artery next to the preceding branch, and it divides into three branches, the last lumbar artery, last sacral artery and the **cranial gluteal artery**. The last one passes out through the greater sciatic (ischiatic) foramen and supply the gluteal muscles.

3. The **urogenital artery in the male** arises from the internal face of the internal iliac artery and supplies branches to urinary bladder, ureter, vas deferens, seminal vesicles, prostate and the urethra.

The **urogenital artery in the female** follows a short course along the lateral surface of the vagina and divides into cranial and caudal branch. The cranial branch is relatively large and gives off the following branches.

- The **caudal uterine artery** anastomoses with the middle uterine artery and supplies the body and cervix of the uterus.
- The **caudal vesicular artery** supplies the neck of the urinary bladder and the adjacent part of the ureter.
- The **urethral branch** supplies the major part of the pelvic urethra.
- The caudal branch of the urogenital in female supplies the branches to vagina, vulva and the rectum.

4. Caudal gluteal artery

The caudal gluteal artery, the first of the terminal branches of internal iliac artery, passes out of the pelvis through the lesser sciatic (ischiatic) foramen and supplies the biceps femoris and middle gluteus muscles of the hip and thigh of the pelvic limb.

5. Internal pudendal artery

The internal pudendal artery is the second and the larger of the two terminal branches of the internal iliac artery. It runs down obliquely on the medial surface of the sacrosciatic ligament towards the floor of the pelvis, supplies branches to the urinary bladder, urethra, obturator internus, levator ani, coccygeus and the ventral perineal branches and then continues down the ischial arch. Here the artery **in** the **male** divides into **dorsal and deep arteries of the penis**. The dorsal artery of penis runs superficially over the dorsum penis as the caudal dorsal artery of the penis and anastomoses with the branches of the cranial dorsal artery of penis. The deep artery of penis supplies the corpus cavernosum of the penis. In the **female**, the internal pudendal artery gives off a large **caudal uterine artery** to the uterus and vagina and terminates as the **artery of the clitoris**. A branch from it passes out of the ischial arch as the **perineal artery** which supplies cutaneus skin in the perineal region and continues as the **caudal mammary artery** for the mammary glands.

External iliac artery

The external iliac artery arises from the abdominal aorta most commonly ventral to the body of the sixth lumbar vertebra or sometimes under the body of the fifth lumbar vertebra. The two, right and left, external iliac arteries are the external branches of the iliac quadrification. Each artery passes caudoventrally parallel to the psoas minor muscle in the sublumbar region, reaches by the side of the pelvic inlet and then to the cranial border of the pubis. Beyond this, it descends in the thigh as femoral artery to supply the pelvic limb. Before its continuation as femoral, during its intrapelvic course from the sublumbar region to the cranial border of pubis, it furnishes the following branches supplying the viscera and the wall of the pelvis.

1. The **deep circumflex iliac artery** arises from external iliac artery close to its origin and passes laterally towards the external angle of the ilium supplying branches to psoas major and iliacus and divides into cranial and caudal branch. The cranial branch runs ventrally and cranially on the transversus abdominis, then gets under the internal oblique muscle, perforates it, gets under the external oblique muscle and finally reaches the skin of the flank. It supplies all these muscles and skin The caudal branch also supplies branches to the ilio-psoas, penetrates the abdominal wall, descends on the tensor fascia lata, supplies branches to these muscles, the prefemoral lymph nodes and the skin on the thigh. Thus, the deep circumflex artery supply mainly to the abdominal wall.

2. The **deep femoral artery** arises from the cranial face of the external iliac artery and divides into two branches, the pudendoepigastric artery and the medial circumflex femoral artery.

- The **pudendoepigastric artery** passes cranially from its origin, crosses the prepubic tendon and divides at the internal inguinal ring into external pudendal and caudal epigastric arteries.
- The **caudal epigastric artery** courses between the obliquus internus abdominis and rectus abdominis muscles furnishes branches to these muscles and anastomoses with the cranial epigastric artery.
- The **external pudendal artery** descends the inguinal canal in the caudal part of the spermatic cord, passes out of the canal at the superficial (external) inguinal ring and divides into subcutaneous abdominal and the

cranial dorsal artery of penis in male and caudal mammary in the female. The subcutaneous abdominal artery passes cranially on the tunica abdominalis, supplies branches to the, superficial inguinal lymph gland and skin in the inguinal region.

- In the **male** it sends branches to the scrotum and in female to the mammary glands. The **cranial dorsal artery of penis** supplies branches to the scrotum gains the dorsal face of the penis and divides into cranial and caudal branches. The cranial branch courses cranially along the dorsum penis, reaches the cranial extremity of penis and terminates at the glans penis. The caudal branch runs caudally along the dorsum penis and anastomoses with the branches of the caudal dorsal artery of penis.
- In **female,** the external pudendal artery, after emerging through the inguinal canal, divides into the **cranial subcutaneous abdominal** artery and the **caudal mammary artery**. The caudal epigastric artery after supplying branches to the superficial inguinal lymph nodes and the muscles around the inguinal region, continues as the **cranial mammary artery** and anastomoses with the branches of the caudal mammary artery to supply the mammary glands.

70

Comparative Anatomy of Arteries of Abdomen and Pelvis

Horse

The **visceral branches** of the abdominal aorta are the coeliac, cranial mesenteric, renal, caudal mesenteric and testicular or ovarian.

The **coeliac artery** in horse is shorter than that in ox. It arises from ventral surface of the aorta and reaches the dorsal surface of the pancreas where it divides into three branches, the left gastric, hepatic and splenic.

The **left gastric artery** passes ventrally and cranially in the gastrophrenic ligament, gives off pancreatic and oesophageal branches and divides dorsal and caudal to the cardia into parietal and visceral branches. The parietal branch crosses the lesser curvature of the stomach just to the right of the cardia and ramifies on its parietal surface. The visceral branch is distributed in the similar manner on the visceral surface of the stomach. A long but narrow oesophageal branch arises from the parietal branch of the left gastric, passes cranially through the hiatus oesophageus and enters the thoracic cavity dorsal to the oesophagus and anastomoses with the oesophageal branch of broncho-oesophageal artery.

The **hepatic artery** is larger than the left gastric. It passes dorsal to the pancreas and reaches medial to the portal vein, divides into right and left branches from which the terminal branches enter the liver through portal fissure. Its collateral branches are the pancreatic, right gastric and the gastroduodenal arteries. The gastroduodenal artery further divides into right gastroepiploic and the cranial pancreaticoduodenal arteries.

The **splenic artery** is the largest branch of the coeliac. It passes on the left border of the pancreas, crosses the saccus caecus of the stomach and then reaches the hilus of the spleen to enter the gland. It gives out the pancreatic, splenic short gastric and left gastroepiploic arteries in its course.

The **cranial mesenteric artery** after arising from the aorta passes ventrally between the caudal vena cava and the left adrenal gland into the root of the mesentery and divides into the caudal pancreaticoduodenal, jejunal, and colic branches. The colic branch further divides into right colic and middle colic arteries.

The **renal arteries** are relatively large and arise from the aorta near the cranial mesenteric artery. The right renal artery is longer of the two. It crosses over the dorsal surface of the caudal vena cava and reach the hilus of the right kidney. The left renal is shorter and arises slightly caudal to the right artery and passes directly to the hilus of the left kidney.

The **caudal mesenteric artery** arises from the aorta at the level of fourth lumbar vertebra about 12 to 15 cm caudal to the cranial mesenteric artery. It passes in the mesocolon and divides into the left colic artery for descending colon and cranial rectal artery for the cranial portion of the rectum.

The **testicular artery** is similar to that of the ox and the **ovarian artery** is similar to that of a cow.

The **lumbar (parietal) arteries** are six pairs and they are similar to those of ox in their disposition and distribution.

The **internal iliac arteries** are shorter than those of ox. It passes caudally under the wing of the sacrum, inclines ventrally on the pelvic surface of the body of the ilium and divides ventral to the lumbosacral articulation into the **caudal gluteal** and **internal pudendal** arteries.

Dog

The **coeliac artery** is very short and is related to stomach on the left, liver and adrenal gland on the right the left pancreatic lobe caudally. A small caudal phrenic and pancreatic branch arises from it before its division into the left gastric, hepatic and splenic arteries. The course and distribution of the **left gastric artery** in dog more or less resembles the artery in horse. The **hepatic artery** passes to the right under the right crus of the diaphragm and reaches to the portal fissure of the liver. Here it divides into three major branches. The **right lateral branch** supplies the right lateral lobe and the caudate lobe. The **right medial branch** supplies to the right and left medial lobes and the quadrate lobe. The **left lateral branch** supplies to the large left lateral lobe. After this division, the hepatic artery gives off right gastric artery and further continues as gastroduodenal artery. The **right gastric artery** anastomoses with the left gastric artery and supply the stomach. The **splenic artery** after its origin from the coeliac, passes to the left and lies in a groove of the left lobe of the pancreas. It supplies the skin, stomach, pancreas and the greater omentum.

The **cranial mesenteric artery**, soon after its origin from the abdominal aorta curves with its convexity facing caudally and divides into a common trunk of **middle colic**, **right colic** and **ileo-caeco-colic arteries**; and the continuing trunk the artery of small intestine thus supplies most of the parts of the small and large intestine.

The **phrenicoabdominal artery** is a paired artery and it arises from the abdominal aorta somewhere between the cranial mesenteric artery and the renal arteries. Each of these arteries soon divides into **caudal phrenic** and **abdominal arteries**. The caudal phrenic artery passes ventrally along the abdominal face extending from the corresponding crus to the sternal end of the diaphragm. The abdominal artery passes laterad crossing the psoas muscles, reaches the abdominal wall and ramifies between the external and internal oblique muscles thus supplying the abdominal wall.

The **lumbar arteries**, the parietal branches of abdominal aorta, are seven pairs in number. Of these, first six pairs arise from the dorsal surface of aorta and the seventh from the internal iliac artery. The first two or three arise from the aorta close to the hiatus aorticus of the diaphragm towards its thoracic side. The remaining arise from the abdominal side of the aorta. The course and disposition of lumbar arteries in dog is similar to that in ox and horse.

The **caudal mesenteric artery** arises from the abdominal aorta at the level of fifth lumbar vertebra. It passes caudally and ventrally and divides into the cranial and caudal branch. The cranial branch continues as **left colic artery** and supplies the middle and caudal portions of descending colon. The caudal branch continues as **cranial rectal artery** and supplies the cranial portion of the rectum.

The **renal, testicular** and **ovarian arteries** of dog resemble those of ox. The **deep circumflex iliac artery** arises from the aorta just caudal to the origin of caudal mesenteric artery at the level of sixth lumbar vertebra. Its course and distribution is same as in horse.

The internal iliac artery arises from the abdominal aorta at the level of seventh lumbar vertebra and after a short course divides into **caudal gluteal** and **internal pudendal** arteries. The further course and distribution of these arteries is similar to that of ox and horse.

Sheep and Goat

The **coeliac artery** arises from the ventral surface of the aorta between the crura of the diaphragm at the level of first lumbar vertebra in sheep and at the level of second lumbar vertebra in goat. A common trunk of coeliac and cranial mesenteric arteries occurs more often in sheep than in the goat. The hepatic artery originates from the left gastric artery. The pancreatic branches arise from hepatic, coeliac, splenic and left gastric arteries. The splenic artery arises frequently with the right ruminal artery. The epiploic branch passes from common trunk of splenic and right ruminal arteries or pancreatic branch in sheep and from splenic in goat. The left ruminal artery arises either from the left gastric or splenic artery in goat and from left gastric or right ruminal in sheep. The reticular artery arises from left ruminal or left gastric or from splenic artery both in sheep and goat. The left gastric artery is the continuation of the coeliac artery and it gives out accessory reticular artery.

The **cranial mesenteric artery** arises usually in a common trunk with the coeliac but sometimes it may have a separate origin just caudal to the origin of cranial mesenteric artery from the aorta. The distribution of branches from cranial mesenteric artery is more or less similar to that in ox.

The **caudal mesenteric artery** arises from the aorta at the level between the fifth and sixth lumbar vertebra. It supplies the descending colon and rectum similar to that in ox.

The **renal arteries** originate from the aorta between second and third lumbar vertebrae in sheep and between the third and fourth lumbar vertebrae in goat. The right renal artery arises slightly cranial to the left artery. Before entering the hilus of the kidney, each renal artery gives off the caudal adrenal and the ureteric branches.

The **testicular** or **ovarian arteries** arise from the aorta ventral to the third or fourth lumbar vertebra. The arteries in sheep arise slightly cranial to the caudal mesenteric artery and in goat they arise slightly caudal to the caudal mesenteric artery.

The **internal iliac artery**, its origin, course and distribution in sheep and goat is almost similar to that in ox.

The **lumbar (parietal) arteries** are six pairs in number and they follow the same course and distribution as that of ox.

Pig

The **coeliac artery** arises from the aorta at the level of last thoracic and first lumbar vertebrae between the crura of the diaphragm. It primarily divides into hepatic and splenic artery. The left gastric artery in pig originates as a branch of splenic as against its origin from the coeliac artery in other species. The caudal phrenic artery originates as a branch of coeliac before its division.

Hepatic artery extends to lesser curvature of stomach between the cardia and pylorus and divides into several branches which include the pancreatic branch, right lateral hepatic branch, the gastroduodenal artery, right medial hepatic branch, left hepatic branch and the right gastric artery.

The **gastroduodenal artery** after coursing ventrally through the pancreas and supplying numerous branches to it, reaches the lesser curvature of the stomach and furnishes several branches to the pyloric part of the stomach and divides into cranial pancreaticoduodenal artery and the right gastroepiploic artery.

The **right gastric artery** shortly after its origin furnishes two to four branches to the parietal surface of the stomach and extends to oesophagus.

The **splenic artery** passes to the dorsal extremity of the spleen and after furnishing several branches to spleen, gives out the **left gastric artery**, the **pancreatic branch**, and the **left gastroepiploic artery**,

The **cranial mesenteric artery** arises from the aorta ar the level of first lumbar vertebra and passes caudoventrally to the left and gives off many primary branches which includes the caudal pancreaticoduodenal artery, jejunal arteries, ileal arteries and the ileocoecocolic artery are similar to those of ox.

The **renal, testicular or ovarian** arteries, **caudal mesenteric** and the **internal iliac** arteries in pig are more or less similar to those of ox.

In addition, there is one more artery arising from the abdominal aorta in pig and it is named as the **cranial abdominal artery**. It arises on either side slightly cranial to the corresponding renal artery about the level of third lumbar vertebra. It passes to the lateral abdominal wall lying on the sublumbar muscles and divides into cranial and caudal branches. After furnishing branches to the transversus abdominis and the internal and external oblique abdominal muscles, the cranial branch anastomoses with the cranial epigastric artery and the caudal branch anastomoses with the caudal epigastric artery.

Fowl

In the absence of diaphragm, there is no demarcation between the thoracic and abdominal part of the aorta in fowl. The aorta passes caudally ventral to the vertebral column initially to the left of the median line and after reaching the cranial extremity of the kidneys it inclines to median line and continues caudally in this position. On reaching the sacrum, it divides into three branches. Two of these, (one each) are for the pelvic limbs and the third is the middle sacral artery to supply the tail region.

The **descending aorta** in its course gives out the parietal and visceral branches. The **parietal arteries** are the paired **dorsal intercostal** arteries and **lumbar intersegmental arteries**. These arteries supply the spinal cord, vertebral column, dorsal axial musculature and the overlying skin. The **ventrolateral rami** of these arteries supply the muscles of the body wall and the bones and skin in the abdominal, pelvic and tail region.

In the fowl, there are three major arteries for abdominal viscera, the coeliac and cranial mesenteric and the caudal mesenteric artery.

The **coeliac artery** begins at about the middle of the ventral surface of the lung, runs obliquely ventrad and caudad to reach the caudal aspect of the liver and divides into three branches namely the left gastric, hepatic and splenic. The left gastric artery supply the glandular and muscular stomach. The hepatic artery supplies the liver and the splenic artery supplies the spleen. The main trunk then continues as a long pancreaticoduodenal artery which supplies the pancreas and the duodenum.

The **cranial mesenteric** artery arises a little caudal to the coeliac artery, passes caudally in the mesentery and supplies the mesentery and most of the parts of the small intestine.

The paired **renal arteries** are short and enter the respective kidneys. The **testicular arteries** supply the testicles in male and the **ovarian arteries** supply the ovaries in female.

The **caudal mesenteric** artery gives out several branches to the large intestine, colon, caeca and the cloaca.

71

Caudal Vena Cava and Veins of Abdomen and Pelvis

The **caudal vena cava** is a large unpaired vein which receives blood from the pelvis, pelvic limbs, mammary glands (in females) and scrotum (in males), the abdominal walls, and the viscera of the abdomen and pelvis. It is formed under the body of the fifth or sixth lumbar vertebra by the union of two common iliac veins which in their turn are formed by the union of the internal iliac and external iliac veins of the corresponding side. It passes cranially in the sublumbar region lying slightly to the right of the median plane and to the right of the abdominal aorta. In the cranial part of the abdomen, it follows the abdominal surface of the diaphragm and is embedded in the liver prior to its entry into the thorax through the foramen vena cava in the diaphragm.

In its abdominal course, the caudal vena cava is related dorsally to the sublumbar muscles and right crus of the diaphragm, ventrally to the colon, pancreas and the liver, on its right to the right kidney and the right adrenal and on its left to the abdominal part of the aorta.

Tributaries of caudal vena cava

The **common iliac veins** are short vessels formed by the union of the internal and the external iliac veins. These are located at the level of the fifth or sixth lumbar vertebra. The left vein crosses the dorsal surface of the aorta to reach the vena cava.

The paired **middle sacral veins** are the satellites of the single middle sacral artery. These are formed by the union of the coccygeal veins and receive the sacral spinal veins along their course. They join the vena cava near its origin. Sometimes, the middle sacral veins join the internal iliac vein instead of the vena cava.

The **testicular (spermatic) veins** in male receive blood from the testicles and spermatic cords. Each of the testicular veins arises from the pampiniform plexus at the upper extremity of the testicle. It ascends through the inguinal canal along with other components of the spermatic cord, accompanies the testicular artery to the sublumbar region and join the ventral surface of the caudal vena cava about 25 mm cranial to the preceding veins. The veins of the opposite sides join the ventral surface of the vena cava separately but in close association.

The **ovarian (utero-ovarian) vein** in female is the homologue of the testicular vein of the male. It receives blood from the ovary, the cranial part of the uterine horn and the uterine tube. From the region of the ovary, the vein passes laterally in the broad ligament of the uterus near its free border and then along the abdominal wall to the sublumbar region to join the ventral surface of the vena cava.

The **renal veins** are large and thick walled. Each renal vein is formed at the hilus of the kidney by the union of several tributaries. The short right vein passes medially, cranial to the artery and enters the lateral surface of the caudal vena cava. The longer left renal vein leaves the hilus of the left kidney, passes cranially and dorsally to join the left surface of the vena cava opposite the termination of the right renal vein. The veins from the adrenal glands join the renal veins in their course.

The **hepatic veins** are entirely within the substance of the liver and reach the fossa for vena cava situated on the parietal surface of the gland and directly join the vena cava. These veins receive blood carried to liver by the portal vein and hepatic artery. During its course through the liver, a large number of small and two or three large hepatic veins open into it.

The paired **phrenic veins** are formed on the thoracic surface of the tendinous part of the diaphragm. These are horizontal and are covered by the pleura. Each of these veins is formed by tributaries from the costal part of the diaphragm. The left vein is longer than the right one. Both the veins open in the vena cava while it passes through the foramen vena cava in the diaphragm.

The **lumbar (spinal) veins** are six pairs of veins joining the dorsal surface of the caudal vena cava. The sixth pair of these veins often join the internal iliac or the common iliac artery. The lumbar veins receive blood from the loin (spinal) region.

Portal vein

The portal vein is a large venous trunk carrying blood charged with digested nutrients from stomach, intestines, pancreas and spleen to the liver. It is formed by the union of two trunks, the gastric and intestinal. The **gastric trunk** is formed by the union of right ruminal, left ruminal, splenic, reticular, left gastric (omaso-abomasal) and pancreatico-duodenal veins. **The intestinal trunk** is formed by the union of cranial and caudal mesenteric veins. After the union of gastric and intestinal trunks, the portal vein runs ventrad and craniad to the right, passes through the pancreatic notch, gains the portal fissure of the liver and divides into branches to supply the parenchyma with functional blood.

Tributaries of the gastric trunk

The **splenic vein** is a large vessel whose course except at its termination is similar to the homonymous artery. It originates in the pulp of the spleen, emerges through the hilus of the gland, passes to the right over the dorsal curvature of the rumen, receives right ruminal vein and join the gastric trunk of the portal vein.

The **right ruminal vein** originates at the cranial transverse groove on the left surface of the rumen, receives the left dorsal and ventral coronary veins and passes to the right side of the rumen with the satellite artery, is joined by the right dorsal and ventral coronary veins and also several other small veins from the right surface of the rumen and then unite with the splenic vein before its joining with the gastric trunk.

The **left gastric (omaso-abomasal) vein** is a large vessel on the cranial part of the right surface of the rumen. It begins as a small radical on the lesser curvature of the abomasum, is joined by the right gastric vein, passes dorsally and caudally towards the dorsal curvature of the omasum, runs cranially towards the reticulum, receives the gastro-epiploic vein and then the left ruminal vein and finally join the gastric trunk of the portal vein.

The **reticular vein** follows the course of the reticular artery and joins the left gastric artery.

The **left ruminal vein** originates at the caudal transverse groove on the left surface of the rumen. It passes cranially along the left longitudinal groove with its satellite artery, turns to the right surface of the rumen to join the left gastric (omaso-abomasal) vein to further unite with the gastric trunk of the portal vein.

The **pancreatic veins** join the portal vein as it passes through the gland. Some smaller veins from the pancreas form a radical that join the duodenal vein and form the pancreatico-duodenal vein that unite with the gastric trunk of the portal just before it reaches the portal fissure.

The **cranial mesenteric vein** is formed by the union of jejuno-ileal and the ileo- caeco-colic veins. A large vein thus formed follows the course of the cranial mesenteric artery. It drains the jejunum, ileum, caecum and colon and also the intestinal lymph glands.

The **caudal mesenteric vein** extends from the caudal part of the rectum to the termination of the cranial mesenteric vein. It follows the course of the cranial vesicular artery in the mesorectum and the terminal part of the colon in the colic mesentery. In the sublumbar region it passes to the right surface of the colon and terminates in the cranial mesenteric vein. It drains out the rectum, the part of the colon and the colic lymph glands.

Internal iliac vein

The internal iliac vein is the chief vein of the pelvis. It is formed at the lesser sciatic (ischiatic) foramen by the union of the internal pudendal and the caudal gluteal veins. It accompanies the internal pudendal artery and is directed cranially and dorsally on the lateral wall of the pelvis to the sublumbar region where it joins the external iliac to form the common iliac vein. It receives blood from the genital organs and the gluteal muscles.

Tributaries of the internal iliac vein

The **uterine (**middle uterine) **vein** is the chief vein for drainage of venous blood from the uterus. It is joined at its origin by the cranial uterine and caudal uterine veins thus forming a large vein that passes laterally through the broad ligament of uterus and then dorsally on the abdominal wall to its termination near the sacral promontory. During its course, it closely accompanies the uterine (middle uterine) artery.

The **cranial gluteal vein** is formed by the tributaries from the biceps femoris and gluteal muscles in the hip region of the pelvic limb that unite into one or more veins and enter the pelvic cavity through the greater sciatic foramen and join the internal iliac vein at the level of the ischiatic spine.

The **urogenital vein** joins the internal iliac near the ischiatic spine. Its tributaries are satellites of the urogenital artery. In the female it receives blood from urethra, bladder, cervix and vagina. In the male its tributaries are from bladder, pelvic urethra, prostate gland and seminal vesicles.

The **caudal gluteal vein** is formed by several veins from the biceps femoris and gluteal muscles and the external ischiatic lymph glands. It enters the pelvic cavity through the lesser sciatic (ischiatic) foramen, runs cranially and dorsally on the medial surface of the sacrosciatic ligament to join the internal iliac vein.

The **internal pudendal vein** in male begins in the perineal region, reaches the ischial arch, is joined by the dorsal vein of the penis, enters the pelvic cavity, passes along the lateral face of the levator ani and coccygeus muscle, and reaches the mid of the sacral region above the ischiatic spine to join the internal iliac nerve. In female the perineal vein is joined by the caudal mammary vein before entering the pelvic cavity. It receives tributaries from the vulva and vagina in its course to join the internal iliac vein.

Vena azygos

The left vena azygos is termed as vena hemiazygos in the ox. The right azygos is inconsistent and may occur only occasionally. It starts in the muscles of the sublumbar region at the level of the first lumbar vertebra or ventral to the last thoracic vertebra. It is joined by a branch of the first lumbar vein and then it courses cranially along the dorsal surface of the aorta and enters the thorax along with the aorta through the hiatus aorticus.

72

Comparative Anatomy of Veins of the Abdomen and Pelvis

Horse

The **caudal vena cava** in horse is largely embedded in the substance of the liver on its diaphragmatic surface. Here its free surface is covered only by the peritoneum. After crossing the liver, the caudal vena cava continues caudally along the right side of the abdominal aorta. During its course it gives off several branches from the dorsal and lateral surface.

The **lumbar veins** (parietal) are five or six pairs in number. The last one or two of these often join the internal iliac veins.

The **renal veins** are thin walled. The right renal vein is shorter than the left one.

The **phrenic veins** are two or three in number. The **circumflex iliac veins** join either the caudal vena cava or the internal iliac vein.

The **portal vein** is formed by the union of cranial and caudal mesenteric and the splenic veins in the cranial part of the sublumbar region at about the level of second lumbar vertebra. It passes cranially and to the right of the median plane continues through the portal ring of the pancreas and reaches to the portal fissure of the liver. Before entering the portal ring of the pancreas, the portal vein receives right gastroepiploic vein, right gastric vein and cranial pancreaticoduodenal vein. The cranial mesenteric, caudal mesenteric and the splenic veins are formed by the tributaries from the veins which are satellites of the branches of the respective arteries. After its entry into the hepatic portal, the portal vein divides into three principal branches. These include the right branch for right lobe, the middle branch also for the right lobe and the left branch for the left and the quadrate lobe.

The **vena azygos** is unpaired. It begins at the first lumbar vertebra and enters the thorax along the dorsal face of the aorta. The **vena hemiazygos** when present begins from the branch of the first lumbar vein and is joined by the branches from the crura of diaphragm.

Dog

The **caudal vena cava** in dog is formed by the common iliac veins at the level of the seventh lumbar vertebra. It passes cranially for a short distance along the right side of the abdominal aorta. At about the level of the second or third lumbar vertebra it leaves the company of the aorta, turns ventrally and caudally and passes between the diaphragm and the dorsal border of the liver embedded in the gland substance. As it passes along the liver, it receives two or three large and numerous small hepatic veins and then passes into the thorax through the foramen vena cava.

The **portal vein** is formed by the union of two large trunks, the gastrosplenic and the common mesenteric. The gastrosplenic trunk is formed by the union of gastric and splenic veins. The common mesenteric trunk is formed by the cranial and caudal mesenteric veins. The tributaries of these trunks and the veins are satellites of the corresponding arteries. At the portal fissure the portal vein is joined by the gastroduodenal and pancreatic veins.

The **vena azygos** begins in the abdomen by the union of the first and second lumbar veins, pass cranially on the right side of the dorsal surface of the abdominal aorta and enters the thorax.

The rest of the veins in the abdomen and pelvis of the dog are similar in the origin, course and termination as that of the ox.

Sheep and Goat

The **caudal vena cava** in sheep and goat runs parallel with and embedded completely in the dorsal border of the liver, partially resembling the caudal vena cava of the ox. Numerous veins of different calibre are received by the caudal vena cava while it passes through the substance of the liver similar to that in horse. Thereafter it passes through the foramen vena cava and enters the thorax.

The formation, tributaries and the course of different veins including the portal vein and the azygos vein in sheep and goat are more or less similar to that of ox.

Pig

The **caudal vena cava** in pig is formed by the union of left and right common iliac veins at the level of seventh lumbar vertebra. It passes cranially on the right side of the aorta, is joined by the tributaries from the viscera of the abdomen and pelvis in same manner as that in other domestic animals. After reaching at the level of first lumbar vertebra it deviates from the company of the aorta and passes ventrally and cranially and reaches the dorsal border of the liver which forms a groove for the passage of the caudal vena cava. However, this groove is comparatively shorter in pig. It is relatively shallow in its initial part. As the caudal vena cava passes through this groove, as if it passes through the tunnel of the liver. About three large and five small hepatic veins join the caudal vena cava as it passes through the liver. Immediately cranial to this, the caudal vena cava passes through the foramen vena cava and enters the thoracic cavity.

The **portal vein** in pig begins with the union of the caudal mesenteric and cranial mesenteric veins. It then traverses to the wide pancreatic ring at the portal fissure. Here it gives out the cystic vein gets itself wider and enters the liver through the portal fissure. Before traversing the pancreatic ring, the portal vein forms the ventral boundary of the epiploic foramen and receives the right gastric and gastroduodenal veins.

The **renal veins**, **testicular or ovarian veins** and the **internal iliac veins** are more or less similar to those of ox.

The left **azygos vein** in pig begins at the sublumbar region at the level of the second lumbar vertebra. At its origin it receives a branch each from the first two or three lumbar veins. It passes cranially and ventrally to the dorsal face of the aorta, receives a branch from the right and left crura of the diaphragm and continues to pass cranially through the hiatus aorticus along the dorsal face of aorta and enters the thoracic cavity. During its thoracic course it receives branches from intercostal veins and opens into the coronary sinus. Occasionally the right vena azygos also occurs in pigs. In that case it runs along the right part of the dorsal surface of aorta and joins the left azygos before its opening into the coronary sinus.

Fowl

The caudal vena cava in fowl is a very short trunk, It begins medial to the cranial extremity of the kidneys by the union of right and left common iliac veins, passes cranially embedded in the substance of the right portion of the liver, receives hepatic veins and then opens into the right atrium of the heart. It is joined by the coccygeal, internal iliac, femoral, coeco-colico-cloacal, and renal veins,

The **common iliac vein** is formed by the union of the coccygeal and the coeco-colico-cloacal veins. The median coccygeal vein passes cranially along the median line under the coccygeal vertebrae and unite with the coeco-colico-cloacal vein which conveys blood from the caeca, colon and cloaca. The trunk thus formed divides into two branches. Each of these, pass cranially and is buried deep in the substance of the caudal and middle lobes of the corresponding kidney. It then emerges through the groove between the middle and cranial lobes of the respective kidney and is joined by the internal iliac vein of the corresponding side and forms the common iliac vein. The right and left common iliac trunks thus formed receive the renal veins of the respective sides and then unite to form the caudal vena cava.

The **portal vein** is formed by the union of cranial and caudal mesenteric veins. The common mesenteric vein thus formed is then joined by the pancreatico duodenal and gastro-splenic veins and then divides into right and left branches which enter the corresponding lobe of the liver.

The vena azygos is absent in fowl.

73

Lymphatics of the Abdomen and Pelvis

The lymph nodes of the abdomen and pelvis are in two major divisions, lymph nodes of the wall of the abdomen and pelvis and those of the viscera of abdomen and pelvis. The lymph from all the lymph nodes is collected by different lymph ducts which carry and pour their contents (lymph) in the cisterna chyli near the hiatus aorticus on the abdominal surface of the diaphragm.

Lymph nodes of the wall of abdomen and pelvis

The **lumbar aortic lymph nodes** are a chain of small lymph nodes situated along the caudal part of the abdominal aorta. These lymph nodes receive afferents from the peritoneum, sublumbar, spinal and abdominal muscles and the lumbar vertebrae. The efferents from these lymph nodes join each other and form two lumbar trunks which later on unite in a single lumbar lymphatic trunk that opens into the cisterna chyli.

The **medial iliac lymph nodes** are situated near the origins of the deep circumflex iliac and the internal external iliac arteries. The afferents for these lymph nodes are received from the internal iliac, tuberal, gluteal coxal, lateral iliac, subiliac, superficial inguinal and popliteal lymph nodes. The efferents from these lymph nodes either form a lumbar trunk or join any of the lumbar aortic lymph nodes.

Lateral iliac lymph nodes are small lymph nodes which are situated in the angle between the two internal iliac arteries. In many cases they are absent. The afferents to these lymph nodes come from the coxal and subiliac lymph nodes and the efferent from this node joins the medial iliac lymph nodes.

The internal iliac lymph nodes are situated on the medial surface of the broad sacrotuberal ligament in association with the internal iliac artery and vein. The afferents of these lymph nodes are received from the sublumbar, deep inguinal, pelvic and thigh regions and the efferents from these lymph nodes open into the lumbar trunk.

The **sacral lymph nodes** are one or two small lymph nodes situated near the angle between the two internal iliac arteries ventral to psoas muscles and the sacrum. They receive afferents from these structures and the efferent from this lymph node joins the lumbar lymph trunk.

The **anorectal lymph nodes** are two or three lymph nodes of a medium size and these are situated on each side near the cranial border of the coccygeus muscle and the dorsal and lateral side of the wall of the rectum. The afferents for these nodes come from rectum, anus and the terminal part of the descending colon. The efferent goes to the medial iliac lymph nodes.

The **superficial inguinal iliac lymph nodes in female** are named as the **mammary lymph nodes.** These are large lymph nodes, situated cranial, caudal and caudodorsal to the udder.. The afferents of these lymph nodes are received from the skin of the udder and the inguinal area and the part of the vulva. **In the male**, these are named as **scrotal lymph nodes**. These are two or three glands of considerable size and are situated dorsolateral to the penis, caudal to the cremaster muscle near the external pudendal artery and vein. The afferents of these lymph nodes come from the prepuce, skin of the caudolateral and caudoventral portions of the abdomen and from the scrotum. The efferents from these lymph nodes join the medial iliac lymph nodes.

The **subiliac lymph node** is a single large lymph node situated on the cranial border of the tensor fasciae latae muscle somewhere between the tuber coxae and the patella. The afferents of this lymph node come from the skin and subcutis of the pelvis, part of the abdomen and the thigh regions. The efferent from this lymph node join the lateral and medial iliac lymph nodes.

The **coxal lymph node** is also a single large lymph node situated on the medial face of tensor fasciae latae muscle, ventral to the tuber coxae and cranial to the proximal part of quadriceps femoris muscle. The afferents for this lymph node come from the skin and subcutis of the hip region and its efferent join the medial or lateral iliac lymph node.

The **gluteal lymph node** is a large usually single lymph node situated on the lateral face of the broad sacrotuberal ligament, dorsal to the caudal gluteal vessels. It receives afferents from the biceps femoris and the gluteal muscles and the adjoining area and its efferent join the medial iliac lymph node.

The **tuberal lymph node** is inconsistent and if present is situated on the medial side of the ischiatic tuber near the attachment of broad sacrotuberal ligament. The afferents of this lymph node comes from the tail and the skin near the tuber ischii. The efferent join the medial and internal iliac lymph nodes.

The **ischiatic lymph nodes** are small one to three lymph nodes situated near the greater sciatic foramen on the medial face of the middle gluteus muscle. The afferents of these lymph nodes are received from the gluteal muscles and other muscles, in that area. The efferents from these nodes join the medial iliac lymph nodes.

Lymph nodes of the Viscera of abdomen and pelvis

The **atrial lymph nodes** are situated on the visceral surface of the atrium ruminis just caudal to the cardia of the rumen.

The **ruminal lymph nodes** are present at three different locations on the rumen. These include two or three small **right ruminal lymph nodes** present in the right ruminal groove. Another two or three small **left ruminal lymph nodes** present in the left ruminal groove and the third group of **cranial ruminal lymph nodes** present in the cranial transverse groove of the rumen. All these lymph nodes are connected with each other by small lymphatics which finally join the gastric trunk.

The **reticular lymph nodes** are small one or two nodes situated on the reticulo-omasal junction. Its efferent is connected to the omasal lymph node.

The **omasal lymph nodes** are one or two small lymph nodes situated in the omasum along the course of the left gastric vessels. Their efferents join the gastric trunk.

The **abomasal lymph nodes** are the dorsal abomasal lymph nodes situated along the greater curvature and the ventral abomasal lymph nodes are situated along the lesser curvature of the abomasum. The efferents from these join the gastric lymphatic trunk.

The **pancreatico duodenal** lymph nodes are situated on the ventral surface of the pancreas and along its right part in relation to the duodenum. The efferents from these lymph nodes join the hepatic lymph nodes.

The **hepatic lymph nodes** are situated in the portal fissure. These are a group of two to four small nodes around the hepatic portal vein. The efferents from these lymph nodes join the gastric lymphatic trunk which finally opens into the cisterna chyli.

The **jejunal lymph nodes** are two or three large, long and narrow lymph nodes in the peripheral part of the mesentery. In addition, there is a chain of numerous small lymph nodes which lie in the mesentery and extend from there to the coils of the jejunum. The afferents for these lymph nodes are received from the jejunum and ilium and the efferents from these form the jejunal lymphatic trunk.

The **caecal lymph nodes** are small two or three lymph nodes situated on the ilio-caecal ligament. The afferents for these nodes come from the ileum and caecum. The efferents from these join the jejunal trunk.

The **colic lymph nodes** include a group of small lymph nodes placed at two locations. One of these is on the right side of the spiral mass of the colon and the other is situated deeply between the coils. The afferents are from the colon, caecum and ilium and the efferents join the jejunal trunk.

The caudal mesenteric lymphocentre is connected with two to three small elongated **caudal mesenteric lymph nodes** situated near the origin of the caudal mesenteric artery. In addition, there are a few small lymph nodes lying in the mesentery along the branches of the caudal mesenteric artery. The afferents for these lymph nodes come from the descending colon and their efferents open into the lumbar aortic and medial iliac lymph nodes.

Lymphatic trunk and ducts in abdomen and pelvis

The lumbar lymphatic trunks are formed by the union of the efferent lymph vessels from the lumbar aortic and the iliosacral lymphocentres at the level of iliac quadrification. From here, the right and the left lumbar trunk pass cranially along the ventral surface of the caudal vena cava and the abdominal aorta and join the cisterna chyli on the dorsal surface of the aorta at the hiatus aorticus. During their course towards the cisterna chyli, these trunks are joined by the caudal mesenteric, jejunal, cranial mesenteric, renal, hepatic and gastric (coeliac) trunks.

Cisterna chyli

The cisterna chyli is a reservoir for the lymph and is formed by the union of lumbar aortic and the gastro-duodenal lymphatic trunks. It is an elongated, fusiform dilatation situated at the hiatus aorticus dorsal to the aorta and ventral to the last thoracic or first lumbar vertebra. It is about 1.5 to 2.0 cm wide. Cranially it continues as thoracic duct which opens into the common jugular vein or the cranial vena cava.

74

Comparative Anatomy of Lymphatics of Abdomen and Pelvis

Horse

Lymph nodes of the wall of abdomen and pelvis

The **lumbar aortic lymph nodes** extend from kidneys to the deep circumflex iliac vessels. These are not clearly distinguishable from the cranial and caudal mesenteric, renal, testicular or ovarian, uterine and iliac lymph nodes.

The **internal iliac lymph nodes** are placed at about the origin of the iliac arteries. The external iliac lymph nodes are several small nodes situated in the triangular space between the cranial and caudal branches of the circumflex iliac artery.

The **deep (internal) inguinal lymph node** is not abdominal in position. It is not situated at the pelvic brim. It is one of the group of the lymph nodes of the hind limb.

The **superficial (external) inguinal lymph nodes** are on either side of the penis and in front of the superficial inguinal ring in male and above the mammary glands as the supramammary lymph nodes in female.

The **prefemoral lymph nodes** are about a dozen small glands arranged in an elongated mass placed on the medial aspect of the cranial border of tensor fasciae lata and on the caudal branch of circumflex iliac artery.

The **sacral lymph nodes** are small and lie along the ventral face of the lateral border of the sacrum.

Lymph nodes of the viscera of abdomen and pelvis

The **coeliac lymph nodes** are situated on the coeliac artery and they extend along the branches of this artery. There are three main groups of these lymph nodes. These are the gastric, hepatic and splenic. The gastric lymph nodes are present on the lesser curvature below the cardia, on the saccus caecus under the pancreas and below the pylorus. The efferents from these go to the common gastric trunk or join the splenic lymph node. The hepatic lymph nodes are similar in position to those of ox. The splenic lymph nodes are lodged in the hilus of the spleen along the course of the splenic artery. The pancreatic and duodenal lymph nodes are associated with the right gastric and the gastroepiploic arteries. The efferents from these lymph nodes join the gastric trunk which open into the cisterna chyli.

The **mesenteric or jejuno-ileal lymph nodes** are present along the parietal border or the root of the mesentery. The caecal and colic lymph nodes are present on the corresponding arteries. The efferents from these lymph nodes join the common intestinal trunk which opens into the cisterna chyli.

The **anorectal lymph nodes** are placed along the dorsal face of the rectum. The efferent from these nodes join the intestinal trunk.

Dog

Lymph nodes of the wall of abdomen and pelvis

The **lumbar aortic lymph nodes** are number of small lymph nodes placed in the sublumbar region around the abdominal aorta and caudal vena cava. Most of these are embedded in fat.

The **internal iliac lymph nodes** are paired. The right nodes are placed in relation to the right common iliac vein and caudal to the caudal vena cava. The left one are placed along the abdominal aorta and the left common iliac vein.

The **external iliac lymph nodes** are placed on the ventral face of psoas minor between the external and internal iliac veins of corresponding side.

The **deep (internal) inguinal, prefemoral and ischiatic lymph nodes are absent in dog**.

The **superficial (external) inguinal lymph nodes** in male are called the scrotal lymph nodes and are placed on either side of the penis and cranial to the spermatic cord. In the female, these are called the mammary lymph nodes and are situated on the dorsolateral side of the mammary glands.

The **anorectal lymph nodes** are absent and the **sacral lymph nodes** are situated along the middle sacral artery.

Lymph nodes of the viscera of abdomen and pelvis

The **gastric lymph nodes** are placed on the lesser curvature of the stomach near the pylorus. The **duodenal lymph nodes** are present along the gastroduodenal vein at its origin in relation with the cranial angle of the pancreas. The **hepatic lymph node** is placed on the left side of the portal vein. The **splenic lymph node** lies on the splenic vein or on its root. The **pancreaticoduodenal lymph nodes** are small and appear inconsistently on the first flexure of the duodenum.

The **mesenteric lymph nodes** are elongated and they lie on the cranial mesenteric artery and vein. The **caecal lymph node** is present on the caecal vein and the small **colic lymph nodes** lie on the mesocolon along the transverse colic and left colic veins.

The **renal lymph nodes** are placed on the corresponding side of the aorta close to the origin of the renal artery of the corresponding side.

Sheep and Goat

Lymph nodes of the wall of abdomen and pelvis

The **lumbar aortic lymph nodes** are several small lymph nodes scattered on the dorsolateral aspect of the abdominal aorta and the dorsal surface of caudal vena cava ventral to the bodies of the lumbar vertebrae, lateral to the lumbar arteries, and between the psoas minor and abdominal aorta.

The **internal iliac lymph nodes** are placed in the angle between the external iliac vessels, abdominal aorta and caudal vena cava.

The **anorectal lymph nodes** are two or three lying ventrally on the retroperitoneal part of the rectum.

The **hypogastric lymph nodes** are placed along the course of internal iliac vessels caudal to the wing of ilium extending between the greater and lesser ischiatic notches. The afferents of these lymph nodes come from the pelvic wall and the pelvic organs. The efferents join the iliac lymph nodes or the lumbar trunk.

The **superficial inguinal** and **deep inguinal** lymph nodes are similar to those of ox.

The **ischiatic lymph nodes** are inconsistent. When present, they are placed along the broad sacrotuberal ligament.

The **tuberal lymph node** is variably present along the medial aspect of the tuber ischi.

Lymph nodes of the viscera of abdomen and pelvis

Coeliac lymph nodes are two or three and they lie along the coeliac artery close to its origin from the aorta.

The **atrial lymph nodes** are present on the visceral surface of atrium ruminis, immediately caudal to the cardia of the rumen. These receive afferents from the rumen, reticulum, spleen, omasum, abomasum and pancreas. The efferents open into the gastric trunk or directly into the cisterna chyli.

The **right ruminal, left ruminal, reticular, omasal and the dorsal and ventral abomasal** lymph nodes are similar to those of ox.

The **cranial ruminal** and **rumino-abomasa**l lymph nodes are absent.

The **hepatic lymph nodes** lie close to the hilus of the liver, between the caudate and papillary processes. They are related to the portal vein and hepatic artery. The accessory hepatic lymph nodes are absent. The pancreatico-duodenal lymph nodes are similar to those of the ox.

The **cranial mesenteric and caudal mesenteric lymph nodes** of sheep and goat resemble to those of ox.

Pig

Lymph nodes of the wall of abdomen and pelvis

The **lumbar aortic lymph nodes** are several small lymph nodes spread along the ventral and lateral sides of the abdominal aorta and caudal vena cava. These are difficult to distinguish cranially from the renal lymph nodes and caudally from the medial iliac lymph nodes. The afferents for these lymph nodes come from the muscles of lumbosacral region and the dorsal half of the abdominal wall, the peritoneum, the urogenital organs, the renal, phrenicoabdominal, caudal mesenteric and the lateral and medial iliac lymph nodes. The efferents join the lumbar trunk or directly to the cisterna chyli.

The **renal lymph nodes** occur in association with the renal vessels close to their origin from the aorta.

The **phrenico-abdominal lymph nodes** lie caudal to the caudal branch of phrenico-abdominal artery and vein. The afferents come from the peritoneum, abdominal muscles and lateral iliac lymph nodes. The efferents open into the lumbar aortic or the renal lymph nodes.

The **testicular lymph nodes are** located along the spermatic cord in association with the testicular vessels. Some of these are on the pampiniform plexus.

The **medial and lateral iliac lymph nodes** are situated cranial and caudal to the origin of deep circumflex iliac artery along the medial and lateral aspects of the internal and external iliac vessels.

The **anorectal lymph nodes** are present on the dorsolateral surface of the retroperitoneal part of the rectum. The uterine lymph node is present in the cranial part of the broad ligament of uterus associated with the utero-ovarian vessels.

The **superficial inguinal lymph nodes** of male are named as scrotal lymph nodes and those of female are called the mammary lymph nodes. The scrotal lymph nodes are situated on the ventral side of the abdominal wall, lateral to the penis. The mammary lymph nodes are located ventral to the cranial branches of the external pudendal vessels.

The **ischiatic lymph node** is situated on the lateral side of the broad sacrotuberal ligament.

The **sacral lymph nodes** are located in the angle formed by the internal iliac vessels near the origin of the medial sacral artery.

Lymph nodes of the viscera of abdomen and pelvis

The **gastric, lymph nodes** are situated at the cardia of the stomach and are associated with the right gastric artery. The **hepatic lymph nodes** are situated about the portal vein at the portal fissure. The **splenic lymph nodes** are associated with the splenic vessels. The **pancreaticoduodenal lymph nodes** are associated with the pancreaticoduodenal artery and are located between the duodenum and pancreas. The **coeliac lymph nodes** are present along the coeliac artery near its origin from the aorta,

The **cranial mesenteric lymph nodes** are located along the cranial mesenteric artery. These are associated with the **jejunal, ileo-caeco-colic** and **right colic lymph nodes**. The **caudal mesenteric lymph nodes** are located along the descending colon to the rectogenital fold of peritoneum.

FOWL

The lymph nodes are absent in fowl.

SECTION-D

NERVES

75

Nerves of the Wall of Abdomen and Pelvis

Lumbar nerves

There are **six pairs** of lumbar spinal nerves. Each of these, after emerging out of the intervertebral foramen, gives out firstly a **meningeal branch** which reenters the vertebral canal through the intervertebral foramen and supplies the meninges. Next to this it furnishes the **ramus communicans** to the sympathetic chain ganglion. After this, the lumbar spinal nerves divide into dorsal and ventral branches. The **dorsal branches** are smaller and they supply the muscles and skin on the loins and croup. The **ventral branches** are larger and they slightly differ from each other in their course and distribution. In their initial course, they pass under the psoas minor and psoas major muscles emerge at the lateral border of the psoas major and supply branches to the sublumbar muscles. Hereafter, they differ in their course and distribution.

The **ventral branch of the first lumbar nerve** passes on the medial face of the quadratus lumborum, runs down the medial face of the transversus abdominis, the obliquus abdominis internus and externus and finally reaches the rectus abdominis, supply all these muscles and the skin on the lateral wall and the floor of the abdomen.

The **ventral branch of the second lumbar nerve** has two divisions. The cranial division passes ventrally and caudally to reach the external angle of the ilium, supplies branches to the oblique muscles of the abdomen and the skin over this region and terminates in the rectus abdominis muscle. The caudal division passes caudally and laterally under the quadratus lumborum, supplies branches to the muscles and skin at the flank region and then crosses the circumflex iliac vessels. Here it joins a similar branch of the third lumbar nerve and forms the **genitofemoral nerve**.

The **ventral branch of third lumbar nerve** penetrates the psoas muscles, passes caudally under the quadratus lumborum, arrives at the level of the bifurcation of circumflex iliac vessels, gives off muscular branches to the iliopsoas, obliquus internus and cremaster muscles, crosses the circumflex iliac vessels and then passes ventrally in front of the external iliac vessel and is joined by the caudal branch of the second lumbar nerve with which it forms the **genitofemoral nerve**.

The **genitofemoral nerve** formed by the union of branches of the second and third lumbar nerves at the medial face of the circumflex iliac vessels passes caudoventrally in front of the external iliac vessels and divides into cranial and caudal branches. The **caudal branch** continues along the femoral vessels and become the lateral cutaneous muscle of the thigh. The **cranial branch** runs ventrally on the external surface of the peritoneum and reaches the deep inguinal ring on the floor of the abdomen. Here it passes through the inguinal canal and emerges through the superficial inguinal ring as the external genital nerve. This nerve **in male** supplies the scrotum, superficial inguinal lymph node, prepuce and skin. **In the female**, it supplies the mammary glands and the mammary lymph nodes.

The **ventral branch of the fourth lumbar nerve** penetrates the psoas minor muscle and divides into the cranial and caudal branch. The cranial branch passes caudally on the iliopsoas and is continued as the lateral cutaneous nerve of the thigh. The caudal branch passes caudally and ventrally under the psoas major and contributes to the formation of the lumbosacral plexus.

The **ventral branch of the fifth and sixth lumbar nerves** chiefly contributes to the formation of the lumbosacral plexus along the medial aspect of the iliopsoas muscle. In addition, a branch from each of the fourth, fifth and sixth nerves contribute to form the **great crural** and **obturator nerves**.

Sacral nerves

There are **five pairs** of sacral spinal nerves. These nerves divide into dorsal and ventral branches within the vertebral canal. The **dorsal branches** of these nerves exit through the dorsal sacral foramina and they supply the muscles and skin of the croup. A branch (dorsolateral) each from the first, second and third nerve innervate the medial part of the gluteal region by their cutaneous branches and these are called as the **middle clunial nerves.** The branches from the fourth and fifth nerves innervate the base of the tail and the tail region. The **ventral branches** of the sacral spinal nerves pass through the ventral sacral foramina and the space between the last sacral segment and the first coccygeal vertebra. These nerves give off the **rami communicantes** to the sympathetic chain ganglia of the sacral part of the sympathetic trunk. The ventral branches of the first and second sacral nerves are large and they pass towards the greater sciatic foramen and converge to form a wide band that joins the caudal part of the lumbosacral plexus. The ventral division of third sacral nerve occasionally joins this plexus. The ventral branches of third, fourth and fifth sacral nerves unite together and form the **pudendal** and the **caudal rectal nerves**.

The **pudendal nerve** passes caudally and ventrally on the medial surface of the sacrosciatic (sacroischiatic) ligament towards the ischiatic arch, gives off branches to the urinary bladder, urethra and the rectum and the muscles and skin around the anus. On reaching the ischial arch, the distribution and further course of pudendal nerve differs in the male and female animals. In the male, it supplies branches to the erecter penis muscle, corpus cavernosum and urethra, then turns around the ischial arch, lies here close to the nerve of the opposite side, descends in a flexuous manner on the dorsum of the penis as the dorsal nerve of the penis, reaches the glans penis. In this course, the nerve breaks into numerous branches to supply its erectile tissue and the skin around the penis. In the female, it supplies branches to the vulva and terminates in the clitoris. Before its termination, it gives off the mammary branch that turns round the ischial arch, passes through the perineal region and reaches to the mammary glands (udder) to supply the muscles and skin around the udder.

The **caudal rectal nerve** passes ventrally and caudally above the pudendal nerve and supplies the rectum and then terminates in the muscles and skin of the anus.

Coccygeal nerves

The coccygeal nerves are five or six pairs which arise from the terminal part of the spinal cord at about the middle of the sacrum. The division of the coccygeal nerves in the dorsal and ventral branches occurs in the subarachnoid space. Both the divisions run caudally inside the sacral canal along with the sacral nerves and gets exit through the caudal intervertebral foramina caudal to the corresponding coccygeal vertebra. After emerging through the foramina, the dorsal and ventral branches connect with each other forming a dorsal and ventral caudal plexus extending to the tip of the tail. These plexuses supply the branches to the dorsal and ventral coccygeal muscles. The coccygeal nerves are not connected with the sympathetic chain.

76

Autonomic Nerves of Viscera of Abdomen and Pelvis

Abdominal part

The sympathetic trunks enter the abdominal cavity between the psoas minor and the crus of the diaphragm of the corresponding side. They run caudally on the ventrolateral surfaces of the lumbar vertebrae and the ventral common vertebral ligament. The left trunk is ventrally related to the abdominal aorta and the right trunk to the caudal vena cava. The sympathetic trunks of the opposite sides in the cranial half of the lumbar part lie rather close to each other and as they pass caudally, they gradually divert from each other. The lumbar sympathetic ganglia are small spindle shaped usually six in number and are present one in each lumbar segment. The first two are larger than the rests. Each is connected with the ventral division of the corresponding lumbar spinal nerve by the ramus communicans. The interganglionic segments of the sympathetic trunk are usually single but some times they split.

Splanchnic nerves

The **greater (major) splanchnic nerve** is formed by the contribution of sympathetic nerve fibres from fifth or sixth thoracic to thirteenth thoracic sympathetic ganglia. It becomes larger and larger as it passes caudally along with the sympathetic trunk. It enters the abdomen at the level of the first lumbar vertebra gets separated from it, passes ventrally and laterally across the aorta (left trunk) and vena cava (right trunk) to join the coeliacomesenteric autonomic plexus on and around the coeliac and cranial mesenteric arteries.

The **lesser (minor) splanchnic nerve** is recognized as the **cranial lumbar splanchnic nerve** and is formed bilaterally by the sympathetic fibres extending from first two lumbar sympathetic ganglia. The sympathetic fibres from the first lumbar sympathetic ganglion, joins the fibres from the second lumbar sympathetic ganglion and a single trunk thus formed crosses the dorsolateral surface of the aorta (left nerve) and the caudal vena cava (right nerve) and the nerves of the two sides unite and join the major splanchnic nerve on and around the coeliac and cranial mesenteric arteries.

The **caudal lumbar splanchnic nerve** is formed by the fibres received from the third, fourth and fifth lumbar sympathetic ganglia. The nerves from each of these ganglia run caudally and ventrally along the abdominal aorta (on left side) and caudal vena cava (on right side) and reach the caudal mesenteric artery to join the caudal mesenteric autonomic plexus.

The **splanchnic nerve** fibres **from the sixth lumbar sympathetic ganglion** on either side run caudally along with the sympathetic trunk and deviate from it laterally at the level of first sacral segment to join the pelvic plexus.

Abdominal autonomic plexuses

The major autonomic plexuses in the abdominal cavity are the coeliac, cranial mesenteric or the coeliacomesenteric and caudal mesenteric plexuses. In addition, there are some specific small plexuses in the abdominal cavity. These are the renal plexus, aorticorenal plexus, adrenal plexus, testicular (in male), ovarian (in female) and the intermesenteric or the abdominal aortic plexus.

Coeliacomesenteric plexus

The coeliacomesenteric plexus is the largest of the autonomic plexuses in the abdominal cavity. It is a defused mass of dense fibrous network surrounding the origins of the coeliac and cranial mesenteric arteries. The paired round coeliac ganglia and a single elongated cranial mesenteric ganglion are enmeshed in this plexus. These three ganglia are connected to each other by ganglionated cords. The greater and lesser splanchnic nerves join this plexus and contribute the sympathetic fibres for this plexus and its ganglia. The parasympathetic fibres reach to this plexus through the vagus nerve. The dorsal and ventral vagal trunks enter the abdomen along with the oesophagus, reach the atrium ruminis of the rumen, gets separated from the oesophagus, turns upward, reach the coeliac and cranial mesenteric arteries and join the coeliacomesenteric autonomic plexus. The sympathetic and parasympathetic nerve fibres from this plexus are distributed to run along the branches of the coeliac and cranial mesenteric arteries and supply most of the visceral organs in the abdominal cavity. The autonomic nerves from this plexus are supplied to rumen, reticulum, omasum, abomasum, duodenum, jejunum, ileum, caecum, colon, liver, spleen **and pancreas.**

Renal plexus

The renal plexus is an extensive loosely dispersed fibrous network surrounding bilaterally the renal arteries. The part of this plexus extends to the adrenal glands of the corresponding side. The renal plexus receives fibres from the coeliacomesenteric plexus and coeliac and cranial mesenteric ganglia, the lesser splanchnic nerve. The nerve fibres from this plexus accompany the renal vessels to the hilus of the kidney and the ureter.

Aorticorenal plexus

The aorticorenal plexus and ganglia is an extension of the renal plexus and it extends along the renal arteries and the part of the aorta at the place of origin of the renal arteries.

Testicular plexus

The testicular plexus (in male) lies along the testicular arteries and it receives contribution from second to fifth lumbar splanchnic nerves. A distinct testicular ganglion is enmeshed inside this plexus. The autonomic nerves from this plexus are supplied to the testes, epididymis and the vas deferens.

Ovarian plexus

The ovarian plexus (in female) is the homologue of the testicular plexus that is formed on the ovarian (uteroovarian) artery and receives contribution from the sources almost similar to those of the testicular plexus. The visceral branches from this plexus accompany the corresponding arterial branches and form the subplexuses as ovarian plexus, tubal plexus and cranial uterine plexus.

Caudal mesenteric plexus

The caudal mesenteric plexus is a dense fibrous network of autonomic nerves around the caudal mesenteric artery. It receives nerve fibres from the third to fifth lumbar spinal nerves, lesser splanchnic nerve, testicular plexus and coeliacomesenteric plexus. The parasympathetic nerve fibres reach this plexus from the vagus nerve through the fibres extending from the coeliacomesenteric plexus. The caudal mesenteric ganglion is small but a distinct ganglion situated caudal to the caudal mesenteric artery. The distribution of autonomic nerves from this plexus is by way of the arterial branches of the caudal mesenteric artery. This comprise the innervation to the terminal part of the large intestine, the hypogastric nerve to the pelvic plexus, intermesenteric plexus connecting the cranial mesenteric ganglion, nerve fibres to the external and internal iliac plexuses and some fibres to testicular or ovarian plexus. The fibres from the internal iliac plexus extend to the cranial vesicular, middle uterine and ureteric plexuses.

Pelvic part

The pelvic (sacral) part of the sympathetic trunk is the caudal continuation of the abdominal part and it gradually diminishes in thickness from first to fifth sacral segment. The trunks of the opposite sides become more and more close to each other as they course along the pelvic surface of the sacrum, medial to the ventral sacral foramina. The interganglionic segments of the trunk are usually split. The sacral sympathetic ganglia are five in number on each side. They are relatively large and round or oblong shaped. The first ganglion is largest and the remaining ganglia gradually diminish in size from second to fifth. The rami communicantes arise from the external surface of each ganglion and after coursing slightly obliquely join the ventral division of the corresponding sacral spinal nerve at the ventral sacral foramina. The transverse branches form connections between the ganglia of the opposite sides.

Pelvic autonomic plexuses

The pelvic plexus is an extensive network of autonomic nerve fibres formed on the ventrolateral aspect of the rectogenital pouch. The ganglionic cells are scattered throughout the meshwork of the plexus. The pelvic nerves extend from each ganglion and after coursing a short distance caudally with the interganglionic trunk divert ventrolaterally, coalesce and form two or three pelvic nerves of considerable size that join the pelvic plexus on the rectogenital pouch. In addition, the right and left hypogastric nerves extend from the caudal mesenteric plexus and ganglion, pass medial to the umbilical artery and after reaching at the level of first or second sacral segment splits and joins the pelvic sympathetic nerves to reach the pelvic plexus. The nerve fibres from the pelvic plexus are distributed to the caudal uterine, caudal ureteric and the urogenital plexuses.

Coccygeal part

The coccygeal (caudal) part of the sympathetic trunk passes caudally along the median coccygeal artery. The left and right trunks pass almost parallel and close to each other on the ventral surface of the coccygeal vertebrae and finally join each other at the impar ganglion at the fourth coccygeal vertebra. Each trunk bears at least four small ganglia one each at each segment. Beyond this a single trunk continues caudal to the impar ganglion up to the level of sixth coccygeal vertebra but it does not bear any ganglion. The rami communicantes from the coccygeal ganglia extend transversely or obliquely from the lateral aspect of each coccygeal ganglion and join the ventral division of the corresponding coccygeal spinal nerve. The visceral nerve fibres from these ganglia form the ventral coccygeal plexus.

77

Comparative Anatomy of Nerves of Abdomen and Pelvis

Horse

There are six pairs of lumbar, five pairs of sacral and five pairs of coccygeal spinal nerves in horse. Their origin, course and distribution is in general similar to those in ox.

The number of sympathetic lumbar and coccygeal ganglia is just the same in horse as that of ox. However, the number of sacral sympathetic ganglia is four in horse as against five ganglia of ox.

The **greater (major) splanchnic nerve** in horse is formed by the fibres received from sixth or seventh to fourteenth or fifteenth thoracic sympathetic ganglia. It is smaller in its cranial thoracic part but as it proceeds caudally it gradually increases in size so much that it becomes larger than the thoracic sympathetic trunk in the caudal thoracic part. It receives a communicating branch from the lesser splanchnic nerve before terminating in the coeliacomesenteric ganglion.

The **lesser (minor) splanchnic nerve** is formed by fibres received from the last three or four thoracic and the first two lumbar sympathetic ganglia. It communicates with the greater splanchnic nerve and the renal and adrenal plexuses and terminates in the coeliac plexus and ganglion.

The rest of the features of spinal nerves and autonomic plexuses of the abdomen and pelvis in horse are almost similar to those of ox except those related to the distribution of fibres to the parts of ruminant versus simple stomach.

Dog

There are seven pairs of lumbar, three pairs of sacral and three pairs of coccygeal nerves in dog. Their origin, course and distribution is in general same as that of ox and horse.

There are seven lumbar and three sacral sympathetic ganglia in dog.

The **greater splanchnic nerve** arise from the twelfth or thirteenth thoracic ganglion, enters the abdomen between the lumbar parts of the diaphragm and the psoas minor and joins the adrenal ganglion which is placed above and in continuation with the coeliac ganglion.

The **lesser splanchnic nerve** is contributed by the fibres from last thoracic and first lumbar sympathetic ganglia and terminates in the adrenal plexus.

The rest of the features are similar to those of ox except those related to the differences due to simple stomach.

Sheep and Goat

The origin, disposition and distribution of lumbar, sacral and coccygeal spinal nerves in sheep and goat is similar to that of ox.

The sympathetic as well as parasympathetic (autonomic) nerve supply to the wall and the viscera of the abdomen and pelvis almost resembles to that in ox.

Pig

There are six pairs of lumbar, four pairs of sacral and six pairs of coccygeal nerves in pig. Their origin, course and distribution is in general same as that of ox and horse.

The **sympathetic trunk** enters the abdominal cavity after traversing the lumbocostal arch.

The abdominal segment of the trunk is fairly uniform in thickness throughout its length. The interganglionic trunk is single. Usually there are six lumbar, four sacral and three coccygeal sympathetic ganglia.

The **greater splanchnic nerve** is formed by the fibres contributed by sixth or seventh to fourteenth or fifteenth thoracic ganglia. It separates distinctly from sympathetic trunk at the level of fourteenth or fifteenth thoracic vertebra, enters the abdominal cavity along the aorta and terminates at the adrenal and coeliacomesenteric plexus. The **lumbar splanchnic nerves** from the first two lumbar sympathetic ganglia extend to join the coeliacomesenteric plexus. There is no **lesser splanchnic nerve** in pig.

The rest of the features of abdominal and pelvic plexuses in pig are similar to those in ox.

Fowl

There are fourteen lumbosacral spinal nerves in fowl. The formation, course and distribution of these nerves and their communication with the sympathetic trunks by rami communicantes is similar to that in mammals. Though the coccygeal nerves are present, they are very small and not so well developed like that in mammals.

The **sympathetic trunks** run bilaterally ventral to the synsacrum. The sympathetic **ganglia** of the trunk are connected with the spinal nerves of the corresponding segments. The sympathetic chains are connected with the **plexuses** from which branches are distributed to the circulatory, digestive, respiratory, urinary and genital organs.

SECTION-E
APPLIED ANATOMY

78

Applied Anatomy of Abdomen and Pelvis

Surface anatomy of the organs of left side of abdominal cavity

Rumen

Topography of the rumen: The left side of the abdomen in cow is completely occupied by the rumen except for a small area occupied by the reticulum at its cranial end and the spleen on the craniodorsal aspect sandwiched between the dorsal border of rumen and the diaphragm. The rumen lies in contact with the left abdominal wall extending from seventh or eight intercostal space where it touches the diaphragm to the transverse plane of the tuber coxae where it almost touches the pelvic inlet.

Palpation of rumen: The rumen can be palpated in the left flank of the abdomen and is usually palpated in the dorsal third of the flank region. In ruminants, the contraction begins at reticulum and it continues in rumen in succession and hence is considered as ruminoreticular contraction cycle. It begins with double contraction of reticulum followed immediately by the contraction of rumen. The rumen contraction begins in the cranial sac and progresses to the dorsal sac and then to the ventral sac. During the contraction of the ventral sac, the dorsal sac is forced out which appears as a bulging at the paralumbar fossa. After this, there is a pause of 30 seconds and thereafter the second ruminal contraction begins which is usually associated with eructation. The ruminoreticular contraction cycle ends with the end of second ruminal contraction. Following this, the second cycle begins. Thus there are two palpable rumen contractions per minute. This rate of contraction increases to 2.8 contractions per minute during the act of feeding of the animal.

Percussion and Auscultation: The percussion at the upper third of the left flank gives a slight resonance while in the middle third it becomes dull. During auscultation, a churning sound is heard at the end of each rumen contraction. This sound gradually reaches to peak and then recedes.

Surgical intervention: **Ruminotomy** is performed in the left paralumbar fossa usually under local anaesthetic infiltration. The incision goes through the skin, fascia and the obliquus abdominis externus, obliquus abdominis internus and the transversus abdominis muscles and lastly the peritoneum (omentum) in that sequence from outside to inside. Cutting through these layers will open the abdominal cavity. After reaching the abdominal cavity, the ruminal wall is incised to open the dorsal sac of the rumen.

Site for skin incision: A vertical incision of about 20 cm in length (height) is made beginning at about 3 to 4 cm below the transverse process of lumbar vertebra and about 3 to 5 cm caudal and parallel to the last rib in the left paralumbar fossa (left flank).

Reticulum

Topography of reticulum

The reticulum lies between the diaphragm and rumen extending from sixth to eighth rib. The mucous membrane of the reticulum is raised into folds of about 1.5 cm and encloses within them 4 to 6 sided cells giving the mucous membrane the honey comb like appearance. This organ can not be palpated. It is in contact with the left abdominal wall at the ventral ends of the sixth and seventh intercostal spaces. In traumatic gastritis, pain is indicated after applying deep pressure in the area of left xiphoid region. In auscultation of reticulum, a sound of liquid or gas in motion can be heard in the left xiphoid region at the ventral end of sixth and seventh intercostal spaces. In traumatic reticulitis a grunt of pain is associated with contraction of reticulum.

Applications of anatomical position and structure in case of TRP in cow

The traumatic reticulopericarditis (TRP) is usually caused by ingestion of sharp metallic objects. The sharp metal objects such as nails or pieces of wire are ingested along with feed travels to rumen and then are pushed into the reticulum. These objects are trapped and settled into the honeycomb like mucous membrane of the wall of the reticulum. The contraction of the reticulum causes these objects to perforate its wall and reach the peritoneum resulting in irritation and then inflammation of peritoneum. In some cases, further contraction of the reticulum causes to push the object deep into the diaphragm and then pierces the pericardium which is in close contact with the thoracic surface of the diaphragm. This leads to pericarditis. Since this type of pericarditis is developed due to injury to pericardium that is caused by sharp object reaching there through reticulum, this syndrome is called the traumatic reticulopericarditis. The indications of this syndrome are fever, anorexia and lethargy. Auscultation of abdomen indicates ruminoreticular atony. The treatment of this syndrome includes removal of the sharp objects physically from the reticular wall accessing it through rumen by surgical procedure of ruminotomy.

Spleen

Topography of spleen

The spleen, **in ox,** extends from the dorsal end of the last two ribs to the costochondral junction of the seventh and eight rib on the left abdominal wall. Clinical examination from outside the body wall (percussion, auscultation and palpation) of spleen is difficult. In exceptional cases it may be explored at the costochondral junction of the seventh and eight ribs. The splenic puncture is performed in the left twelth intercostal space at the level of tuber coxae.

In **horse,** the spleen can be examined by percussion and auscultation at the area extending from dorsal end of left seventeenth intercostal space to the middle and ventral thirds of tenth intercostal space.

Surface anatomy of the organs of right side of the abdominal cavity

Omasum

The omasum is in contact with the right abdominal wall at the ventral part of seventh to eleventh ribs and on the abdominal floor at a small area between the xiphoid cartilage and costochondral cartilages.

Palpation of omasum can not be done because of its position inside the rib cage between seventh to eleventh ribs of the right abdominal wall. However, it can be palpated through the wall of the rumen during ruminotomy. In the condition of traumatic peritonitis, pain can be marked by deep pressure in the area of right xiphoid region and at the ventral part of right seventh to ninth intercostal spaces. **Percussion** in these areas indicates dullness which is distinguished from that of the liver in the dorsal part of these landmarks. In the **auscultation** at the ventral part of seventh to eleventh intercostal spaces, slight noise is heard. Liquid sound indicates accumulation of backup fluid as a result of atony of abomasum. The auscultation of the pylorus can be done in the ventral part of the eleventh intercostal space.

Abomasum

The abomasum in cow lies on the floor of the abdominal cavity behind the xiphoid cartilage. The fundus lies in the xiphoid region, the body on the ventral midline with more than half of it inclining to the left of the medial plane and the pyloric part curving round to the right behind the omasum and the pylorus at the ventral end of the ninth or tenth intercostal space. The position of the abomasum varies according to the relative size and weight of the rumen. In pregnant cow, the uterus pushes the pylorus to the left. The **percussion and auscultation** of abomasum can be done through the ventral abdominal wall. Percussion indicates muffled resonance.

Displacement of abomasum to the left is diagnosed by auscultation. Gurgle or tinkle sound at left eleventh intercostal space indicates abnormality.

The **stomach in horse** lies on the dorsal part of the abdominal cavity behind the diaphragm and liver with its major part lying to the left of the median line. In case of bloat, it can be punctured on left side at the seventeenth intercostal space at the level of tuber coxae.

The **stomach of dog** lies between ninth to twelth ribs, behind the diaphragm and liver. On the left side it is in contact with the diaphragm and the ventral abdominal wall and on right side with the liver. The fundus can be palpated at the left ventral abdominal floor at the level of ninth to twelth ribs. The pylorus can be palpated, particularly in the case of congenital pyloric stenosis through a paracostal incision.

Intestines

The intestines **in cow** can be examined over the right abdominal wall by percussion and auscultation caudal to the costal arch. The upper half of the wall is the area for examination of duodenum, caecum and colon while the festoon of jejunal coils can be examined in the lower half of the wall. It may be noted that the greater omentum intervenes between the intestines, except the descending duodenum, and the wall of the abdomen. Some times, due to distention the ventral sac of rumen encroaches on the right side resulting into displacement of intestines to caudodorsal part of the abdominal cavity.

In horse, the surface area for examination of intestines is both, on the left and right abdominal wall. The area for examination of small intestine and small colon is on left side. The small colon is cranial to tuber coxae and the small intestine is ventral to the area of small colon. The rest of the parts of small and large intestines are examined on the right abdominal wall. The base of the caecum is in contact with the right paralumbar fossa. The body of the caecum is in contact with the caudal border of the right abdominal wall. The caecum can be trocarized at a point equidistant from the last rib, lumbar transverse processes and tuber coxae. The small intestine lies behind the caecum. The greater colon is in contact with the cranioventral part of the right abdominal wall.

In dog, the descending duodenum and the ileocoecocolic junction are palpable at the right paralumbar fossa by pressing dorsally the sublumbar muscles and rolling them from medial to lateral side. The descending colon can be palpated in the left paralumbar fossa.

Liver

The liver lies on the right side of the abdominal surface of the diaphragm extending obliquely craniad and ventrad from the right lumbocostal angle to the eleventh intercostal space. It can be palpated on the right abdominal wall at the lumbocostal angle and last three intercostal spaces. In case of liver abscess, severe pain is indicated on palpation. Percussion of liver is also possible at the same level as that for palpation. Dullness of the liver along the basal border of lung is normal but in case of enlargement of liver, the dullness expands caudoventrally towards the costal arch.

In horse, the light percussion of liver is possible at the right tenth to seventeeth and the left seventh to tenth intercostal spaces. Palpation of liver is possible at ventral to the costal arch.

In dog, the liver is not palpable over the abdominal wall. However, its enlargement due to disease conditions enables it to be palpated caudal to the costal arch. Although the normal liver extends beyond the costal arch ventrally, the rectus abdominis muscle prevents palpation in this area.

Kidneys

The left kidney **in ox** usually lies ventral to third, fourth and fifth lumbar vertebrae, a little caudal and ventral to the right kidney. When rumen is full, it is pushed slightly to the right side. In this state it can be examined by palpation with finger tips by pressing the fingers ventral to sublumbar muscles at the right paralumbar fossa. However, when the rumen is not full, the left kidney is to the left of the median plane and is difficult to examine by palpation through right flank.. The right kidney lies ventral to the last costovertebral joint and the first two or three lumbar transverse processes. Its cranial extremity is lodged in the renal fossa (renal impression) on the visceral surface of the liver. The right kidney can be easily palpated at the right paralumbar fossa.

In horse, the left kidney is ventral to seventeenth or eighteenth thoracic vertebra and the first two lumbar vertebrae and is palpable through the left paralumbar fossa. The right kidney extends from fifteenth or sixteenth rib to first lumbar vertebra and can be examined by percussion at the dorsal end of the sixteenth and seventeenth intercostal space and by palpation of its caudal end at the right paralumbar fossa.

In dog, the left kidney lies ventral to the second, third and fourth lumbar vertebrae and is palpated at the left paralumbar fossa while the right kidney lies under the twelth or thirteenth rib and the first two or three lumbar vertebrae and is palpable at the right paralumbar fossa.

Site for Laparotomy

The laparotomy is a surgical procedure applied to open the abdominal cavity for surgical interventions on the abdominal and pelvic organs such as cesarean section etc. In cattle, it is performed at the paralumbar fossa like the one described above for ruminotomy. A vertical incision is given about 3 to 5 cm caudal and parallel to the last rib in the left or the right as per the need. In cattle, only rumen and reticulum are approached through laparotomy at the left paralumbar fossa while all other organs in the abdominal and pelvic cavity are approached through laparotomy at the right paralumbar fossa. In the laparotomy for cesarean section in cow and mare, usually a high vertical flank incision or a low ventrolateral flank incision is made. The higher vertical flank incision begins higher in the paralumbar fossa and extends vertically for about 20 to 25 cm. In the low ventrolateral flank method, the craniocaudal incision of about 25 to 35 cm length is made in oblique direction in the skin of right flank region in front of the stifle joint The incision passes deep through the skin, fascia, obliquus abdominis externus, obliquus abdominis internus and transversus abdominis muscles just lateral to the rectus abdominis muscle and the peritoneum. The uterus lies just beneath the incision and provides good enough exposure for performing the cesarean section. The procedure for laparotomy is done under the local anaesthesia while that for cesarean section the epidural anaesthetic block is performed.

Site for epidural anaesthesia

The epidural anaesthesia is indicated in the surgical procedures in the region of abdomen, pelvis and perineum. It is mostly performed for the operative interventions on the organs of lower intestinal and genital tracts including the mammary glands (udder). The sensory nerve fibres to these parts are supplied by way of the lumbar, sacral and coccygeal spinal nerves. Blocking of these nerves is possible by injecting anaesthetic solution in the epidural space without injury to the spinal cord. Two sites are identified for this purpose, the high epidural and low epidural.

The **high (lumbar) epidural anaesthesia** is performed at the space between the spinous processes of L-1 and L-2. To locate this space, a transverse line is drawn across the cranial edges of the transverse processes of L-2. The needle is inserted at the right border of the supraspinous ligament and through the interarcuate space inclining at the angle of 12 degree from the median plane. The needle first pierces the ligamentum flavum and then reaches the epidural space. The anaesthetic solution infiltrates the spinal roots of T-13, L-1 and L-2.

The **low (sacrococcygeal) epidural anaesthesia** is usually performed at the first intercoccygeal space. In order to locate the point of injection, the tail is moved up and down. The first movable joint is between the first and second coccygeal vertebra. The first prominence caudal to sacral crest is the first coccygeal spine. A transverse plane about 10 to 11 cm cranial to tuber ischii intersects the first coccygeal space. The needle is inserted perpendicular to the skin in the middle of this space. Just prior to entry into the epidural space, the needle can be felt to penetrate the interarcuate ligament.

Site for pudendal nerve block

The pudendal nerve block is indicated for surgical intervention on the vagina, vulva, labium, and mammary glands in female and on the urethra penis and the glans in male. It is formed by the union of fibres from ventral branch of third and fourth sacral nerves. It passes on the medial surface of the ligament, crosses the lesser sciatic foramen and reaches to ischial arch to supply the structures mentioned above. It detaches the hemorrhoidal branch which supplies the skin and the muscles in the perineal region. The pudendal nerve is located per rectal in the following manner.

First the lesser sciatic notch and foramen are located by palpation per rectal. Next, the internal iliac (pudendal) artery is located by palpation at the cranial border of the lesser sciatic foramen. The pudendal nerve can be palpated just craniodorsal to the pudendal artery. After locating the nerve, the needle is inserted about 1 to 2 cm deep from the ischiorectal fossa.

PART-2.2: ANATOMY OF FORE LIMB

SECTION-A

MUSCULO-SKELETAL COMPONENT

79

Skeleton of Fore Limb

The **fore limb** is termed as **pectoral limb** or **thoracic limb (Fig. 5-1)**. It is attached to the thorax by means of muscles of pectoral girdle (shoulder girdle). It is composed of four major segments, the **shoulder girdle, arm**, **forearm** and **manus**. The skeleton of shoulder girdle is formed by the **shoulder bone**, the **scapula.** The arm is formed by the **arm bone** the **humerus.** The forearm is formed by two bones the **radius and ulna**; and the manus is formed by the **carpus** consisting of six short bones –the **carpal bones** arranged in two layers, the **metacarpus** consisting of one **large and** one **small metacarpal bones** and the **digits** consisting of six short bones the **phalanges** and six small **sesamoids** arranged in two rows for each limb.

Shoulder girdle

The shoulder girdle (thoracic girdle or pectoral girdle) in general is composed of the **scapula, coracoid and clavicle**. In ruminants the **scapula** is well developed, the **coracoid** is in the form of a small rounded process fused with the ventral end of the scapula and the **clavicle** is absent or in some subjects it occurs embedded in the brachiocephalicus muscle cranial to the point of the shoulder. But this possibility is very rare. Hence, in ox only scapula is considered as the bone of shoulder girdle.

Scapula

The scapula is a flat triangular bone applied obliquely ventrad and craniad against the cranial part of the lateral wall of thorax. Its long axis extends from the fourth thoracic spine to the sternal end of the first rib. It presents two surfaces, three borders and three angles.

The **lateral surface** (Fig. 5-1 A) is wide above and narrow below. It is divided into two unequal areas by a long vertical ridge the **spine** of the scapula. The spine extends from the dorsal border to the ventral narrow constricted part the neck of the scapula. It is quite prominent and sharp in outline, bent caudally in its middle and rostrally in the ventral part. Its free border is thick in the middle where the trapezoid muscle is attached. The ventral end of the spine is prolonged into a pointed projection the **acromion process**. The muscle deltoideus arises from the acromion process. The area cranial to the spine is about one fourth of the lateral surface of the scapula. It is called the **supraspinous fossa**. The muscle supraspinatus is attached to this area. The area caudal to the spine is larger and forms about three fourth of the lateral surface of scapula. This area is called the **infraspinous fossa** and it is occupied by the infraspinatus muscle. The lower third of this area is roughened and provides attachment to teres minor muscle. The **medial or costal surface of scapula (Fig. 5-1 B)** is wider dorsally and narrow ventrally and it presents a shallow smooth area called the **subscapular fossa** in the middle and it gives attachment to subscapularis muscle. The proximal third of this surface presents cranially a rough triangular area for the insertion of serratus cervicis muscle while caudally it presents a rough line for insertion of serratus thoracis muscle.

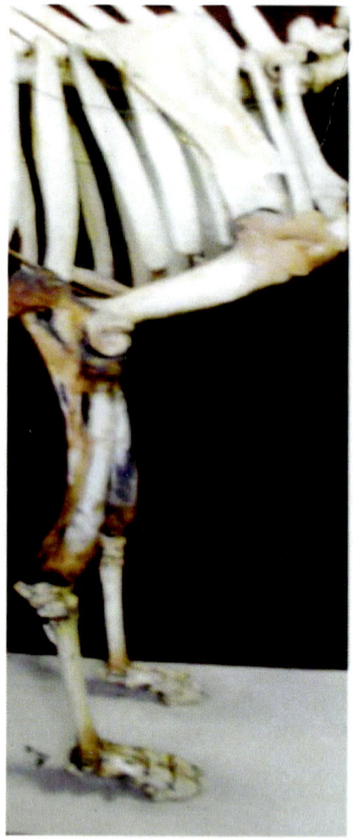

Fig. 5 – 1: Skeleton of forelimb of Ox

The **cranial border** is thin, sharp and convex in the dorsal two thirds of its length and rounded and concave in the remaining part of its extent. The **caudal border** is thick and slightly concave. On the lower third of this border is the **nutrient foramen**. The **dorsal** or **vertebral border** is thick and pitted by impressions into which the **scapular cartilage** fits. Caudally, the dorsal border extends beyond the bone and forms a rounded projection.

The **cranial angle** is thin and is formed at the junction of the cranial and dorsal borders. It lies opposite the second thoracic spine. The **caudal angle** is thick and tuberous and is formed by the junction of caudal and dorsal borders. The **ventral** or **glenoid angle** is joined to the body of the bone by a constriction called the **neck** of the scapula. It is composed of **a** glenoid cavity and tuber scapulae. The **glenoid cavity** is a shallow depression, nearly circular in outline with a thin rim which is cut laterally into a notch called the glenoid notch. The glenoid cavity forms articulation with the head of the humerus. The **glenoid notch** provides passage for the tendon of origin of teres minor muscle. Just dorsal to the caudolateral part of the glenoid cavity is a tubercle to which is attached the tendon of origin of teres minor muscle. Just cranial to the glenoid cavity is a rough eminence the **tuber scapulae** or **supraglenoid tubercle**. This tubercle provides attachment to the tendon of origin of the biceps brachii muscle. A short rounded **coracoid process** projects from the medial side of the tuber scapulae and it gives origin to the coraco-brachialis muscle.

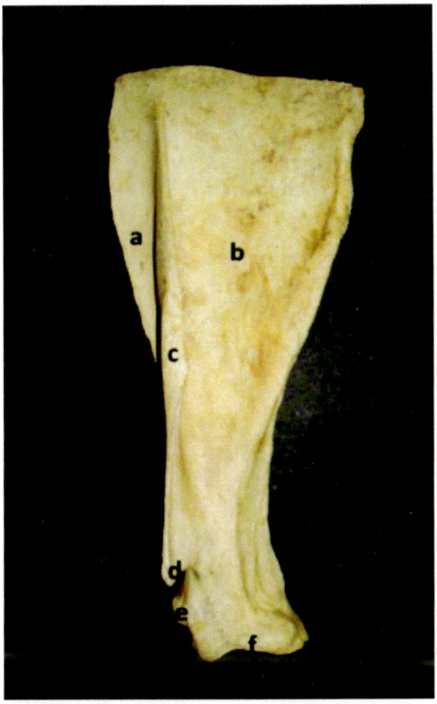

Fig. 5 – 1 A: Scapula of Ox (Lateral surface) a. Supraspinous fossa b. Infraspinous fossa c. Spine d. Acromion process e. Tuber scapulae f. Rim of glenoid cavity

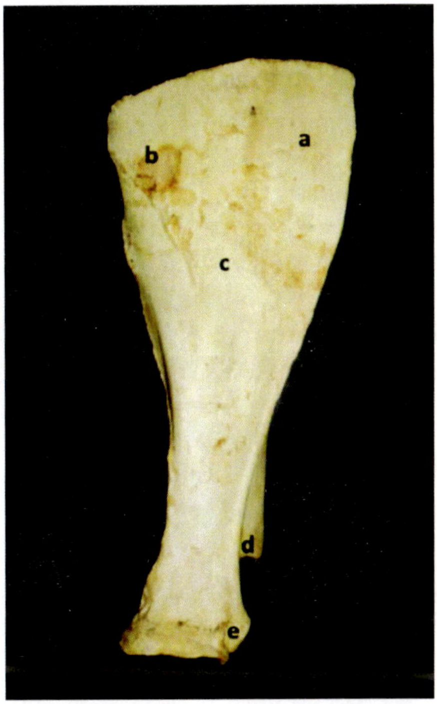

Fig. 5 – 1 B: Scapula of Ox (Medial surface) a. Area for insertion of serratus cervicis muscle b. Area for insertion of serratus thoracis muscle c. Subscapularis muscle d. Acromion process e. Tuber scapulae

Arm

The arm is the second segment of fore limb. It is between the thoracic girdle and fore arm. It is composed of a single strong and large long bone the humerus.

Humerus

The humerus (Fig. 5-1 C and D) is a long bone placed obliquely caudad and ventrad extending from the shoulder joint at the proximal end to the elbow joint at the distal end. It consists of a shaft and two extremities.

The **shaft** of the humerus is irregularly cylindrical and twisted. It has four surfaces. The **cranial surface** (Fig. 5-1 C) is triangular, wide and smooth proximally and narrow and roughened distally. The **caudal surface** is smooth and rounded from side to side and it blends with the medial and lateral surfaces. About the middle of the distal third of this surface is the **nutrient foramen**. The **medial surface** is smooth and nearly straight. It blends with the cranial and caudal surfaces. It presents about its middle the **teres tubercle** which provides attachment for the tendon of insertion of teres major muscle. The **lateral surface** (Fig. 5-1 D) is smooth and is spirally curved, forming a **musculospiral groove** which is occupied by the brachialis muscle. The lateral surface is separated from the cranial surface by a distinct border the crest of the humerus called the **deltoid ridge** which bears in its middle the **deltoid tuberosity**. It provides attachment to the tendon of insertion of the deltoid muscle. Extending from the deltoid tuberosity to the head of the humerus is a curved line to which the triceps brachii muscle is attached. Behind this curved line lying on the dorsal part of lateral surface is a prominent tuber or the nodule for attachment of insertion of teres minor muscle.

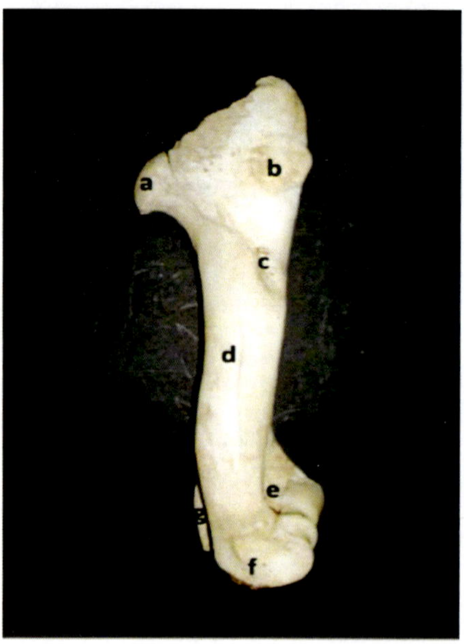

Fig. 5 – 1 C: Humerus of OX (Lateral surface)

a. Head b. Rough round area for tendon of infraspinatus c. Deltoid tuberosity d. Musculo spiral groove e. Coronoid (radial) fossa f. Lateral epicondyle g. Olecranon fossa

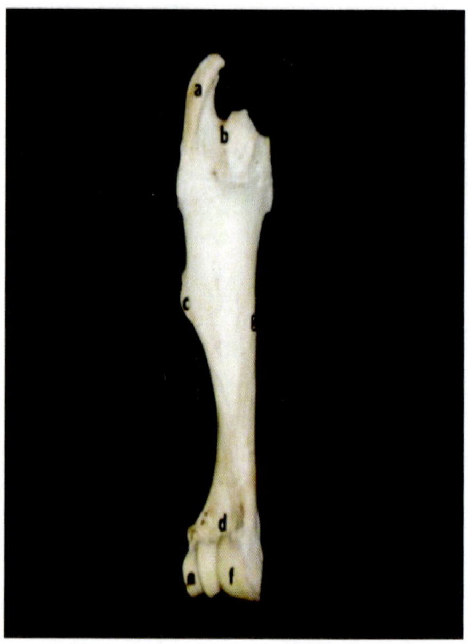

Fig. 5 – 1 D: Humerus of Ox (Cranial surface)

a. Lateral tuberosity b. Bicipital groove c. Deltoid tuberosity d. Radial fossa e. Lateral condyle f. Medial condyle g. Teres tubercle

The **proximal extremity** consists of the head, neck, two tuberosities and the intertuberal (bisipital) groove. The **head** is large, rounded and convex. It presents a circular and convex articular area that is almost double the size of the glenoid cavity of scapula with which it articulates to form the shoulder joint. The **neck** is a constriction just below the head. It is well defined and distinctly visible caudally. The two tuberosities are the lateral and medial tuberosities. The **lateral tuberosity** is larger and is termed as **greater tuberosity**. It is situated on the craniolateral part of the head. It rises about 3 cm proximal to the level of the head and forms the point of shoulder. It has two parts, the summit and the convexity. The **summit** forms the lateral boundary of the intertuberal groove. Lateral to the summit is a large circular rough area for attachment of the tendon of insertion of the infraspinatus muscle and over the summit is attached the lateral tendon of insertion of supraspinatus muscle. The **convexity** of the lateral tuberosity is the proximal end of the lateral tuberosity. It curves inward and overhangs the intertuberal groove. The **medial tuberosity** is termed as **lesser tuberosity** and it is much smaller than the lateral tuberosity. It has two parts, the cranial and caudal. The **cranial part** forms the medial boundary of intertuberal groove and curves over it. It presents attachment to the medial tendon of insertion of supraspinatus muscle dorsally and to the deep pectoral muscle ventrally. The **caudal part** presents attachment to the tendon of insertion of subscapularis muscle. The **intertuberal (bisipital) groove** is situated on the cranial part of proximal extremity and is bounded by the cranial parts of the two tuberosities. In fresh state, this groove is covered by a fibrocartilage over which the tendon of biceps brachii muscle passes.

The **distal extremity** has oblique surface which is divided by a craniocaudal ridge into two condyles. The **medial condyle** is much larger than the lateral condyle and is traversed by craniocaudal deep groove which extends into the olecranon fossa and articulates with the semilunar notch of the ulna. The **lateral condyle** is much smaller than the medial condyle and is placed lower in level because of which this extremity appears oblique. Cranially, above the articular area is a depression called the **coronoid fossa** which receives the **coronoid process** of radius during extreme flexion of elbow joint. Caudally above the articular area is much deeper olecranon fossa which receives the **olecranon process** of the ulna during extreme extension of the joint. The **olecranon fossa** is bounded on either side by prominent ridge the epicondyle. The **medial epicondyle** gives origin to all the flexor muscles of carpus and digits except the ulnaris lateralis. The **lateral epicondyle** at its tuberous portion gives origin to ulnaris lateralis muscle. The lateral epicondyle on its lateral aspect marks the **condyloid crest** which forms the boundary of the musculospiral groove and gives origin to the extensors of carpus and digits.

Forearm

The forearm is the third segment of fore limb. It is between the arm and the manus. It is composed of two long bones the radius and ulna.

Radius

The radius (Fig. 5-1 E and F) is the larger and shorter of the two bones of the fore arm. It is a long bone that extends in an oblique direction from elbow where it articulates with the humerus to the carpus where it articulates with the carpal bones. Its proximal end is little outward and the distal end correspondingly inward. It has a shaft and two extremities.

The **shaft** of the radius is curved in its length and is flattened craniocaudally. It presents four surfaces. The **cranial surface** (Fig. 5-1 E) is slightly convex in its length. It is smooth and is covered by the extensors of metacarpus and digits. Ventrally it presents three grooves for the passage of the tendons of extensors. The **caudal surface** (Fig. 5-1 F) is concave in its length. It presents all along its lateral border a long narrow rough area for articulation with the

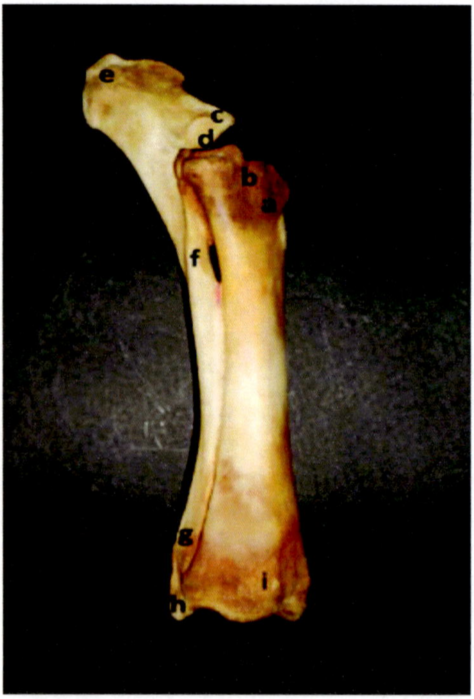

Fig. 5 – 1 E: Radius and Ulna of Ox; Cranial surface

a. Radial tuberosity b. Coronoid process c. Anconeus process d. Semilunar notch e. Olecranon process f. Proximal interosseous space g. Distal interosseous space h. Styloid process of Ulna i. Groove for extensor tendons

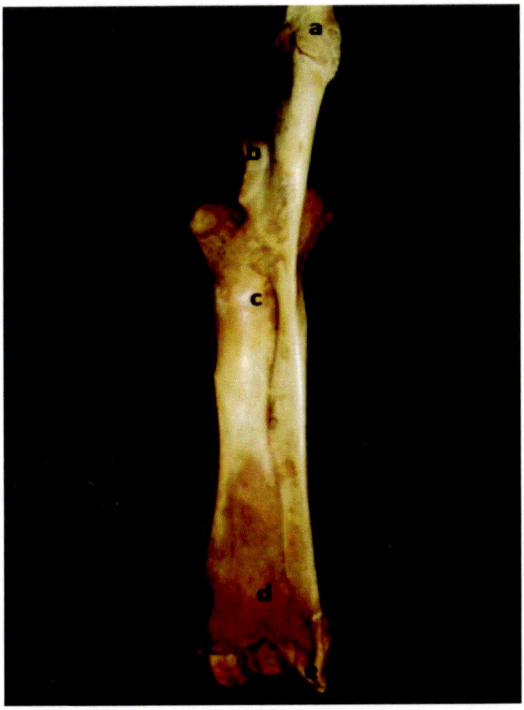

Fig. 5 – 1 F: Radius and ulna; Caudal surface

a. Olecranon process b. Anconeus process c. Proximal interosseous space d. Distal interosseous space e. Styloid process

shaft of ulna. The rough area is interrupted by two smooth areas, one in its proximal third and the other in its caudal third. These are called the **interosseous spaces** or the **radioulnar arches** which are connected laterally with the radioulnar groove. The **nutrient foramen** is placed just lateral to the proximal interosseous space. The radioulnar interosseous groove provides passage for the interosseous vessels. The **medial surface** is for the most part subcutaneous and presents at its proximal end a smooth area for the attachment of the tendon of brachialis muscle and distal to this is a small rough area for attachment of the medial ligament of the elbow joint. The **lateral surface** is rounded in its proximal third and wide and flat in the distal part. It blends with the cranial and caudal surfaces.

The proximal extremity is flattened craniocaudally and wide transversely. It presents an articular area which is divided by a craniocaudal sagittal groove into two divisions, the medial being larger than the lateral articular area. The articular area articulates with distal extremity of the humerus and is surrounded by a rim which bears the coronoid process at about the middle of its cranial part. The coronoid process fits into the coronoid fossa of the humerus during extreme flexion of the elbow. Caudally, just below the articular surface, there are two facets for articulation with similar facets of the ulna. Between the articular facets and the proximal interosseous space is a quadrilateral rough area to which the ulna is attached. At the craniomedial aspect of the proximal extremity is a large radial tuberosity for the insertion of the tendon of biceps brachii muscle. On either side of this extremity are two roughened tubular areas the medial and lateral tubercles to which the medial and lateral ligaments of the elbow joint are attached.

The distal extremity is thick and wide. Ventrally it presents three oblique facets for articulations with the carpal bones of the upper row of the carpus. The medial facet is largest and is for the radial carpal. The middle facet is intermediate in size and it is wide and concave cranially and is narrow and pointed caudally. It articulates with the intermediate carpal. The lateral facet is saddle shaped and its lateral part is completed by ulna. It articulates with the ulnar carpal. The cranial surface of the distal extremity presents three shallow grooves separated by ridges. The medial groove gives passage to the tendon of medial digital extensor. The middle groove is for the passage of extensor carpi radialis and the lateral groove is for the passage of common digital extensor. The caudal surface of the distal extremity is crossed by a rough transverse crest. Distal to this crest are three depressions. On either side of the distal extremity are the **tuberosities**. The medial and lateral collateral ligaments of elbow joint are attached to these medial and lateral tuberosities. The lateral tuberosity presents a small vertical groove for the passage of the tendon of lateral digital extensor muscle.

Ulna

The ulna (Fig. 5-1 E and F) is an aborted long bone fused to and longer than the radius, It is strongly curved and is situated on the caudolateral aspect of the radius. It presents a shaft and two extremities.

The **shaft** is three sided and a little curved. It is fused with the shaft of the radius except at two places, the proximal and distal interosseous spaces. It is three sided. Its **cranial surfac**e lies against the lateral side of the caudal surface of the radius. This surface of the shaft of ulna is rough and is fused with the corresponding caudal surface of the radius except at the site of **interosseous spaces** (**radioulnar arches**) where it is smooth. The **proximal interosseous space** is about 5.0 cm ventral to the proximal extremity while the **distal interosseous space** is about 3.5 cm above the distal extremity. Lateral to the proximal interosseous space is the **nutrient foramen**. The **medial surface** of the shaft is narrower and slightly concave while the lateral surface is narrower and nearly flat. The **lateral surface** subscribes the interosseous (radioulnar) groove with the shaft of the radius.

The **proximal extremity** forms the major part of the bone and is composed of the olecranon process and semilunar notch. The **olecranon process** is quadrilateral in shape and is directed dorsad and caudad. Its medial surface is concave while the lateral surface is convex. The **cranial border** is concave and terminates ventrally in the **anconeus process** or the beak. It fits into the olecranon fossa of the humerus during extreme flexion of the elbow joint. The caudal border is thick and concave. The free dorsal end of the olecranon process is called the **summit.** It forms the point of elbow. It gives attachment to the tendons of insertion of the extensor muscles of the elbow joint. The **semilunar notch** is present ventral to the anconeus process and articulates with the caudal part of the medial division of the articular area of the humerus. Ventral to the notch are two facets which articulates with similar facets on the caudal surface of the proximal extremity of radius.

The **distal extremity** of the ulna is fused with the radius and forms the **styloid process** of the ulna. It contributes for completing the periphery of the facet for ulnar carpal.

Manus

The manus is the fourth and the middle and lowermost segment of the forelimb. It consists of three sub-segments, the carpus, metacarpus and digits.

Carpus

The carpus is the first of the three sub-sections of manus and it is composed of six short bones compounded and arranged in two layers, one above the other. The individual short bones of this part are called the carpal bones. The bones of the proximal row from medial to lateral side are the radial carpal, intermediate carpal, ulnar carpal and the accessory carpal. The bones of the distal row are the second and third fused carpal and the fourth carpal. The first carpal is absent in ox.

The **radial carpal** (Fig. 5-1 G) is the largest of the bones of the proximal row. Its **dorsal surface** is convexo-concave in cranio-caudal direction and it articulates with the medial oblique facet of the distal extremity of the radius. The **ventral surface** of the radial carpal articulates with the second and third fused carpal. The **lateral surface** of the radial carpus bears four facets which articulate with similar facets on the medial surface of the intermediate carpal. The **cranial, medial and caudal surfaces** are continuous and rough for the attachment of muscles and ligaments.

The **intermediate carpal** is wedge shaped. Its **cranial surface** is wide and rough and forms the base of this bone. The narrow **caudal surface** forms the apex. The **medial surface** has four facets for articulation with similar facets on the lateral surface of the radial carpal. The **lateral surface** of the intermediate carpal articulates with the ulnar carpal. The **dorsal surface** is convexo-concave in cranio-caudal direction and articulates with the middle oblique facet of the distal extremity of the radius. The **ventral surface** is divided by sagittal ridge into two facets. One (medial) of these articulates with the second and third fused carpal and the other (lateral) articulates with the fourth carpal.

The **ulnar carpal** is very irregular in form. It is situated lateral to the intermediate carpal and is the outermost bone of the first row of carpus. Its **dorsal surface** is oblique and is directed caudally and laterally. It encroaches on the lateral surface and articulates with the ulna. The **ventral surface** is small and obliquely concave. It articulates with the lateral facet on the dorsal surface of the fourth carpal. The **medial surface** presents two facets on its cranial part which articulates with the intermediate carpal. The **lateral and cranial surfaces** are continuous and rough. The **caudal surface** is oblique and has an oval facet for articulation with the accessory carpal.

The **accessory carpal** is short, thick and rounded. It is a **sesamoids bone** situated behind the ulnar carpal. Its **dorsal surface** is narrow and rough. It is interposed in the course of the tendons of flexor carpi ulnaris and the ulnaris lateralis muscles. The **ventral surface** is broad and rough. The **cranial surface** has a facet for articulation with the ulnar carpal. The **medial surface** is vertically grooved close to the cranial facet.

The **second and third carpal** bones are fused into a single, thick short bone. It is situated medially and is the larger of the two bones of the distal row of carpus. Its **dorsal surface** is wide and it is divided by a ridge into two unequal facets. The medial of these is larger and it articulates with the radial carpal bone. The lateral facet is smaller and it articulates with the medial facet on the ventral surface of intermediate carpal bone. The **ventral surface** is undulating and articulates with the large metacarpal bone. The **lateral surface** has three facets for articulation with the fourth carpal. The **cranial and medial surfaces** are continuous and the caudal surface is narrow.

The **fourth carpal** bone is smaller of the two bones of distal row of carpus and it is placed on the lateral side. It is quadrilateral and is thicker cranially than its caudal part. Its **dorsal surface** has two oblique facets divided by a craniocaudal ridge. The medial facet is oblong shaped and is craniocaudally cocavo-convex. It articulates with lateral facet on the ventral surface of intermediate carpal. The lateral facet articulates with the ulnar carpal. The **ventral surface** of the fourth carpal articulates with the small metacarpal bone. The **medial surface** has two small facets for articulation with second and third fused carpal bone.

The **lateral and cranial surfaces** are rough, convex and are continuous with each other. The **caudal surface** is rough and tuberous.

Metacarpus

The metacarpus is the middle sub-segment of the manus. It consists of a large metacarpal bone and a small metacarpal bone.

Large metacarpal bone

The large metacarpal bone (Fig. 5-1 H) is a fused bone of third and fourth metacarpals. It is a long bone placed vertically between the carpus proximally and fetlock distally. It has a shaft and two extremities.

The **shaft** is semi-cylindrical and has two surfaces and two borders. The **cranial (dorsal) surface** is convex transversely and is traversed vertically in the center of this surface the **vertical vascular groove** for the passage of the vessels. The vascular groove lodges two **foramina**, one proximal and the other distal foramen. These foramina traverse the thickness of the shaft and communicate with similar foramina on the caudal (palmer) surface. The **caudal (palmer) surface** is flat and presents a **shallow vertical groove** which marks the fusion of the third and fourth metacarpal bones. This groove communicates with the cranial (dorsal) groove through the proximal and distal foramina. The caudal (palmer) surface is in contact and supports the suspensory ligament. The **borders**

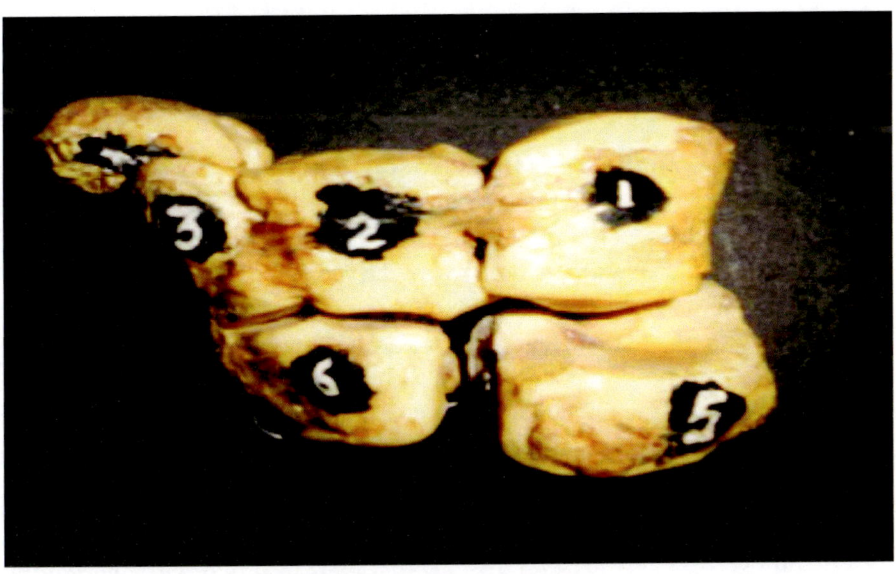

Fig. 5 – 1 G: Carpal bones of ox

1. Radial carpal 2. Intermediate carpal 3. Ulnar carpal 4. Accessory carpal 5. 2nd & 3rd fused carpal 6. Fourth carpal

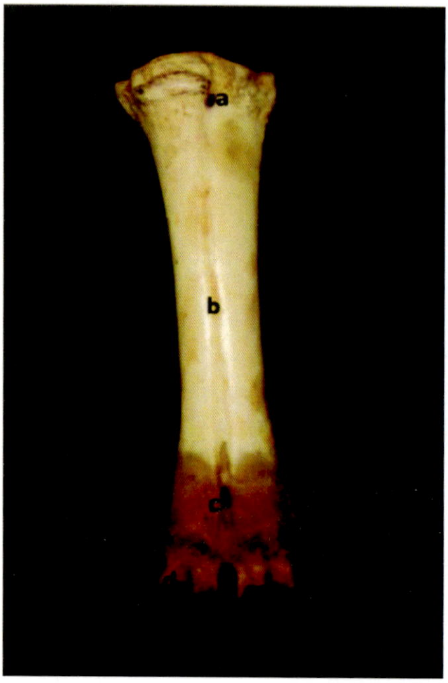

Fig. 5 – 1H: Large Metacarpal bone of Ox (Dorsal surface)
a. Proximal foramen b. Cranial vascular groove c. Distal foramen d. Condyle e. Condyloid ridge f. Intercondyloid cleft

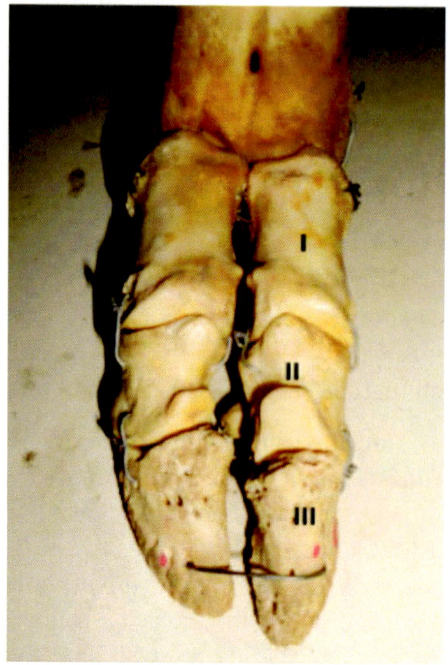

Fig. 5 – 1 I: Bones of digits of Ox; Phalanges
I. First phalanx II. Second phalanx III. Third phalanx

are **medial and lateral**. These are smooth and rounded. The lateral border in its proximal third is attached to the small metacarpal bone.

The **proximal extremity** has two concave **facets** separated by a median ridge in front and deep notch behind. The **medial facet** is larger of the two and it articulates with the second and third fused carpal bone. The **lateral facet** is smaller and articulates with the fourth carpal bone. On the lateral aspect of the proximal extremity just below its articular surface, is a small convex facet for articulation with the small metacarpal bone At the cranio-medial (dorso-medial) aspect of the proximal extremity is an obtuse eminence the **metacarpal tuberosity** for the attachment of extensor carpi radialis muscle. On the cranial (dorsal) aspect of the proximal extremity is a roughened elevation for attachment of ulnaris lateralis muscle while on its caudal (palmer) aspect is a nodule for attachment of flexor carpi radialis muscle.

The **distal extremity** is divided by a sagittal cleft into two parts the **medial and lateral condyle**. Each condyle represents the distal extremity of one metacarpal bone. A craniocaudal (dorso-caudal) sagittal ridge divides each condyle into two articular areas for articulation with the first phalanx ventrally and two sesamoids caudally (on the palmer side).

Small metacarpal bone

The small metacarpal is an aborted long bone of about 4.0 to 5.0 cm length and is situated at the proximal part of the lateral border of the large metacarpal bone. The **shaft** is attached to the proximal part of the shaft of the large metacarpal bone. The **proximal extremity** is rounded and bears a small facet on the cranial (dorsal) surface for attachment with the large metacarpal bone. The **distal extremity** is pointed.

Digits

The digit (Fig. 5-1 I) is the most distal segment of the forelimb. In ox, there are four digits for each limb. Two of these, the third and fourth digits, are **fully developed** and the remaining two, the second and fifth digits, are **vestiges** which are placed caudal (palmer) to the fetlock joint as **dew claws**. Each dew claw has one or two very short bony pieces within the cornified tissue of the skin but these bony pieces do not articulate with the skeleton of the limb. The first digit is absent in ox. As a result, apparently there are only two well developed digits the third and fourth digits for each limb in ox. Each of these fully developed third and fourth digits is composed of three **phalanges** and three **sesamoids.**

Phalanges

The three phalanges (Fig. 5-1 I) of each of the two digits are arranged vertically in three layers as proximal, middle and distal phalanx.

The **proximal phalanx** (first phalanx) is a long bone placed obliquely ventrad and craniad between the large metacarpal proximally and second phalanx distally. The **shaft** is four sided. The **cranial (dorsal) surface** is convex and blends with the **lateral surface**. The **caudal surface** is flat and bears two tubercles one each on either side at about the middle of its borders for the attachment of ligaments. The **medial (interdigital) surface** is flat and rough for the attachment of digital ligament. The **proximal extremity** is larger than the distal extremity. Its articular surface is concave craniocaudally and is divided by a sagittal groove into two unequal areas. The lateral area is larger and a little higher in position than the medial area. These areas articulate with the condyle of the distal extremity of the large metacarpal bone. Caudal to these areas are two small facets for the proximal sesamoids. On the caudal aspect of the proximal extremity are two tubercles for the attachment of the ligaments of the digits. The **distal extremity** is smaller and its articular surface is divided by a sagittal groove into two condyles which articulate with the proximal extremity of the second phalanx.

The **middle phalanx** (second phalanx) is also a long bone but is shorter than the proximal phalanx. It is about two thirds of the length of the proximal phalanx. It is placed obliquely craniad and ventrad between the proximal and distal phalanges. The ventral half of each middle phalanx is included within the hoof of the limb. The **shaft** of the middle phalanx is three sided. The **lateral surface** is convex, rounded and rough for the attachment of ligaments. The **medial or interdigital surface** is flat and depressed. The **caudal (palmer) surface** is nearly flat and is encroached up on by the distal articular surface. The **proximal extremity** is composed of two glenoid cavities separated by a sagittal ridge. The lateral glenoid cavity is larger than the medial one. The lateral and medial **glenoid cavities** articulate with the lateral and medial condyles of the distal extremity of the proximal phalanx respectively. The sagittal ridge between the two glenoid cavities lodges into the sagittal groove between the two condyles of the distal extremity of the proximal phalanx. The caudal aspect of the articular surface of the proximal extremity presents two **tubercles** for the attachment of tendons of superficial digital flexor. The **distal extremity** is smaller and is divided by a sagittal groove into two condyles the lateral condyle is larger than the medial condyle. It articulates with the third phalanx distally and distal sesamoids caudally (palmerly).

The **distal phalanx** (third phalanx) is a terminal short bone of the digit. It is entirely enclosed within the hoof. It presents four surfaces divided by six borders. The **proximal or articular surface** is narrow from side to side. It is concave craniocaudally and slopes distally and palmerly. It is oblique transversely with its axial side at a lower level. This surface is adapted to the distal extremity of the middle phalanx. On the caudal aspect of this surface, is a small facet for distal sesamoid. The **parietal or lateral surface** slopes from above downward and becomes steep caudally (palmerly). It is marked in its distal part by a shallow groove with several foramina, the most caudal (palmer) of these being largest. It conducts to a canal in the interior of the bone. Distal to this groove, the parietal surface is prominent, rough and porous. In life, this surface is covered by the sensitive laminae. **The distal or solar surface** is nearly flat, wide in the middle and narrow in the front. It presents two or three foramina of considerable size. It is separated from parietal surface by a border which is sharp dorsally and rounded palmerly. It is in contact with the sensitive sole in life. The **axial (interdigital surface)** is smooth and grooved distally and rough and porous proximally. This surface is separated from the parietal surface by a rounded border and from the solar surface by a sharp edge. The **cranial proximal border** is slightly concave and sharp and it bears a central eminence, the **extensor process**, to which the tendon of insertion of common digital extensor muscle is attached. On either side of this eminence is a depression for attachment of the collateral ligament. The **dorso-lateral border** is convex and separates the lateral (parietal) and articular surfaces. The **dorso-medial border** is concave and sharp and separates the interdigital and articular surfaces. The **ventrolateral border** is convex and separates the ventral (solar) and lateral (parietal) surfaces. The **ventromedial border** is nearly straight and sharp and separates the ventral (solar) and medial (interdigital) surfaces. The **caudal (palmer) border** is thick and rounded and it provides attachment to the tendon of insertion of the deep digital flexor muscle.

Sessamoids

The sesamoids are small elongated or oval short bones resembling the nuts interposed between the tendons of the flexors of the digits and the palmer aspect of the phalanges. These are provided to reduce the friction of the tendons as well as to increase the leverage to the flexors of the digits. There are two sets of sesamoids designated as proximal and distal sesamoids according to their location.

The **proximal sesamoids** are four in number in each limb and are arranged in pairs as one pair for each digit in ox. The bones of the medial pair are slightly larger than those of lateral pair. Of the two bones of each pair, the lateral one is wider and less elongated than the medial. These are situated on the caudal aspect of the distal extremity of the large metacarpal bone. Each sesamoid has a form of pyramid with its base directed distally and the apex proximally. The **cranial surface** of each sesamoid is concave and is divided into two unequal areas by a faint vertical ridge. This surface articulates with the caudal aspect of the distal extremity of the large metacarpal. The **caudal surface** is rough and convex for the attachment of ligament. The opposing surface is flat and presents a facet for articulation with its fellow in the same pair. It is covered in life by fibrocartilage and forms a groove in association with its fellow for the passage of one of the tendons of the deep digital flexor muscle. The intersesamoidean ligament is also attached to this surface. The **base** is drawn forward to present a facet for the first phalanx. It gives attachment to the distal sesamoidean ligament. The **apex** faces dorsally and gives attachment to one of the slips of the suspensory ligament.

The **distal sesamoids** are two in number for each limb, one for each digit of the limb. It is a short bone like the proximal sesamoid but is placed transversely on the caudal aspect of the distal inter-phalangeal articulation. It is flattened craniocaudally and presents two surfaces, two borders and two extremities. The **cranial or articular surface** faces dorsally and cranially and presents two facets for the second phalanx. **The caudal** or **flexor surface** is broader and in fresh state is covered by fibrocartilage for the passage of the tendon of insertion of deep digital flexor. The **dorsal border** is grooved for attachment of the ligament. The **ventral border** bears a small facet about its middle for third phalanx. Both the extremities (medial and lateral) are rounded and smooth.

Hoof

The hoof is the protective covering of the distal part of the digit. It resembles the shape of the distal phalanx and firmly encloses the same. In ox, each limb has two hooves, one for each digit. The hoof is a modification of the epidermis. It is composed of the wall, sole and bulb (frog).

The **wall** of the hoof is that part which is visible when the foot is in its natural position on the ground. It covers the front and sites of the foot and is separated from the distal phalanx by the pododerm or corium of the hoof. Its abaxial surface is convex from side to side and is marked by ridges parallel with the coronary border. The axial or interdigital surface is concave and is marked by grooves. It forms an angle of about 30 degrees with the ground. The basal or ground surface has two parts, the slightly concave sole which is pointed caudally or palmerly (or plantarly in case of hind limb) and a prominent bulb or soft thin horn which is continuous above with the skin. The cranial part of the wall is called the toe, the sides as the quarters and the caudal part, the heel. The internal surface of the wall presents large number of laminae extending from dorsal to ventral end.

The **sole** forms the ground surface and is slightly concave. It is placed in the angle of the reflection of the wall and is continuous without demarcation with the periople of the bulb. Its internal surface is convex and presents numerous fine openings as in the coronary groove. The external or ground surface is concave. The cranial border is convex and is joined to the wall. The caudal border is deeply notched and the bars and apex of the bulb are situated in these angles. The part between the bars and wall is the angle of the sole.

The **bulb or frog** is a wedge shaped mass placed in the angle between the bars. The internal surface presents a central ridge, the bulb stay. On either side of this is a deep depression. This surface presents openings for the corium. The ground surface presents a central sulcus bordered by two ridges, the crura. The medial and lateral surfaces are united at the upper part with the bars and sole but are free below. The base is depressed centrally and prominent at the sides where it unites with the angles of the wall. The apex lies in the central angle of the concave border of the sole and is blunt.

80

Comparative Anatomy of Skeleton of Fore Limb

Horse

The **scapula** of horse is a flat triangular bone placed at the shoulder region applied against the cranial part of the lateral wall of thorax similar to that in ox. The **scapular spine** is placed a little further caudad from the cranial border so that the proportion of the area of supraspinous to infraspinous fossa is one third to two third of the lateral surface of the scapula. The **subscapular fossa** is deeper and presents well marked vascular impressions. The **nutrient foramen** is placed at the distal third of the infraspinous fossa. The **tuber scapulae** and the **glenoid cavity** are placed further apart. The **glenoid cavity** is oval in outline and its rim has a distinct notch on its craniomedial aspect. The **coronoid process** is better developed and the **acromion process** is absent.

The **humerus** in horse is directed obliquely distally and caudally forming an angle of about 55 degrees with the horizontal plane almost equaling to that in ox. The **musculospiral groove** on the shaft is deeper and more spirally curved. The **nutrient foramen** is placed on the distal third of the medial surface. The **deltoid tuberosity** is better developed. The **medial and lateral tuberosities** of the proximal extremity are more prominent. The **intertuberal (bisipital) groove** is divided by an intermediate ridge. The summit of the lateral tuberosity does not arch inward. The head is smaller than that in ox. The **coronoid and olecranon fossae** of the distal extremity are shallower than those in ox.

The **radius** of the horse is larger and longer of the two bones of the forearm. Close to the medial border of the caudal surface in the lower third of the shaft is a **rough elevation for** attachment of the **superior check ligament** (an accessory ligament of the superficial digital flexor). The **caudal surface of the shaft** towards its lateral border presents a rough triangular area which tapers to a point in the distal third of this surface. This is for attachment of the ulna. The **distal interosseous space** is absent because the shaft of ulna is shorter and does not reach to the distal part of the shaft of radius. The grooves on the cranial surface of the distal part of the shaft are better marked. The **radial tuberosity** at the craniomedial aspect of the proximal extremity is larger and more prominent than in ox. The **distal articular surfaces** are not oblique. It presents two tubercles one on each side, for ligamentous attachment. The tubercle on the lateral aspect is grooved for passage of tendon of lateral digital extensor.

The **ulna** of horse is less developed and shorter than that of ox. It extends only to the distal third of the radius. It forms with radius only the proximal radioulnar arch. The distal radioulnar arch is absent. The semilunar notch is more triangular in outline. The facets placed below the notch for articulation with radius are convex in horse as against the nearly flat facets of ox.

The **carpus** of horse consists of seven or eight carpal bones, four in the proximal row and three or four in the distal row. The bones of proximal row are larger and they resemble the bones of ox. The **radial carpal** is larger. The **intermediate carpal** bears a concave facet for articulation with the radius. The lateral angle of its articular face is more pointed. The **ulnar carpal** is the smallest bone of the proximal row. The proximal articular surface of this carpal articulates only with the radius. The accessory carpal is flat and discoid. Its medial surface is concave. The lateral surface is convex and rough. It is grooved for the passage of tendon of ulnaris lateralis. The cranial border has two facets, the dorsal concave facet for the radius and the ventral convex facet for ulnar carpal. The **first carpal** bone of the distal row is inconstant. When present, it is placed caudal to the second carpal. The **second carpal** is the smallest of the bones of distal row and it is placed on the medial side of the carpus. It is hemispherical in shape. Its proximal articular surface has a convex facet for articulation with the radial carpal. The distal articular surface is flat and it articulates with the second (medial small metacarpal) and third metacarpal bone (large metacarpal). The **third carpal** bone is the largest and is placed centrally. It is compressed proximo-distally. It is triangular in shape with its base cranially. The proximal articular surface articulates with radial and intermediate carpal and the distal surface with the third (large metacarpal) and fourth metacarpal bone (lateral small metacarpal). The **fourth carpal** is the lateral most bone of the distal row of carpus. Its proximal surface is convex and articular and it encroaches up on the lateral face. The distal articular surface articulates with the large and lateral small metacarpal bones. The medial surface has two facets for third carpal bone.

The **metacarpus** of horse consists of one large metacarpal and two, medial and lateral, small metacarpal bones. The large metacarpal is formed by fusion of second and third metacarpal bones. The medial small metacarpal is the first metacarpus and the lateral small metacarpal is the fourth metacarpus in horse.

The **large metacarpal** is a long bone with **shaft and two extremities**. The upper two third of the caudal (palmer) surface of the **shaft** is roughened on the medial and lateral sides for attachment with the small metacarpal bones, between which it forms a wide groove for lodgment of suspensory ligament. The vascular grooves on the dorsal (cranial) and palmer (caudal) surfaces are absent. The nutrient foramen is placed on the dorsal two third of the palmer surface. The **proximal extremity** presents palmerly on either side two facets which articulate on the facets of the proximal extremity of small metacarpal bones. The **distal extremity** is not divided and the whole articular area of the of the distal extremity resemble one of the two articular areas on the distal extremity of the large metacarpal of ox. The **small metacarpals** are the **medial and lateral** and they extend to the distal third of the shaft of the large metacarpal on its palmer surface. The **medial small metacarpal** is slightly larger than the lateral. The shaft of the small metacarpal is three sided. The cranial (dorsal) surface is attached to the caudal (palmer) surface of the shaft of large metacarpal by interosseous ligament. The **proximal extremity** is relatively massive and has two facets on its dorsolateral (craniolateral) aspect for large metacarpal. The lateral small metacarpal bears a single facet for articulation with fourth carpal bone while the medial small metacarpal has two facets for articulation with second and third carpal bones. The **distal extremity** is **nodular** and usually forms the **button** of the splint that can be felt in living animal.

The **digits** in horse are composed of only one digit in each limb. Each digit consists of **three phalanges** and **three sesamoids**. Each phalanx appears as a combination of two corresponding phalanges of the ox. The palmer surface of the **first phalanx** presents a 'V' shaped area beginning from the two tubercles and converging distally where the distal sesamoidean ligament is attached. **The proximal articular surface** is divided by a sagittal groove into two concave areas which articulate with the condyles of the distal extremity of the large metacarpus. The medial articular area is larger than the lateral one. The **second phalanx** is a short bone and is more wide. The **third phalanx** though a single bone, appears like a combined third phalanx of ox. It has three surfaces, three borders and two angles. The **proximal articular surface** is adapted to the distal extremity of the second phalanx and the distal sesamoid. The **distal (volar) surface** is divided by a **semilunar crest** into a larger concave **solar surface** and a smaller semilunar **flexor surface**. The volar surface marks the centrally raised rough triangular area on either side of which are two **volar foramina** into which extends the volar groove from the angles. The crest and the rough triangular area furnish attachment to the tendon of insertion of the deep digital flexor. The dorsal or **coronary border** bears about its middle the extensor process for attachment of the tendon of common digital extensor. The ventral or **volar border** is convex and is irregularly notched. The **palmero-proximal**

border is nearly straight and forms the palmer limit of the proximal articular surface. The **angles** for wings project palmerly. The **sesamoids** are three in number in each limb. A pair of **proximal sesamoids** placed vertically on the palmer aspect of the distal extremity of the large metacarpal bone and a single transversely placed **distal sesamoid** placed transversely on the palmer aspect of the second interphalangeal articulation. The proximal sesamoids of horse are much larger than those of ox. Each is distinctly three sided and is pyramidal in shape. The two proximal sesamoids of the pair do not articulate with each other unlike that of ox. The distal sesamoid is shuttle shaped. It is larger and longer than that of the ox. The extremities are pointed and directed slightly upward.

Dog

The **scapula** in dog is a flat triangular bone of shoulder region similar to that in ox. The **scapular spine** lies in the middle of the lateral surface dividing it into two equal parts, the **supraspinous and infraspinous fossae**. The **spine** gradually increases in height from above downward to the level of glenoid cavity and terminates in the acromion process. The **acromion process** is short, blunt and overhangs the glenoid cavity. The **subscapular fossa** is very shallow. The **cranial border** is thin and convex. The **caudal border** is thick and nearly straight. The **vertebral border** is convex. The **scapular cartilage** is in the form of a thin band. The **glenoid cavity** extends to the ventral face of the tuber scapulae. The **tuber scapulae** is blunt and the **coracoid process** is absent. The **clavicle** is inconsistent. When present, it is a very small cartilaginous or bony plate in the brachiocephalicus in front of the shoulder joint and does not articulate with rest of the skeleton.

The **humerus** of dog is relatively long and slender. The musculospiral groove on the lateral surface of the shaft is less spiral and is shallow. The deltoid tubercle is in the form of a low ridge. The teres tubercle is in the form of a rough mark. The lateral tuberosity of the proximal extremity is single and the intertuberal (bisipital) groove is undivided. The coronoid and olecranon fossae communicate with each other through a large supra-trochlear foramen.

The **radius and ulna** of dog are relatively long and articulate with each other at their extremities enclosing a narrow interosseous space and permit certain degree of movement. The **proximal extremity of radius** is small and bears dorsally a concave surface for articulation with humerus and caudally a convex area for articulation with the ulna. The **distal extremity** is wide and its medial border projects ventrally forming the styloid process of radius. Laterally there is a concave facet for articulation with ulna.

The **ulna** is well developed and crosses the caudal face of the radius enclosing a narrow interosseous space. The **olecranon process** is grooved and shows three prominences of which the caudal one is large and rounded. Below the **semilunar notch** is a concave surface for radius. The **styloid process** articulates with radius craniomedially and with the ulnar and accessory carpals.

The **carpus** of dog is composed of seven carpal bones, three in the proximal row and four in the distal row. The bones of the **proximal row** are the **intermedio- radial** (a bone formed by fusion of the radial and intermediate carpals) on the medial side and the **ulnar carpal** on the lateral side. The accessory carpal lies behind the ulnar carpal. The bones of the **distal row** from medial to lateral side are the **first carpal, second carpal, third carpal and the fourth carpal.**

The **metacarpal** bones in dog are five in number. The **first** is shortest. The **second** is slightly shorter than the **third and fourth** metacarpal and a little longer than the fifth metacarpal. The **fifth metacarpal** is the thickest of all the metacarpals. The five metacarpal bones articulate proximally with each other by lateral facets and form diarthrodial joints. Each metacarpal bone has a **shaft** and two **extremities**. The shaft is compressed dorso-palmerly. It is nearly quadrilateral in the third and fourth metacarpal, trilateral in the second and fifth and rounded in the first.

There are five **digits** for each limb in dog. The **first digit** is shortest and has **two phalanges** and it does not come in contact with the ground in walking. The **rest of the digits** have **three phalanges** each. The third and fourth digits are longest. The **proximal phalanges** of all the five digits are four sided and these are slightly curved dorsally. The proximal articular surface of the proximal phalanx of all digits is concave and it articulates with the corresponding metacarpal bone. The distal end has a trochlea for articulation with the middle phalanx. The **middle phalanges** are about two thirds of the length of proximal phalanxes. The **distal phalanges** have the form of the **claws** and are **hook like**. The **base** of the distal phalanx has the articular surface which is adapted to the middle phalanx. Its solar surface bears a tubercle. On each side of the tubercle has a foramen. The distal end of the distal phalanx bears the ungula process which is a curved rod with a blunt pointed free end. The two phalanges of the first digit resemble the proximal and distal phalanges of the other four digits. There are **nine sesamoids** for each limb. All of these are proximal sesamoids. These are placed in pairs on the cranial (palmer) aspect of each of the **metacarpo-phalangeal** joint of second to fifth digit. However, the metacarpo-phalangeal joint of the first digit has only one sesamoid. In addition to these nine proximal sesamoid bones, there are five **cartilaginous nodules**, one each on the cranial (dorsal) aspect of the metacarpo-phalangeal articulation of first to fifth digits of the limb. The distal sesamoids are absent in dog.

Sheep and Goat

The **scapula** in sheep and goat in its general form resembles that of ox but differs from it on certain features. Its dorsal border is relatively longer. The neck is narrower. The scapular spine is less sinuous. The subscapular fossa is more extensive. The ventral extremity is relatively long. The tuber scapulae is connected to the rim of the glenoid cavity.

The **humerus** is relatively longer and slender than that of ox. The deltoid tuberosity is nearer to the proximal end of the shaft and is not much prominent. The cranial part of greater tuberosity of proximal extremity is blunt and less curved inwardly. Its caudal part is small.

The **radius and ulna** are relatively longer than those of ox. The **radius** is a little more curved than that of ox. Its cranial (dorsal) surface is more rounded. The shaft of the **ulna** is more slender particularly in its distal half. The fusion of the ulna with radius is less extensive than that in ox.

The **carpal bones** in general resemble those in ox. However, in size they are smaller than those of ox.

The **large metacarpal** bone is long and slender. The lateral **small metacarpal** is often absent and if present, it is in the form of a small ridge on the shaft of the large metacarpal.

The **digits** in sheep and goat resemble in number of those in ox. The **phalanges** are relatively long and narrow. The distal phalanx on its abaxial side is much flattened and its cranial (dorsal) border is more prominent. The proximal **sesamoids** of the abaxial sides of the digits are compressed from side to side and those of axial side are compressed dorso-palmerly. The flexor surface of distal sesamoids forms a shallow groove for the passage of the tendon.

Pig

The **scapula** of pig is relatively very wide. The scapular spine is triangular and thickly wide in the middle. It curves caudally over the infraspinous fossa. It presents a large tubercle. The ventral part of the scapula bears a rudimentary acromion in the form of small projection. The cranial border is strongly convex and sinuous. It is thick and rough in the middle. The caudal border is slightly concave. The dorsal border is convex. The scapular cartilage is not so extensive unlike that of ox and horse. The cranial angle is thin and the caudal angle is thick. The neck is well defined. The rim of the glenoid cavity is rounded. The notch on the rim of glenoid rim is absent. The coronary process on the supraglenoid tubercle is absent.

The **humerus** of pig is relatively longer but slender than that in the ox. Its general form is similar to that of ox. The shaft is compressed from side to side, The medial surface is flattened and is separated from the cranial surface by a distinct border. The teres tubercle is absent. The musculospiral groove on the lateral surface is shallow. The deltoid tubercle is smaller than that in ox. At the proximal extremity, the head is more strongly curved and the neck is better marked than that in the ox and horse. The greater tuberosity is very large and it extends up on the cranial aspect of the proximal extremity. It is divided into two high prominences by a deep groove. It has a third eminence distally and laterally for attachment of supraspinatus muscle. The intertuberal (bisipital) groove is undivided like that of ox but is almost converted into a canal. The lateral groove on the condyle of the distal extremity is shallow. The olecranon fossa is very deep. A bony plate separating the olecranon fossa from the radial fossa is thin and some times perforated.

The **radius** is short and narrow but thick. The most of the caudal surface of the shaft of radius is covered by the shaft of ulna. The radial tuberosity is in the form of a rough area. The distal end or trochlea is relatively large. It possesses concavo-convex facets for articulation with the radial and ulnar carpal bones.

The **ulna** is massive, much longer and considerably heavier than the radius. The shaft of ulna is curved. Its cranial surface is convex and rough for attachment with the radius. The proximal and distal interosseous spaces are wider than those of ox The medial surface is extensive, concave and smooth. The lateral surface is slightly convex and its proximal part presents an oblique rough line or ridge. The proximal extremity is large and is somewhat curved medially. The distal extremity is relatively small and it articulates with the ulnar and accessory carpals.

The **carpus** consists of eight bones, four in the proximal and another four in the distal row. The bones of cranial row resemble those of ox, the accessory carpal, however, is more like that of horse. The bones of the distal row has the first, second, third and fourth carpals. The first carpal is elongated dorso-palmerly. It articulates with the second carpal dorsally (cranially). The second carpal is high and narrow and articulates distally with second and third metacarpal bone. The third carpal articulates with the radial and intermediate carpals proximally and the third metacarpal bone distally. The fourth metacarpal is the largest of the bones of distal row. It articulates with intermediate and ulnar carpals proximally and the fourth and fifth metacarpal bones distally. It bears a tuberosity on its caudal (palmer) aspect.

The **metacarpals** in pig are four in number. The first metacarpal is absent. The **third** and **fourth** metacarpals are large and they constitute the **chief digits** and the **second** and **fifth** metacarpals are much smaller and they constitute the **accessory digits**. The **proximal extremities** of all the four digits articulate with each other .and with the carpals. The **shafts** of the third and fourth metacarpals are flattened dorso-palmerly and three sided. The third metacarpal is wider of the two and it articulates with all the bones of the distal row of carpus except the first carpal. The fourth metacarpal articulates mainly with the fourth carpal and partly with the third carpal. The second and fifth metacarpals are placed farther palmerly than the third and fourth metacarpals. The **distal extremity** is relatively large and its articular surface is condyloid dorsally and trochlear palmerly.

The **digits** in pig constitute **two major or chief digits** and **two accessory digits**. The chief digits are composed of three phalanges and three sesamoids each. The phalanges of chief digits resemble those of ox in form. The foramen on the axial surface of the extensor process is, however, absent. The phalanges of the accessory digits are similar to those of chief digits in form but are much smaller and hence the accessory digits are shorter and they do not reach the ground. The proximal sesamoids are narrow and ridged palmerly.

Fowl

The **shoulder girdle** (thoracic or pectoral girdle) of fowl is specially designed and developed to support the wings for flight. It is composed of all the three components, the scapula, coracoid and clavicle equally and fully developed. The **scapula** is a narrow, thin, elongated and flat long bone. It is slightly curved and it extends caudally from the shoulder joint along and parallel to the vertebral column reaching almost to the pelvis. Its cranial extremity is thick and articular and it articulates with the coracoid, humerus and the furculum. It participates in the formation of glenoid cavity for articulation with head of humerus at the shoulder joint. It presents a pneumatic foramen near the acromion process. The caudal end is thin, free and non-articular. The **coracoid** is the strongest of the three bones of pectoral girdle in fowl. It extends caudally and ventrally from the shoulder joint to the coracoidal sulcus of the sternum. The coracoid is a hollow pneumatic long bone and it communicates with the clavicular air sac. The proximal extremity of coracoid prolongs into a hook like process which completes the formation of foramen triosseum with scapula and clavicle. Its distal extremity is expanded and flattened and presents a saddle shaped articular surface for articulation with the sacrum. The **clavicle** is a slender, rod like bone. Its proximal end rests against the scapula and coracoid while the distal ends of the bones of opposite side unite and gets fused ventrally into a flattened plate, the hypocleidium or the furculum which is attached to the cranial apex of the sternum by a hypocleidial ligament. The **humerus** is the largest of the bones of the wing (fore limb) of birds. Its shaft is a little curved. The deltoid tubercle is in the form of the crest and is called the deltoid crest. A strong pectoralis muscle inserts on this crest. The proximal extremity has an oval large convex head which fits into the glenoid fossa (cavity) formed by the scapula and coracoid. The pneumatic foramen is placed medially below the head and through it the cavity of the bone communicates with the clavicular air sac. The distal extremity has two condyles which articulate with the radius and ulna. **The radius and ulna** are of equal length but the ulna is larger and more massive than the radius. The radius is placed lateral to ulna. The radius and ulna articulate with each other at their proximal and distal extremities and their shafts are distinctly separated from each other by a large extensive interosseous space.

The **proximal extremity of radius** has an articular facet which articulates with the lateral and smaller of the two condyles of the distal extremity of humerus. The **distal extremity** articulates with the radial carpal and the ulna. The **ulna** is stronger and more massive than radius. Its proximal extremity has a concave surface for articulation with the larger of the condyles of the distal extremity of the humerus. The **olecranon process** is small and short. The **nutrient foramen** is placed about midway on the shaft of the ulna. The **shaft** presents a series of small bony projections which represent the attachment of the secondary feathers of the wing. The **distal extremity of ulna** has two facets one for radial carpal and the other for ulnar carpal. The **carpus** consists of two carpal bones, the radial carpal and the ulnar carpal. The distal row of carpus does not exist because the carpal bones of distal row are fused with the metacarpals. The **metacarpus** in birds is called the **carpo-metacarpus**. It has three bones fused into a single mass. The first metacarpal is a small projection while the second and third are fused at their extremities enclosing a narrow elongated interosseous space between their shafts. The **digits** are three in number and are present at the terminal segment of the wing. The first and second digits have two phalanges each and the third has one. The second digit is the longest of the three.

81

Articulations of Fore Limb

Shoulder joint

The shoulder joint (Fig. 5-2 A) is an enarthrosis formed between the glenoid cavity of scapula and head of humerus.

Ligaments: The shoulder joint is enclosed by the capsular ligament which is loose enough to accommodate the wide range of movements of the joint and is attached about 1.25 cm away from the periarticular area of the two segments of the joint. The capsular ligament is supported externally by the muscles of the shoulder region.

Movements: The shoulder joint performs all kinds of movements but the extension and flexion are best marked.

Elbow joint

The elbow joint (Fig. 5-2 B) is a composite joint consisting of the Humero-radial and the Radioulnar joints.

Humero-Radial articulation

The humero-radial articulation is formed between the condyles of the distal extremity of humerus and the proximal articular area of the radius and ulna which is glenoid.

Ligaments: The joint is covered by the capsular ligament which forms a pouch over the olecranon fossa. The medial and lateral collateral ligaments support the capsule externally. The medial and lateral collateral ligaments are attached above to the tubercle and depression respectively on the distal extremity of the humerus and below to the medial and lateral tuberosities of the proximal extremity of the radius.

Movements: The humero-radial articulation being a hinge joint, performs extension and flexion movements.

Radio-Ulnar articulation

The radio-ulnar articulation is a diarthrosis and amphiarthroses formed between the radius and ulna.

The **diarthrosis** is formed between the facets of the proximal extremity of radius and corresponding facets of the proximal extremity of ulna. This joint is enclosed by capsular ligament of the humero-radial articulation.

The **amphiarthrosis** is formed between the shafts of the radius and ulna which are united by three interosseous ligaments. In addition, there are two arciform ligaments, the medial and lateral. These are attached to the caudal surface of the shaft of radius, blend with the collateral ligaments and are attached to the olecranon process of ulna on the respective side.

The **movements** in these articulations are inappreciable.

Carpal joint

The carpal joint (Fig. 5-2 C) is a composite joint consisting of (1) the radio-ulnar-carpal articulation formed between the distal extremity of radius and ulna and the proximal row of carpus (2) the intercarpal articulation formed between the proximal and distal rows of carpus and (3) the carpo-metacarpal articulation formed between the distal row of carpus and proximal extremity of large metacarpal bone.

Ligaments: These joints have two types of ligaments, the common ligaments and the special ligaments.

The **common ligaments** are the capsular and collateral ligaments.

The **capsular ligament** is large and capacious and it covers the whole of the carpal joint. It is attached proximally to the margin of the distal articular surfaces of the radius and ulna and distally to the margin of the proximal articular surface of the metacarpus. It closely adheres to all the bones and ligaments comprising the carpal joint and the tendons of muscles passing over this joint. The dorsal (cranial) part of this ligament is known as **dorsal carpal ligament**. This part is forms fibrous canals internally for passage of the tendons of extensor muscles of the carpus and digits. The palmer (volar) part of the capsular ligament is known as **palmer carpal ligament**. It is thicker than the dorsal part and it is deeply grooved for passage of the tendons of the flexor muscles of the carpus and digits.

The **collateral ligaments** are medial and lateral collateral ligaments. These are thick and wide bands of ligaments extending from the distal extremity of the radius and ulna to the proximal extremity of the large metacarpal bone. The

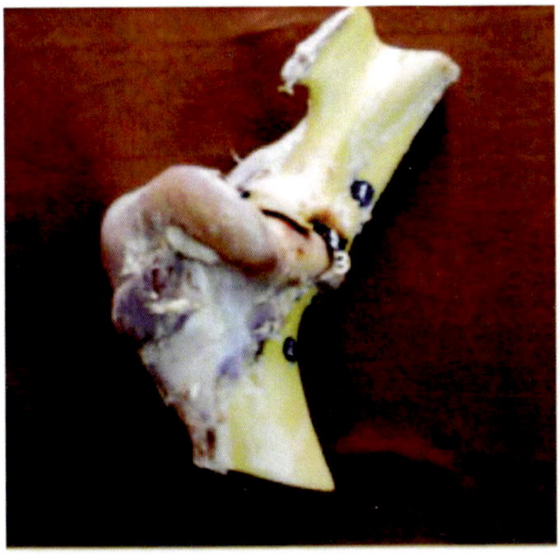

Fig. 5 – 2 A: Shoulder Joint of Ox
1. Scapula 2. Humerus 3. Capsular ligament

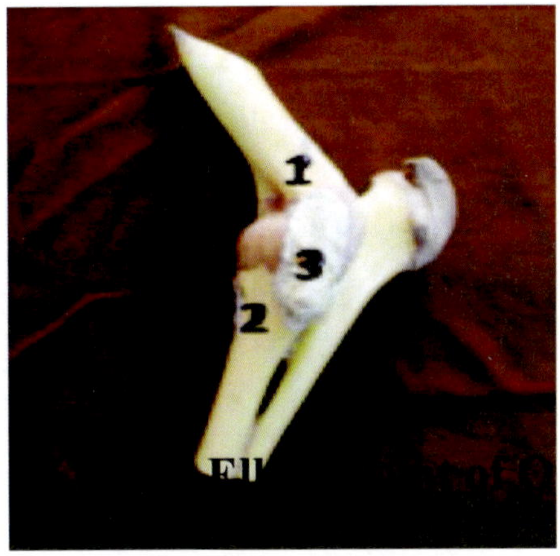

Fig. 5 – 2 B: Elbow Joint of Ox
1. Humerus 2. Radius Ulna 3. Lateral collateral ligament

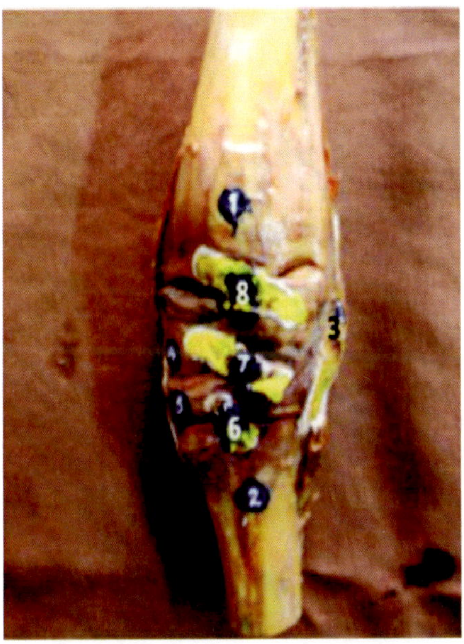

Fig. 5 – 2 C: Carpal Joint of Ox
1. Radius 2. Metacarpal 3. Medial collateral ligament 4. Ulnar carpal bone 5. Fourth carpal 6. Carpometacarpal ligament. 7. Intercarpal ligament. 8. Radiocarpal ligament.

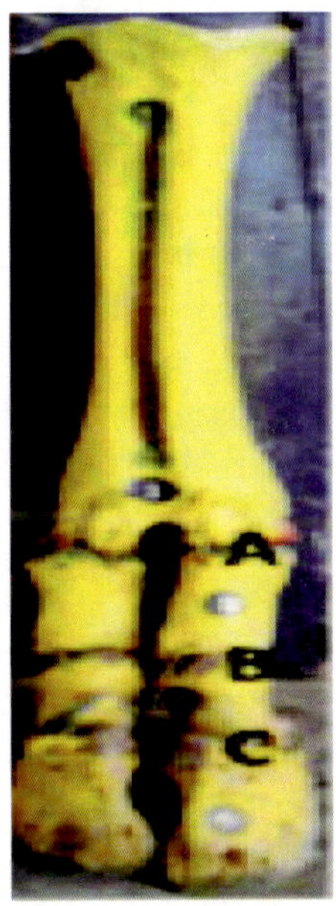

Fig. 5 – 2 D: Joints of Digital bones
A. Fetlock joint; B. Pastern joint and C. Coffin Joint

medial ligament is attached proximally to the medial tuberosity on the distal extremity of radius. It descends on the medial side of the carpus where it gives out two short fasciculi, the superficial and deep, and then terminates distally on the medial aspect of the proximal extremity of large metacarpal bone. The deep fascicle attaches to the radial carpal in the proximal row while the superficial fascicle attaches to the second and third fused carpal in the distal row of carpus. The **lateral ligament** is attached proximally to the lateral tuberosity on the distal extremity of radius and the styloid process of ulna descends vertically on the lateral side of the carpus, gives out the superficial and deep fasciculi and then terminates on the lateral aspect of proximal extremity of the large and small metacarpal bones. The deep fascicle attaches to the ulnar carpal in the proximal row and the superficial fascicle to the fourth carpal in the distal row of the carpus. This ligament is grooved internally for the passage of the tendon of lateral digital extensor.

The **special ligaments** of the carpal joint are large number of thin and short ligamentous fasciculi that connect the individual carpal bones with each other and with the bones of the proximal, middle and the distal segments of the carpal joint..

The **radio-ulnar-carpal articulation** is bound by two oblique and three palmer ligaments. The **oblique ligaments** include the dorsal oblique ligament between the distal extremity of radius and the ulnar carpal bone. The volar (palmer) oblique ligament connects the distal extremity of radius and ulna to the intermediate carpal bone. The **volar (palmer) ligaments** connect the radius with radial carpal; the ulnar bone with accessory carpal and the radius with the ulnar carpal.

The **proximal carpal articulations** are bound by the **dorsal ligaments** between (1) the radial carpal and intermediate carpal (2) the intermediate carpal and ulnar carpal and (3) the ulnar carpal and accessory carpal bones; the **volar (palmer) ligaments** between (4) the ulnar carpal and accessory carpal and (5) the intermediate and ulnar carpal bones and the **interosseous ligaments** between (6) the radial carpal and intermediate carpal (7) the intermediate carpal and ulnar carpal and (8) the ulnar carpal and accessory carpal bones.

The **intercarpal articulation** has the **dorsal oblique ligaments** between (1) the radial carpal and fourth carpal (2) the ulnar carpal and the second and third fused carpal bones; the **volar (palmer) ligaments** between (3) the radial carpal and second and third fused carpal bones and (4) the ulnar carpal and fourth carpal bones and the **accessory ligament** between (5) the accessory carpal and the fourth carpal bones.

The **distal carpal articulations** have (1) the **dorsal ligament** between the second and third fused carpal and the fourth carpal bones and (2) the **interosseous ligament** between the second and third fused carpal and fourth carpal bones.

The **carpo-metacarpal articulation** has two **dorsal ligaments,** two **volar ligaments** and three **interosseous ligaments** connecting the bones of the distal row of the carpus and the proximal extremity of the large and small metacarpal bones.

The synovial membrane of the capsular ligament of carpal joint forms three large and one small sac. The large sacs are for lubrication of radio-ulnar carpal, intercarpal and carpo-metacarpal articulations. The small sac is for lubricating the ulnar carpal-accessory carpal articulation.

The chief **movements** performed at the carpal joint are the **extension and flexion**. These movements are specifically performed at the radio-ulnar-carpal and the intercarpal articulations. However, these movements are not marked much at the carpo-metacarpal articulation where the two segments slightly glide one upon the other.

Intercarpal joints

The intermetacarpal joint is formed at two places, first between the facets at the proximal extremity of the large metacarpal and the rudimentary small metacarpal bones and the second between the shafts of the two bones. The first joint is diarthrosis and the second is the amphiarthrosis.

The **ligaments** of the carpo-metacarpal articulation cover the intermetacarpal articulation of the proximal extremity of the large and small metacarpal bones. The shafts of these two bones however are joined by interosseous ligament.

The **movements** of these joints are restricted to slightly vertical gliding.

Fetlock joint

The fetlock joints (Fig. 5-2 D) are two for each limb, one for each digit, in ox. It is a Ginglymus type of joint formed between the condyles of the distal extremity of large metacarpal bone, the proximal articular surface of the proximal phalanx and a pair of proximal sesamoids. The joint has capsular, collateral and the sesamoidean ligaments.

The **capsular ligament** encloses the joint and is attached proximally to the large metacarpal bone and distally to the proximal phalanx. It blends externally to the collateral ligaments. Its internal surface is lined by the synovial membrane of the joint. The synovial bursa disposes between the capsular ligament and the tendons of the extensor muscles on the dorsal surface of the ligament.

The **collateral ligaments** are two, the medial and lateral. The medial ligament arises from the cleft of the distal extremity of the large metacarpal bone and spreads on the interdigital space of the proximal phalanx. The lateral ligament extends from the depression on the lateral aspect of the distal extremity of the large metacarpal bone, attaches to the lateral face of the lateral proximal sesamoid and then inserts on the lateral aspect of the proximal phalanx.

The **sesamoidean ligaments** are the superior, inferior, collateral and intersesamoidean.

The **intersesamoidean ligaments** are three for each limb and these are placed between four sesamoids. Each of these ligaments connects the opposing surfaces of the adjacent sesamoids.

The **collateral sesamoidean ligaments** are two, the medial and lateral. The medial ligament connects the medial surface of the medial sesamoid to the medial aspect of the proximal extremity of the proximal phalanx. The lateral ligament connects the lateral surface of the lateral sesamoid to the lateral aspect of the proximal extremity of the proximal phalanx.

The **inferior (distal) sesamoidean ligaments** are four for each limb. These are divided into superficial and deep bands. The superficial bands extend from the base of the respective sesamoids to the volar (palmer) surface of the proximal extremity of the proximal phalanx. The deep bands extend from the base of the respective sesamoid and the adjacent bands cross each other before terminating on the volar surface of the proximal phalanx.

The **superior sesamoidean (suspensory) ligament** arises from the palmer surface of the distal row of carpal bones and the proximal extremity of the large metacarpal bone, descends on the palmer surface of the shaft of the metacarpus and divides about its middle into two branches, the cranial (deep) and caudal (superficial). The caudal branch soon bifurcates at the distal third of the metacarpus. Each of these two divisions unites with the corresponding division of the tendon of superficial digital flexor muscle behind the flexor to form a ring for the passage of the one of the divisions of the tendon of deep digital flexor. The cranial branch divides into six branches. Four of these pass to the bases of four sesamoids. The outer two branches (the medial and lateral) detaches a slip which passes ventrally and cranially to join the tendons of medial and lateral digital extensors. The remaining two branches of the cranial division pass into the cleft of the large metacarpus, enter the interdigital space and join the tendons of the common digital extensor. The superior sesamoidean (suspensory) ligament prevents excessive dorsal flexion of the fetlock joint and its slips prevent the excessive volar flexion.

Movements performed at the fetlock joint by the metacarpo-phalangeal articulation are the extension and flexion while the movements performed by the metacarpo-sesamoidean articulations are of gliding type.

Interphalangeal joints

The interphalangeal articulations (Fig. 5-2 D) are two, the proximal interphalangeal and distal interphalangeal articulations.

Proximal interphalangeal articulation (pastern joint)

The proximal interphalangeal articulations are two for each limb. Each is a ginglymus joint formed between the condyloid articular area of the distal extremity of proximal phalanx and the glenoid articular area of proximal extremity of middle phalanx. This joint is bound by the capsular, collateral and volar ligaments.

The **capsular ligament** is attached around the articular areas of two segments of the joint.

The **collateral ligaments** are medial and lateral. These extend from the corresponding surfaces of first phalanx and ends on respective surfaces of the second and third phalanx.

The **volar ligaments** are the caudo-medial and caudo-lateral. These extend from the corresponding borders of the first phalanx to the proximal extremity of second phalanx.

The **movements** performed at this joint are extension and flexion.

Distal interphalangeal articulation (coffin joint)

The distal interphalangeal articulations are also two for each limb and one for each digit of the limb. Each of these is a ginglymus joint formed between the distal end of middle phalanx and proximal end of distal phalanx with the distal sesamoid on the volar (palmer) aspect of the joint.

The **ligaments** of this joint are the capsular, dorsal elastic, collateral, cruciate, superior and inferior navicular and interdigital ligaments.

The **capsular ligament** is attached to the articular margins of two segments of the joint.

The **dorsal elastic ligament** extends from the distal end of the proximal phalanx, crosses the dorsal surface of the middle phalanx and ends on the extensor process of distal phalanx.

The **collateral ligaments** are medial and lateral bands of ligament extending from the medial and lateral borders of the middle phalanx and terminate on the corresponding border of the distal phalanx.

The **cruciate ligaments** are medial and lateral. They extend from the corresponding surface of the proximal extremity of middle phalanx, cross the tendons of deep digital flexor and blend with each other at the interdigital space. They terminate on the distal sesamoids of the opposite side.

The **superior navicular ligament** is formed by the fibres detached from collateral ligaments which unite on and gets attached to the dorsal border of the distal sesamoid. The **inferior navicular ligaments** extend from the ventral border of the distal sesamoid and terminate on the flexor surface of distal phalanx.

The **interdigital ligaments** connect the interdigital opposing sides of the proximal and middle phalanges and those of the middle and distal phalanges.

The **movements** performed at this joint are extension and flexion.

82

Comparative Anatomy of Articulations of Fore Limb

Horse

The **shoulder joint** of horse has same features as those of ox. However, this joint in horse exhibits greater degree of mobility.

The **elbow joint** of horse is almost similar to that of ox except that there is only one interosseous ligament in horse against two in ox.

The **carpal joint** of horse has only minor differences from that of ox. The special feature of the joint in horse is that it has two additional ligaments, the superior check ligament and the inferior check ligament. The superior check ligament starts from the rough elevation on the distal third of the caudal surface, close to the medial border of the radius and is inserted to the tendon of superficial digital flexor above the carpus. The inferior check ligament is the continuation of the caudal (palmer) capsular ligament of the carpus. It joins the tendon of deep digital flexor at about midway on the palmer surface of the metacarpus. The check ligaments assist the tendons of flexor muscles of the digits after severe exertion to keep then tight and prevent flexion.

The **fetlock joint** in horse is composed of only one metacarpo-phalangeal articulation for each limb because it has a single digit. The superior sesamoidean ligament after originating in manner similar to that in ox and reaching a little above the proximal sesamoids, divides into two branches. Each branch passes ventrad and laterad, attaches over the summit and the abaxial surface of the proximal sesamoids (which are two in number for each limb in horse). These further continue running ventrad and craniad to join the tendon of common digital extensor at the cranial (dorsal) aspect of the proximal phalanx. The inferior sesamoidean ligament is made up of three parts, the superficial, middle and deep. The superficial part is 'Y' shaped, the middle part is 'V' shaped and the deep part is 'X' shaped. All the three parts assist in connecting the sesamoids to the palmer surface of the proximal phalanx.

The **proximal and distal interphalangeal articulations** are only one each for each limb in horse. The dorsal elastic and the interdigital ligaments of the distal interphalangeal articulation are absent but it has other three ligaments that connect the lateral cartilages to the phalanges.

Dog

The **shoulder joint** in dog is similar to that in ox. The rim of the glenoid cavity is raised by marginal cartilage. The joint capsule is supported externally by a band of ligament that extends from acromion process.

The **elbow joint** and its capsular ligament in dog is strengthened by an oblique ligament. The collateral ligaments are attached below to the radius and ulna.

In the **radioulnar articulation**, both the extremities of radius and ulna articulate by diarthrodial joint. The joint of the proximal extremity of these bones has, in addition to capsular ligament, the annular ligament. The joint of the distal extremities has a tight capsular ligament.

The **carpal joint** has only minor differences which occur because of the difference of the number and arrangement of carpal bones.

The **intermetacarpal articulations** in dog have four interosseous ligaments which connect the five metacarpal bones with each other.

The **metacarpo-phalangeal articulations** are five for each limb. The suspensory ligament is replaced by interosseous muscles.

The **interphalangeal articulations** (proximal and distal) are in general similar to those in ox except for the number of these joints in each limb. The distal interphalangeal joint has a fibrocartilage on the palmer aspect of the joint that replaces the distal sesamoid which is absent in dog. Each of these joints has capsular and collateral ligaments. In addition, it has elastic ligament.

Sheep and Goat

The articulations of the fore limb in sheep and goat are almost similar to those in ox without any remarkable differences.

Pig

The **shoulder joint** in pig is similar to that in ox with a difference that a rudimentary marginal cartilage is bounds around the rim of the glenoid cavity and the cranial part of the capsule is reinforced by cruciate bands.

In the **elbow joint**, the radius and ulna are firmly united with each other by interosseous ligament and no movements are performed by this joint.

The **carpal joint** of pig has the same general features as those of ox and horse with two special features differentiating from other species. Two oblique elastic bands cross dorsal to radio-carpal and intercarpal joints. The proximal ligament is attached to the distal end of radius and passes distally and laterally to the ulnar carpal bone. The other ligament is the distal ligament that connects the radial carpal with the fourth carpal bone. The other variations are concerned with the ligaments which vary because of the variation in the number and arrangement of carpal bones.

In the **intermetacarpal joint**, the chief metacarpal bones articulate with each other at their proximal ends and are connected by interosseous ligaments.

The **metacarpo-phalangeal joints** are four in each limb of pig. Each of these joints is covered by a joint capsule and collateral ligaments. In addition, there are intersesamoidean and phalangeo-sesamoid ligaments. The suspensory ligaments are absent. The **Interphalangeal joints** of chief digits of pig resemble those of ox. There are special ligaments which connect the small digits with each other and with chief digits.

83

Muscles of Fore Limb

The muscles of fore limb (Fig. 5-3 A and B) are distributed in different regions of fore limb as muscles of shoulder girdle, shoulder, arm and those of forearm and manus. By means of the muscles of shoulder girdle the forelimb is attached with the trunk of the body by synsarcosis and bears the weight of the body. The rest of the groups of muscles act on different joints of the fore limb as extensors or flexors of these joints. The group of muscles acting on these joints originates on the bone of the proximal segment and insert on the bone of distal segment of the concerned joint.

Muscles of shoulder girdle

The muscles of shoulder girdle have been described with the muscles of thorax.

Muscles of shoulder

The muscles of shoulder arise on the scapula, act on shoulder joint and end on the humerus. These muscles are in two groups as the lateral group of muscles and the medial group of muscles.

Lateral group (FIG. 5-3 A) Deltoideus

The deltoideus is a flat triangular muscle on the lateral surface of the shoulder. It has two parts, the acromial and scapular. Both parts join and forms a fleshy belly.

Origin: The acromial part originates on the acromion and adjacent part of scapular spine and the scapular part originates on the proximal half of the caudal border of the scapula by aponeurosis.

Insertion: The distal part of the muscle forms a tendon for insertion on the deltoid tuberosity and fascia covering the arm region.

Action: To flex the shoulder joint and abduct the arm.

Blood supply: Through the circumflex scapular, subscapular and caudal circumflex humeral artery.

Nerve supply: Through axillary nerve.

Teres minor

The teres minor muscle is small and it lies on the deep surface of the deltoideus. The muscle is fleshy except near its insertion where the fibres attach to a tendon on the deep surface of the muscle.

Origin: The muscle originates on the distal half of the caudal border of the scapula.

Insertion: On a tubercle distal and caudal to the greater tuberosity of the humerus.

Action: To flex the shoulder joint.

Blood supply: The caudal circumflex humeral artery.

Nerve supply: The axillary nerve.

Supraspinatus

The supraspinatus is a powerful muscle in ox. It forms a slightly flattened conical mass that occupies the whole of the supraspinous fossa and extends cranial to the fossa and covers the tuber scapulae.

Origin: The supraspinous fossa, the scapular spine and the ventral part of the cartilage of the scapula.

Insertion: The cranial portion of the greater and lesser tuberosities of the proximal extremity of the humerus.

Action: To extend the shoulder joint.

Blood supply: The suprascapular and superficial cervical arteries.

Nerve supply: The suprascapular nerve.

Infraspinatus

The infraspinatus is a heavy powerful muscle of the shoulder and it occupies the whole of the infraspinous fossa.

Origin: It originates on the infraspinous fossa, scapular spine and scapular cartilage.

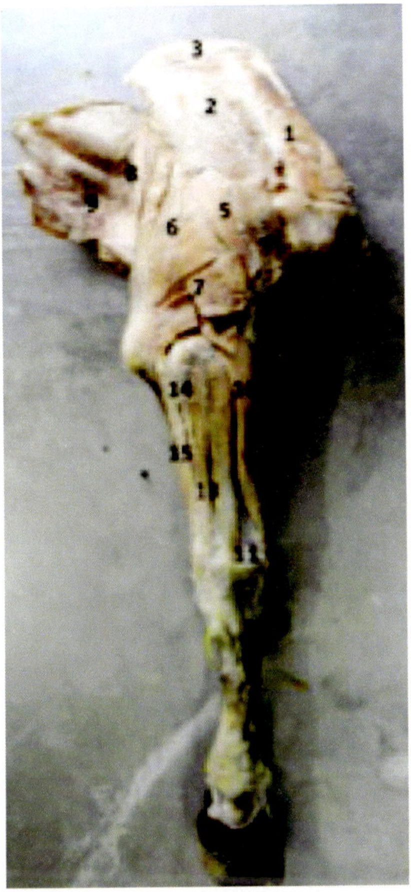

Fig. 5 – 3 A: Muscles of Forelimb of Ox (Lateral aspect)
1. Supraspinatus M. 2. Infraspinatus M. 3. Scapular Cartilage 4. Deltoideus M. 5. Teres Minor M. 6. Long head of Triceps 7. Lateral head of Triceps 8. Tensor Facia Antibrachi M. 9. Latissimus Dorsi M. 10. Extensor Carpi Radialis M. 11. Extensor Carpi Obliqus M. 12. Medial Digital Extensor M. 13. Common Digital Extensor M. 14. Lateral Digital Extensor M. 15. Ulnaris Lateralis M.

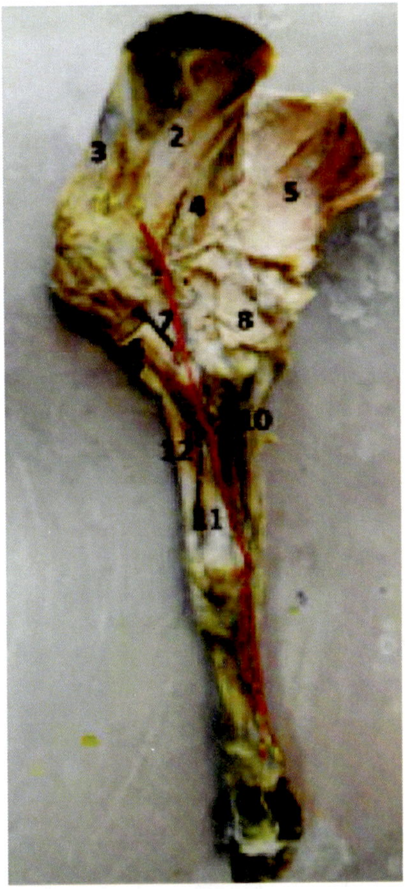

Fig. 5 – 3 B: Muscle of shoulder, arm and forearm of Ox; Medial view
1. Scapular cartilage 2. Subscapularis m 3. Supraspinatus m 4. Teres major m 5. Latissimus dorsi 6. Biceps brachii m 7. Coracobrachialis m 8. Medial head of Triceps m 9. Flexor carpi radialis m 10. Flexor carpii ulnaris m 11. Radius bone 12. Extensor carpi radialis m

Insertion: The muscle inserts on the medial aspect of the caudal part of greater tuberosity and a circular rough area below the cranial part of the greater tuberosity of humerus.

Action: To abduct the arm and to rotate it laterad. This muscle also acts as a lateral collateral ligament of the shoulder.

Blood supply: The circumflex scapular and caudal circumflex humeral artery.

Nerve supply: The suprascapular nerve.

Medial group (FIG. 5-3 B) Subscapularis

The subscapularis is a flat and triangular muscle and it lies on the medial surface of the scapula. It follows the exact contour of the costal surface of the scapula. It is composed of three parts. The cranial part is fleshy, the middle part is infiltrated with tendinous fibres and the caudal part extends a little behind the caudal border of the scapula.

Origin: The subscapular fossa and scapular cartilage on the costal surface of the scapula.

Insertion: The lesser tuberosity of the humerus.

Action: To adduct the limb.

Blood supply: Subscapular, suprascapular, circumflex scapular and superficial cervical arteries.

Nerve supply: The subscapular and axillary nerves.

Coracobrachialis

The coracobrachialis is a flat muscle that lies on the medial surface of the shoulder joint and arm and it obliquely crosses the shoulder joint before its termination on the medial side of humerus.

Origin: The coracoid process of the scapula.

Insertion: The medial surface of humerus between the lesser tuberosity and teres tubercle and the medial border and adjacent cranial and medial surfaces of the shaft as far down as the medial condyle of the humerus.

Action: To adduct the arm and flex the shoulder joint.

Blood supply: The cranial circumflex humeral and subscapular arteries.

Nerve supply: The musculocutaneous nerve.

Muscles of arm

The muscles of arm are grouped in two major groups around the humerus. They arise from the humerus and scapula, act upon the elbow joint and insert on the radius and ulna (forearm). The two groups are the flexors and the extensors of elbow. The flexors serve to retract the limb while the extensors serve to support the weight of the cranial part of the body.

Flexors of elbow

Biceps brachii

The biceps brachii is a strong cylindrical muscle and it lies on the cranial surface of the humerus. The muscle extends from the tuber scapulae in the form of a strong, thick and flat tendon that passes through the intertuberal (bisipital) groove, runs down over the cranial surface of humerus and then the elbow joint and terminates below this joint.

Origin: The tuber scapulae on the scapula.

Insertion: The muscle has three prominent tendons of insertion. One of these is the tendon that terminates on the radial tuberosity on the medial aspect of the proximal extremity of the radius. The second tendon of insertion terminates along the medial collateral ligament of the elbow and the third tendon passes along with the tendon of the pronator teres and the antibrachial fascia.

Action: To flex the elbow joint, to extend and fix the shoulder joint.

Blood supply: The muscular branch of brachial artery and the cranial circumflex humeral artery.

Nerve supply: The musculocutaneous nerve.

Brachialis

The brachialis is a large fleshy muscle that occupies the musculospiral groove on the lateral surface of the shaft of humerus.

Origin: The proximal third of the musculospiral groove of humerus.

Insertion: A rough area on the medial border and volar surface of radius below the radial tuberosity.

Action: to flex the elbow joint.

Blood supply: The caudal circumflex humeral and collateral radial arteries.

Nerve supply: The musculocutaneous nerve and a small branch of the radial nerve.

Pronator teres

The pronator teres is a small, week, narrow band of muscle situated on the medial surface of the elbow and extending to the medial border of the radius.

Origin: On the medial epicondyle of the humerus in close proximity with the medial collateral ligament of elbow joint.

Insertion: The medial border of the radius

Action: Flexion of elbow.

Blood supply: Branches of the brachial and the median arteries.

Nerve supply: The median nerve.

Extensors of elbow

Tensor fasciae antibrachii

The tensor fasciae antibrachii is a slender muscle that lies on the caudal border and somewhat medial to the long head of triceps brachii. It extends from the caudal angle of scapula to the medial surface of the olecranon. The muscle has a thin, long and narrow belly.

Origin: It originates on the caudal aspect of the scapula.

Insertion: On the medial surface of olecranon process of ulna and the antibrachial fascia.

Action: To flex the shoulder and extend the elbow joint.

Blood supply: The Thoracodorsal artery.

Nerve supply: The radial nerve.

Triceps brachii

The triceps is a large three headed muscle that occupies the angle formed by the scapula and humerus. The **lateral head** is broad and flat, and has a considerable thickness in the middle of its length. It is separated from the long head by a groove which is deeper and prominent towards scapular side than the humeral side where it is shallow and negligible. The **long head** is the largest of the three heads and its caudal border forms the margin of the omobrachial region. The **medial head** is the smallest and is covered to some extent by the long head.

Origin: The long head from the caudal border of the scapula, the lateral head from the curved muscular line above the deltoid tuberosity of the humerus and the medial head from the medial surface of the humerus.

Insertion: The medial, lateral and caudal surface of the olecranon process of ulna and the antibrachial fascia.

Action: The long head flexes the shoulder joint. All the three heads extend the elbow joint. The main action of this muscle is to extend the elbow.

Blood supply: The subscapular, the triceps branch of caudal circumflex humeral and deep brachial arteries.

Nerve supply: The radial nerve.

Anconeus

The anconeus is a small fleshy and slightly thick muscle that covers the olecranon fossa.

Origin: On the caudal surface of the distal third of the shaft of humerus and the ridges forming the boundaries of olecranon fossa.

Insertion: On the cranial border and lateral surface of the olecranon process of ulna.

Action: To extend the elbow joint.

Blood supply: The triceps branch of subscapular artery.

Nerve supply: The radial nerve.

Muscles of forearm and manus

The muscles of forearm and manus cover these regions on three sides, the dorsal (cranial), lateral and the volar (caudal) sides while the medial side is subcutaneous. The dorsal and lateral surfaces are covered by the extensors and the volar surface is covered by flexor muscles.

Extensors of carpus

Extensor carpi radialis

The extensor carpi radialis is the largest and most medial of the muscles of the extensor group. It extends from the distal part of humerus to the metacarpus and it lies entirely on the dorsal (cranial) surface of forearm. The belly of the muscle is irregularly circular except at its origin.

Origin: The condyloid crest and coronoid fossa of the humerus.

Insertion: The metacarpal tuberosity.

Action: To extend the carpus and flex the elbow.

Blood supply: The radial artery.

Nerve supply: The radial nerve.

Extensor carpi obliquus

The extensor carpi obliquus is a small muscle which crosses obliquely the distal half of the radius and the carpus passing from lateral to medial side.

Origin: The distal half of the lateral surface of ulna and triangular area on the adjacent part of the dorsal surface of the radius.

Insertion: The medio-volar angle of the proximal extremity of the large metacarpal bone.

Action: To extend and to slightly rotate outwardly the carpal joint.

Blood supply: The dorsal interosseous artery.

Nerve supply: The radial nerve.

Extensors of digit

Medial digital extensor

The medial digital extensor muscle is situated lateral to the extensor carpi radialis. It extends from distal extremity of humerus to the third phalanx. The belly of this muscle is narrow and a little larger than the next muscle. The muscular belly passes down the forearm by a long narrow tendon which passes through the lateral groove on the dorsal surface of the distal extremity of the radius with the tendon of common digital extensor, crosses the carpus and metacarpus medial and close to the tendon of common digital extensor muscle. Near the distal third of the metacarpus, the tendon inclines medially, crosses the medial surface of the fetlock joint, receives two slips from the suspensory ligament and then divides into two branches that terminate on the second and third phalanges.

Origin: The cranial aspect of the lateral epicondyle of humerus with the origin of common digital extensor muscle.

Insertion: The cranial border of proximal extremity of the middle and distal phalanx.

Action: To extend the joints of medial digit and to abduct the digit.

Blood supply: The radial artery.

Nerve supply: The radial nerve.

Common digital extensor

The common digital extensor is a long slender muscle that extends from the distal end of the humerus to the distal phalanx of both, medial and lateral digits. The muscle has two heads of origin, the humeral and the ulnar heads. These two heads fuse about the middle of the forearm and the single belly thus formed is succeeded by a single strong and flat tendon above the distal third of the forearm. The tendon passes through the lateral groove on the dorsal surface of the distal extremity of radius with the tendon of medial digital extensor, crosses the carpus and metacarpus inclining towards the median plane of the limb and divides above the distal extremity of metacarpus into two branches, one for each digit. Each of the two branches runs down along the cranial border of the proximal and middle phalanx and terminates on the extensor process of the distal phalanx.

Origin: Cranial aspect of the lateral epicondyle of humerus and the lateral surface of the shaft of ulna proximal to the interosseous space.

Insertion: The extensor process of the distal phalanx of each digit.

Action: To extend the digit, flex the elbow and indirectly to extend the carpus.

Blood supply: The radial artery.

Nerve supply: The radial nerve.

Lateral digital extensor

The lateral digital extensor is a long slender muscle that extends from the proximal extremity of radius to the distal phalanx of the lateral digit. This muscle lies lateral to the preceding muscle. Its fleshy belly tapers from its origin at the lateral tuberosity of radius to its distal extremity. The tendon appears to about the middle of the forearm and the muscle fibres join it till it reaches near the carpus. The tendon passes through a synovial sheath on the lateral aspect of the carpus along with the tendon of common digital extensor, passes down the metacarpal region behind the tendon of the preceding muscle, receives two slips from suspensory ligament near the distal extremity of the metacarpus and terminates on the proximal and middle phalanx of the lateral digit.

Origin: The lateral tuberosity of radius and adjacent part of ulna. Lateral collateral ligament of the elbow and the lateral surface of ulna between the proximal and distal interosseous spaces.

Insertion: The cranial part of the proximal extremity of the middle and distal phalanx.

Action: To extend the phalangeal joints of the lateral digit and to abduct them.

Blood supply: The common interosseous artery of forearm.

Nerve supply: The radial nerve.

Flexors of carpus

Flexor carpi radialis

The flexor carpi radialis is the medial flexor of the carpus. It is narrow and fusiform in shape. It lies on the medial aspect of the forearm. At its origin, the muscle is tendinous and subsequently it becomes flat and fleshy and then it tapers to the tendon of insertion. Before its termination, it passes through the volar carpal ligament and is surrounded by the synovial sheath of the capsular ligament.

Origin: Medial epicondyle of humerus, caudal to the medial collateral ligament of elbow.

Insertion: The caudomedial angle of the proximal extremity of the large metacarpus.

Action: To flex the carpal joint.

Blood supply: The median artery.

Nerve supply: The median nerve.

Flexor carpi ulnaris

The flexor carpi ulnaris is the middle or oblique flexor of the carpus. It crosses the volar (caudal) surface of the carpal region obliquely to reach the accessory carpal. The muscle has two heads of origin. The humeral head forms the major part of the muscle. The ulnar head is narrow oblique band that joins the caudal border of the humeral head in the proximal part of the forearm. The fleshy belly of the muscle contains considerable amount of tendinous tissue which appears on the superficial as well as deep surface of the muscle. The deep part of the muscle forms a separate tendon for insertion of muscle on the accessory carpal bone.

Origin: The medial epicondyle of the humerus behind the origin of the flexor carpi radialis muscle and the medial surface of the olecranon process.

Insertion: The accessory carpal bone.

Action: To flex the carpus and slightly extend the elbow.

Blood supply: The median and ulnar arteries.

Nerve supply: The ulnar nerve.

Ulnaris lateralis

The ulnaris lateralis muscle is the lateral flexor of the carpus. It lies on the lateral surface of the forearm behind the lateral digital extensor muscle. The origin of the muscle is small and tendinous. The belly is flat fleshy and is continued by two tendons near the carpus. The caudal tendon is attached to the accessory carpal while the cranial tendon crosses the lateral collateral ligament to reach the dorsal surface of the metacarpus.

Origin: The lateral epicondyle of the humerus.

Insertion: The lateral surface of the accessory carpal and a tubercle on the dorsolateral aspect of the proximal extremity of the large metacarpus.

Action: To flex the carpal joint and to slightly extend the elbow joint.

Blood supply: The interosseous artery.

Nerve supply: The radial nerve.

Pronator teres

The pronator teres is a small feeble fibromuscular band of muscle situated along the medial aspect of the elbow joint closely blended with the medial collateral ligament.

Origin: The medial epicondyle of the humerus with the medial collateral ligament of the elbow joint.

Insertion: The medial border of the radius.

Action: No action is appreciable of this muscle, since it is a vestigial.

Blood supply: The median artery.

Nerve supply: The median nerve.

Flexors of digit

Superficial digital flexor

The superficial digital flexor muscle lies under cover of the flexor carpi radialis muscle. It extends from the distal extremity of the humerus to the phalangeal joints of the limb. The belly of the muscle is in the forearm, is largely covered by the flexors of the carpus up to the middle of the radius. At this level, the muscle splits into superficial and deep parts with a separate tendon for each part. The tendon of the superficial part passes over the carpal sheath. The tendon of the deep part passes through the carpal sheath in company with the deep digital flexor and is connected to it by a strong fibrous band. The tendons of the two parts unite about the middle of the metacarpus. The common (single) tendon thus formed divides just above the fetlock joint into two branches. Each of these two branches forms along with the caudal division of suspensory ligament a ring (canal) through which passes the tendon of deep digital flexor muscle.

Origin: The medial epicondyle of humerus.

Insertion: The caudal (volar) aspect of the upper extremity of the middle phalanx.

Action: To flex the digits and carpus and extend the elbow.

Blood supply: The median artery.

Nerve supply: The ulnar nerve.

Deep digital flexor

The deep digital flexor is larger of the two digital flexors and it lies mostly under cover of the superficial digital flexor. It extends from the distal part of humerus and proximal part of ulna to the distal phalanx of each digit. It has three heads of origin, the humeral, radial and ulnar. The humeral head is the largest and is divided in two parts of about equal size. They originate from the medial epicondyle of humerus. The radial head is the deepest and smallest and arises from the lateral part of the caudal surface of radius at its proximal half. The ulnar head is the most superficial and is situated between the flexor carpi ulnaris and ulnaris lateralis. It arises from the medial and lateral faces of the olecranon process of ulna. Each head is succeeded by a tendon. All the three tendons unite and form a common tendon just proximal to the carpus. It passes through the carpal sheath and then in the metacarpal region it passes between the suspensory ligament in front and the tendon of superficial flexor behind. Just proximal to fetlock it divides into two divisions which pass through the rings formed by the superficial digital flexor muscle and the suspensory ligament and terminate on the caudal surface of distal phalanx of the two digits.

Origin: The medial epicondyle of humerus, the proximal half of the caudal surface of radius and the olecranon process of ulna.

Insertion: The caudal surface of distal phalanx of both the digits.

Action: Primarily to flex the digits, partly to flex the carpus and and secondarily to extend the elbow.

Blood supply: The medial and common interosseous arteries.

Nerve supply: The median nerve.

84

Comparative Anatomy of Muscles of Fore Limb

Horse

The **muscles of shoulder region** namely the **supraspinatus, infraspinatus, teres major, teres minor and coracobrachialis** in horse resemble those of ox. The **subscapularis** muscle has only a single head of origin in horse as against three heads in ox. The **deltoideus** muscle has two parts of origin as that of ox but in horse its acromial part is named as cranial part and it arises from scapular spine and the scapular fascia instead of the acromion process. In addition to these muscles, the shoulder in horse is composed of one more muscle named as capsularis. The **capsularis** is a very fine narrow muscle arising from the caudal part of the rim of the glenoid cavity of scapula and is inserted on the caudal part of the neck below the head of the humerus by insinuating itself between the fibres of brachialis muscle. This muscle is peculiar to solipeds and it raises the capsular ligament of shoulder joint during flexion of the joint.

The **muscles of arm** in horse are in general similar to those of ox except the following minor differences. The tendon of origin of **biceps brachii** is adapted to the intertuberal (bisipital) groove. The **tensor fasciae antibrachii** is thin in front and wide below. The medial head of **triceps brachii** is less developed and extends from the middle of the medial surface of shaft of humerus. The **anconeus** is smaller and less voluminous.

Amongst the **muscles of forearm and manus**, the flexors of carpus especially the **flexor carpi radialis, flexor carpi ulnaris and the ulnaris lateralis** resemble those of ox. The pronator teres is either vestigial or completely absent. The **medial digital extensor** is absent. The **extensor carpi radialis** resembles that of ox. The **common digital extensor** arises in common with the extensor carpi radialis. Its tendon descends over the synovial capsule of the carpus, passes down the metacarpus and at the fetlock it receives two slips from suspensory ligament to form the broad ligament which is inserted to the pyramidal extensor process of the distal phalanx. The **lateral digital extensor**

is smaller. It arises from humerus and radius. Its tendon is inserted to the prominence on the dorsal (cranial) aspect of the proximal extremity of the proximal phalanx. The **extensor carpi obliquus** is inserted to the head of the medial small metacarpal bone. The **superficial digital flexor** does not divide into two parts. Its tendon is reinforced above the carpus by a strong fibrous band- the superior check ligament. The ring for the deep digital flexor is formed entirely by the tendon of superficial digital flexor. The **deep digital flexor** has same heads of origin as those of ox. Its tendon receives about half way down the metacarpus the inferior check ligament. It is inserted to the semilunar crest and tendinous surface of the distal phalanx.

Dog

Amongst the **muscles of shoulder** region, the **supraspinatus** in dog is in general similar to that of ox. However it extends beyond the limit of the cranial border of scapula. The **infraspinatus** is smaller but longer than supraspinatus. The **deltoideus** is well developed. Its acromial part is short, thick and distinct. The scapular part of this muscle is triangular. The **teres major** is comparatively thicker and more developed. The **subscapularis** resembles that of ox. The **coracobrachialis** is relatively smaller. The capsular muscle which appears in horse is absent in dog.

Amongst the **muscles of arm**, the **biceps brachii** is very prominent. It is tendinous both at its origin as well as at the insertion. The **tensor fasciae antibrachii** is closely associated with the latissimus dorsi at its origin and separates from it before joining the olecranon. The **triceps brachii** is massive and voluminous. It has an additional accessory head of origin that arises from below the head of humerus. The tendon of insertions of brachialis and biceps brachii are wrapped into a common sheath near their insertion.

The **muscles of forearm and manus** in dog have some major differences owing to the difference of digits in this species. The **extensor carpi radialis** is triangular with its base above and the apex tapering into the tendon of insertion below. The insertion of this muscle is in two divisions on the proximal ends of second and third metacarpal bones. The one that ends on second metacarpal is named as **extensor carpi radialis brevis** and the other ending on third metacarpal is named as **extensor carpi radialis longus**. The **extensor carpi obliquus** is only slightly oblique and it ends on first metacarpal bone. It abducts the first digit and the manus region. An additional muscle of forearm namely the **brachio-radialis** is inconstantly present in dog. When present, it extends from the lateral epicondyle of humerus and ends on the medial border of radius. The **ulnaris lateralis** and **pronator teres** are same as those of ox. The **flexor carpi radialis** is slender and conical and its tendon is thin and long. The **flexor**

carpi ulnaris has two heads of origin, the humeral and ulnar. The **common digital extensor** has a very short muscular belly which is continued from the middle of the forearm into the tendon of insertion that divides into four divisions for insertion on the distal phalanx of second to fifth digits. The **lateral digital extensor** is an inconstant small muscle that is attached to the distal phalanx of the third and fourth digits. It is named as the **extensor of the third and fourth digits**. The **extensor of the first and second digits** is a small muscle placed between the common digital and lateral digital extensors. It arises from the shaft of the ulna and terminates by joining the tendon of common digital extensor and by giving slips to the first and second digits. The **superficial digital flexor** arises by a single head of origin on the medial condyle of the humerus, its muscular belly runs on the palmer surface of the carpus, is strengthened by receiving slips from the accessory carpal and the carpal sesamoids and then divides into four divisions for termination on the middle phalanx of the second to fifth digits. The **deep digital flexor** originates in three heads, the humeral, radial and ulnar. It has two tendons of insertion. The medial one inserts on the first digit and the lateral division sub divides into four branches for insertion on the distal phalanx of second to fifth digits.

Sheep and Goat

The gross anatomical features of the muscles of fore limb in sheep and goat are almost similar to those in ox except that (1) the tendon of insertion of **biceps brachii** in goat splits into two divisions, the larger one of these inserts on the radial tuberosity while the smaller one inserts on the coronoid process of ulna. (2) the **brachialis muscle** in goat inserts in two parts, one on the caudal surface of radius and the other on the medial surface of coronoid process of ulna as against the insertion on radial tuberosity in ox and (3) the superficial and deep divisions of the lateral belly of the **common digital extensor** unite at about the distal fourth of the forearm in sheep and goat instead of their union at the middle of the forearm in ox.

Pig

The **muscles of shoulder** region of the fore limb of pig resemble those of ox in their general disposition with the following special features. (1) The **deltoid muscle** is undivided. It arises by aponeurosis with the fascia covering the infraspinatus and terminates chiefly on the deltoid ridge with a small part inserting on the fascia on the arm region. (2) The **supraspinatus** is relatively large and ends on both, the lesser and greater tubercles of the proximal extremity of humerus. (3) The **infraspinatus** is wide and it ends on a depression ventral to the caudal division of greater tubercle. (4) The **teres minor** is large and rounded and it terminates on a tubercle between the greater tuberosity and the deltoid tubercle. (4) The **subscapularis** is very broad at its dorsal part extending to almost the caudal end of the scapula. (5) The **coracobrachialis** is short, wide and undivided. (6) The **capsularis** is inconsistently present but when present, it is very small.

The special features of the **muscles of arm** region are as below. (1) The **biceps brachii** is fusiform. Its tendon of origin is rounded and when it passes through the intertuberal (bisipital) groove it is bound by a small band of synovial membrane. For insertion, there are two tendons one ends on the ulna and the other on radius. (2) The **brachialis** is large and its tendon of insertion is divided. And these insert on radius and ulna.(3) The long head of **triceps brachii** inserts by two tendons on the olecranon process and between the two tendons lies the synovial bursa. The medial and lateral heads of triceps brachii end on the respective surfaces of olecranon process of ulna.

The **muscles of forearm and manus** have following special features. (1) The **extensor carpi radialis** is strong and fleshy muscle. It inserts on the third metacarpal. (2) The **extensor carpi obliquus** is well developed. It originates on the distal two thirds of the lateral surface of radius and ulna and terminates on second metacarpal bone. (3) The **common digital extensor** arises on the lateral epicondyle of humerus and lateral collateral ligament of elbow and divides into three parts, the medial, middle and lateral. The medial division terminates on the third (chief) digit and gives a small branch to the second digit. The tendon of middle division splits into two sub parts which terminate one each on the third and fourth (chief) digits. The lateral division ends on the fifth digit. (4) The **lateral digital extensor** has two tendons of insertion. One inserts on the fourth (chief) digit and the other on the fifth digit. (6) The **flexor carpi radialis** is well developed; the flexor carpi ulnaris is narrow and usually does not have the ulnar head and the ulnaris lateralis ends on the proximal end of fifth metacarpal bone. (7) The **superficial digital flexor** ends by two branches on the middle phalanx of the fourth digit. (8) The common tendon of insertion formed by the union of the three heads of the **deep digital flexor** divides into four branches, of which the middle two (central pair) ends on the distal phalanx of the third and fourth (chief) digits and the outer two (abaxial pair) ends on the second and fifth (accessory) digits.

Fowl

The **wing muscles** (muscles of pectoral or fore limb) of fowl are specifically designed to produce aerodynamic power needed to support the weight of the body in the air. This requirement is fulfilled mainly by two muscles, the large pectoralis and a smaller supracoracoideus. The **pectoralis** is a large muscle of the pectoral girdle. It has three parts. The largest one is the **sterno-brachialis** which originates on the elongated sternal keel. The second part, **thoraco-brachialis** is smaller than the first and it originates on the dorsal part of the ribs. The third part, the **clavico-brachialis** is the smallest one which originates on the furculum of the clavicle. All the three parts unite over the keel, pass over the shoulder joint and insert on the deltoid crest of the humerus. The other muscle which is antagonistic to the pectoralis is the **supracoracoideus.** It is much smaller (about one fifth) than and lies deep to the pectoralis muscle originating on the keel and inserting on the deltoid crest of the humerus. It helps in elevation of the wing. The other major muscles of the pectoral limb (wing) of the fowl are the **coracobrachialis cranialis** and **caudalis, deltoideus, biceps brachii** and **triceps brachii** in brachial region and the extensors and flexors of the antibrachium and manus region.

SECTION-B

BLOOD VESSELS AND LYMPHATICS

85

Arteries of Fore Limb

Subclavian artery

The fore limb is chiefly supplied by the **subclavian artery (Fig. 5-4 A)**. It originates from the brachiocephalic trunk within the thoracic cavity. The **left subclavian** detaches from the brachiocephalic trunk opposite the second rib, passes craniodorsally towards the thoracic inlet winds around the cranial border of the first rib and then courses caudoventrally through the axillary space between the subscapular and teres major muscles as the **axillary artery**. It gives off the subscapular branch and continues as the **brachial artery.** The **right subclavian** is the direct continuation of the brachiocephalic trunk after the later gives off the bicarotid trunk opposite the first rib. It gets exit through the thoracic inlet, winds around the cranial border of the first rib and then continues as the right axillary artery and thereafter as the brachial artery similar to the artery of the left side.

Axillary artery

The axillary artery is the continuation of the subclavian after the later reaches the axillary space. During its course through the space between the subscapularis and teres major, it gives off three major branches, the external thoracic, the suprascapular artery and the subscapular artery and then after reaching at the ventral end of the teres major muscle it continues as the brachial artery.

1. The **external thoracic artery** has a variable origin. It usually arises from the axillary artery lateral to the first rib and passes ventrally on the medial surface of the deep pectoral muscle to the junction of this muscle with the superficial pectoral. Here it supplies branches to the deltoideus, the superficial and deep pectorals, the biceps brachii and the brachialis muscles,

2. The **suprascapular artery** arises from the dorsal face of the axillary artery and passes with suprascapular vein and suprascapular nerve dorsally across the insertion of the subscapularis muscle. It gives branches to supraspinatus and subscapularis muscles.

3. The **subscapular artery** is the largest branch of the axillary. It arises from the axillary, caudal to the shoulder joint, runs dorsad parallel to the caudal border of scapula and reaches to its caudal angle, turns laterally and ends in the infraspinatus muscle. The major part of this artery lies on the origin of long head of triceps brachii and is covered by the caudal part of subscapularis muscle. During its course, the subscapular artery gives off three major branches the caudal circumflex humeral artery, the thoracodorsal artery and the circumflex artery of scapula.

- The **caudal circumflex humeral artery** arises from lateral face of the subscapular passes laterally behind the shoulder joint to the deep surface of the deltoid muscle and furnishes branches to deltoideus, teres minor and infraspinatus muscles. Prior to these, a large branch is given off by this artery near its origin to the triceps brachii muscle.

- The **thoracodorsal artery** which arises from the subscapular artery next to the preceding branch crosses the teres major muscle and then passes caudad and dorsad on the deep face of the latissimus dorsi muscle and furnishes branches to the latissimus dorsi, long head of triceps and the tensor fasciae antibrachii muscles.

- The **circumflex artery of scapula** arises from the cranial border of the subscapular artery at the level of the neck of the scapula. It may arise either as a common trunk of medial and lateral branches or as two separate arteries. The medial branch passes to the medial surface of scapula and supplies the subscapularis muscle. The lateral branch reaches the infraspinatus fossa and supplies the infraspinatus muscle.

Brachial artery (Fig. 5-4 A & Fig. 5-4 B)

The brachial artery is the continuation of the axillary artery in the arm region. It courses distally along with the medial nerve and reaches the flexor surface of the elbow joint where it passes beneath the tendons of insertion of biceps brachii and pronator teres muscles and gives out common interosseous artery distal to the elbow joint. It then continues down as the median artery. Before its continuation as median artery, the brachial artery gives out the following branches.

1. The **cranial circumflex humeral artery** is the first branch of the brachial artery and it arises from the cranial face of brachial artery close to or just next to the origin of subscapular branch of axillary artery. It passes cranially on the medial surface of the arm. The artery along with the vein and nerve passes between the two parts of the coracobrachialis muscle and ends in the biceps brachii muscle. It furnishes branches to these muscles and the medial aspect of the shoulder joint.

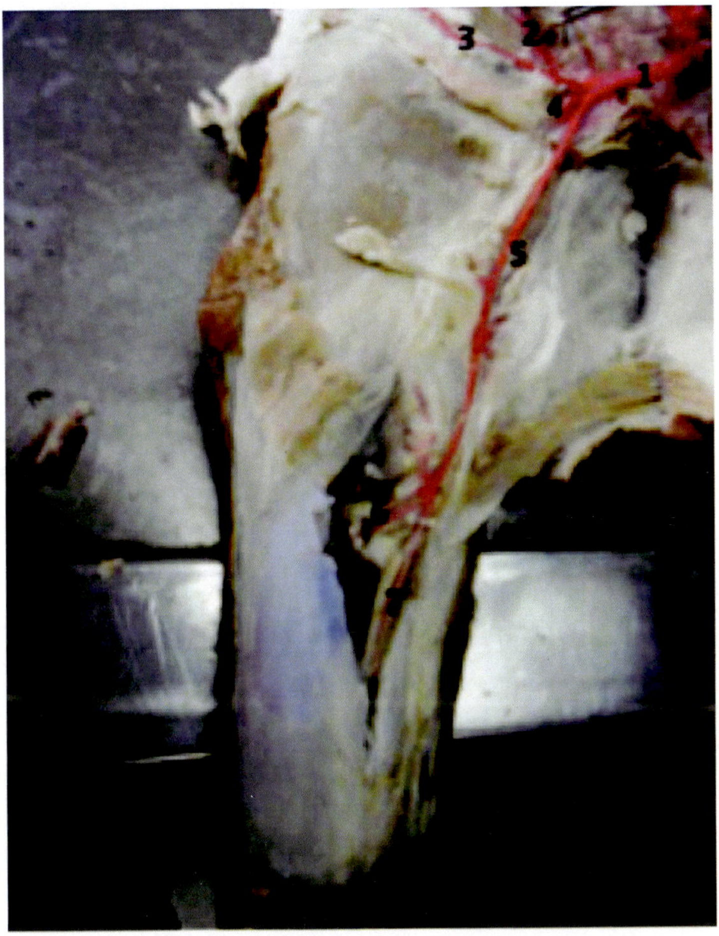

Fig. 5 – 4 A: Blood vessels of forelimb of Ox

1. Axillary Artery 2. Subscapular Artery 3. Thoraco dorsal Artery 4. Anterior circumflex humoral Artery 5. Brachial Artery 6. Interosseous Artery 7. Median Artery

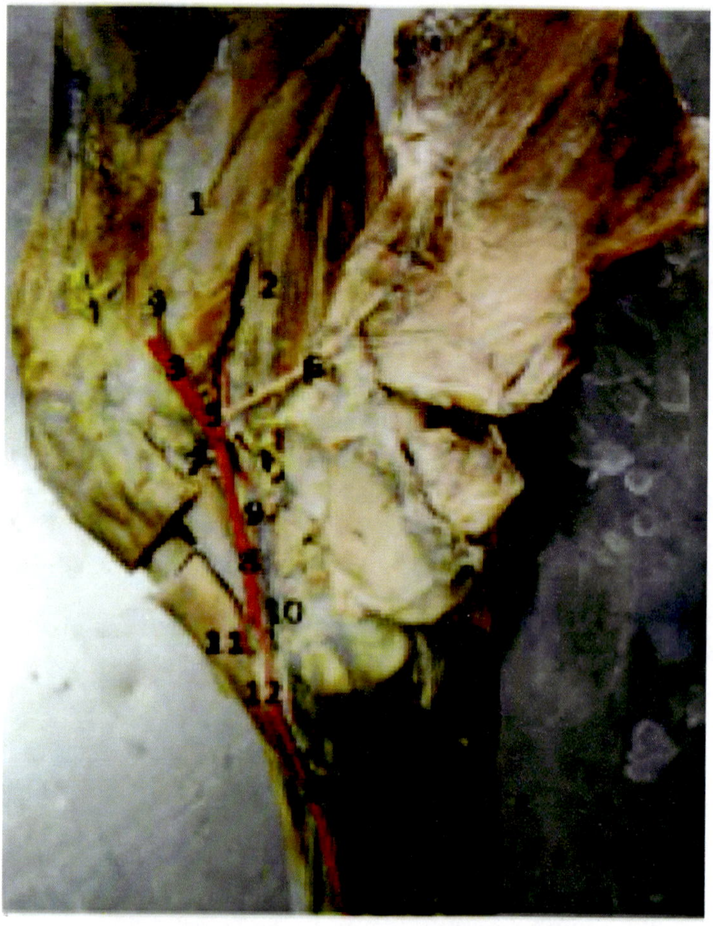

Fig. 5 – 4 B: Blood vessels of forelimb of Ox

1. Subscapular m. 2. Teres major m. 3. Axillary artery 4. Suprascapular artery 5. Subscapular artery 6. Thoraco-dorsal artery 7. Anterior circumflex artery 8. Brachial artery 9. Deep humeral artery 10. collateral ulnar artery 11. Collateral radial artery 12. Median artery 13. Common interosseous artery

2. The **deep brachial artery** is a small vessel arising from the caudal surface of the brachial near the middle of the arm. It supplies to the long head of the triceps brachii muscle.

3. The **collateral ulnar artery** arises from the caudal aspect of the brachial artery slightly dorsal to the medial condyle of the humerus. It passes caudad and ventrad on the medial surface of the arm, crosses the medial epicondyle and turns ventrad between the epicondyle and the olecranon process of ulna under cover of the ulnar head of flexor carpi ulnaris. It furnishes branches to the superficial pectoral, the medial and long heads of triceps brachii, flexor carpi ulnaris and the superficial and deep digital flexor muscles.

4. The **transverse cubital artery** arises from the brachial on the flexor surface of elbow joint and after passing between this joint and the biceps brachii and brachialis muscles divides into proximal and distal branches. During this course it furnishes branches to coracobrachialis, brachialis, brachiocephalicus and pectoral muscles. The proximal branch anastomoses with the branches of collateral ulnar and supplies to extensor carpi radialis, biceps brachii, brachialis and brachiocephalicus muscles. The distal branch supplies to extensor carpi radialis, common digital extensor and the medial and the lateral digital extensors.

5. The **common interosseous artery** is the last collateral branch of brachial artery before its continuation as median artery distal to the elbow joint. It arises from brachial at the level of proximal interosseous space, furnishes muscular branches to the deep digital flexor, ulnaris lateralis and other adjoining muscles and then divides into the cranial and caudal interosseous arteries. The **cranial interosseous artery** descends along the interosseous groove between the shaft of the radius and ulna and at about the distal half of the forearm divides into dorsal and palmer branches. The dorsal interosseous artery contributes the dorsal carpal rete while the palmer interosseous artery passes through distal interosseous space of forearm and contributes the palmer carpal rete. The **caudal interosseous artery** is very slender and it supplies the superficial and deep digital flexors.

Median artery

The median artery is the distal continuation of the brachial artery distal to the elbow joint. At the elbow it crosses the insertion of biceps brachii, passes under the pronator teres and continues distally covered by flexor carpi radialis. It descends along the medial aspect of the caudal surface of the radius in association with the median nerve, and at a variable distance down the forearm divides into radial and ulnar arteries.

Radial artery

The radial artery is the smaller of the two terminal branches of the median artery. It descends along the caudomedial aspect of radius under the flexor carpi radialis, passes down subcutaneously over the carpal sheath on the palmer aspect of the carpus. Here the artery lies covered by fascia but outside the carpal sheath. The radial artery further continues down as the **medial deep palmer metacarpal artery.** Before this, the radial artery gives out a branch each to the dorsal carpal rete and palmer carpal rete and two other large branches which pass between the suspensory ligament and the large metacarpal bone as **middle deep palmer metacarpal artery** and the **lateral deep palmer metacarpal artery**.. These arteries descend down the caudal longitudinal groove of the large metacarpal bone and join the medial deep palmer metacarpal to form the **deep palmer metacarpal arch** above the fetlock joint.

Ulnar artery

The ulnar artery is the larger of the two terminal branches of the median artery. It descends under the flexor carpi radialis, passes through the carpal sheath on the medial face of the tendon of deep digital flexor and continues down as the **palmer superficial large metacarpal artery**. This vessel passes underneath the deep fascia of the metacarpus along the medial border of the tendon of deep digital flexor in company with the median nerve. At the distal third of the metacarpus it gives off a branch to form a **superficial palmer metacarpal arch** and is continued as the **palmer common digital artery** which enters the interdigital space and divides into two **palmer axial digital arteries**, one for each digit. Each of these two arteries reach the extensor process of the distal phalanx, passes through the foramen and enter the sinus in the interior of the bone (distal phalanx) forming arterial circle inside the sinus from which the branches are supplied to the corium of the foot.

The **dorsal metacarpal artery** is a small artery that arises from the dorsal carpal rete, passes down the dorsal metacarpal groove and after reaching the interdigital space at the fetlock joint continues down as the dorsal common digital artery. The later receives a branch from the **palmer common digital** and divides into two **dorsal proper digital arteries** one for each digit.

86

Veins of Fore Limb

The venous drainage of the fore limb of ox is conducted by two independent routes, the superficial and deep routes, in the fore limb. The major vein of the superficial route is the cephalic vein and that of the deep route is the axillary vein. The venous drainage of the fore limb begins at the digits and is carried by branches of both the routes intermingling or confluent with each other up to the level of elbow joint. From the elbow upwards the journey of the two paths is completely independent of each other. The superficial veins join the cephalic vein while the deep veins join the axillary vein to open into the cranial vena cava.

Superficial veins

The superficial veins begin in the form of **distal deep and distal superficial palmer arch** just above the fetlock joint. These venous arches are formed by the union of **axial and abaxial digital veins**. From these venous arches extend the dorsal metacarpal vein ascending first through the interdigital space and then winding around the large metacarpal bone. In this course it anastomoses with the branches of radial vein on the dorsomedial aspect of the carpometacarpal region and passes further upward as accessory cephalic vein.

The **accessory cephalic vein** lies on the dorsal surface of the carpus and distal part of the radius. It receives venous branches from the dorsal metacarpal and the carpal joint and the skin in that region. In the region of the forearm, the accessory cephalic vein forms anastomosis with the branches of the median vein and from these anastomoses extend upwards the **medial cubital (metacarpal) vein** which passes craniodorsally under the pronator teres muscle, crosses the insertion of brachialis muscle and joins the cephalic vein.

The **cephalic vein** is a subcutaneous vein on the dorsomedial aspect of the arm and forearm regions of the fore limb. It is the upward continuation of the medial metacarpal (cubital) vein near the distal extremity of the radius. Starting at this point the vein passes dorsad and craniad to the tendon of extensor carpi radialis and then upward on this muscle to the elbow. Just above (proximal to) the distal extremity of radius it forms anastomosis with the branches of the median vein and then enters the groove formed by the superficial pectoral and brachiocephalic muscles. It traverses through this groove to the cranial border of the first rib and terminates in the jugular vein.

Deep veins

The deep division of the venous drainage of fore limb is larger and major of the two. It is comprised of the palmer lateral, palmer middle and palmer medial deep metacarpal veins, the radial vein, the ulnar vein, the median vein the brachial vein and the axillary vein. The main vessel of this group is the axillary vein. The venous drainage begins at the distal superficial and deep palmer venous arches at the fetlock joint. These arches are formed by the anastomotic branches of the medial and lateral digital veins.

Metacarpal veins

The palmer medial, palmer middle and palmer lateral deep metacarpal veins ascend the respective side of the metacarpal bone under cover of the suspensory ligament.

The **palmer medial deep metacarpal vein** is the upward continuation of the medial digital vein. It gives anastomotic branch to the palmer lateral deep metacarpal vein to form the palmer deep distal metacarpal arch just above the fetlock joint. From here it courses upward between the suspensory ligament and large metacarpal bone along the medial border of the bone, communicates with the palmer middle deep metacarpal vein, ascends the palmer medial aspect of the carpus passing superficially over the carpal sheath in company with the radial artery and divides in the distal third of the forearm into two, the cranial and caudal branches. The cranial vein join the cephalic vein of the superficial group of veins and the caudal branch continues upward as the radial vein.

The **palmer lateral deep metacarpal vein** is the upward continuation of the lateral deep digital vein. After reaching at the distal end of the metacarpus, it contributes to the formation of the palmer deep distal metacarpal arch with the palmer medial deep metacarpal vein and also furnishes a branch that passes craniad and dorsad to join the dorsal superficial metacarpal vein. It then passes between the two divisions of the suspensory ligament furnishes a branch for the distal superficial metacarpal arch and then ascends along the lateral border of the palmer surface of the large metacarpus. At about the proximal extremity of the metacarpus it unites with the palmer middle deep metacarpal vein. A common trunk of these two receives a branch from the palmer aspect of the carpus and then unites with the palmer medial deep metacarpal vein to form the proximal deep palmer metacarpal arch.

The **palmer deep middle metacarpal vein** arises from the palmer deep distal metacarpal arch and follows the upward course on the palmer surface of metacarpus lying between the palmer medial and lateral deep metacarpal veins. It then joins these veins in the formation of the proximal deep palmer metacarpal arch.

Radial vein

The radial vein is the upward continuation of the palmer medial deep metacarpal vein at about the distal third of the forearm. From here it passes along the medial border of the caudal surface of the radius running in association with the radial artery between the radius and the flexor carpi radialis muscles. After reaching at about the level of distal attachment of the pronator teres muscle it is joined by the medial ulnar vein forming the **radio-ulnar vein**. The later vein courses upward in front of the median artery, is joined by the lateral ulnar vein and then is continued as the **median vein**. The radial vein at its origin from the medial palmer deep metacarpal vein in the lower third of the forearm is joined by the palmer carpal vein. The later is formed by the palmer medial and the palmer lateral carpal veins. These two veins emerge from the respective sides of the carpus.

Ulnar vein

The ulnar veins, medial and lateral, are the upward continuation of the medial and lateral palmer superficial metacarpal veins. These veins ascend through the carpal sheath along with the ulnar artery. After reaching at the distal end of the forearm, the medial ulnar vein ascends the forearm region lying between the radius and the flexor carpi radialis and joins the radial vein to form the **radio-ulnar vein** at the proximal third of the forearm. The lateral ulnar vein ascends the forearm region along with the ulnar artery and median nerve and then joins the radioulnar vein which later on continues as the **median vein.**

Median vein

The median vein is formed by the radial and ulnar veins at the point of emergence of the median artery and nerve from under the pronator teres muscle on the medial aspect of the elbow joint. From here it courses upwards on the medial aspect of the forearm covered by the flexor carpi radialis muscle, receives the common interosseous vein and a muscular branch formed by the small veins coming from the flexors of carpus and digits. After reaching at the proximal extremity of the radius, the median vein crosses over the tendon of insertion of the biceps brachii, continues upward along with the median artery and median nerve and divides into two branches at the level of medial condyle of humerus. The two branches thus formed continue further upward as **brachial veins.**

Brachial veins

The brachial veins are the upward continuation of the two divisions of the median veins at the level of the medial condyle of the humerus. These two veins ascend for a short distance together lying one in front and the other behind the brachial artery crossing over the lower part of the coracobrachialis and the medial head of the triceps brachii muscles. At this stage, the vein on the front of the artery slips to the back side of the artery and thus both the branches of the brachial veins come close together in their further course and then unite to form a single large brachial vein which receives a deep humeral branch from brachialis and then at the level just distal to the caudal aspect of the shoulder joint continues as the **axillary vein.**

Axillary vein

The axillary vein is the continuation of the brachial vein and it courses as a satellite of the axillary artery through the axillary space between the arm and the lateral wall of the thorax from the level of third rib to first rib. It begins as a large venous trunk on the medial aspect of the arm just distal to the caudal aspect of the shoulder joint. From here it ascends the arm lying ventral to the axillary artery and after reaching the distal part of the first rib crosses its cranial border turns up as subclavian vein which join the common jugular vein to open into the cranial vena cava. During its course the axillary vein receives the **external thoracic, suprascapular** and **subscapular veins.**

87

Lymphatics of Fore Limb

The lymph from the fore limb is collected and carried into the circulation through two main lymph nodes, the prescapular and the axillary lymph nodes. There may be two more lymph nodes in fore limb but those are inconsistent and only occasionally found in ox. These include the accessory axillary lymph node and infraspinous lymph nodes and their afferents are mostly from the thoracic wall.

The **prescapular lymph node** is an elongated large lymph node. It is about 10 cm to 13 cm long and 2.5 cm wide. It is embedded in fat cranial and dorsal to the shoulder joint. It is covered on its dorsal two thirds by omotransversus and on the ventral third by brachiocephalicus muscles. Its deep face is in contact with the supraspinatus and a part of serratus cervicis muscles. The afferents of this lymph node come from a series of haemal lymph nodes which extends from the prescapular lymph node to the cranial angle of the scapula under cover of the trapezious muscle. The major afferents for this lymph node are received from the bones and muscles of the shoulder and arm region of the fore limb along with the serratus ventralis and the superficial and deep pectoral muscles. The efferent of the right prescapular lymph node opens into the right tracheal lymph duct while that of the left lymph node opens into the left tracheal lymph duct.

The **axillary lymph node** is the major lymph node of the fore limb. It lies on the medial surface of the distal portion of the teres major muscle about 6 to 10 cm caudal to the shoulder joint. It is oval in out line and measures about 2.5 to 3.5 cm in length. The afferents for this lymph node come from the muscles of shoulder, arm, forearm, elbow and carpal joints. Its efferent vessel opens into the prescapular lymph node or directly into the jugular vein of the corresponding side.

88

Comparative Anatomy of Blood Vessels and Lymphatics of Fore Limb

Horse

The **arteries** of fore limb of horse are more or less similar in their course and distribution. However, there are some special features in respect of some of these arteries as described below.

1. The **brachial artery** descends vertically on the medial aspect of humerus to its distal extremity, crosses it obliquely and descends along the joint capsule and medial lateral ligament of elbow joint, gives off common interosseous artery at the proximal third of the forearm and then continues distally as median artery.
2. The **median artery** descends along the caudomedial aspect of the radius covered by flexor carpi radialis muscle and divides just proximal to medial condyle into radial and collateral ulnar (ulnar) arteries.
3. The collateral **ulnar artery** is smaller of the two terminal branches of median artery. It descends along the cranial surface of radius under cover of the extensor carpi radialis and terminates a little above the carpus by anastomosing with a branch of radial artery.
4. The **radial artery** is the larger of the two terminal branches of the median artery. It descends on the medial aspect of the caudal surface of radius between the flexor carpi radialis muscle and the radius and after forming anastomosis with caudal collateral ulnar artery just above the carpus terminates by dividing into medial palmer metacarpal and lateral palmer metacarpal arteries.
5. The **lateral palmer metacarpal artery** descends along the palmer surface of the large metacarpus on the side of the lateral small metacarpal bone and enters into formation of superficial palmer arch above the fetlock joint.

6. The **medial palmer metacarpal artery** descends along the medial aspect of the metacarpus and at the level of fetlock joint divides into **medial and lateral palmer proper digital arteries** which diverge from each other and descend on the abaxial surfaces of the proximal, middle and distal phalanges along with the corresponding branches of the tendons of superficial and deep digital arteries.

The **veins** in the fore limb of horse are arranged in two groups, the **superficial and deep group of veins** similar to that in ox. The **superficial venous group** is comprised of the accessory cephalic, median cubital and cephalic veins.

1. The **cephalic vein** is the upward continuation of palmer medial metacarpal vein. It begins on the medial side of the carpus and ascends the forearm in the groove between the radius and flexor carpi radialis muscle. It passes obliquely craniad on the medial face of the radius, reaches the level of the insertion of biceps brachii, receives a branch from the brachial vein, continues to pass through the groove between the superficial pectoral and brachiocephalicus muscles and finally opens into the jugular vein in front of the cranial border of the first rib.
2. The **accessory cephalic vein** is a small vein arising at the fascia over the carpus, runs upward along the cranial face of the forearm and joins the cephalic vein at the level of proximal extremity of the radius.
3. The **deep veins of the fore limb** of horse are comprised of the digital and metacarpal veins which slightly differ in disposition from that of ox and the radial, ulnar, median, and brachial and finally the axillary vein which are almost similar to those of ox.
4. The **medial and lateral digital veins** arise from the venous network formed on the cartilage of the foot and ascend along the medial and lateral abaxial (outer) sides of the three phalanges of the digit to unite above the sesamoids between the tendon of deep digital flexor muscle and the suspensory ligament and to form the sesamoidean venous arch. From this venous arch arise three metacarpal veins.
5. The **medial and lateral deep metacarpal** veins and the common deep metacarpal veins ascend the palmer surface of the metacarpus lying between the bone and the suspensory ligament. The rest of the disposition of these veins is similar to that of ox.

The **lymphatics** of fore limb of horse are almost similar to those of ox and needs no special description.

Dog

The blood supply to fore limb of dog is through the subclavian artery which continues as axillary artery and further down as brachial and then the **median artery.** The course, disposition and distribution of branches of these arteries in the shoulder, arm and forearm regions of the fore limb of dog is mostly similar to that of ox. However, beyond the carpus especially in the metacarpal and digital regions it differs substantially owing to the major difference in the number of digits of these two species. There are five digits in dog as against two digits in ox. The major artery supplying the metacarpus and digits is the medial artery.

The **median artery** in dog gives out a connecting branch to the radial artery just proximal to the carpus and then descends along the medial border of the deep digital flexor muscle lying between the tendons of superficial and deep digital flexor muscles. In the middle of the metacarpus it joins the superficial palmer branch of **radial artery** and forms the **superficial palmer arch**. From this arch arise five branches. One of these is the **lateral palmer digital artery V** for the lateral abaxial digit and the remaining four arteries are the **palmer common digital arteries I, II, III and IV**. These arteries descend in the respective intermetacarpal spaces and join the corresponding **palmer metacarpal arteries**, the branches of the **radial and ulnar arteries** at the metacarpo-phalangeal joints. Further down the palmer common digital arteries divide into two each and descend along the opposite surfaces at the adjacent metacarpus and digits.

The **veins** of the fore limb of dog follow the same pattern of **superficial and deep veins** as that of ox except in the metacarpal and digital regions. The cephalic vein is the major vein of the superficial division.

The **cephalic vein** begins in the digital region as the dorsal lateral digital vein at the metacarpo-phalangeal joint and receives palmer medial metacarpal vein in the metacarpal region. It then ascends the craniomedial aspect of the forearm along the superficial branch of radial nerve and reaches the flexor (caudal) aspect of the elbow. Here it receives a branch from the median vein and continues upward passing through a groove between the brachiocephalicus and brachialis muscles and divides into two branches the cranial and the caudal. The cranial branch is larger and is the main trunk of the cephalic vein. It passes upward in a groove between the acromial part of deltoid and superficial pectoral muscles and join the jugular vein. The caudal branch, the **accessory cephalic vein** passes along the cranial border of the lateral head of triceps brachii muscle, passes on the caudal aspect of shoulder joint and opens into the subscapular vein.

The **deep veins** begin as **dorsal and palmer digital veins** and continue upward as **palmer common digital veins I to V**. In their upward continuation, these veins continue as **palmer medial, palmer middle and palmer lateral metacarpal veins**. The rest of the veins namely the **radial, ulnar, median, brachial and axillary veins** in dog follow the same pattern of course and distribution as that of ox and horse.

The **lymphatics** of fore limb of dog present the same gross anatomical features as those in ox and horse.

Sheep and Goat

The **arteries** of fore limb of sheep and goat in general follows the same pattern of gross anatomical features like course, disposition and branching as that of ox except a few minor differences cited below.

1. The **suprascapular artery**, a branch of axillary artery in ox arises from the prescapular branch of superficial cervical artery in sheep and goat.
2. The **cranial circumflex humeral artery**, a branch of axillary artery in ox arises from the caudal circumflex humeral artery in sheep and from thoracodorsal artery in goat.
3. The **collateral ulnar (ulnar) artery** in sheep forms anastomoses with a branch of subscapular artery and also with the cranial circumflex humeral artery.
4. The **transverse cubital artery** in sheep anastomoses with recurrent interosseous artery and in goat it anastomoses with recurrent interosseous and collateral radial artery.

The **veins** are the satellites of the arteries and follow the same pattern as that of ox.

The **lymphatics** of the fore limb of sheep and goat resemble those of ox.

Pig

The **arteries** of the fore limb of pig are similar to those of the ox except those in the metacarpal and digital regions owing to the presence of additional two accessory digits in pig.

The **veins and lymph nodes** of fore limb of pig also resemble those of ox.

Fowl

The **arteries** of the wings (fore limbs) of fowl have following special features in fowl.

1. The **subclavian artery** of each side divides into pectoral and axillary artery. However, the pectoral artery in some birds may arise from the brachial artery.
2. The **axillary artery** passes dorsally and cranially, bends around the cranial border of the first rib and continues caudally on the ventral face of the wing and supplies the muscles of the wing.
3. The **brachial artery** is the continuation of the axillary artery in the arm region. It passes down the arm with the ulnar nerve between the biceps and triceps muscles and at the mid of the arm divides into the radial and ulnar arteries.
4. The **radial artery** is mainly distributed to the deep muscles on the flexor aspect of forearm. Its perforating branches furnish small twigs to the extensor muscles, skin and the feather muscles of the wing.
5. The **ulnar artery** passes subcutaneously in the ventral aspect of the forearm and reaches the carpus. It serves as the main artery of the carpus.

The **venous blood from the fore limb** is collected and carried to the jugular vein by the axillary vein along with the branches of subclavian and thoracic veins.

The **lymph nodes** are absent in birds. However the lymph is carried through very minute lymph ducts accompanying the veins of the body. The **lymphatic ducts** in the wing (fore limb) of fowl accompany the basilic vein, deep ulnar vein and the deep radial vein. In addition, some minor vessels accompany the deep brachial and the brachial veins which open into the axillary and the subclavian vein that finally join the jugular vein.

SECTION-C

NERVES

89

Nerves of Fore Limb

Brachial plexus (FIG. 5-5 A)

The fore limb is supplied by nerves that extend from the brachial plexus. The brachial plexus is a large wide, flat and thick fascicular anastomosis of nerves formed by the convergence of ventral branches of last three cervical and first two thoracic spinal nerves in ox. It is placed between the scalenus muscle on the lateral wall of thorax and subscapularis and deep pectoral muscles on the costal (medial) surface of the scapula. From this plexus extend the following eleven branches (nerves) which are distributed mainly to the fore limb (thoracic limb) and most of the muscles of the thoracic girdle.

1. The **suprascapular nerve** is derived from the cranial part of this plexus. It passes cranially on the medial side of the limb, continues to pass between the subscapular and supraspinatus muscles, crosses the cranial border of scapula, turns caudad on the neck of the scapula below the scapular spine and terminates in the infraspinatus muscle.

2. The **subscapular nerve** arises from the cranial part of the plexus just caudal to the suprascapular nerve. It is a short nerve that may divide into two or three small branches passing cranially across the subscapularis muscle in the middle of the shoulder and terminate into this muscle near the cranial border of the scapula.

3. The **axillary nerve** arises from the plexus just caudal to the origin of subscapular nerve. After coursing ventrally across the medial face of subscapularis muscle it gains the space between the teres major muscle and the subscapular artery, runs caudal to the shoulder joint in company with the caudal circumflex vessels and reaches the lateral surface of shoulder joint. It further passes between the long head and lateral head of the triceps brachii and reaches the deltoideus muscle. The nerve divides here into several branches supplying the deltoid, teres major, teres minor muscles, and the humeral portion of the brachiocephalic muscle. In addition to these, the axillary nerve gives out the cutaneous branch below the

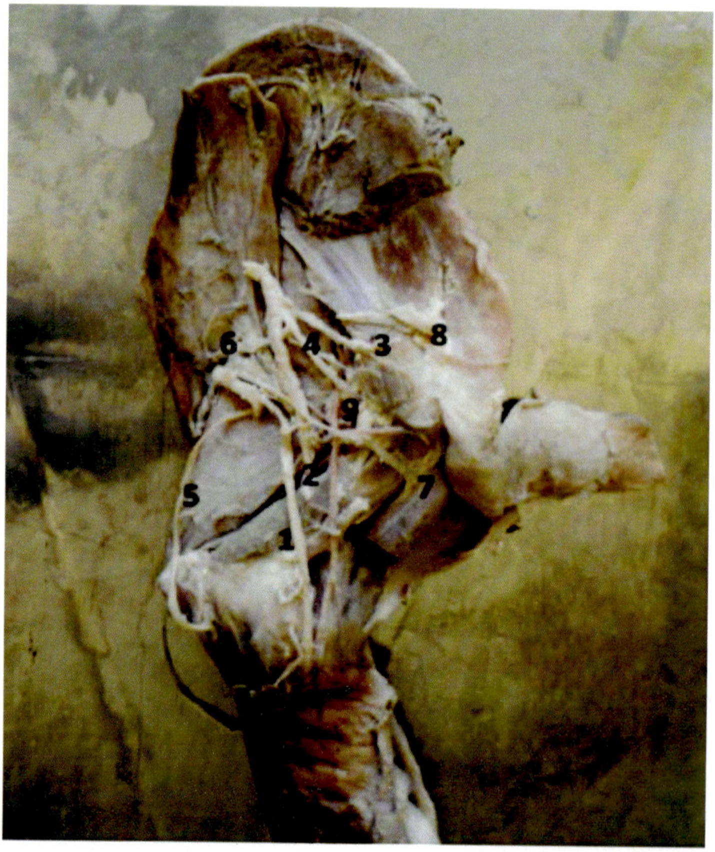

Fig. 5 – 5 A: Brachial plexus and nerves of forelimb of Ox
1: Median N 2: Radial N 3: Subscapular N 4: Nerve to teres major 5: ulnar N 6: Thoraco dorsal N 7: Musculo cutaneous N 8: External thoracic N 9: Axillary N.

deltoid tuberosity and after giving anastomotic branch to cutaneous branch of radial nerve, it supplies the skin on the cranial surface of forearm.

4. The cranial and caudal **pectoral nerves** arise from the caudal portion of the brachial plexus medial to the musculocutaneous and median nerves. They pass ventrally on either side of the brachial artery, gives out small interconnecting branches forming anastomosis in the form of a loop deep to the brachial artery. Several small nerve branches extend from this loop and they supply the cranial (cervical) and caudal (thoracic) parts of superficial and deep pectoral muscles.

5. The **external (lateral) thoracic nerve** (subcutaneous thoracic nerve) is a unique nerve arising from the caudal portion of the brachial plexus by a common trunk with ulnar nerve. In the beginning, it is placed medial to

the ulnar nerve but soon leaves its company, passes caudally to the medial surface of long head of triceps brachii muscle. From here it runs ventrally across the humeral insertion of cutaneous muscle and then along its deep face in company with the subcutaneous thoracic vein and supply several branches to the deep pectoral and cutaneous muscle before terminating in the skin over the lateral thoracic and abdominal wall at its flank region. One of its branch unites with perforating second, third and fourth intercostal nerves, winds around the ventral border of latissimus dorsi, courses cranially and ramifies in the scapulo-humeral part of the cutaneous muscle.

6. The **long thoracic nerve** is a thin and wide nerve. It arises from the cranial part of the brachial plexus, passes caudally under the deep face of the serratus ventralis muscle and supplies this muscle.

7. The **thoracodorsal nerve** extends from the caudal portion of the plexus, passes caudally over the deep surface of the latissimus dorsi muscle and ramifies in this muscle.

8. The **musculocutaneous nerve** arises from the cranial portion of the plexus closely caudal to the suprascapular nerve. It descends the medial surface of the shoulder joint and just distal to this joint, it joins the medial nerve by a large short branch to form a loop in which the axillary artery passes. One or two small branches are supplied to pectoral muscles from the loop or directly from this nerve, It then courses in the space between the two divisions of insertion of the coracobrachialis muscle in company with the cranial circumflex vessels, gives off a branch to supply the coracobrachialis muscle and finally terminates into the biceps brachii muscle.

9. The **radial nerve** is the largest of all nerves of the brachial plexus. It extends from the caudal portion of the plexus, passes down caudally and ventrally across the subscapularis and teres major muscles, and deeps into the space between the scapula, humerus and the long head of triceps brachii muscle. After emerging through this space at the proximal part of the lateral surface of the humerus it passes through the musculospiral groove between the brachialis and triceps brachii and reaches the cranial aspect of the elbow joint between the brachialis and extensor carpi radialis muscles. Here it gives off a large cutaneous branch and terminates by supplying several branches to the extensors of the carpus and digits. The **cutaneous branch** of the radius descends under the deep fascia on the dorsal surface of forearm and crosses the dorsal surface of carpus and metacarpus. On reaching proximal to the fetlock joint, it divides into three

dorsal digital nerves. During this course, the cutaneous branch of the radial nerve supplies branches to the skin and fascia on the dorsal aspect of the forearm, carpus and metacarpus.

10. The **ulnar nerve** arises with the median nerve by a short common trunk from the caudal portion of the plexus. It first lies caudal to the axillary vessels and after a short course deviates from these vessels and continue to pass ventrally in company with the median nerve till the middle of the arm region. Here it gives off a long cutaneous branch to the skin on the medial surface of the forearm. It then leaves the company of the median nerve, reaches the space between the olecranon process of elbow and the medial condyle of the humerus, gains the company of the collateral ulnar artery and vein, gives out a branch to elbow joint and then deeps between the two heads of flexor carpi ulnaris muscle. Here it furnishes branches to flexor carpi ulnaris, superficial digital flexor and the ulnar head of the deep digital flexor muscles. The nerve then continues ventrally between the flexor carpi ulnaris and superficial digital flexor muscles and then between the superficial digital flexor and the flexor carpi radialis muscles, supplies branches to these muscles and divides at about the distal third of the forearm into superficial and deep branches.

    i. The **superficial branch** passes ventrally caudal to the tendon of insertion of ulnaris lateralis, runs superficially over the carpal sheath, courses down ventrad and laterad to the metacarpal region and is continued as **dorsal lateral digital nerve** on the lateral (abaxial) aspect of the lateral (outer) digit.

    ii. The **deep branch** descends deeply under the deep fascia on the palmer aspect of the carpus over the carpal sheath, furnishes a branch to the suspensory ligament distal to the carpus and runs down subcutaneously as **palmer lateral digital nerve** on the abaxial side of the lateral digit.

11. The **median nerve** arises with the ulnar nerve from the caudal portion of the brachial plexus and is enclosed in a connective tissue sheath with the later nerve up to the middle of the arm. A large branch of the musculocutaneous nerve joins the median nerve and forms a loop over which the axillary artery is suspended. The median nerve separates from the ulnar nerve near the middle of the arm and inclines caudally and ventrally. It then crosses the cranial border of the artery obliquely and continues in this position to the elbow joint. Here it crosses the artery, passes under the pronator teres muscle and continues ventrally along the caudal surface of radial covered by the flexor carpi radialis muscle to the

distal part of the forearm. It passes vertically through the carpal sheath, descends to the distal third of the metacarpus on its palmer surface between the bone and the suspensory ligament and divides into two, the medial and lateral branches.

Before this division, the median nerve during its course through the arm and forearm gives out first the musculocutaneous branch then the muscular branch and then the interosseous branch.

- The **musculocutaneous branch** leaves the cranial border of the median nerve near the middle of the arm, passes under cover of the biceps brachii and divides into muscular and cutaneous branches. The muscular branches are supplied to the brachialis and biceps brachii muscles. The cutaneous branch supplies the skin on the cranial aspect of the forearm.
- The **muscular branches** extend from the median nerve immediately distal to the elbow pronator teres, flexor carpi radialis and the humeral and radial heads of the deep digital flexor muscles.
- The **interosseous branch** from this nerve passes in company with the common interosseous artery and passes down through the interosseous groove between the radius and ulna. From this nerve extends a delicate cutaneous branch a little above the carpus to join the cutaneous branch of the radial nerve.

The **medial and lateral terminal divisions of the median nerve** after a short course at the distal third of the palmer surface of the metacarpus again divide into two branches each as medial and lateral branch. The medial branch of the medial division supplies a branch to the medial accessory digit and then continues ventrally at the fetlock joint on the medial aspect of medial digit as **palmer medial digital nerve**. The lateral branch of the medial division joins the medial branch of lateral division and passes through the interdigital space as **palmer common digital nerve**. The lateral branch of the lateral division joins the deep branch of the ulnar nerve, supplies a branch to the lateral accessory digit and then passes down on the lateral aspect of the lateral digit as **palmer lateral digital nerve**. The palmer common digital nerve descends along the interdigital aspect of the two digits and divides into **medial and lateral proper digital nerves** to supply the respective digits of the limb.

90

Comparative Anatomy of Nerves of Fore Limb

Horse

The brachial plexus in horse is formed by ventral branches of the last three thoracic and first two thoracic spinal nerves similar to that in ox. The disposition and distribution of nerve branches extending from the plexus is almost similar to that of the ox except the following two.

1. The **radial nerve** after reaching the musculospiral groove gives out a **cutaneous branch** that passes through the lateral head of triceps and is distributed to the skin on the lateral aspect of forearm. The main trunk of the radial nerve after crossing the carpus descends along the medial aspect of the palmer surface of metacarpus as **palmer medial metacarpal nerve** and further down on the medial digit as **palmer medial digital nerve.**

2. The **ulnar nerve** descends the carpus and after reaching the metacarpal region joins the lateral branch of the median nerve, descends first along the lateral aspect of the palmer surface of metacarpus as **palmer lateral metacarpal nerve** and then along the lateral (abaxial) aspect of the lateral digit as **palmer lateral digital nerve.**

Dog

The brachial plexus in dog is formed by the ventral branches of last four cervical and first thoracic spinal nerves. Out of eleven branches distributed from this plexus, four branches namely the musculocutaneous, radial, ulnar and median nerves have distinct characteristics which differ from those of the ox and horse.

1. The **musculocutaneous nerve** does not join the median nerve to form a loop for suspending the axillary artery. Instead, it gives out a branch at about the distal third of arm which passes down and connects it with the median nerve. The main nerve furnishes branches to biceps brachii and coracobrachialis and then descends the arm, furnishes a communicating

branch to median nerve and divides into **muscular and cutaneous branches**.

2. The **radial nerve,** while leaving the plexus establishes connections with ulnar, median and axillary nerves through small communicating branches. It supplies branches to triceps brachii and anconeus muscles and then passes between the brachialis and lateral head of triceps brachii muscles and after emerging through this passage at the proximal part of the forearm, divides into two branches. Of these, the deep branch is the muscular branch. It passes over the dorsolateral face of the forearm and supplies the muscles in that region. The other, superficial branch is the cutaneous branch. It divides into medial and lateral branches. The medial branch distributes **proper digital nerves to first four digits** while the lateral branch unites with the ulnar nerve to supply the **proper digital nerve to fifth digit**.

3. The **ulnar nerve** unites with the median at the distal third of the arm region and after a short course gets separated from it, descends the arm region and then the extensor aspect of the elbow joint and at about the middle of forearm it divides into dorsal (cranial) and palmer (caudal) branches. The dorsal branch runs down the lateral aspect of the forearm, carpus and metacarpus supplying the skin and cutaneous muscle on these regions and ends as the **lateral dorsal proper digital nerve for the fifth digit**. The palmer branch passes through the carpal sheath and at the proximal third of the palmer surface of the metacarpus divides into superficial and deep branches. The deep branch further divides into **three palmer common digital nerves** that pass through the intermetacarpal spaces second to fourth and join the corresponding palmer metacarpal branches of the median nerve contributes for the formation of **palmer proper digital nerves**. The superficial branch descends along the tendons of flexors of digits and divides into two branches. One of these terminates as **lateral palmer digital nerve of the fifth digit** and the other joins the deep branch in the intermetacarpal sheath between the fourth and fifth digits.

4. The **median nerve** after reaching the proximal third of the palmer surface of the metacarpus divides into three palmer metacarpal nerves which contribute the formation of **palmer proper digital nerves** of the first four digits. The palmer proper digital nerve of the fifth digit is supplied by a branch from ulnar nerve.

Sheep and Goat

The brachial plexus in sheep and goat is formed by the ventral branches of last three thoracic and first thoracic spinal nerves. The distribution of nerves from the plexus and their further disposition in sheep and goat is almost similar to that in ox except the following few difference.

1. The superficial branch of **radial nerve** divides into dorsal common digital nerve for the medial and lateral digit on the dorsal aspect of the carpometacarpal articulation in sheep and at the proximal one fourth of the metacarpus in the goat.

2. The medial branch of the **median nerve** in sheep divides into palmer medial accessory common digital nerve and palmer medial proper common digital (axial) nerve. Whereas, in goat it divides into palmer medial accessory and proper common digital nerves and the later further divides into palmer medial and lateral proper digital nerves.

3. The lateral branch of the **median nerve** in goat joins directly the superficial branch of the palmer division of the ulnar nerve.

Pig

The brachial plexus in pig is formed by the ventral branches of last four cervical and first thoracic spinal nerves. The distribution of nerves from the plexus is in general similar to that in ox except the following special features in respect of the radial, ulnar and median nerves, especially the digital nerves constituted by these nerves.

1. **Radial nerve** divides into superficial and deep branches at the level of condyle of the humerus. The superficial branch at about the middle of the dorsal surface of metacarpus divides into **medial and lateral branch**. The medial branch after a short course divides into medial (abaxial) dorsal accessory digital nerve which ends at the proximal phalanx and the dorsal common accessory digital nerve which after a short course gives rise to the dorsal medial accessory digital and dorsal medial proper digital nerve. The lateral branch gives rise to the **dorsal medial common digital nerve** and the **dorsal lateral common digital nerve**. The deep branch of the radial nerve supplies to the extensor muscles of carpus and digits along with the ulnaris lateralis muscle.

2. The **ulnar nerve** after coursing along the caudolateral aspect of the arm and forearm divides at the middle of forearm into the dorsal and palmer branches. The dorsal branch divides into **medial and lateral branch** near the carpus. The medial branch later on becomes **dorsal lateral**

common digital nerve which finally divides into dorsal lateral proper digital nerve and dorsal lateral accessory digital nerve. The palmer branch of ulnar nerve also divides into medial and lateral branch. The medial branch becomes **palmer lateral common digital nerve** and with further division gives rise to **palmer lateral proper digital nerve** and **palmer lateral accessory digital nerve**. The lateral branch of the palmer division continues as **palmer lateral accessory digital nerve**

3. The **median nerve** after coursing through the arm, forearm and carpus regions and furnishing branches to the muscles in these regions reaches near the fetlock region and divide into **palmer medial common digital nerve** and **palmer lateral common digital nerve**. These two nerves finally give rise to **palmer medial** and **lateral accessory digital nerves** and **palmer medial and lateral proper digital nerves.**

Fowl

The brachial plexus in fowl is formed by the ventral branches of the last three cervical (twelfth, thirteenth and fourteenth) and the first thoracic spinal nerves. Some times the eleventh cervical or second thoracic spinal nerves also join the brachial plexus in fowl. The plexus is formed in two parts connected with each other by anastomotic branches. From the cranial part of the plexus extend the **ulnar, musculocutaneous** and **median nerves.** From the caudal division extend the **radial** and the **circumflex (axilary) nerves**.

SECTION-D

APPLIED ANATOMY

91

Applied Anatomy of Fore Limb

Site for nerve block

Brachial plexus block

The brachial plexus is the key source of nerve supply to the fore limb. Loss of sensation below the elbow is achieved by blocking the nerve roots contributing to this plexus. In ox it is formed by the ventral branches of 6th to 8th cervical and 1st and 2nd thoracic spinal nerves. These nerve roots pass over the lateral aspect of the middle third of the first rib before anastomosing to form the plexus. All these nerve roots can be blocked by injecting anaesthetic solution on these nerves at the middle third of the lateral surface of the first rib. To reach this site, the needle is inserted between the thoracic wall and the medial face of the shoulder at the level of acromion process of the scapula about 12 to 14 cm cranial to it horizontally in the caudal direction.

The blocking of brachial plexus is indicated for operations for reducing the fractures of the bones of fore arm and manus.

Median and Ulnar nerve block

The median and ulnar nerve block is recommended for operative procedures on the caudomedial aspect of metacarpus and the volar (palmer) aspect of digits. These nerves are located beneath the superficial fascia at the medial epicondyle of humerus. The median nerve is just cranial to and the ulnar nerve is just caudal to the medial epicondyle of humerus at the elbow joint..

To block these nerves the needle is inserted subcutaneously beneath the superficial fascia at these sites.

Digital nerve blocks

For induction of anaesthesia in the digital region, it is necessary to block the dorsal metacarpal branches of the radial, musculocutaneous and ulnar nerves in addition to the median and ulnar nerves.

The dorsal metacarpal nerve is the continuation of the radial nerve in the metacarpal and digital region. It is joined by the cutaneous branch of musculocutaneous nerve or the two nerves may run separately. These nerves can be palpated medial to the tendon of medial digital extensor on the dorsal surface of middle of the metacarpus.

The volar (palmer) metacarpal nerve is a continuation of the median nerve. It divides into three branches, the volar digital nerves in the mid metacarpal region. This nerve is blocked at about hands breadth ventral to the carpus at a place before its division.

Hygroma of carpal joint

Hygroma is a localized synovial swelling of the joints of the limb. It more commonly affects the carpal joint in cattle. It leads to bursitis as a result of trauma at the carpus. The tendons of extensor carpi radialis and common digital extensor muscles may also be involved in this condition.

Surgical approach to the carpal joint usually necessitates complete dorsal exposure of the carpal joint. This is best accomplished using a dorsal skin incision over the carpus extending from the distal part of the radius to the proximal part of the large metacarpal bone. Deep incision exposes and enables retraction of the tendons of common digital extensor and extensor carpi radialis muscles.

Transverse arthrotomy incision allows exposure of radial and ulnar carpal bones and that at the middle of the carpus exposes the first carpal, second and third fused carpal and the fourth carpal bones.

Site for puncture or injection at the joints of fore limb

Arthritis (inflammation of joints) is the most common clinical disorder in the forelimb of dairy cattle. Traumatic capsulitis and synuvitis (inflammation of synovial membrane and fibrous capsule) is associated with this condition. The cause of the disease in most of these cases is injury caused due to hard floor of the cow sheds or because of agricultural implements in draught animals. What ever the cause may be, the injury leads to synuvitis and capsulitis of the joint. As a remedy in these cases, it is necessary to drain out the synovial fluid and inject the medicines into the joint capsule. Sites for puncture of the different joints of forelimb are as below.

Shoulder joint

For the puncture of shoulder joint the scapular spine is traced down to its distal end and the lateral tuberosity of the humerus is identified by palpation. The needle is penetrated horizontally from the craniolateral aspect of the joint just in front of the tendon of infraspinatus muscle.

Elbow joint

The site for puncture of the joint capsule of elbow joint is close to the cranial or caudal aspect of the lateral collateral ligament just proximal to the lateral tuberosity of the radius. The needle is inserted horizontally close to the cranial border of the lateral collateral ligament and is pushed along the bone obliquely inward to reach the synovial cavity.

Carpal joint

For puncture of the joint capsule of the carpal joint, the needle is inserted from craniolateral aspect of the joint between the common digital extensor and the extensor carpi radialis muscles.

Fetlock joint

The site for puncture of joint capsule of fetlock joint is in the triangle formed by suspensory ligament, the lateral sesamoid bone and the large metacarpal bone, The needle is inserted horizontally through the skin and then pushed obliquely inward and downward till it reaches the middle of the joint capsule.

PART- 2.3: ANATOMY OF HIND LIMB

SECTION-A

MUSCULO-SKELETAL COMPONENT

92

Skeleton of Hind Limb

The hind limb (Fig. 6-1) is termed as pelvic limb and it consists of four segments- the pelvic or hip region, thigh, leg and the pes region. The skeleton of pelvic region is formed by the pelvic girdle (os coxae). The skeleton of thigh region is mainly formed by a long bone (thigh bone) the femur and at its lower extremity is a short sesamoid bone, the patella. The leg region is formed by two long bones, the larger one the tibia and the smaller one the fibula. The last segment, the pes has three subdivisions as tarsus, metatarsus and digits. The tarsus has five short bones arranged in two rows on par with the carpus of fore limb. The metatarsus is constituted by two bones of which one is a long bone called the large metatarsal and the other a short small rudimentary bone the small metatarsal bone. The last part of the hind limb is the digits which are constituted by six phalanges and six sesamoids like those of the forelimb.

Pelvic bone

The pelvic bones (os coxae) or hip bones of the two sides along with the sacrum participate in the constitution of pelvic cavity. Each pelvic bone has three parts- the ilium, ischium and pelvis which are completely fused and meet with each other at the cotyloid cavity the acetabulum. The later forms a joint (hip joint) with the head of the femur and through this joint the hind limb (pelvic limb) is connected with the trunk (body) of the animal. Since the pelvic bone plays major role in the constitution of pelvic region (part of abdomen and pelvis), it is described in detail under the chapter on skeleton of abdomen and pelvis.

Femur (Thigh bone)

The femur (Fig. 6-1 A and B) is the largest and most massive of the long bones of the body. It is placed obliquely craniad and ventrad between the hip joint proximally and stifle joint distally. It has a shaft and two extremities.

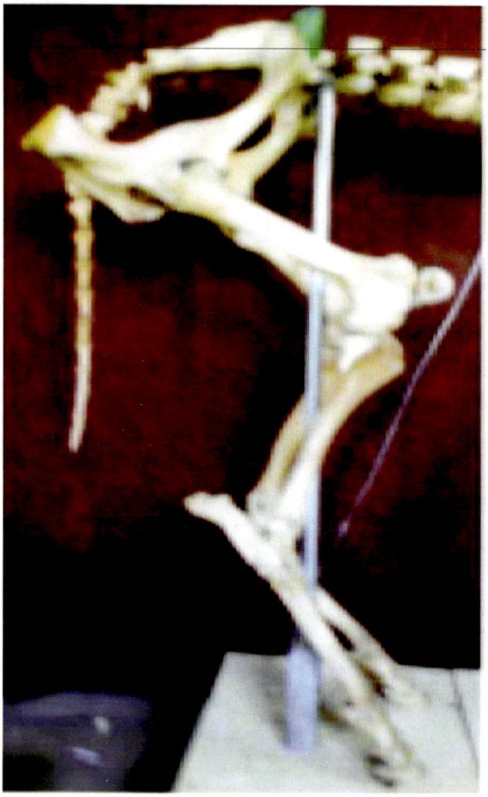

Fig. 6 – 1: Skeleton of Hind limb of Ox

The **shaft** of femur is long and cylindrical and becomes prismatic in the distal third. The cranial, medial and lateral surfaces are smooth and continuous with each other and they are strongly convex from side to side. These surfaces are covered by quadriceps femoris muscle. The caudal surface is rough and narrow in its middle where it provides attachment to adductor muscle. Below this, there is an oblique vascular impression that marks the course of the femoral vessels running ventrally and laterally. The medial border of this surface presents in its proximal third a rough ridge called the **trochanter minor.** It presents attachment to quadratus femoris and iliopsoas muscles. Extending obliquely dorsad from the trochanter minor is the **trochanteric ridge** which forms the caudolateral boundary of the **trochanteric fossa**. The middle gluteus muscle is attached to the trochanteric ridge and the obturator externus, obturator internus and gemmelus muscles are attached at the trochanteric fossa. The distal third of the medial border is the **medial supracondyloid crest** on which the medial head of the gastrocnemius muscle is attached. The rest of the part of this border distal to the trochanter minor presents the attachment to the pectineus muscle. The lateral border in its distal third presents the **lateral supracondyloid crest** over which the lateral head of the gastrocnemius muscle is attached. Medial to this crest and between the medial and lateral supracondyloid crests is supracondyloid fossa. The superior flexor of the digits arises from the **supracondyloid fossa.**

The **proximal extremity** of the femur contains the **head** on the medial side and the **trochanter major** on its lateral side. The **head** is a round tuberous projection directed dorsally and medially from the proximal extremity and it is distinctly marked from its lower part, the neck. It articulates with the acetabulum of the pelvic bone. There is a small nonarticular sulcus in the middle of the head for the attachment of round ligament of the hip joint. The **trochanter major** is placed on the lateral aspect of the head at the proximal extremity of the femur. Its cranial part (lateral surface) is opposite to the head and it rises higher than the head. It is convex and In fresh state it is covered by cartilage over which pass the tendon of insertion of medial and deep gluteus muscles before their insertion on the trochanteric ridge (crest) and the trochanteric fossa respectively. The caudal part (medial surface) of the trochanter major is concave and forms the lateral boundary of the **trochanteric fossa**. The trochanter major is connected with the trochanter minor by an oblique **trochanteric ridge.** Medial to the trochanteric ridge is the deep trochanteric fossa in which the obturator externus, obturator internus and gemmelus muscles are inserted.

The **distal extremity** is large and comprises the **trochlea** cranially and **condyles** caudally. The **trochlea** is composed of two ridges separated by a groove. It presents an extensive area for articulation with the patella. The medial ridge is larger, more prominent and extends higher than the lateral one. The two ridges, medial and lateral, converge very slightly distally. There is a thin rim around the trochlea for attachment of the capsular ligament of the femoro-patellar articulation. The **condyles** are medial and lateral and are separated by the deep intercondyloid fossa. The condyles of the femur articulate with the condyles of the tibia through cartilaginous discs the menisci at the stifle joint. The **intercondyloid fossa** lodges the tibial spine and the cruciate ligament of the femoro-tibial articulation. The **medial condyle** on its medial surface presents an eminence for the attachment of medial collateral ligament of the stifle joint. The **lateral condyle** presents two depressions on its lateral surface. The upper depression is for attachment of lateral collateral ligament of the stifle joint and the lower depression is for the attachment of popliteus muscle. Between the lateral condyle and the lateral ridge of the trochlea is the extensor fossa for the attachment of complexus muscle. On the outer surfaces of the medial and lateral condyles are small eminences called the medial and lateral epicondyles on which are attached the medial and lateral collateral ligaments of stifle joint.

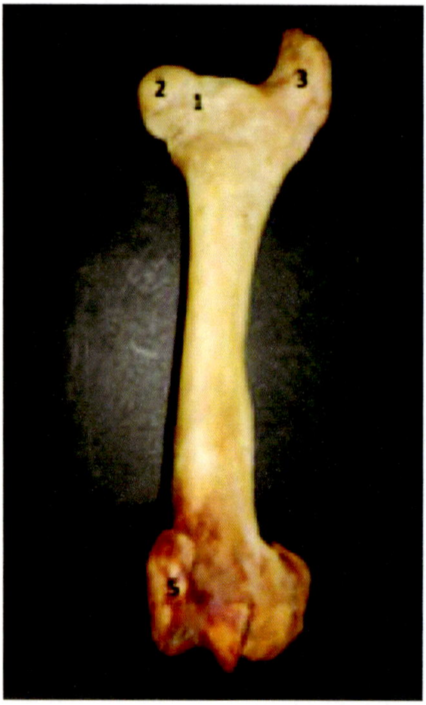

Fig. 6 – 1 A: Femur of ox; Cranial view 1. Head 2. Fovea capitis 3. Trochanter major 4. Trochlea 5. Medial ridge of trochlea

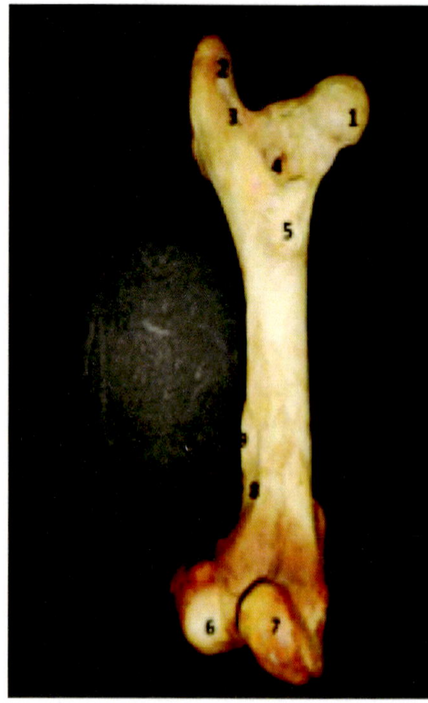

Fig. 6 – 1B: Femur of Ox; Caudal view 1. Head 2. Trochanter Major 3. Trochanteric ridge 4. Trochanteric fossa 5. Trochanter minor 6. Lateral condyle 7. Medial condyle 8. Supracondyloid fossa 9. Lateral supracondyloid crest

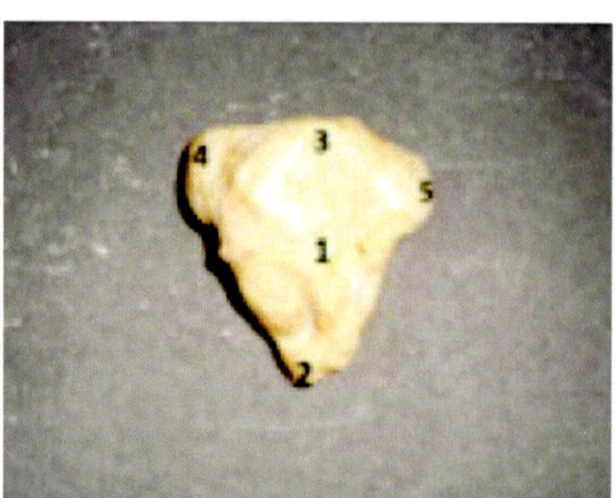

Fig. 6 – 1 C: Patella of Ox; Cranial surface 1. Cranial surface 2. Apex 3. Base 4. Medial angle 5. Lateral angle

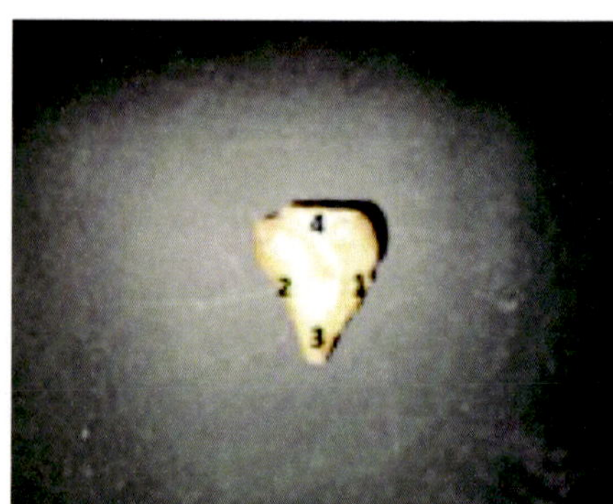

Fig. 6 – 1 D: Patella of Ox; Caudal surface 1. Lateral border 2. Medial border 3. Apex 4. Base

Patella

The patella (Fig. 6-1 C and D) is a large sesamoid bone applied against the trochlea of the femur. It is irregularly triangular and presents two surfaces, two borders, a base and an apex. The base faces upward and the apex faces downward. The **cranial surface** is convex and rough for the attachment of muscles and ligaments. The extensors of the leg pass over this surface which provides leverage for these muscles. The **caudal or the articular surface** is divided by a vertical ridge into two, medial and lateral concave areas which are applied against the medial and lateral ridges of the trochlea of femur and thus creates a pulley like arrangement for the upward and downward sliding mechanism for the patella. The two **borders** converge distally at the apex. The **lateral border** is convex. The **medial border** is concave and it forms an angle at the base and gives attachment to the fibrocartilage of the patella. The **base** is wide and convex. The **apex** is narrow and pointed.

Tibia (Leg bone)

The tibia (Fig. 6-1 E and F) is a long bone placed in the leg region of the hind limb. It extends obliquely distally and caudally from stifle joint to the hock joint. It has a shaft and two extremities. The **shaft** is three sided in the proximal two thirds and flattened craniocaudally in the distal third. It has three surfaces and three borders. The **lateral surface** (Fig. 6-1 E) is spiral. It is wide and facing laterally in its proximal part and inclines gradually to the cranial side of the bone in its distal part. It is covered by tibialis anticus muscle. The **medial surface** is broad and rough in its proximal part and gives attachment to Sartorius, gracilis and semimembranosus muscles. The distal part of the medial surface is narrow, smooth and subcutaneous. The **caudal surface** (Fig. 6-1 F) of the shaft is flat. The proximal fourth of this surface, towards the medial border possesses a narrow triangular area marked by **popliteal line** for the attachment of popliteus muscle. The rest of the part of this surface is marked by rough lines for the origin of flexor muscles of the hock joint. The **cranial border** is prominent in its proximal third and is called the **tibial crest.** The rest of the extent of the cranial border is rounded and indistinct. On the medial aspect of the tibial crest is rough prominence for the insertion of semitendinosus muscle. The **lateral border** is concave and in life the fibrous part of fibula is attached to this border. **The medial border** is rounded and thick in its proximal half for the attachment of popliteus muscle.

The **proximal extremity** is large and three sided. It is formed by tuberosity on its cranial aspect and two condyles, one each on medial and lateral side. The **tuberosity** is a large eminence on the cranial side. It continues distally with the tibial crest on the cranial border of the shaft of the tibia. A small median vertical groove on the cranial surface of the tuberosity and the tibial crest presents attachment to the middle patellar ligament. Each **condyle** bears a saddle shaped articular surface for articulation with the condyle of the femur and the meniscus. The articular surfaces of the condyles continue upward centrally into **spine of the tibia**. The summit of the spine is bifid and it fits into the intercondyloid fossa of the femur. On the cranial and caudal sides of the spine at its base are small depressions for the attachment of cruciate ligaments and the menisci. The **condyles** are separated caudally by the **popliteal notch** on the medial aspect of which is a tubercle for attachment of caudal cruciate ligament. The lateral condyle on its lateral surface (outer surface) has a small articular facet for articulation with the head of the rudimentary fibula. There is a smooth semicircular notch between the lateral condyle and the tuberosity which provides passage to the tendon of origin of the long digital extensor muscle.

The **distal extremity** of tibia is much smaller than the proximal extremity. Its articular (ventral) surface has two craniocaudally **sagittal deep grooves** separated by an osseous ridge. The **medial groove** is bounded on its medial (outer) side by the **medial malleolus** while the **lateral groove** is bounded laterally (on outer side) by the **lateral malleolus**. The cranial part of the medial malleolus is prolonged ventrally and it ends in a blunt point..

Fibula

The fibula is a **rudimentary bone**. In young subjects it is in the form of a **fibrous cord** extending from the lateral side of the lateral condyle of tibia to the lateral malleolus at its distal extremity. As the age advances, the fibrous cord becomes receding in the middle of its length. In the middle aged animal, the proximal and distal ends of the fibrous cord becomes ossified and the rest of the fibrous cord reduces to a short, tapering and blunt prolongation extending ventrally from the proximal ossified end of the cord. The ossified **proximal end** gets fused with the lateral condyle of the tibia while the ossified **distal end** of the cord remains separated from the distal extremity of the tibia but participates in completing the lateral boundary of the lateral groove of tibia. Thus the fibula is represented by only the **proximal head** of the fibula and the **distal lateral malleolus**. The **lateral malleolus** is quadrilateral in outline and is compressed from side to side.

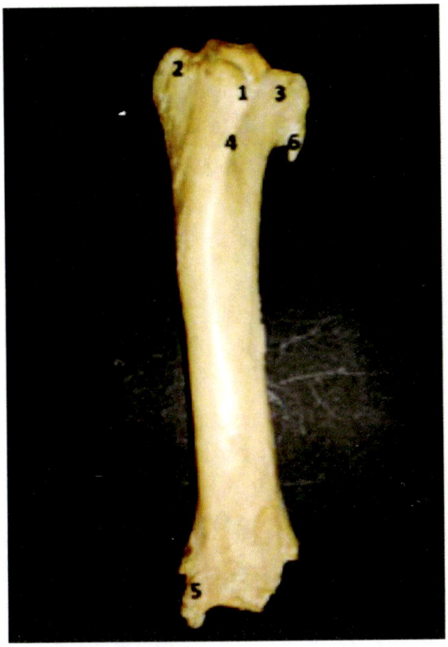

Fig. 6 – 1 E: Tibia fibula of Ox; Dorsal surface
1. Cranial tuberosity 2. Medial tuberosity 3. lateral tuberosity 4. Cranial tibial crest 5.Lateral malleolus 6. Fibula

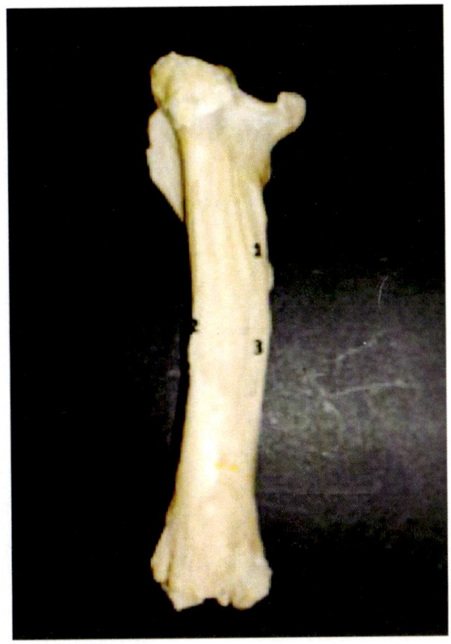

Fig. 6 – 1F: Tibia of Ox; Caudal surface
1. Linia muscularis 2. Lateral border 3. Medial border

Tarsus (Hock)

The tarsus or hock in ox (Fig. 6-1 G) consists of five bones arranged in two rows, the proximal and distal. The bones of the proximal row are the tibial tarsal (talus) and the fibular tarsal (calcaneus). The bones of the distal row are the central and fourth fused tarsal (scapho-cuboid), first tarsal (cuneiform parvun) and the second and third fused tarsal (cuneiform magnum).

Tibial tarsal

The tibial tarsal (talus) is the medial bone of the proximal row of tarsus. It is compressed craniocaudally. It has six surfaces. The **cranial and dorsal surfaces** are continuous and form a trochlea with two vertical ridges separated by a wide deep groove between them. The **trochlea** articulates with the distal extremity of tibia craniodorsally. The ventral surface of the tibial tarsal articulates with the central and fourth fused tarsal (scapho-cuboid). The **caudal surface** is articular for most of its part except a small elongated rough area. The articular area is for articulation with the fibular tarsal and the rough elongated area is for attachment of interosseous ligament. The **lateral surface** has two facets for articulation with the lateral malleolus. The **medial surface** is slightly depressed in its proximal third and below this it is nearly flat. It presents a small tubercle beneath the depression for attachment of the ligament. The **ventral surface** is composed of two condyles separated by a groove. The condyles articulate with the central and fourth fused tarsal. On the caudal side of the ventral surface is a rough area for attachment of interosseous ligament.

Fibular tarsal

The fibular tarsal (calcaneus) is the largest bone of the tarsus (hock). It is elongated and flattened from side to side and is placed caudal and lateral to the tibial tarsal. It consists of a body and a process called the sustentaculum tali. The **body** is elongated and flattened compressed from side to side. It has two surfaces, two borders, and two extremities, the distal extremity as the base and the proximal extremity as the tuber calcis. The **medial surface** of the body is concave while the lateral surface is convex. The **cranial (dorsal) border** is slightly concave, smooth and rounded. The **caudal (plantar) border** is straight and rough for attachment of calcaneo-metatarsal (plantar) ligament. The **proximal extremity (tuber calcis)** is enlarged, rounded and tuberous summit of the body. It forms the point of hock. It presents a depression (sulcus) in the centre for attachment of the tendon of insertion of gastrocnemius muscle. Cranial to this sulcus is convexity over which rests the tendon of the gastrocnemius muscle during the flexion of the hock. Caudal to the central sulcus is a groove which in fresh state appears to be covered by fibrocartilage that enables the passage of the tendon of insertion of superficial digital flexor muscle. The lateral and medial sides of the tuber calcis present insertion to the tendons of biceps femoris and semitendinosus muscles. Thus the tuber calcis provides attachment to the flexor muscles of the hock joint. The **distal extremity of the body** is irregular and bears a concave facet for articulation with the central and fourth fused tarsal bone. From the medial aspect of the distal extremity of the body extends a strong blunt process the **sustentaculum tali**. On its cranioventral aspect, the sustentaculum tali possess a large oval and slightly concave facet for articulation with the tibial tarsal. On its caudal (plantar) surface it forms a deep groove with the medial surface of the body through which the tendon of deep digital extensor muscle passes and on its medial surface it possesses a rough area for attachment of the medial collateral ligament of the hock joint. The **lateral surface** of the body of the fibular tarsal is flattened except a part of its distal extremity which bears a rough prominence for attachment of the lateral collateral ligament of the hock joint. On the cranial (dorsal) surface of the distal extremity of the body is a projection which articulates with the lateral malleolus of tibia. The medial surface of the process bears two facets one on the proximal part and the other on its distal part for articulation with similar facets on the lateral surface of tibial tarsal. The area between the two facets is rough and excavated.

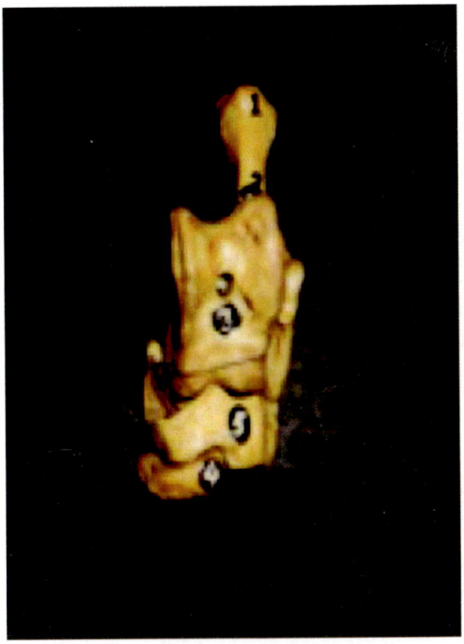

Fig. 6 – 1 G: Tarsal Bones of Ox
1. Calcaneal tuber/ tuber calcis 2. Fibular tarsal 3. Tibial tarsal 4. Second & third fused carpal 5. Central and fourth fused carpal

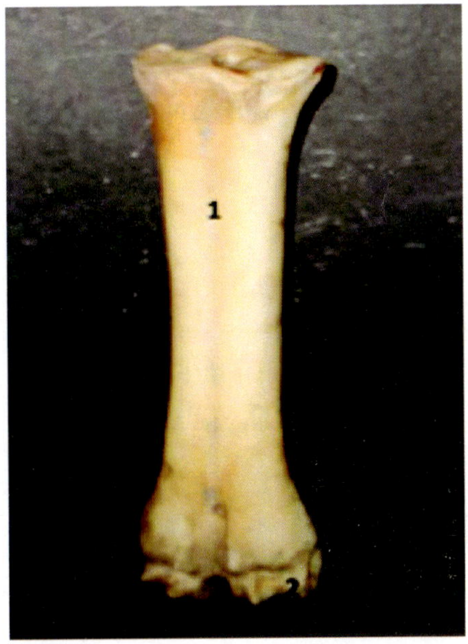

Fig. 6 – 1 H: Large Metatarsal bone of Ox; Dorsal surface
1. Cranial longitudinal vascular groove 2. Condyle

Central and fourth fused tarsal

The central and fourth tarsals are fused to form a single large bone the central and fourth fused tarsal which occupies the entire width of the tarsus and articulates with all the bones of the hock joint. Its **proximal (upper) surface** is smooth and concave. It is divided into two equal parts by a craniocaudal ridge. These two parts adapt themselves to apply against the trochlea of the tibial tarsal. The **distal (ventral or lower) surface** is uneven in level. The medial part is at a higher level than the lateral part and it bears a convex facet cranially for articulation with second and third fused tarsal bone and caudally for articulation with the first tarsal. The lateral part of this surface is at a lower level and it presents a large convexo-concave facet cranially and a small slightly concave facet caudally. Between the two facets is a deep groove through which passes the tendon of peroneus longus muscle. This lateral part of the distal surface of the central and fourth fused tarsal articulates with the lateral part of the proximal extremity of the large metatarsal bone. The **cranial and medial surfaces** are continuous with each other and are convex and rough for attachment of ligaments. The **lateral surface** is slightly over hanged by proximal surface and is rough for muscular and ligamentous attachment. The **caudal surface** is irregular and has two tubercles separated by a depression.

First tarsal

The first tarsal bone is the smallest among the all the tarsal bones in ox. It is quadrilateral in shape and is placed at the caudomedial aspect of the tarsus. It is articulated proximally with the central and fourth fused tarsal bone, distally with the large metatarsal bone and cranially with the second and third fused tarsal bone.

Second and third fused tarsal

The second and third fused tarsal is a small flattened piece of bone ventral to the central and fourth fused tarsal bone. Its **dorsal (cranial) surface** is continuous with the **medial surface** and it is convex and rough. The **planter (caudal) surface** is narrow and it bears a small facet for articulation with the first tarsal. The **lateral surface** presents a small facet for articulation with the central and fourth fused tarsal bone. The **proximal (upper) surface** is concave and articulates with the medial part of the ventral (distal) surface of the central and fourth fused tarsal bone. The **distal (lower) surface** is concavo-convex and articulates with the medial facet on the proximal articular surface of the large metatarsal bone.

Metatarsals

The metatarsal bones of hind limb are just the counter parts of metacarpals of fore limb. In ox there are two metatarsals, one large and one small metacarpal. The general arrangement of the metatarsals is similar to that of the metacarpals except the following features which differ from those of the metacarpals.

Large metatarsal bone

The large metatarsal bone (Fig. 6-1 H) is longer than the large metacarpal and it is quadrilateral in form as against the cylindrical and two sided metacarpal. The **shaft** of the large metatarsal is compressed from side to side. The dorsal (cranial) surface presents a deep vertical median vascular groove. This groove of the large metatarsus is wider and deeper than that of the large metacarpal bone. The foramen at the proximal end of the groove as appears in the metacarpus is absent in the metatarsus. The plantar (caudal) surface of the shaft is flat and is in contact with the suspensory ligament. A shallow median vertical groove on the plantar surface marks the union of the third and fourth metatarsal bones fused to form the large metatarsal bone. At the proximal end of the vascular groove is a foramen that passes obliquely upward and opens into the caudal part of the proximal articular surface (proximal extremity) of the large metatarsal bone as against its passing through the shaft and opening on the dorsal (cranial) surface of the metacarpus. The medial surface of the shaft is flat and wide above. At the proximal end of this surface is a metatarsal tuberosity to which the tendons of peroneus tertius and tibialis anticus muscles are attached. The lateral surface is nearly flat and smooth. The **proximal extremity** has two the medial and lateral articular areas separated by a nonarticular groove. The medial articular area is larger and oval in shape. It bears two facets one is cranial in position and it articulates with the second and third fused tarsal. The other one is smaller, slightly convex and is placed caudally. This is for articulation with the first tarsal. The lateral articular area of the proximal extremity of the large metatarsus is oval and concave and it articulates with the central and fourth fused tarsal bone. The **distal extremity** of large metatarsus is smaller than that of the large metacarpus but the rest of the features are same. It comprises the medial and lateral condyles separated by the intercondyloid cleft. The medial and lateral condyles represent the third and fourth metatarsals and these articulate with the medial and lateral digits of the limb.

Small metatarsal bone

The small metatarsal bone is a small quadrilateral, dorsoventrally compressed disc of bone measuring about 2.5 cm both in length and breadth. It is situated on the caudomedial aspect of the proximal extremity of the large metatarsal bone. It has a small facet on its cranial face for articulation with the large metatarsal bone. Other than this facet, the rest of the area of this bone is rough and irregular.

Digits

The digits of the hind limb are similar to the digits of fore limb. The two digits of each limb are composed of six phalanges and six sesamoids and their arrangement is also similar to that in fore limb except for slight differences in their size. The first phalanx of the digit of hind limb is slightly longer, the second is longer and narrower and the third is shorter and thinner. The proximal sesamoids are smaller and the distal sesamoids are shorter and narrower.

93

Comparative Anatomy of Skeleton of Hind Limb

Horse

The **femur** of horse is more massive than that in ox. The proximal third of the caudal surface of **shaft** of femur presents a rough eminence for attachment of biceps femoris muscle. The **trochanter minor** is a rough ridge like structure. The proximal third of the **lateral border** of shaft presents trochanter tertius for attachment of superficial gluteus muscle. The **trochanter major** is comprised of a convexity, a summit and a crest. The **trochanteric ridge** is vertical and it connects the trochanter major with the **third trochanter**. The **lateral supracondyloid crest** and the **supracondyloid fossa** are better developed in horse than that in ox. The **patella** of horse is wider and longer than that of ox.

The **tibia** in horse is relatively longer than that in ox. The **popliteal line** is prominent. It extends from the proximal third of the medial border, obliquely crosses the caudal surface and ends at the middle of the lateral border of the shaft of tibia. The **medial border** in its proximal third bears a small popliteal tubercle for attachment of popliteus muscle. The **lateral border** is attached to the shaft of the fibula and encloses an interosseous tibiofibular arch with the fibula. At the **proximal extremity**, the cranial tuberosity is vertically grooved. The lateral condyle on its lateral side presents facet for articulation with the proximal extremity of fibula. At the **distal extremity**, the grooves are oblique. The **lateral malleolus** is fused with the distal extremity of tibia, The **medial malleolus** is more prominent than the lateral one.

The **fibula** in horse is better developed than that in ox and is placed along the lateral border of tibia. The **shaft** of the fibula is a slender rod that runs down to about the middle of the lateral edge of the shaft of the tibia and the two enclose between them an interosseous tibiofibular arch. The **proximal extremity** of fibula is large and flattened from side to side. Its medial surface has a facet through which it articulates with tibia. The lateral surface is convex and rough for attachment of ligaments. The cranial and caudal borders are blunt and rounded. The **distal extremity** is tapering and pointed and it terminates at about the distal third of the shaft of tibia.

The **tarsus or hock** of the horse is made of six tarsal bones. These are the tibial tarsal, fibular tarsal, central tarsal, first and second fused tarsal, third tarsal and the fourth tarsal. The **tibial tarsal** is relatively shorter and wider. The ridges of the trochlea along with the groove between them are oblique and are directed obliquely ventrad and laterad. The lateral surface of tibial tarsal has no articulation with the fibular tarsal and hence the facet on its lateral surface is absent. The **fibular tarsal** is short and thick. It does not articulate with tibial tarsal. The medial process (sustentaculum tali) is larger and stronger in horse than that of ox. It bears a facet on its cranial side for articulation with tibial tarsal. The **central tarsal** is not fused with fourth tarsal unlike that in ox. It is flat and irregularly quadrilateral in form. Its proximal surface is concave and articulates with tibial tarsal. The distal surface is convex and articulates with the first and second fused tarsal and the third tarsal. The dorsal (cranial) and the medial borders are continuous and rough for ligamentous attachment. The lateral border is oblique and has two facets for articulation with fourth tarsal. The **first and second fused tarsal** is smallest and most irregular of all the tarsals in horse. Its medial surface is convex while the lateral surface is concave. The proximal surface is concave and has two facets for articulation with the central tarsal. The distal surface articulates with the large and medial small metatarsal bones. The caudal (palmer) end projects downward into a nodule. The **third tarsal** is triangular in outline. Its proximal surface is concave and articulates with central tarsal. The distal face is convex and it articulates with large metatarsal bone. The medial border has a facet for articulation with first and second fused tarsal and the lateral border has two facets for articulation with the fourth tarsal bone. The **fourth tarsal** is brick shaped with six surfaces. The proximal surface is convex transversely and it articulates with tibial and fibular tarsals. The distal surface has two facets separated by a sagittal ridge. The facets articulate with the large and small metatarsal bones. The medial face bears a facet for articulation with the first and second fused tarsal and the central tarsal. The cranial (dorsal) lateral and caudal (palmer) surfaces are convex and rough for attachment of ligaments.

The **metatarsals** in horse are three, one large and two small as against two, one large and one small in ox. The small metatarsals are one medial and one lateral and they lie on the corresponding side of the plantar surface of large metatarsal bone. The **medial small metatarsal** is slightly longer than the lateral small metatarsal. Each one of these has two facets on the cranial (dorsal) face of their proximal extremity for articulation with the large metatarsal bone. The proximal surface of the proximal extremity of medial small metatarsal has two facets for articulation with first and second fused tarsal and the third tarsal while the **lateral small metatarsal** also has two facets for articulation with the fourth tarsal bone. The shaft of the **large metatarsal** of horse is cylindrical as against the quadrilateral shaft of large metatarsal of ox. The **vascular grooves** on the dorsal and plantar surfaces of the shaft occurring in ox are absent in horse. The large metatarsal in many respects resemble the metacarpus of the same species.

The **digits** of hind limb of horse resemble those of the fore limb of horse. However, in differentiating with ox, the **third phalanx** of horse has a more pointed toe and more concave sole surface.

Dog

The **femur** of dog is relatively larger. The shaft is strongly curved facing cranially. The supracondyloid fossa is absent. The trochanteric fossa is deep and rounded. The ridges of the trochlea are sagittal and equal. The intercondyloid fossa is wide. On the caudal aspect of distal extremity, just above each condyle is a facet for articulation with the sesamoid the fabella. The patella is long and narrow.

The **tibia** in dog has the same length as that of the fibula. The shaft forms a double curve, the proximal half is convex medially while the distal half is convex laterally. The tibial crest is more prominent but shorter. The facet for fibula is on the caudolateral aspect of the lateral condyle. The distal extremity has a facet on lateral side for fibula.

The **fibula** in dog is as long as tibia. It is slender, somewhat twisted and enlarged at both the extremities. The proximal extremity has a facet on its medial aspect for the tibia. The distal extremity forms lateral malleolus which articulates with tibia and tibial tarsal medially.

The **tarsus** in dog is made of seven bones. These are the tibial tarsal, Fibular tarsal, central tarsal, first tarsal, second tarsal, third tarsal and fourth tarsal. Thus all the tarsal bones are separate and none of them are fused unlike in other species.

The **metatarsals** in dog are five in number. The first is small and pea like. The rest of the metatarsals resemble the metacarpals.

The **digits** of the hind limb are similar to those of fore limb. The first is short with two phalanges and does not come in contact with the ground. The other four digits have three phalanges each. The third and fourth digits are longest.

Sheep and Goat

The shaft of **femur** of sheep and goat is slightly curved with convexity facing cranially. The caudal surface is separated from the lateral surface by a distinct line. The supracondyloid fossa is shallow. The sulcus in the centre of the head is shallow and the neck is distinct. The trochanter major is slightly higher in position than the head of the femur. The ridges of the trochlea are relatively less oblique. The **patella** is relatively longer and narrower than that in ox.

The **tibia** is long and slender. The rest of the features of the tibia are similar to those of ox. The **fibula** is in the form of a small osseous prominence ventral to the lateral margin of lateral condyle of tibia. The distal end of fibula is marked by lateral malleolus similar to that in ox.

The **tarsal bones** resemble those of ox however they are smaller in size. The **metatarsus** and **digits** of hind limb are similar to the metacarpus and digits of fore limb.

Pig

The **femur** of pig is relatively large and massive. The caudal surface of the shaft is wide. Its lateral border is marked by a ridge that extends from the trochanter major to the lateral supracondyloid tuberosity. The supracondyloid fossa is absent. The head of the femur is strongly curved to medial side and bears a large tuberosity for attachment of the ligament of the head. The neck is distinct. The trochanter major rises only to the level of the head and does not exceed it. The trochanteric crest between the trochanter major and trochanter minor is oblique, similar to that of ox. The trochanteric fossa also resembles that of ox. There is no third trochanter. The ridges of the trochlea at the distal extremity are similar and almost sagittal. The patella is nearly compressed from side to side and has three surfaces.

The shaft of the **tibia** is slightly curved. The cranial tuberosity of the proximal extremity is grooved vertically. It is separated from the lateral condyle by a narrow sulcus. The caudal border of the lateral condyle bears a facet for articulation with the head of the fibula. The cranial border of the proximal extremity is very prominent and is slightly curved laterally. The distal extremity of the tibia of pig resembles that of ox.

The **fibula** in pig is fully ossified in its entire length and is separated from tibia by a wide interosseous space. The shaft is flattened from side to side. Its proximal portion is wider and presents a deep groove on lateral side. Its distal portion is narrow and thicker than the proximal part. The proximal extremity of fibula is flattened and articulates medially with the lateral condyle of tibia. The distal extremity forms the lateral malleolus. It is grooved laterally and articulates with the tibia and tibial tarsal medially and the fibular tarsal distally.

The **tarsus** of pig is comprised of seven bones similar to that of the dog. The tibial and fibular tarsals in general resemble those of ox. The central tarsal is thick and is narrow transversely. Its proximal surface is deeply concave for articulation with tibial tarsal. Its plantar surface has a tubercle. The first tarsal is high and narrow. The second tarsal is small and prismatic. The third tarsal is large and is compressed proximodistally. The fourth tarsal is large and has a oblique groove on its lateral surface.

The **metatarsal bones** in pig are four for each limb and they in general resemble the metacarpals of fore limb. The metatarsals are, however, are longer than the metacarpals.

The **digits** of hind limb resemble those of fore limb. The proximal and middle phalanges are, however, a bit longer than those of fore limb.

Fowl

The **femur** of fowl is relatively short. The shaft is cylindrical and slightly curved. The head is prominent and is much smaller than the acetabulum. The distal extremity has a deep pulley like articular area for patella and two condyles for head of the tibia and fibula. The patella is wide and thin.

The **tibia** in fowl becomes **tibio-tarsus** because of the fusion of distal extremity of tibia with the tarsal bones of the proximal row of tarsus. The shaft of the tibia is nearly straight. The proximal extremity has a small lateral and large medial condyle for articulation with the condyles of the femur. The distal extremity is composed of a trochlea is condyloid with a trochlea caudally and two condyles cranially formed by the bones of the proximal row of tarsus fused with this part of the tibia. It articulates with the tarso-metatarsus.

The **fibula** of fowl is an elongated slender rod of bone. The head of the fibula is massive and flattened from side to side. It presents a facet on its medial aspect for the lateral condyle of femur. It gradually tappers and ends into a pointed distal extremity at about the distal third of the shaft of tibia.

The **tarsus** as such is absent in fowl because of the fusion of the proximal row of tarsal bones with the tibia making it tibio-tarsus and the fusion of distal row of tarsal bones with the metatarsal bones making it the **tarso-metatarsus**.

The **metatarsus** is a single bone formed by fusion of three bones, the second, third and fourth metatarsal bones. Its proximal extremity is formed by fusion of the bones of distal row of tarsus. It is very irregular and has two concavities for articulation with tibia. The distal extremity is divided into three articular projections that support the corresponding digits. In male, a conical curved projection at the distal third of the metatarsus serves as support to the horny spur.

The **digits** in fowl are four in number. The three principal digits are directed cranially and these are arranged in a radiating manner. The fifth digit is rudimentary. It is directed caudally and medially extending from the caudal aspect of the metatarsal bone with which it is attached by a fibrous cord. The first and second digits have three phalanges each, the third digit has four phalanges and the fourth digit has five phalanges.

94

Articulations of Hind Limb

The articulations of hind limb (pelvic limb) comprises the joints of pelvic region which include the sacro-iliac articulation, pelvic symphysis and the hip joint; the articulation of thigh region named as stifle joint; the articulation of tarsal or hock joint and the articulations of digits which include the metatarso-phalangeal joint (fetlock) joint, the proximal interphalangeal joint (pastern joint) and the distal interphalangeal joint (coffin joint). The joints of pelvic region especially the sacro-iliac joint and the pelvic symphysis have been described with the articulations of abdomen and pelvis.

Hip joint

The hip joint or coxo-femoral articulation (Fig. 6-2 A) is an enarthrosis formed between the acetabulum of the pelvic bone and the head of femur. The cotyloid cavity (acetabulum) is rather shallow and smaller in diameter than the head of femur. However, the rim of the acetabulum is lined by a fibrocartilage called the **cotyloid ligament** which because of its elasticity and larger diameter than the cavity itself allows the greater size of head of femur to accommodate into the acetabular cavity. A part of the cotyloid ligament which passes over the notch into the rim of the acetabulum is named as the **transverse acetabular ligament.**

The ligaments of the hip joint are the capsular ligament and the round ligament other than the cotyloid ligament and the transverse acetabular ligament described above.

The **capsular ligament** is attached to the rim of the acetabulum proximally and the rim around the head of the femur distally. The medial surface of the capsular ligament is lined by the synovial membrane which reflects over the round ligament and covers the acetabular fossa. It reflects around the round ligament.

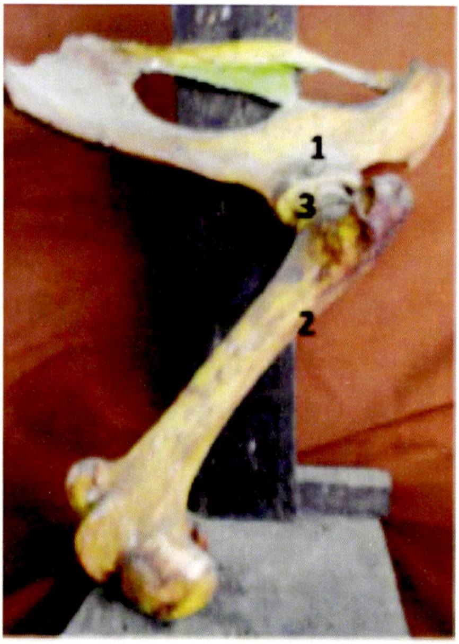

Fig. 6 – 2 A: Hip Joint of Ox
1. Os coxae 2. Femur 3. Capsular ligament

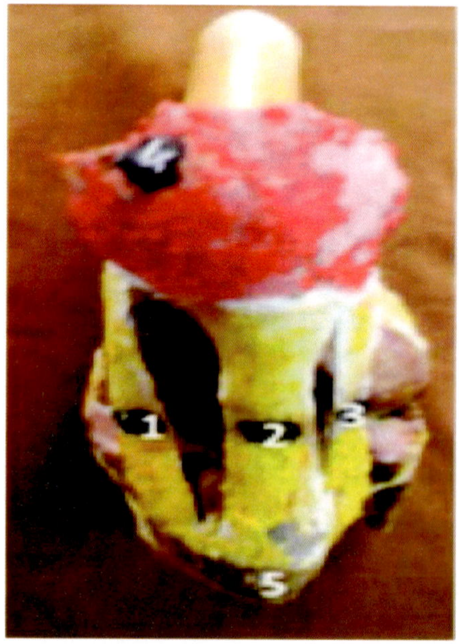

Fig.6 – 2 B: Stifle joint Femoro-patellar articulation
1. Lateral patellar ligament 2. Middle patellar ligament 3. Medial patellar ligament 4. Patella 5. Tibia

The **round ligament** is a small, short but strong band which extends from the nonarticular part of acetabulum the acetabular fossa and ends at the central sulcus the fovea capitis on the head of the femur.

The hip joint is covered externally on its cranial aspect by the rectus femoris, on caudal aspect by gemelli and obturator internus, on lateral side by obturator externus and on medial side by a common tendon of iliacus and psoas major muscles.

Movements: The hip joint, being a ball and socket joint can perform all types of movements viz- extension, flexion, adduction, abduction, rotation and circumduction. However, the extension and flexion are most marked.

Stifle joint

The stifle joint (Fig. 6-2 B) is a most extensive and elaborate joint amongst the articulations in the animal body. It is a composite joint consisting of a femoro-tibial and femoro-patellar articulations formed between the condyles at the distal extremity of femur and proximal extremity of tibia and between the trochlea of femur and the patellar bone respectively.

Femoro-patellar articulation (Fig. 6-2 B)

The femoro-patellar articulation is a gliding type of joint formed between the trochlea on the cranial aspect of the distal extremity of femur and the articular surface of the patella. The trochlea is a pair of asymmetrical nearly vertical ridges separated by a groove. The medial ridge is larger than the lateral ridge. The two ridges partially converge ventrally. The articular surface of the patella presents a vertical ridge in its middle which separates the two nearly vertical concave areas, the medial being larger than the lateral one. The articular area of the patella is smaller than that of the trochlea of femur.

The ligaments of the femoro-patellar articulation include the capsular, collateral and patellar ligaments.

The **capsular ligament** is attached to the margin of articular surface of the trochlea of femur and that of the patella. The ligament is lined internally by the synovial membrane. The synovial sac of this membrane continues with the synovial membrane of femoro-tibial articulation through one or two openings on the ventral side.

The **collateral ligaments** are two, medial and lateral. These are thin flat bands that support the joint from outside the capsule of the joint. The **medial collateral ligament** is attached to the medial epicondyle of the femur and the fibrocartilage on the medial border of the patella. The **lateral collateral ligament** is attached to the lateral condyle of femur and the lateral border of the patella.

The **patellar ligaments** are three large, flat strong bands of ligament which attach the patella with the tibial crest and the cranial tuberosity of the proximal extremity of tibia. The three ligaments are the medial patellar, middle patellar and the lateral patellar ligaments. The **medial patellar ligament** extends from the medial part of the cranial surface and the medial border of the patella to the medial aspect of the cranial tuberosity of the patella. It partly blends by aponeurosis with the tendon of gracilis and Sartorius muscles and with e few fibres of the vastus internus part of the rectus femoris muscle of the thigh. The **middle patellar ligament** extends from the apex of the patella to the cranial tuberosity and the tibial crest of the tibia. It lies between the medial and lateral patellar ligaments. The **lateral patellar ligament** is the largest and most powerful of the three patellar ligaments. It extends from the lateral part of the cranial surface and the fibrocartilage on the lateral border of the patella to the lateral side of the cranial tuberosity and the tibial crest of the tibia. It completely fuses with the tendon of insertion of the biceps femoris and a large **synovial bursa** is interposed between this ligament and the lateral condyle of tibia. Another bursa is interposed between the middle patellar ligament and the dorsal part of the trochlea. In addition, a small bursa appears between the apex of the patella and the middle patellar ligament.

Movements of the joint are gliding type. The patella glides upward and downward over the trochlea of the femur with the help of the muscles on one side and the patellar ligaments on the other.

Femoro-tibial articulation (Fig. 6-2 C)

The femoro-tibial articulation is a ginglymus type of joint. It is formed between the condyles of the distal extremity of femur, the articular surface of the proximal extremity of tibia and the intervening interarticular cartilaginous pieces the menisci. The condyles of the femur are slightly oblique in direction. The articular surfaces of the condyles of tibia are saddle shaped and these are not adapted to the condyles of the femur. The articular surfaces of the femur and tibia are thus not in contact with each other except a small area occupied by the tibial spine that fits into the intercondyloid fossa of the femur. To make the articular surfaces suitable for articulation, small semilunar pieces of cartilage called menisci are interposed between them.

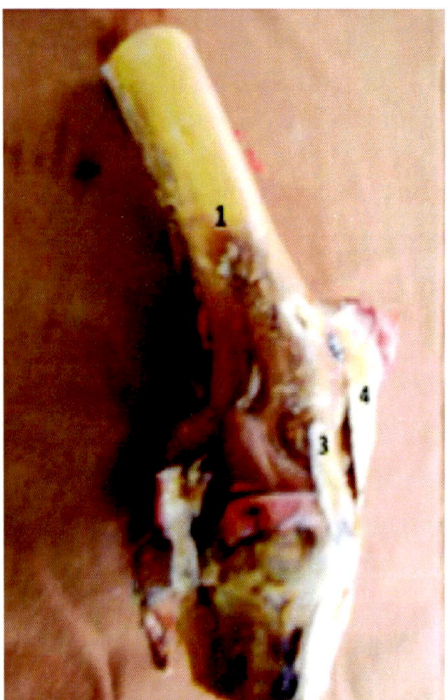

Fig. 6 – 2 C: Stifle joint; Femoro-tibial articulation
1. Femur 2. Tibia 3 . Lateral collateral ligament 4. Lateral patellar ligament

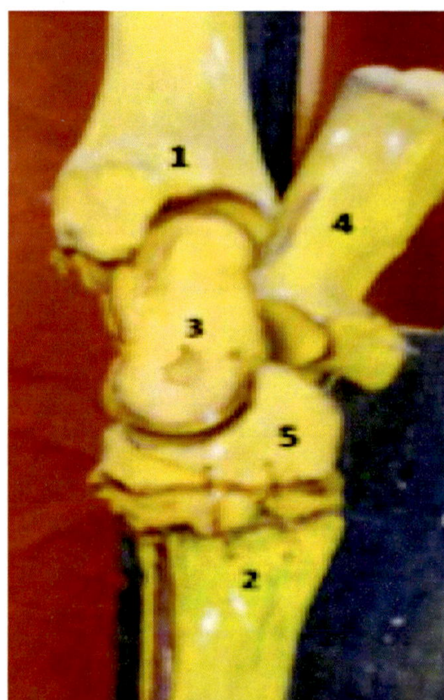

Fig. 6 – 2 D: Hock Joint of Ox
1. Tibia 2. Metatarsal 3. Tibial tarsal 4. Fibular tarsal 5. Central and fourth fused tarsal

The **menisci** are two, medial and lateral. These are dorsoventrally compressed 'C' shaped plates of fibrocartilage interposed between the condyles of femur and tibia. They are thick along their margins and thin centrally. Their dorsal surface is concave to accommodate the convex articular surface of the condyles of the femur. The ventral surface is flat and articulates with the flat articular surface of the tibial condyles. The menisci are kept attached to the tibial articular surface by the cranial and caudal coronary ligaments that are attached to the respective side of the tibial spine.

The **ligaments** of the femoro-tibial articulation are the capsular, collateral and cruciate ligaments.

The **capsular ligament** surrounds the entire stifle joint. It is attached to the margin of the articular surface of the distal extremity of femur proximally and proximal extremity of tibia distally. The caudal part of the ligament extends above the condyles of femur proximally and below the condyles of tibia distally. The ligamentous capsule is thin in front and thick behind. It is lined by a thin synovial membrane internally. The synovial membrane completely covers the articular surfaces, the menisci and the cruciate ligaments. The caudal surface of the capsule is covered by the gracilis muscle and is vertically crossed by popliteal vessels and nerve. The interarticular septum of the synovial membrane divides the synovial cavity of femoro-tibial articulation into two compartments and they communicate with the femoro-patellar synovial membrane.

The **collateral ligaments** are two, the medial and lateral. The medial ligament extends from a small tubercle on the medial condyle of femur, descends over the medial aspect of the joint capsule and ends on a rough area below the medial margin of the medial tuberosity of tibia. The lateral ligament is attached proximally to the higher of the two depressions on the lateral condyle of femur. From here the lateral ligament runs down crossing the tendon of origin of the popliteus muscle and ends on the lateral aspect of the lateral tuberosity of tibia. On the deeper side of this ligament is a synovial bursa at the origin of popliteus muscle.

The **cruciate ligaments** are cranial and caudal lying on the respective side of the femoro-tibial articulation. These are strong intercrossing bands lodged in the intercondyloid groove of the femur. The cranial ligament extends from tibial spine, runs obliquely upward and ends on the lateral wall of the intercondyloid groove of the femur. The caudal ligament begins at a tubercle ventral to the rim of the tibial articular surface, runs upwards obliquely craniad and terminates on the cranial part of the intercondyloid groove of the femur.

The **movements** of this joint are mainly the extension and flexion with a little degree of rotation.

Tibio-fibular articulation

The tibio-fibular articulation as such does not occur. This is because the fibula is just a rudimentary bone in the form of its head which is fused with the lateral condyle of the tibia. The shaft of fibula does not exist and the distal extremity (lower end) is ossified as a separate piece of bone called the lateral malleolus that forms a diarthrodial joint with the lateral surface of the distal extremity of tibia.

Tarsal joint (Hock joint)

The tarsal articulation or hock joint (Fig. 6-2 D) is a composite joint comprising the (1) tibio-tarsal articulation (2) intertarsal articulations and (3) tarsometatarsal articulation. The bones of these joints are binded by small ligaments which are specific to that particular joint and are called the **special ligaments** of the corresponding joint. In addition, there are some common ligaments that bind the whole of the hock joint and these are called the **common ligaments.**

Tibio-tarsal articulation

The tibio-tarsal articulation is a ginglymus type of joint formed between the distal extremity of tibia and fibula and the tibial and fibular tarsal bones. The articular surfaces are the trochlea of the tibial tarsal and the corresponding grooves on the distal extremity of the tibia. The grooves of the tibia are slightly oblique and so the corresponding ridges of the trochlea of tibial tarsal are also slightly oblique in direction. The articular surfaces of the trochlea are more extensive than that of the grooves of the tibia. The tibio-tarsal articulation has **one special ligament** called the transverse ligament. It connects the lateral malleolus to the caudal aspect of tibial tarsal.

Proximal tarsal articulation

The proximal tarsal articulation is formed between the tibial and fibular tarsals and the central and fourth fused tarsal. The articular surfaces of both the segments of the joint are flat. This joint is binded by the dorsal ligament, medial and lateral collateral ligaments and the interosseous ligament as **special ligaments** of this joint. The dorsal ligament connects the dorsal border of the tibial tarsal to the fibular tarsal. The collateral ligaments bind this joint on medial and lateral sides. The interosseous ligament connects the ventral surface of tibial tarsal to the roughened depression on the medial surface of the fibular tarsal.

Distal tarsal articulation

The distal tarsal articulation is formed between the first tarsal, second and third fused tarsal and central and fourth fused tarsal bones proximally and the articular surface on the proximal extremity of the large metatarsal bone distally. This joint is supported by one cranial (dorsal) ligament and three interosseous ligaments as **special ligaments** of this joint. The cranial (dorsal) ligament is a flat band that connects all the bones in the distal row of the tarsus. The first interosseous ligament connects the ventral surface of the central and fourth fused tarsal to the synovial fossa on the proximal extremity of large metatarsal bone. The second interosseous ligament connects the central and fourth tarsal to the second and third fused tarsal bone. The third interosseous ligament connects the first tarsal to the second and third fused tarsal bone.

The **common ligaments** of the tarsal or hock joint as a whole are the capsular ligament, medial and lateral collateral ligaments, dorsal ligament and the plantar ligament.

The **capsular ligament** is attached to the margin of the articular surface of tibia proximally and that of the metatarsal bone distally. It is also attached to the outer surfaces of the other bones constituting this joint and is blended with the medial and lateral collateral ligaments. The dorsal (cranial) part of this ligament is thin and distended. It is related externally to the tendons of peroneus tertius, tibialis anticus, and the medial and lateral digital extensor muscles and the cranial tibial vessels and deep peroneal nerve. The plantar (caudal) part of the capsular ligament is very thick and is intimately attached to the tarsal bones. This part of the capsular ligament becomes cartilaginous and forms smooth surface for the passage of tendons of deep digital flexor muscle over it. The fibrous layer of the capsule is lined internally by a thin synovial membrane. The synovial membrane of the capsular ligament forms four sacs. The tibio-tarsal sac is the largest and it lubricates the structures of tibio-tarsal articulation, the proximal intertarsal sac lubricates bones of the first layer of tarsals, the distal intertarsal sac lubricates the joint formed by the bones of distal layer of tarsals and the tarsometatarsal sac lubricates the joints formed between the tarsal and metatarsal bones.

The **collateral ligaments** are the lateral and medial. The **lateral collateral ligament** has two bands, the superficial and deep. The superficial band of this ligament is longer. It arises from the caudal part of the lateral malleolus, extends vertically downward over the capsular ligament and ends on the tibial tarsal, fibular tarsal, lateral part of the central and fourth fused tarsal and the lateral side of the proximal extremity of the metatarsal bone. The deep band is short and it arises from the dorsal (cranial) part of lateral malleolus, descends obliquely ventrad and caudad over the capsular ligament and ends on the fibular and tibial tarsal bones. The **medial collateral ligament** has three parts. The superficial band arises from the caudal part of the medial malleolus, extends ventrally and ends on the tibial tarsal, large metatarsal and small metatarsal bones. The middle and deep bands extend from the cranial part of the medial malleolus, runs obliquely ventrad and caudad and the deep band terminates on tibial tarsal while the middle band ends on the sustentaculum tali.

The **dorsal ligament** is a narrow triangular band placed on the dorso-medial aspect of the tarsal joint. It extends from the distal tuberosity on the medial face of tibial tarsal passes obliquely ventrad and ends on the central and fourth fused tarsal and proximal extremity of large metatarsal bone.

The **plantar ligament** is very strong flat band which covers the lateral part of the plantar surface of the tarsus. It is attached to the caudal border of the tuber calcis of the fibular tarsal, central and fourth fused tarsal and the large metatarsal bones.

The **movements** of hock joint are mainly the extension and flexion performed at the tibio-tarsal joint. The segments of the rest of the articulations of the hock joint perform gliding movements.

Articulations of digits

The articulations of the digits of hind limb include the metatarso-phalangeal articulation (fetlock joint), proximal interphalangeal articulation (pastern joint) and the distal interphalangeal articulation (coffin joint). These joints of hind limb resemble those of fore limb.

95

Comparative Anatomy of Articulations of Hind Limb

Horse

The **hip joint** has an additional ligament called the pubio-femoral ligament. It arises from the prepubic tendon, passes dorsally and laterally and then caudally and lodges into the subpubic (pubio-femoral) groove, penetrates the capsular ligament, passes through the acetabular notch and is inserted into the fovea capitis behind the round ligament on the head of femur. This ligament is peculiar to solipeds and it prevents the side kicking. The absence of this ligament in ruminants allows them abduction freely and that is how the ruminants can kick sideways. As against this, the equines can kick only back way. The other difference about the hip joint in horse is that the cotyloid ligament is narrower because of the deeper acetabulum.

The **stifle joint** of horse in general resembles that of ox except that the middle patellar ligament is not so prominent as that in ox.

The **tibio-fibular articulation** in horse is a diarthrosis and an amphiarthrosis. The diarthrosis is formed between the lateral condyle of tibia and the head of the fibula. It has intimate capsular ligament. The amphiarthrosis is formed between the shafts of the tibia and the fibula. The shafts of the two bones are binded by the proximal and distal interosseous ligaments.

The **hock joint** of horse has minor differences with those of ox owing to the difference in the number of tarsal bones and their arrangement. The synovial membrane is supported everywhere except at the dorsomedial (craniomedial) aspect where it bulges out in the cases of bog-spavin. If there is a distension of tarsal sheath, it bulges out as two rounded swellings on either sides of the tendon of deep digital flexor. The movements at the hock joint are very limited.

Dog

The **hip joint** of dog resembles that of ox.

The **stifle joint** of dog has a single patellar ligament at the femoro-patellar articulation. The capsular ligament and synovial membranc is single and common for both, the femoro-patellar and the femoro-tibial articulations.

The **tibio-fibular articulations** are three, one each at the proximal and distal extremities and the third at the shafts of the tibia and fibula. The articulations at the extremities are diarthrodial joints and are covered by joint capsules. The shafts of tibia and fibula are united with each other throughout their length and are binded by the interosseous ligament.

The **hock joint** of dog resembles that of ox except for the differences because of the difference of the number and arrangement of the tarsal bones. The collateral ligaments are comparatively small. The plantar ligament is not developed as better as that of ox and the dorsal (oblique) ligament is not so distinct as that of ox.

Sheep and Goat

The articulations of the hind limb in sheep and goat resemble those of the ox.

Pig

The hip joint in pig has no remarkable differences.

At the stifle joint, the capsule of the femoro-patellar articulation is reinforced by the collateral ligaments of the femoro-tibial articulation. The patellar ligament is single and strong. Under the distal part of this ligament is the synovial bursa. The cranial faces of the menisci are connected by a small transverse ligament.

The tibio-fibular articulations are formed between the proximal extremities, the shafts and the distal extremities of the tibia and fibula. The articulation of the proximal extremities of the two bones is covered under a separate joint capsule which is reinforced cranially and caudally by fibrous tissue. The joint between the shafts of two bones has the interosseous ligament as the binding medium. The joint of the distal extremities of tibia and fibula is enclosed under the joint capsule of the hock joint and is strengthened by the dorsal and plantar ligaments.

The hock joint of pig almost resembles in respect of the number of tarsal bones and their arrangement with that of the ox.

Fowl

At the **hip joint**, the acetabulum of pelvic bone is perforated and the head of the femur is freely accommodated within it. The rotating movements are performed at this joint.

The **stifle** joint is formed between the distal extremity of femur and the proximal extremity of tibiotarsus. The small patella is accommodated into a large rotular groove at the distal extremity of the femur.

At the **tarsal joint**, the tarsal bones of the proximal row are fused with the distal extremity of the tibia making it the tibiotarsal bone. Similarly the tarsal bones of the distal row of tarsus are fused with the metatarsal bone. The distal extremity of tibiotarsus presents prominent condyles for articulation with the tarsometatarsus. The joint is binded by medial and lateral ligaments.

At the **digits**, the three tarsometatarsal bones are joined with the proximal phalanges of the three principal digits.

96

Muscles of Hind Limb

The **fascia** covering the hind limb is the superficial and deep fascia. The superficial fascia is very scanty lies beneath the skin. It has the same general disposition as in other regions of the body. The deep fascia is in the form of a thick strong sheet covering the superficial layer of muscles over the medial aspect of the hind limb. From this sheet extend several septa that pass between different muscles or muscle groups in the thigh region. The deep fascia of the leg region continues cranially with the fascia of the thoracolumbar region. Caudally it is attached to the aponeurotic tendon of insertion of sartorius and gracilis muscles. The part of the deep fascia that continues on the lateral aspect of the thigh is the fascia lata which is continuous with the gluteal fascia dorsally.

The **muscles** of the hind limb (Fig. 6-3 A and B) are arranged into different regional, positional as well as functional groups. The muscles of hip and thigh region are arranged in the lateral, medial and cranial groups. The muscles of leg and foot are arranged in dorsolateral and plantar groups. The dorsolateral muscles are generally the extensors of tarsus and digits while the plantar muscles are the flexors of tarsus and digits.

Lateral muscles of hip and thigh (FIG. 6-3 A)

Tensor fasciae latae

The tensor fasciae latae is the most superficial muscle that lies beneath the skin and the fascia on the cranial and craniolateral aspect of the hip and thigh region of the hind limb. It is a triangular muscle with its base below and apex above. It originates as a narrow aponeurotic tendon at the external angle of ilium (tuber coxae) and as it passes down widens at about the middle of its course and after reaching proximal to the stifle joint, divides into superficial and deep layers which form aponeurosis with the fascia lata.

Origin: This muscle originates on the external angle of the ilium (tuber coxae).

Insertion: The insertion of this muscle is by aponeurosis on the fascia lata and the lateral patellar ligament.

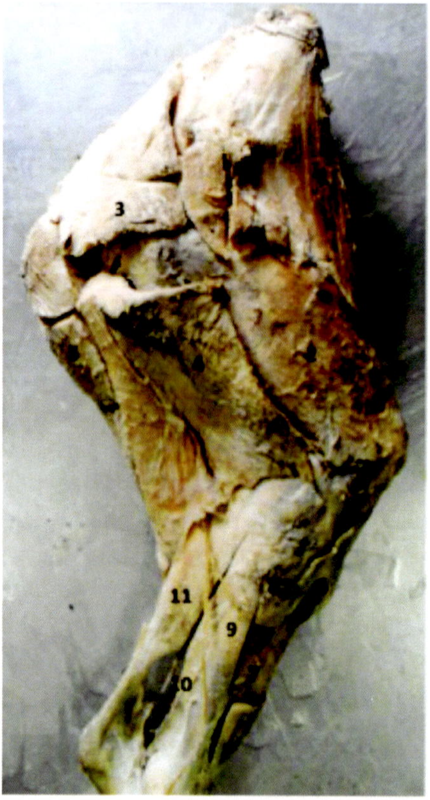

Fig. 6 – 3 A: Muscles of Hind limb (Lateral View)
1. Tensor Fascia Lata M. 2. Quadriceps Femoris M. 3. Middle Gluteus M. 4. Biceps Femoris M. 5. Semitendinosus M. 6. Tibialis Anticus M. 7. Complex M. 8. Peroneus Longus M. 9. Lateral Digital Extensor M. 10. Deep Digital Flexor M. 11. Gastrocnemius M.

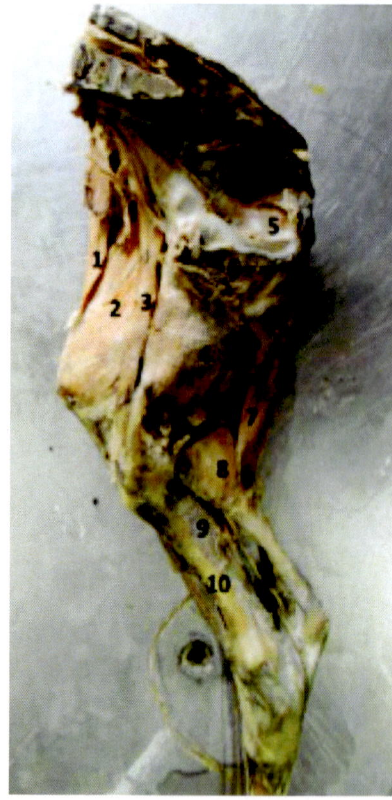

Fig. 6 – 3 B: Muscles of Hind limb (Medial View)
1. Tensor Fascia Lata M. 2. Vastus Medialis 3. Sartorius M. 4. Gracilis M. 5. Obturator Internus M. 6. Obturator Externus M. 7. Semimembranosus M. 8. Gastrocnemius M. 9. Popliteus M. 10. Tibia bone

Action: The muscle acts to tense the fascia lata by way of which it participates in flexion of hip joint and extension of stifle joint.

Blood supply: Circumflex iliac artery

Nerve supply: Cranial gluteal nerve.

Biceps femoris (gluteobiceps)

The biceps femoris is a vast expansive muscle situated on the lateral aspect of the hip and thigh extending from the sacral spines to the proximal end of the leg. It covers the middle gluteus (gluteus medius) muscle. The superficial gluteus (gluteus superficialis) is merged with the biceps and hence the name gluteobiceps. The muscle appears nearly quadrilateral in form. It is very much thick in the middle and thinner in its proximal part. The distal part is tendinous in nature. It is covered laterally by the skin and fascia of the lateral surface of thigh. Medially it is related to iliosacral and sacrosciatic ligaments, tuber ischii and trochanter major; middle gluteus, gemelli, quadratus femoris, adductor, semimembranosus, semitendinosus and vastus externus muscles; the caudal gluteal vessels and nerves, the sciatic nerve and its branches, external popliteal and external saphenous nerves and the femoral and deep femoral vessels.

Origin: The origin of this muscle is at multiple locations. It originates on the sacral spines, sacrosciatic ligament, tuber ischii, curved ridge and the tubercle on the ventral surface of ischium and the gluteal fascia.

Insertion: The muscle divides distally into three parts before its insertion. The cranial division inserts on the patella, the middle division inserts on the lateral patellar ligament and the tibial crest while the caudal division inserts on the fascia lata and through it on the fibular tarsal (os calcis).

Action: It causes extension and adduction of the hind limb. The cranial part of the muscle extends the stifle joint, the middle part extends the hip joint and the caudal part flex the stifle and abducts the limb.

Blood supply: The blood supply to this vast muscle is through multiple sources. It is supplied by cranial and caudal gluteal, medial circumflex femoral, caudal femoral and popliteal arteries.

Nerve supply: It is supplied by caudal gluteal and ischiatic or tibial nerves.

Gluteus muscles

The gluteus is a set of three muscles in domestic animals. These are the superficial, middle and deep gluteus. However, in ruminants the cranial part of superficial gluteus muscle is merged with the tensor fascia lata and its caudal part is merged with the biceps femoris muscle. Thus, the superficial gluteus muscle as a separate muscle is altogether absent in ruminants. The middle gluteus and deep gluteus muscles exists separately medial to the biceps muscle in the thigh region.

Middle gluteus

The middle gluteus (gluteus medius) is thick fleshy muscle lying in the space between the trochanter major and tuber coxae. It covers the gluteal (lateral) surface of the ilium and the lateral wall of the pelvis and extends on the lumbar part of the longissimus dorsi up to the fourth lumbar vertebra. It is covered laterally in its cranial part by the tensor fascia lata and in the caudal part by the biceps femoris muscle along with the skin and the gluteal and lumbodorsal fascia.

Origin: The middle gluteus muscle originates on the gluteal surface along with its lateral angle (tuber coxae) and medial angle (tuber sacrale), the sacrosciatic ligament. And the aponeurosis of the longissimus dorsi muscle as far up to the fourth lumbar vertebra.

Insertion: The muscle is inserted by three tendons. The cranial tendon inserts ventral to the trochanter major of femur, the middle tendon inserts on the dorsal border of trochanter major and the caudal tendon inserts on the trochanteric ridge.

Action: To extend the hip joint and abduct the limb.

Blood supply: The blood supply to medial gluteus muscle is through the cranial gluteal, deep circumflex iliac, and the medial and lateral circumflex femoral arteries.

Nerve supply: Through the cranial gluteal and ischiatic nerves.

Deep gluteus

The deep gluteus (gluteus profundus) muscle lies under cover of the middle gluteus. It is thinner and smaller than later one. It is irregularly quadrilateral and its fibres course caudoventrally spreading in fan shaped manner directly over the hip joint.

Origin: The wide base of this fan shaped muscle originates on the lateral angle of the ilium (tuber coxae), the gluteal surface and the gluteal line of the ilium, the ischiatic spine and the broad sacrosciatic ligament.

Insertion: The apex of this fan shaped muscle is inserted on the small tubercle below the trochanter major just cranial to the insertion of the middle gluteus muscle at the proximal extremity of the femur.

Action: The muscle causes the abduction and inward rotation of the thigh.
Blood supply: Cranial gluteal and lateral circumflex femoral arteries.

Nerve supply: Cranial gluteal nerve.

Semitendinosus

The semitendinosus is a long fleshy muscle extending from the tuber ischii to the proximal third of the medial surface of the tibia. In its course, it lies first between the biceps femoris and semimembranosus and then between the biceps femoris and gracilis muscles.

Origin: It originates at the caudoventral surface of the lateral angle of the ischium (tuber ischii).

Insertion: It inserts on the tibial crest, the fascia lata and the fibular tarsal (os calcis).

Action: To extend the hip joint and hock joint, to flex the stifle joint and to rotate the leg medially.

Blood supply: Deep femoral and medial circumflex femoral arteries

Nerve supply: Caudal gluteal, ischiatic or tibial nerves.

Semimembranosus

The semimembranosus is a long thick fleshy muscle lying deeply on the caudodorsal aspect of hip and thigh. It extends from the tuber ischii, passes obliquely ventrad and craniad to the medial face of the proximal third of the tibia (leg). The muscle is elongated dorsoventrally. It is expanded at the proximal and distal portions and is constricted in the middle.

Origin: The semimembranosus muscle originates on the ventral surface of the tuber ischii, the ventral surface of the caudal portion of the ischium and the caudal part of the pelvic symphysis.

Insertion: The muscle has two tendons for insertion. The large proximal tendon of insertion is attached to the medial epicondyle of femur and the small distal tendon inserts on a small area distal to the medial articular margin of tibia just caudal to the medial collateral ligament.

Action: To extend the hip joint and to abduct the limb.

Blood supply: Deep femoral, medial circumflex femoral, saphenous, popliteal, cranial tibial and the femoral arteries.

Nerve supply: Ischiatic or tibial nerve.

Medial muscles of hip and thigh (FIG. 6-3 B)

Medial to the hip region is the pelvic cavity and there are no muscles on this side of the hip except one, the obturator internus which lies on the floor of pelvis and for the purpose of convenience has been included in the group of medial muscles of thigh. The muscles of the medial side of the thigh are arranged in three layers, the superficial, middle and deep layer. The superficial layer consists of two muscles, the sartorius and gracilis, the middle layer has three muscles the pectineus, adductor and semimembranosus, while the deeper layer consists of four muscles the quadratus femoris, obturator externus, obturator internus and the gemellus.

Sartorius

The sartorius is a long, thin and flat strap like muscle that extends obliquely ventrad and caudad from the sublumbar region just cranial to the pelvic brim, courses across the craniomedial aspect of the thigh to the medial aspect of the thigh. It is covered superficially by the skin and subcutaneous muscle on the medial surface of thigh. It is related on its deep (lateral) surface to the iliacus and psoas major muscle in its initial course and to the vastus medialis and semimembranosus muscles at its insertion. On its caudal aspect lies the gracilis and pectineus muscle. The sartorius muscle forms the cranial boundary of the femoral canal through which passes the vessels and nerves of the hind limb.

Origin: The origin of this muscle is in two parts. The cranial part originates on the tendon of psoas minor and iliac fascia while the caudal part originates on the shaft of the ilium.

Insertion: the muscle inserts by aponeurosis on the medial aspect of the proximal third of the tibia and on the medial patellar ligament.

Action: To flex the hip joint and to adduct the limb.

Blood supply: Deep circumflex iliac, femoral and saphenous arteries.

Nerve supply: Saphenous or femoral nerve.

Gracilis

The gracilis muscle is the larger and caudal of the two muscles of the superficial layer of the medial group of thigh muscles. It is a broad, thin, flat and quadrilateral muscle lying superficially on the caudal portion of the medial aspect of the thigh. It has extensive attachment in the subpelvic area and its insertion is wide and aponeurotic. It is related superficially to skin and fascia and deeply to semimembranosus, semitendinosus, adductor, and pectineus muscles.

Origin: The gracilis muscle has an extensive origin on the ventral median raphe of the pelvic symphysis, ventral surface of pubis and the prepubic tendon.

Insertion: The insertion of this muscle is by aponeurosis on the medial patellar ligament, the medial aspect of proximal part of tibia and the fascia lata.

Action: To adduct the limb, to flex the stifle joint and to extend the hock joint.

Blood supply: Saphenous and medial circumflex femoral arteries

Nerve supply: Saphenous and obturator nerves.

Pectineus

The pectineus is a large thick conical muscle. It is situated beneath the sartorius and gracilis muscles. It extends obliquely craniad and laterad from the cranial border of the pubis to the proximal extremity of the tibia. It is somewhat triangular in shape. At its origin it is single and massive but at its insertion it tapers and divides into two heads of insertion. The muscle is related laterally to the vastus medialis, adductor and iliopsoas, medially to gracilis, cranially to sartorius and iliacus and caudally to adductor and obturator externus.

Origin: on the cranial border of pubis and the prepubic tendon

Insertion: Medial border of the caudal surface of shaft of femur and the medial epicondyle of femur.

Action: To adduct the limb and flex the hip joint.

Blood supply: Medial circumflex femoral, deep femoral, saphenous and the femoral arteries.

Nerve supply: Saphenous and obturator nerves.

Adductor

The adductor is a thick and fleshy muscle lying caudal to the pectineus and vastus internus muscles. It is very extensive in its origin and insertion. It extends from the ventral surface of the pubis and ischium, passes obliquely ventrad, laterad and craniad to the medial aspect of the thigh.

Origin: It originates on the ventral surface of the pubis and ischium and the tendon of origin of the gracilis muscle.

Insertion: The large scale of the distal end of the this muscle inserts on the lateral border of the caudal surface of femur and a small portion inserts on the tendon of origin of the medial head of gastrocnemius muscle.

Action: To adduct the limb and extend the hip joint.

Blood supply: Medial circumflex femoral and femoral arteries.

Nerve supply: Obturator and ischiatic nerve.

Obturator externus

The obturator externus (obturatorius externus) is a short, thick, flat fan shaped muscle lying on the ventral surface of the pubis and ischium. It extends from the ventral surface of ischium and pubis to the trochanteric fossa of the femur.

Origin: On the ventral surface of ischium and pubis and the ventrolateral part of the margin of obturator foramen.

Insertion: It inserts by a flat tendon on the trochanteric fossa along with the gemelli muscle.

Action: To adduct the thigh and rotate it laterally.

Blood supply: Medial circumflex femoral artery and its obturator branch.

Nerve supply: Obturator nerve.

Obturator internus

This is a thin fan shaped muscle lying on the floor of the pelvic cavity, dorsal and caudal to or partly over the obturator foramen. The muscle arises on the pelvic symphysis, passes laterally on both sides in the craniolateral direction to reach the caudolateral border of the obturator foramen. On reaching this foramen, it becomes tendinous and leaves the pelvic floor by passing out through the obturator foramen, unites with the tendon of insertion of obturator externus to terminate at the trochanteric fossa at the proximal extremity of the femur.

Origin: Pelvic surface of ischium and pubis.

Insertion: Trochanteric fossa at the proximal extremity of the femur

Action: To rotate the femur laterally

Blood supply: Internal iliac or internal pudendal and obturator branch of medial circumflex femoral artery.

Nerve supply: Obturator nerve.

Gemellus

The gemellus is a thin triangular muscle extending from the ventrolateral aspect of the ischium to the trochanteric fossa of the femur. The muscle has a wide fleshy origin in a fan like manner, course in a cranioventral direction and turns into a tendinous insertion that converges with the obturator externus muscle to insert on the trochanteric fossa of the femur.

Origin: Ventrolateral part of the ischium at the level of the lesser sciatic notch and the medial surface of the tuber ischii.

Insertion: At the trochanteric fossa with insertion of obturator externus.

Action: To rotate the femur laterally.

Blood supply: Caudal gluteal artery

Nerve supply: Sciatic nerve.

Quadratus femoris

The quadratus femoris is a small short fleshy muscle lying on the caudal surface of the ischio-femoral region. It is covered by the adductor and semimembranosus muscles. It extends from ventral surface of ischium, passes obliquely cranio ventral and lateral to reach the trochanter minor of the femur.

Origin: The ventral surface of ischium near the caudolateral angle of the obturator foramen.

Insertion: The upper part of trochanter minor and the adjacent caudal surface of the femur.

Action: To extend the hip and adduct the thigh.

Blood supply: Medial circumflex femoral artery.

Nerve supply: Obturator and ischiatic nerves.

Femoral canal

The muscles of the medial group of thigh forms and enclose between them a long canal called the femoral canal. The canal is formed by the sartorius muscle cranially, the pectineus muscle caudally, the gracilis medially and the iliacus, psoas major, and vastus internus muscles laterally. The femoral canal at its proximal end opens into the abdomen is bounded by the inguinal ligament cranially, the cranial border of pubis caudally and the tendon of psoas minor laterally. This opening is called the femoral ring. The canal at its distal end opens at the distal part of the thigh near the insertion of the pectineus muscle. The canal provides a passage for the femoral artery vessels and the saphenous nerve.

Cranial muscles of thigh (FIG. 6-3 C)

The cranial group of muscles of thigh includes one large and massive muscle the quadriceps femoris and the other very small muscle the articularis genu.

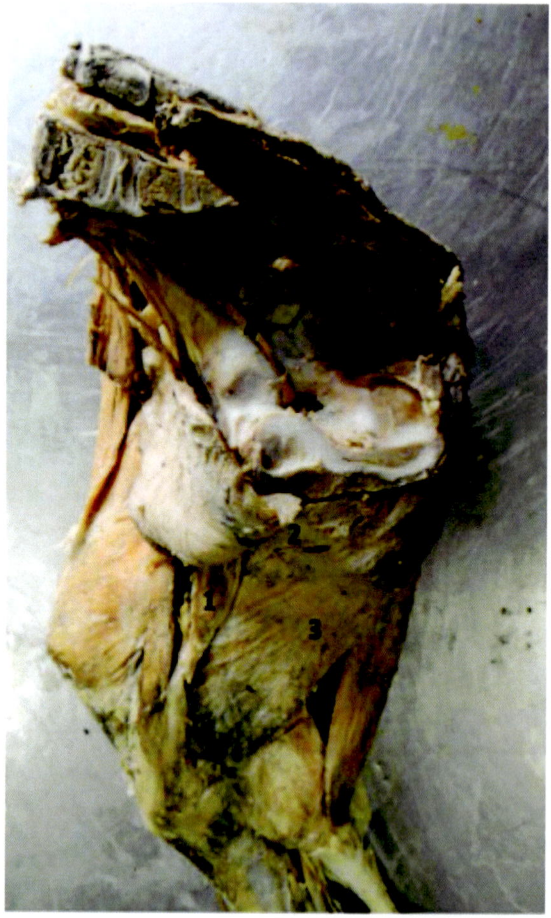

Fig. 6 – 3 C: Muscles of Hip and Thigh of Ox; Deep Dissection
1. Pectineus M. 2. Adductor M. 3. Semimebranosus M. 4. Obturator Nerve

Quadriceps femoris

The quadriceps femoris muscle, as the name indicates, is composed of four parts. These parts are the rectus femoris, vastus externus, vastus internus, and the vastus intermedius. These parts cover the cranial, medial and lateral aspects of the femur. Of these, the rectus femoris extends from the ilium of the pelvic bone while the other three parts arise from the femur. All the four parts, however, terminate on the patella at the stifle joint.

Rectus femoris

The rectus femoris muscle is lodged for most of its extent between the vastus internus and vastus externus. It extends from the cotyloid angle of ilium to the patella. It is nearly rounded in form being thick in the middle and narrow at the extremities. The muscular belly of this muscle is composed of closely placed fasciculi and is lodged in a groove formed by other three components of the quadriceps femoris muscle.

Origin: On a rough depression on the inner side and a ridge on the outer side of the rim of the acetabulum.

Insertion: On the cranial surface of the patella.

Action: To extend the stifle and flex the hip joint.

Blood supply: Deep circumflex iliac and lateral circumflex femoral artery.

Nerve supply: Femoral nerve.

Vastus externus (vastus lateralis)

The vastus externus (lateralis) is placed on the lateral side of the rectus femoris muscle and on the lateral surface of the shaft of the femur. This muscle is thicker and larger than the vastus internus. It is wider in the middle and narrow at its proximal and distal ends. A synovial bursa is interposed between the tendon of insertion and the patella.

Origin: The lateral surface of the shaft of femur, the supracondyloid fossa and the trochanter major of the femur.

Insertion: The lateral border of patella and the lateral patellar ligament

Action: To extend the stifle joint

Blood supply: Lateral circumflex femoral, caudal femoral and popliteal arteries.

Nerve supply: Femoral nerve.

Vastus internus (vastus medialis)

The vastus internus (medialis) is thinner and narrower than the vastus externus muscle. It lies on the medial surface of the shaft of femur extending from its neck to the patella. It forms a deep groove with the preceding muscle into which the rectus femoris muscle is lodged. Between the terminal part of this muscle and the patella lies a synovial bursa.

Origin: Caudal surface of femur on its medial aspect extending from the neck to the middle of the shaft. Some fibres of tendon of origin are received from the vastus intermedius.

Insertion: Craniomedial surface of the patella and the medial patellar ligament.

Action: In association with vastus externus and rectus femoris, it causes extension of the stifle joint.

Blood supply: Lateral circumflex femoral and the femoral arteries.

Nerve supply: Femoral nerve.

Vastus intermedius

The vastus intermedius lies deeply on the cranial surface of the shaft of the femur and is completely covered by the other three muscles of this group of rectus femoris muscle. It is clearly separable from the other three muscles and it itself has two divisions. It is narrow in its proximal part, thick in the middle and slightly flattened in its distal part.

Origin: The origin of this muscle is very much extensive and the fibres of this muscle originate on the cranial, lateral and medial surfaces of the shaft of the femur.

Insertion: The medial and lateral side of the base and the cranial surface of the patella.

Action: To extend the stifle joint

Blood supply: Lateral circumflex femoral artery.

Nerve supply: Femoral nerve

Articularis genu

The articularis genu is a very small muscle lying under cover of the distal part of the vastus intermedius. It has just a few fascicles which arise one above the other on the cranial surface of the shaft of femur.

Origin: Distal part of the cranial surface of the shaft of femur.

Insertion: The medial patellar ligament and the cartilage of the patella

Action: To tense the femoro-patellar capsule.

Blood supply: Lateral circumflex femoral artery.

Nerve supply: Femoral nerve.

Muscles of leg and pes

The muscles of this group cover the entire tibia except its medial surface which remains subcutaneous. These muscles are arranged in two groups, the craniolateral (dorsolateral) group and the caudal (plantar) group. The muscles of craniolateral group are extensors of the digits and flexors of the hock. The muscles of the caudal group are flexors of the digits and extensors of stifle.

Craniolateral group

Peroneus tertius

The peroneus tertius is a large, superficial muscle extending along the craniomedial (dorsomedial) aspect of the leg from the stifle joint to the tarsal joint. It originates in a common tendon with the common digital extensor and medial digital extensor muscles at the extensor fossa of the femur. The thick flat muscular belly of this muscle runs down in association with the other two muscles on the medial aspect of the cranial surface of the tibia till the middle of the leg, gets separated from them after a short course and forms a flat tendon at the distal third of the tibia. This tendon is perforated for the passage of tibialis anticus near the hock joint and then divides into two branches. The larger branch passes down and is inserted on the rough eminence at the craniomedial part of the proximal extremity of the large metatarsal bone. The smaller short branch passes down caudally and medially under the tendon of insertion of the tibialis anticus and is inserted to the medial surface of the second and third fused tarsal bone.

Origin: The extensor fossa situated between the trochlea and the lateral condyle at the distal extremity of the femur.

Insertion: The craniomedial aspect of the proximal extremity of large metatarsal bone and the medial surface of the second and third fused tarsal bone.

Action: To flex the hock joint

Blood supply: Cranial tibial artery.

Nerve supply: Deep peroneal nerve.

Common digital extensor

The common digital extensor is a large and long muscle with flattened and somewhat fusiform belly lying on the craniolateral aspect of the tibia. It extends from the extensor fossa situated between the trochlea and the lateral condyle of the femur, passes down the leg with other muscles of the group, separates from them by transforming in a strong tendon that passes vertically down the dorsolateral aspect of the tarsus and metatarsus, divides at the metatarso-phalangeal joint into two, the medial and lateral divisions that terminates on the third phalanx of the medial and lateral digits of the limb.

Origin: The extensor fossa of femur in common with the origin of medial digital extensor and peroneus tertius muscle.

Insertion: Extensor process of the third phalanx of both the digits of the limb.

Action: To extend the digits and flex the hock.

Blood supply: Cranial tibial artery

Nerve supply: Deep peroneal nerve.

Medial digital extensor

The medial digital extensor is a three sided muscle under cover of the common digital extensor and the peroneal muscles. It extends from the extensor fossa situated between the trochlea and the lateral condyle at the distal extremity of the femur in a common tendon of origin with the common digital extensor and peroneal tertius muscles, runs down with these muscles up to the middle of the leg, gets separated from them, becomes narrower and then forms a tendon. This tendon together with that of the common digital extensor passes down on the cranial (dorsal) capsular ligament of the tarsal joint. On reaching the proximal part of the metatarsal region it receives the tendon of insertion of extensor bravis. At the distal third of metatarsal bone it gates separated from the company of the common digital extensor and lies on the medial side of that muscle. It then passes down on the craniomedial (dorsomedial) aspect of the metatarso-phalangeal articulation, receives two branches from the suspensory ligament at about the middle of the first phalanx, passes down over the craniomedial (dorsomedial) aspect of the proximal interphalangeal articulation and finally inserts on the cranial (dorsal) aspect of the second phalanx and the lateral face of the third phalanx of the medial digit.

Origin: Extensor fossa of the femur in common with the common digital extensor and the peroneal muscles.

Insertion: Cranial (dorsal) surface of the second phalanx and lateral surface of third phalanx of the medial digit of the limb.

Action: To extend the metatarso-phalangeal and proximal interphalangeal articulations of the medial digit.

Blood supply: Cranial tibial artery

Nerve supply: Deep peroneal nerve.

The peroneus tertius, common digital extensor and medial digital extensor, these three muscles have a common tendon of origin, and in the proximal part of their bellies are closely attached to each other. The general appearance, constitution and the disposition of these muscles is also more or less similar. Because of these characters they are considered as one single muscle with three branches and is commonly termed as **complex muscle or complexus.**

Tibialis anticus (tibialis cranialis)

The tibialis anticus is the deepest of the extensor group of muscles of the leg and foot. It is a thin and triangular muscle situated on the craniolateral surface of the tibia. It has a very thin belly. The muscle arises by two heads. Both the heads originate on the proximal part of the lateral surface of tibia. The cranial head is larger and almost entirely muscular while the caudal head is smaller and it is mostly fleshy and partly fibrous. The two heads soon combine to form a thin flat belly. After a short course on the proximal part of cranial surface of tibia, the muscle tapers to a tendon near the middle of the shaft of the tibia, crosses its cranial surface obliquely from lateral to medial side passing through a ring formed by the tendon of peroneus tertius, descends the medial surface of the hock and finally inserts on the cranial border of the second and third fused tarsal bone and the medial aspect of the proximal extremity of the large metatarsal bone.

Origin: The cranial head originates from the tibial tuberosity, the cranial border of tibia and the proximal part of the shaft of tibia. The caudal head originates on the lateral condyle of tibia and the vestigial head of the fibula.

Insertion: The second and third fused tarsal bone and the medial aspect of proximal extremity of the large metatarsal bone.

Action: To flex the hock joint.

Blood supply: The cranial tibial artery.

Nerve supply: The deep peroneal nerve.

Peroneus longus

The peroneus longus is a long thin triangular muscle placed superficially on the lateral surface of the leg. It is situated cranial to the lateral digital extensor and caudal to the complex muscle. It arises in the form of a short, conical muscular body at the cranial aspect of the lateral tuberosity of the tibia. The muscular belly tapers to a long, thin, flat tendon of insertion at the distal half of the tibia. The tendon passes ventrally and caudally over the lateral surface of the hock, crosses over the tendon of the lateral digital extensor and under the lateral collateral ligament and terminates on the first tarsal bone and the proximal extremity of large metatarsal bone.

Origin: Lateral condyle of tibia, the fibrous cord representing the body of the fibula and the lateral collateral ligament of the femoro-tibial articulation.

Insertion: Caudal surface of first tarsal and the proximal extremity of large metatarsal bone.

Action: To rotate the hock joint medially.

Blood supply: Cranial tibial artery.

Nerve supply: Deep peroneal nerve.

Lateral digital extensor

The lateral digital extensor lies on the lateral aspect of the leg and is lodged between the muscles of extensor and flexor groups of muscles of leg. It is a thin long strip of muscle that extends from the lateral condyle of tibia and after reaching the middle of the tibia, it narrows into a tapering tendon that passes distally on the lateral surface of the tibia and then courses under the tendon of peroneus longus up to the lateral surface of the tarsus and gets adherent to the capsular ligament of this joint. From here, it passes down first along the craniolateral aspect of the meta tarsus and then along the craniolateral aspect of the lateral digit, receives two branches from the suspensory ligament at the level of the first phalanx, passes down the craniolateral aspect of the proximal interphalangeal articulation and terminates on the cranial face of the second phalanx and the lateral face of the third phalanx of the lateral digit of the limb.

Origin: The lateral tuberosity of tibia, lateral, lateral surface of the rudimentary fibula and lateral collateral ligament of femoro-tibial articulation.

Insertion: The cranial face of the second phalanx and lateral face of third phalanx of the lateral digit.

Action: To extend the lateral digit.

Blood supply: Cranial tibial artery

Nerve supply: Deep peroneal nerve.

Extensor brevis (Extensor digitorum brevis)

The extensor bravis is a very small, thin and flat muscle located on the dorsal surface of the tarsus. The muscle originates in the form of a short flat tendon arising at a groove formed between the cranial and ventral surface of the tibial tarsal bone, transforms into a thin flat fusiform muscular belly on the cranial surface of the tarsus, passes down along the medial part of the cranial surface of the proximal third of the shaft of large metatarsal bone, and terminates somewhere in the middle of the metatarsal bone. It is superficially covered by the skin, fascia and the tendons of common and medial digital extensor muscles and on its deeper surface are the tarsals and the metatarsal bone. Laterally it is covered by the tendon of lateral digital extensor muscle.

Origin: Dorsal surface of the tibial tarsal proximal to the trochlear surface.

Insertion: On the tendon of insertion of the common digital extensor muscle at the middle of the large metatarsal bone.

Action: To assist the common digital extensor muscle in extending the digits.

Blood supply: Dorsal metatarsal artery

Nerve supply: Deep peroneal nerve,

Plantar group

Gastrocnemius

The gastrocnemius is a large, fleshy muscle with two heads of origin and also two separate bellies in its proximal half. Both the bellies are flattened, wider in the middle and narrow at the extremities. Together they form the major portion of the caudal aspect of the leg. The medial and lateral head of origin arises from the respective supracondyloid crest at the distal extremity of the femur. The two heads descend over the plantar aspect of the stifle joint separately wide apart, gain the plantar surface of the tibia runs down this part of the leg and fuse with each other at about its middle. The single mass of this muscle thus formed receives the insertion of soleus muscle at its craniolateral face, runs for a short distance and forms a strong round cord as the tendon of insertion of this muscle at about the distal third of the tibia. This tendon first lies caudal to the tendon of superficial digital flexor, gets twisted with the later and then becomes cranial to it. As they pass down, the two tendons rest over the tuber calcis of the fibular tarsal of the tarsal or hock joint. The tendon of gastrocnemius muscle inserts over the tuber calcis while the tendon of superficial digital flexor continues down to the digits.

Origin: The medial head of origin arises from the medial supracondyloid crest and the lateral head from the lateral supracondyloid crest at the distal extremity of the femur.

Insertion: Tuber calcis of the fibular tarsal of the hock.

Action: To extend the hock.

Blood supply: Femoral, caudal femoral and popliteal arteries.

Nerve supply: Tibial nerve.

Soleus

The soleus is a long, thin, ribbon like strip of muscle lying immediately under the deep fascia of the leg and between the fascia and the deep digital flexor muscle.

It extends from the head of the fibula to the middle of the leg. The muscle originates on the lateral surface of the head of the fibula, passes down the lateral aspect of the plantar surface of the proximal third of the tibia lying between the skin and fascia laterally and the deep digital flexor and lateral digital extensor muscle medially and terminates into the combine mass of the belly of the gastrocnemius muscle at about the middle of the tibia. It joins the tendons of gastrocnemius, biceps femoris, semitendinosus and the superficial digital flexor muscles in constituting the common calcaneal tendon or the hamstring tendon. But the tendon of the gastrocnemius and soleus muscles only is called the calcaneal tendon or the tendon of achille.

Origin: The lateral tuberosity of tibia and the head of the fibula.

Insertion: Gastrocnemius muscle near the middle of the leg.

Action: To assist the gastrocnemius in extending a hock.

Blood supply: Popliteal artery.

Nerve supply: Internal popliteal nerve

Popliteal

The popliteal is a fleshy, thick and triangular muscle extending from the lateral condyle at the distal extremity of femur to about the distal third of caudal surface of the tibia. The muscle originates in the form of a short and strong tendon at the lower depression on the lateral surface of the lateral condyle of the femur under cover of the lateral collateral ligament of the femoro-tibial articulation. The tendon is followed by a thick triangular fleshy belly which courses in a medial and distal direction to insert on the plantar surface of tibia.

Origin: The lower of the two depressions on the lateral condyle of the femur.

Insertion: The triangular area on the proximal half the caudal surface of the tibia and its medial border.

Action: To flex the femoro-tibial articulation and rotate the tibia slightly outwards.

Blood supply: Popliteal and the cranial and caudal tibial arteries.

Nerve supply: The tibial nerve.

Superficial digital flexor

The superficial digital flexor is a well developed fleshy muscle that lies between the two heads of the gastrocnemius muscle extending from the distal part of femur to the middle of the digits. The muscle originates as a short but strong tendon at the supracondyloid fossa of the distal extremity of femur. After a short course over the stifle joint, the tendon transforms into a fleshy belly that descends on the caudal surface of the femoro-tibial articulation and then between the two heads of the gastrocnemius muscle. Running in this position up to the middle of the leg, it tapers to a strong round tendon which initially lies in front of the tendon of the gastrocnemius but at the distal third of the leg winds round the tendon of that muscle, lies on its medial face for a short distance and thereafter on its caudal face. The two tendons together in that position run down towards the tuber calcis, the tendon of the gastrocnemius terminates on the tuber calcis and the tendon of superficial digital flexor passes down through the groove on the summit of the tuber calcis with the synovial bursa lying below it. It then runs down the metatarsal region in company with and caudal to the tendon of deep digital flexor. A little above the proximal sesamoid, the tendon of superficial digital flexor divides into two parts the medial and lateral. Each part meets with the corresponding slip from the caudal division of suspensory ligament and forms the ring at the level of the metatarso-phalangeal articulation for the passage of the corresponding division of the tendon of deep digital flexor muscle. Both the branches then pass down under the annular ligaments of the corresponding side and are inserted by three slips each to the tubercles on the caudal aspect of the middle phalanx of the respective digits, medial and lateral.

Origin: The supracondyloid fossa of the femur.

Insertion: Plantar surface of the middle phalanges of the medial and lateral digits of the limb and partly to the tuber calcis of the fibular tarsal of the hock joint.

Action: To flex the digits and to extend the hock.

Blood supply: Medial plantar, caudal femoral and caudal tibial arteries.

Nerve supply: Tibial nerve.

Deep digital flexor

The deep digital flexor is a complex muscle with three divisions lying on the caudal surface of the tibia. The three divisions are the superficial, deep and the medial. The muscle has a tendinous origin. The tendons of the **superficial and medial divisions** originate on the lateral tuberosity of the tibia and the lateral surface of the head of the fibula. The tendon of the **deep division** arises from the small short fibrous cord that represents the shaft of the fibula and the caudal surface of the tibia except the triangular area for attachment of popliteal muscle. The muscular bellies of all the three divisions run down the caudal surface of tibia and narrows into separate tendons. The tendons of superficial and deep divisions combine and form a common tendon. The later passes through the plantar tarsal sheath and continues down the plantar surface of the metatarsus.

The tendon of **medial division** of this muscle originates in common with the tendon of superficial division on the lateral tuberosity of the tibia, transforms into the fusiform, fleshy muscular belly which occupies the space between the superficial division of this muscle and the popliteus muscle on the caudal surface of the tibia and tapers to the narrow flat tendon at the level of the distal third of the tibia. This tendon then passes over the tarsus, runs down the caudal surface of metatarsus and joins the common tendon of first two divisions at the middle of the metatarsus. The combined tendon of the three divisions of this muscle thus formed divides into the medial and lateral branches which pass through the rings of the corresponding side formed by the superficial digital flexor with the branches of the suspensory ligament, and terminate on the flexor (plantar) surface of the distal phalanx.

Origin: The tendons of superficial and medial divisions originate on the lateral tuberosity of the tibia and the lateral surface of the head of the fibula. The tendon of the deep division originates over the fibrous cord ventral to the head of the rudimentary fibula.

Insertion: Plantar side of the distal phalanx of the medial and lateral digits of the limb.

Action: To flex the metatarso-phalangeal and the proximal and distal interphalangeal articulations of the medial and lateral digits and to extend the hock joint.

Blood supply: The cranial and caudal tibial and the popliteal artery.

Nerve supply: The tibial nerve.

The medial division of the deep digital flexor muscle is considered as a separate muscle and is named as long head of deep digital flexor muscle or long digital flexor muscle by some authors.

97

Comparative Anatomy of Muscles of Hind Limb

Horse

The **tensor fasciae latae** is less extensive.

The **superficial gluteus** exists separately. It is 'V' shaped. It originates from the lateral angle of ilium (tuber coxae) and gluteal fascia and is inserted to the third trochanter. The **middle gluteus** is the largest of the three gluteal muscles and is very extensive. It originates from the aponeurosis of the longissimus dorsi, extends as far forwards up to first lumbar vertebra and is inserted in three heads, to the trochanter major, the crest ventral to trochanter major and the trochanteric ridge. The **deep gluteus** is smaller than the middle gluteus and is inserted to the convexity of the trochanter major.

The **biceps femoris** has an additional insertion to the femur on the rough surface near the trochanter tertius.

The **semitendinosus** arises from the transverse processes of the first two or three coccygeal vertebrae. The semimembranosus is larger and arises from the sacrosciatic ligament also.

The **sartorius** does not arise from the shaft of the ilium.

The **gracilis** is not so extensively fused to its fellow at the origin.

The **obturator internus** has an iliac part- the pisiformis. Its tendon passes through the lesser sciatic foramen and hence does not unite with that of the obturator externus.

Articularis genu is absent

An additional muscle named as **capsularis** occurs in horse but is absent in ox. It arises from ilium above the outer tendon of origin of the rectus femoris. Its tendon of insertion is very narrow, passes between vastus externus and intermedius and is attached to the proximal two thirds of the cranial surface of the shaft of femur. Some of these fibres are attached to the joint capsule. Its action is to raise the joint capsule during the flexion of the hip joint.

The **common digital extensor** arises in common with peroneus tertius. Its tendon receives below the hock on its lateral aspect the tendon of extensor bravis and lateral digital extensor.

The **medial digital extensor** is absent. The lateral digital extensor joins the tendon of common digital extensor in the proximal third of the metatarsal region for insertion into the digit.

The **peroneus longus** is absent and the superficial digital flexor is thinner and less developed.

Dog

The **superficial gluteus** is separate and overlies the middle gluteus caudally. It is inserted by aponeurosis on the rough line in the proximal third of the shaft of femur. The **middle gluteus** has no lumbar part for its origin and it inserts on the trochanter major of femur.

The **biceps femoris** arises on tuber ischii and inserts on patella and tarsus. The **semitendinosus** arises on tuber ischii and inserts on tibial fascia on its medial aspect. The **semimembranosus** is clearly divisible into two parts. The cranial part ends under the attachment of the pectineus. The caudal part is attached to the caudal border of adductor and terminates on the medial condyle of the femur.

The **gracilis** is thinner and narrower. The adductor has two parts, the major and minor and both are inserted on the rough line on the medial aspect of the shaft of femur.

The **tibialis anticus** is larger and it covers the lateral surface of **common digital extensor** at its proximal extremity.

The **soleus** is absent.

Sheep and Goat

The muscles of the hind limb (pelvic limb) of sheep and goat are almost similar to those of ox. There are no distinct differences in the gross origin, disposition and insertion of the muscles of hind limb of sheep and goat and those of ox.

Pig

The **tensor fascia latae** is broad and its fleshy part reaches almost to the patella.

The **superficial gluteus** is separate muscle and has sacral head of origin and it blends with the biceps femoris. The **middle gluteus** has a small lumbar part which dose not extend far cranially in the lumbar region. The **deep gluteus** is extensive and reaches to the tuber coxae for attachment.

The **biceps femoris** has a narrow origin from the broad sacrosciatic ligament and the tuber ischii. The semitendinosus has two heads of origin resembling those in horse.

The **Sartoriu**s originates with two heads of origin. The middle head originates from the tendon of psoas minor and the lateral head from iliac fascia.

The **pectineus** is well developed and is flattened from cranial to caudal ends. The **adductor** is partly fused with the gracilis. It terminates on the femur just dorsal to the origin of gastrocnemius.

The **obturator externus** is similar to that of horse. The obturator internus is extensive.

The **gemellus** is partly fused with obturator internal.

The division of the four parts of **quadriceps femoris** is quite distinct. There is no capsularis muscle.

The **peroneus tertius** is continued distally up to the distal end of leg by a strong tendon which joins the tendons of common digital extensor and tibialis anticus and ends on first and second tarsal and third metatarsal bones. The tendon of tibialis anticus ends on the second tarsal and proximal end of second metatarsal bone. The tendon of the common digital extensor divides into medial and lateral branches. The medial branch ends on the middle and distal phalanges of the medial (chief) digit and the lateral branch ends on the middle and distal phalanges of the lateral (chief) digit.

The **lateral digital extensor** muscle arises from the proximal end (head) of the fibula and its tendon of insertion ends on the lateral (accessory) digit. The tendon of long digital extensor terminates on the medial (accessory) digit.

The **tendon of superficial digital flexor** after reaching the distal part of the plantar surface of the hock divides into medial and lateral branches which terminate on the extensor process of the distal phalanx of the medial and lateral chief digits. From the plantar surface of these parts extend slips to the fascia on the respective accessory digits.

The **deep digital flexor** muscle has three heads of origin and three bellies. The tendons of insertion of the three divisions pass through the tarsal canal on the plantar surface of the tarsus and join each other forming a common tendon which finally end like that of the forelimb.

Fowl

The **biceps femoris** (iliofibularis) is somewhat triangular. It originates on the post acetabular iliac crest and inserts by a strong rounded tendon on proximal end of the shaft of fibula.

The **sartorius** forms the craniolateral border of the thigh. It originates on the preacetabular iliac crest, caudal thoracic vertebrae and the medial dorsal ridge of the synsacrum. It inserts on medial surface of patella and contributes to the formation of medial patellar ligament.

The **semitendinosus** originates on the post acetabular iliac crest and the transverse processes of one or two free coccygeal vertebrae. It inserts by a tendon on the medial surface of proximal end of tibia.

The **semimembranosus** is thin and flat. It originates from the lateral and ventrolateral surface of the ischium and inserts on the medial aspect of the proximal extremity of tibiotarsus.

The **pectineus** (ambiens) originates on the pectineal process of ilium and terminates by thin flat tendons on the flexor surface of second, third and fourth digits.

The **adductor** consists of two parts with two tendons of origin and their muscular bellies but have a common tendon of insertion. The bellies of the two parts lie close to each other. The lateral division of the muscle originates on ventrolateral surface of ischium and the medial division originates just ventral to the origin of lateral division on the ventral surface of the ischium. The insertion of both the divisions is common on the caudal surface of femur.

The **quadriceps femoris** in birds has three divisions instead of four divisions of mammals and is named as femorotibialis muscle.

The **gastrocnemius** has three divisions with three separate origins, two from the the femur and one from the tibia.

The **flexors of the digits** grouped into three morphological units based on their level of insertion. These are named as superficial, intermediate and deep flexors for the second, third and fourth digits. The **extensors** are short muscles.

SECTION-B

BLOOD VESSELS AND LYMPHATICS

98

Arteries of Hind Limb

The main arterial trunk that supplies blood to the hind limb is the **external iliac artery.** As this trunk passes down through different segments (regions) of the limb it is differently named according to that segment or the region. In the abdomen it is named as iliac, in the thigh region as femoral, in the leg region as tibial and popliteal and down that the metatarsal artery and lastly the digital.

External iliac artery

The external iliac artery arises from the abdominal aorta ventral to the fifth or sixth lumbar vertebra. It descends at the side of the pelvic inlet ventrally and caudally along the tendon of psoas minor, crosses the tendon, reaches the cranial border of the pubis, gains the space between the sartorius and pectineus muscles and then continues in the thigh (femoral region) as the femoral artery. In this course it is covered by peritoneum and is related laterally to the psoas minor, sartorius and iliacus muscles, medially to the common iliac vein and caudally to the external iliac vein. The following are the collateral branches of the external iliac artery.

1. The **deep circumflex iliac artery** arises from the external iliac artery close to its origin from the aorta, passes laterally towards the external angle of the ilium (tuber coxae) supplying branches to the psoas major and iliacus muscles and iliac lymph node and divides into two, the cranial and caudal branches. The **cranial branch** passes ventrad and craniad on the transversus abdominis and then under the obliquus abdominis internus muscle, perforates this muscle and gets under the obliquus abdominis externus muscle and finally reaches the skin of the flank region. It supplies all the muscles in its contact in this course. The **caudal branch** supplies small branches to the iliacus and psoas muscles, penetrates the abdominal wall and descends on the deep face of the tensor fasciae latae, gives out several branches to these muscles and terminates in the skin of the thigh region.

2. The **prepubic artery** usually arises in a common trunk with the deep femoral artery from the external iliac artery, passes cranially, crosses the border of the inguinal ligament, reaches the internal inguinal ring and divides into two, the caudal abdominal (caudal epigastric) and external pudic (external pudendal) arteries. The **caudal abdominal (caudal epigastric) artery** crosses the spermatic cord, passes between the obliquus abdominis internus and rectus abdominis muscles, gives branches to these muscles and anastomoses with the branches of cranial abdominal (cranial epigastric) artery. The **external pudic (external pudendal) artery** leaves the abdominal cavity through the internal (deep) inguinal ring and then through the external (superficial) inguinal ring, supplies the scrotum, prepuce and vaginal tunic and finally divides into the subcutaneous abdominal and the cranial dorsal artery of the penis in male and cranial mammary artery in female. The **subcutaneous abdominal artery** passes cranially on the tunica abdominalis and supplies branches to scrotum, superficial inguinal lymph node and the skin. The **cranial dorsal artery of penis** also supplies branches to the scrotum, gains the dorsum penis and divides into cranial and caudal branches. The caudal branches pass caudally over the dorsum penis and anastomose with the branches of the caudal artery of penis. The cranial branch runs cranially over the dorsum penis and terminates as **arteria glandis.** In female, this artery passes through the inguinal canal and divides into the cranial subcutaneous abdominal and the **caudal mammary artery** to supply the mammary gland.

3. The **deep femoral artery** usually arises in a common trunk with the prepubic artery. It passes under the inguinal ligament between the iliacus and pectineus muscles. It then runs ventrally and caudally between the pectineus and obturator externus and then between the biceps femoris and semimembranosus and finally divides into two sets of vessels that supply the biceps femoris and semitendinosus muscles. In this course the deep femoral artery supplies branches to pectineus, gracilis, obturator externus and internus, adductor, semimembranosus, semitendinosus, quadratus femoris, biceps femoris muscles and the hip joint.

4. The **cremasteric artery** or the **artery of the cord** is most variable in origin. It may originate directly from the aorta or the external or internal iliac or from the caudal epigastric artery. What ever the origin may be, it passes through the inguinal canal with the spermatic vessels and the cremaster externus muscle and supplies branches to this muscle, tunica vaginalis and the other structures of the cord. In the female, this artery is represented by the cranial uterine artery which anastomoses with the middle uterine artery.

Femoral artery

The femoral artery is the main arterial trunk in the thigh region of the hind limb. It begins as a distal continuation of the external iliac artery at the level of the cranial border of the pubis, passes caudoventrally in the femoral triangle formed by the iliopsoas, sartorius and pectineus muscles, descends in the femoral canal in company with the femoral vein and saphenous nerve, passes underneath the distal part of the gracilis over the vastus internus below the insertion of the adductor and then passes obliquely ventrad and laterad in the oblique vascular groove and finally deeps between the two heads of the gastrocnemius at the distal extremity of femur to continue as popliteal artery. The collateral branches of femoral artery are as below.

1. The **cranial femoral artery** or the lateral circumflex femoral artery arises from the cranial face of the femoral artery in its initial course. It passes down cranially and laterally to the termination of the iliopsoas muscle under the sartorius, gains the company of the femoral nerve, reaches the space between the rectus femoris and vastus internus and divides into branches to supply the four heads of the quadriceps femoris muscle and the articularis genu.

2. The **saphenous artery** is the most extensive branch of the femoral artery. It arises from the femoral artery at about the middle of its course through the femoral canal. It becomes superficial by emerging between the distal parts of the sartorius and gracilis, passes down in company with the saphenous vein and saphenous nerve on the medial surface of the leg. Here it becomes subcutaneous and furnishes small branches to the skin, fascia and muscles in this region. Hereafter, it gradually passes caudad and on reaching the distal third of the leg it lies cranial to the hamstring tendon or the Achille's tendon of the hock. It then continues distally along the medioplantar aspect of the tarsus (hock) and divides into medial and lateral tarsal arteries. In this course it supplies branches to the sartorius, and gracilis muscles, the tendons of gastrocnemius and superficial digital flexor muscles and the fascia and skin around the leg and hock region.

- The **lateral tarsal artery** is smaller of the two terminal branches of saphenous. It passes caudally under cover of the lateral plantar vein, crosses the lateral face of the tibial nerve, gives out branches to the gastrocnemius muscle and the skin on lateral aspect of the hock and finally contributes to the formation of the rete tarsi dorsale or the superficial and deep plantar arch.

- The **medial tarsal artery** passes down in company with the tibial nerve along the tendon of deep digital flexor muscle and divides into medial and lateral plantar arteries.

i. The **medial plantar artery** is larger and it passes down through the tarsal sheath, gives out the articular branch to the tarsus and a cutaneous branch to the skin of the tarsus and reaches the metatarsal region. On reaching the caudal surface of the proximal extremity of thc metatarsus it passes down between the metatarsal bone and the suspensory ligament. Here it gives off a branch to the **proximal plantar arch** and then continues down first along the medial border of the suspensory ligament and later along the tendon of deep digital flexor muscle as the **caudomedial superficial metatarsal artery**. The later artery, in the distal third of the metatarsal region, furnishes a branch to the **distal plantar arch** and some other branches to the tendons and skin in this region and is continued down as **plantar medial digital artery**.

ii. The **lateral plantar artery** is smaller and it passes down over the tarsal sheath, courses on the lateral side of the caudal surface of the metatarsal region similar to that of the medial plantar artery, contributes branches to the **proximal and distal plantar arch** and the tendons and skin of this region and finally continues as the **plantar lateral digital artery**.

3. The **caudal femoral artery** is a large and the last branch of the femoral artery before its continuation as popliteal artery at the level of lower distal extremity of the femur. It arises from the caudal face of the femoral artery and following a short course it divides into ascending and descending branches. The ascending branch ascends between the semimembranosus and biceps femoris and supplies these muscles. The descending branch accompanies the lateral head of gastrocnemius and supplies this muscle.

Popliteal artery

The popliteal artery is the direct continuation of the femoral beyond the origin of the caudal femoral artery. It first passes down through the two heads of the gastrocnemius muscle and reaches the plantar surface of the tarsal sheath, gives out a branch to the tarsus, passes down through the popliteal region under cover of the popliteus muscle and at a variable level in this region divides into the cranial and caudal tibial arteries.

The **caudal tibial artery** is smaller than the cranial tibial and it passes down on the caudal (plantar) surface of the popliteus muscle and furnishes branches to the popliteus and the deep digital flexor muscle.

The **cranial tibial artery** is the larger of the two terminal branches and is considered as the distal continuation of the popliteal artery. It passes obliquely ventrad and laterad under the popliteus and deep digital flexor muscles, crosses the proximal part of the lateral border of tibia, passes through the tibiofibular arch and then passes successively under the origins of the lateral digital extensor and peroneus longus lying between these muscles and the bone and finally reaches the lateral face of the tibia. Here onward it passes almost in a vertical direction for a short course and then gradually inclines to the dorsal (cranial) surface of tibia. It then runs down along the lateral border of the tibialis anticus and between this muscle and the bone in company with the deep peroneal (fibular) nerve and the vein. After reaching the dorsal (cranial) face of the tibia, the cranial tibial artery passes over the dorsal ligament of the tarsus and divides into the perforating tarsal artery and the dorsal metatarsal artery.

The **perforating tarsal artery** passes caudad through the vascular canal in the tarsal bones, reaches the plantar (caudal) surface of the large metatarsal bone and unites with the branches of the medial and lateral plantar arteries to form the **proximal plantar arch** between the bone and the suspensory ligament in the proximal third of the large metatarsal bone. From the distal face of this arch, a small **middle deep plantar metatarsal artery** descends through the caudal groove of the bone to the **distal plantar arch** which is formed by the union of the branches from the medial and lateral plantar arteries. From the distal face of the distal plantar arch arises the **plantar common digital artery** which enters the inter-digital space and divides into two branches that join the similar branches of the dorsal common digital artery and supply the corresponding, medial and lateral digits of the limb.

The **dorsal metatarsal artery**, although a terminal branch, is considered as the continuation of the cranial tibial artery. It gives out a small branch to the extensor bravis and descends in the cranial longitudinal groove of the metatarsus in company with the peroneal vein and nerve. During this course, in the lower third of the metatarsal bone it detaches a branch called the perforating metatarsal artery that passes caudally through the vascular canal and joins the **distal plantar arch** in the caudal third of the plantar surface of the metatarsal bone. Hereafter, the dorsal metatarsal artery continues down as the **dorsal common digital artery** which enters the inter-digital space and divides into two branches. These branches join the similar branches of the plantar common digital artery to form the two proper digital arteries, one for each digit.

99

Veins of Hind Limb

The venous drainage of hind limb begins from two digital venous plexuses, one for each digit, situated in the corium of the foot. From each of these plexuses extend three digital veins namely the dorsal common digital vein, the medial digital vein and the lateral digital vein. The digital veins in their upward course converge and form the metatarsal veins which in their turn continue upward in the leg region as tibial and popliteal veins and then in the thigh region as femoral vein which finally joins the external iliac vein as the chief vein of the hind limb.

Digital veins

The **dorsal common digital vein** arises from the corresponding digital plexus in the form of proper digital vein.The two proper digital veins ascend along the medial face of the corresponding digit and unite at about the middle of the interdigital space below the metatarso-phalangeal articulation (fetlock joint) and form the dorsal common digital vein. The later, thus formed, ascends through the interdigital space, crosses vertically the metatarso-phalangeal articulation and after reaching the distal extremity of the metatarsal bone continues upward as dorsal metatarsal vein.

The **medial digital vein** after arising from the digital venous plexus ascends along the caudomedial aspect of the medial digit in company with the satellite artery, shares a branch each from the dorsal common digital and lateral digital veins, ascends the medial face of the fetlock joint and is then continued up as the medial plantar metatarsal vein.

The **lateral digital vein** after arising from the digital venous plexus of the lateral digit passes upward in the interdigital space, communicates a branch to the dorsal common digital and medial digital veins and then ascends the lateral face of the fetlock joint and then is continued up as the lateral plantar metatarsal vein.

Metatarsal veins

The **dorsal superficial metatarsal vein** is the ascending continuation of the dorsal common digital vein. It passes up on the dorsal aspect of the distal extremity of the large metatarsus, inclines laterad in the distal third of the metatarsal bone, receives a branch from the caudolateral metatarsal vein and then continues upward along the dorsolateral aspect of the metatarsus. In its further upward course it reaches the dorsolateral aspect of the tarsus, communicates with the cranial tibial vein and divides into cranial and caudal branches at the distal third of the tibia.

The **dorsal deep metatarsal veins** are usually two, the medial and lateral. These arise from the dorsal common digital vein, pass up first in the interdigital space, then in the cleft of the large metatarsal bone and then ascend through the dorsal (cranial) vertical groove of this bone, the two veins lying one each on either side of the dorsal metatarsal artery. In their course through the vertical groove, the medial and lateral arteries communicate with each other by communicating branches. In addition, each of these sends a perforating metatarsal vein to pass through the vascular canal at the distal third of the metatarsus to communicate with the distal deep plantar venous arch. In their further ascending course, the two veins reach the dorsal aspect of the tarsus, receives a branch called the perforating tarsal vein from the proximal deep plantar venous arch and then continue upward in the leg region as cranial tibial veins.

The **medial plantar vein** or the caudomedial metatarsal vein is the upward continuation of the medial digital vein. It passes upward along the medial aspect of the plantar surface of the metatarsus, contributes through a small branch in the formation of the distal superficial plantar venous arch in association with the lateral plantar vein, furnishes another small branch that unites with the perforating metatarsal vein and the similar branch from the lateral plantar vein to form the distal deep plantar venous arch in the distal third of the metatarsal bone. It then continues upward between the medial border of the suspensory ligament and the plantar surface of the large metatarsal bone and after reaching the proximal third of the metatarsus it releases a branch that unites with the similar branch from the lateral plantar vein to form the proximal deep plantar venous arch. Here after, the medial plantar vein continues its upward course along the caudo medial aspect of the tarsus and then that of the leg as the medial saphenous vein.

The lateral plantar metatarsal vein is the upward continuation of the lateral digital vein. After its beginning from the later vein at the distal extremity of the metatarsal bone it releases two branches, the medial and the lateral. The medial branch passes between the two divisions of the suspensory ligament and unites with the similar branch from the medial plantar metatarsal vein to form the distal superficial plantar venous arch. The lateral branch passes proximally laterad and dorsad and joins the dorsal superficial metatarsal vein. It gives another branch immediately above the medial branch. This one passes upward between the suspensory ligament and the bone and join the similar branch from the medial plantar vein and the perforating metatarsal vein to form the distal deep plantar venous arch in the distal third of the metatarsal bone. From here, the lateral plantar artery continues upward and after reaching the proximal third of the metatarsus contributes a branch for the formation of proximal deep plantar venous arch. Here after, the lateral plantar vein continues its upward course along the caudo lateral aspect of the tarsus and then that of the leg as the lateral saphenous vein.

Veins of tibial (leg) region

The **medial saphenous vein** is the upward continuation of the medial plantar (metatarsal) vein. Usually in its initial course this vein is subcutaneously placed and has two roots of origin. The cranial root is the upward continuation of the dorsal superficial metatarsal vein and the caudal root is that of the medial plantar metatarsal vein. The two roots unite after a short course along the craniomedial aspect of the hock and the venous trunk formed by their union ascends obliquely upward and backward in company of the lateral saphenous nerve, passes first between the semitendinosus and biceps femoris and then between the biceps femoris and outer head of the gastrocnemius and terminates by merging into the popliteus muscle.

The **lateral saphenous vein** begins as the upward continuation of the lateral plantar vein on the caudolateral aspect of the distal end of leg, From here it ascends along deep fascia on the medial face of the leg in company with the saphenous artery and nerve, passes for a short distance on the lower part of the gracilis lying between this muscle and the sartorius and finally merges with the femoral vein.

The **cranial tibial veins** are two, the **medial and lateral**. These are the upward continuation of the medial and lateral deep metatarsal veins in the region of the tarsus. They ascend vertically in the leg region lying on either side of the cranial tibial artery, receives a branch from the cranial superficial metatarsal vein in the distal third of the leg, gradually inclines caudolateral and then passes up along the lateral border of the tibialis anticus or between this muscle and the tibia. After reaching the proximal third of the leg, these veins pass upwards under the peroneus longus and the lateral digital extensor muscles, cross the proximal part of the lateral border of the tibial bone and then join each other forming a single trunk. The single trunk of the cranial tibial vein thus formed passes dorsally under the deep digital flexor and popliteus muscles and joins the caudal tibial vein on the caudal aspect of the femoro-tibial articulation to form the **popliteal vein.**

The **caudal tibial vein** is formed by the union of several thin radicles of veins emerging from the deep digital flexor muscle. It ascends the caudal surface of the deep digital flexor muscle, passes between this muscle and the superficial digital flexor, receives a branch from the long head of deep digital flexor and the popliteus muscles while passing between these muscles and joins the cranial tibial vein to form the **popliteal vein.**

Popliteal vein

The popliteal vein is the satellite of the popliteal artery. It is formed by the union of the cranial and caudal tibial veins on the caudal surface of the femoro-tibial articulation. In its short upward course over the caudal surface of this joint it receives a branch from the joint, deeps between the two heads of the gastrocnemius muscle and continues further upward as femoral vein.

Femoral vein

The femoral vein is the satellite of the femoral artery and follows the same course as that of the artery passing through the femoral canal in the thigh region lying parallel to the artery but in ascending manner. In this course it receives several branches which are satellites of the arterial branches of the femoral artery. Of these, the major branches are the cranial femoral and the lateral saphenous veins. On reaching the cranial border of the pubis, it joins the external iliac artery just in front of the pubis.

External iliac vein

The external iliac vein is the upward continuation of the femoral vein. It begins at the cranial border of the pubis lying parallel to the satellite artery in the space between the sartorius and pectineus muscles. It runs obliquely craniad and dorsad in company with the satellite artery, crosses the tendon of insertion of the psoas minor and unites with the internal iliac vein forming the common iliac vein ventral to the fifth or sixth lumbar vertebra at the level of the sacroiliac articulation. During its course, the external iliac artery receives many branches from the muscles and other structures on its way. Of these, the major branches include the deep femoral vein, prepubic vein, external pudic vein, caudal abdominal and subcutaneous abdominal veins and the perineal vein. Most of these are the satellites of the arteries and they follow the same course as that of the arteries.

100

Lymphatics of Hind Limb

The lymphatics of hind limb is comprised of four lymph nodes namely the deep inguinal, epigastric, coxal and popliteal lymph nodes and the afferents and efferent ducts joining and leaving these lymph nodes.

Deep inguinal lymph node

The deep inguinal lymph node is located in the region of deep femoral artery near the origin of the caudal epigastric and the pudic branches from it. The lymph node receives afferents from the muscles in the prepubic and the thigh regions. The efferent vessel from this lymph node joins and opens in the medial iliac lymph node.

Epigastric lymph node

The epigastric lymph node is inconstant. When present, it is located on the course of the caudal epigastric artery near the pubis on the medial surface of the rectus abdominis muscle. The afferents for this lymph node are received from the abdominal muscles and the peritoneum in the vicinity. The efferent vessel of this lymph node joins the medial iliac lymph node.

Coxal lymph node

The coxal lymph node is also inconsistent and exists only in a few subjects. When present, it is situated in front of the rectus femoris and between this muscle and the tensor fasciae latae. It receives afferents from the quadriceps femoris and tensor fasciae latae muscles and the prefemoral lymph node. The efferent from this lymph node goes to internal iliac or deep inguinal lymph node.

Popliteal lymph node

The popliteal lymph node is a large and main lymph node of the hind limb. It is situated deeply embedded in the fat on the gastrocnemius muscle between the biceps femoris and semimembranosus muscle. The afferent vessels of this lymph node come from the skin of the lateral and caudal portions of the leg, the biceps femoris, semitendinosus and the semimembranosus muscles and from all the tendons, muscles and joints distal to the location of this lymph node in the limb. The efferent vessels from this lymph node join usually the deep inguinal lymph node but some of them may join the internal iliac or ischiatic lymph node.

101

Comparative Anatomy of Blood Vessels and Lymphatics of Hind Limb

Horse

The **arteries** of the hind limb of horse have in general similar architecture as that of ox except the special features mentioned below.

The **deep circumflex iliac artery** which is a branch of the external iliac artery in ox has a variable origin in horse. It may originate directly from the aorta or the common iliac trunk just prior to the origin of the external iliac artery. The **prepubic and deep femoral arteries** arise either by a common trunk or separately from the femoral artery. The **obturator artery** is a well developed independent branch of the femoral artery in horse as against its origin as a branch of deep femoral artery in ox. The **saphenous artery** is a small branch of femoral artery and it supplies the skin on the medial aspect of the thigh and leg. The **popliteal artery** terminates by its division into **cranial and caudal tibial arteries** at a lower level in horse than that in ox. The **caudal tibial artery** is larger and longer in horse than that in ox. From the proximal plantar arch extend four caudal metatarsal arteries instead of four, two of them are superficial and the other two deep branches. The **large metatarsal artery** descends along the groove between the large and lateral small metatarsal bone and divides just above the fetlock into lateral and medial digital arteries. Each **digital artery** divides at the middle of the wing of the third phalanx into preplantar and plantar digital arteries. The **preplantar digital arteries** supply the sensitive laminae of the sole. The plantar digital arteries of the opposite sides form anastomosis. Small laminar branches from the anastomosis form the **circumflex artery of the toe** which supplies branches to the sole.

The **veins of the hind limb** are mostly the satellites of the arteries. The **digital veins** of the hind limb are similar to those of the fore limb in respect of their number, origin, course and distribution with the following special features. The two, **medial and lateral digital veins** unite to form the **sesamoidean arch** between the tendon of deep digital flexor muscle and the suspensory ligament just above the fetlock joint. Three **metatarsal veins**, the medial, lateral and deep, extend upward from the sesamoidean venous arch. These veins ascends the metatarsal and then the tarsal region and after reaching the fetlock joint the **medial metatarsal vein** forms the cranial root of the medial saphenous vein and the **lateral metatarsal vein** forms the caudal root of the medial saphenous vein. The **middle metatarsal vein** passes through the tarsal vascular canal as perforating tarsal vein and forms the largest root of the cranial tibial vein. In the leg region, the cranial and caudal roots merge and form the **medial saphenous vein** which passes up between the gracilis and sartorius muscles and join the **femoral vein**. The **external saphenous** vein, after arising at the lateral aspect of the fibular tarsal on the hock joint, ascends the leg passing along the lateral head of gastrocnemius muscle join the **popliteal vein**. The **cranial and caudal tibial, popliteal, femoral and the external iliac veins** have no distinctive differential features.

The **lymphatics** in the hind limb of horse are similar to those in ox except that the **popliteal** and **deep inguinal lymph nodes** are in a mass of three or four elongated small glands. The epigastric and the coxal lymph nodes are, however, totally absent in horse.

Dog

The arteries of the hind limb of dog have significant differences. The **external iliac artery** does not give out any collateral branch. The **circumflex iliac artery** extends directly from the abdominal aorta. The **prepubic artery** and the **common trunk of external pudic and caudal abdominal (epigastric) arteries** are the branches of deep femoral artery and the **deep femoral artery** arises from the external iliac artery The **saphenous artery** is considerably larger in size and it arises from the femoral artery at about the middle of the thigh, descends to the proximal part of the leg and divides into cranial and caudal branches. The **cranial branch of saphenous** descends along the dorsal (cranial) surface of the tibia and after reaching the dorsal aspect of the tarsus, divides into medial and lateral branches. The **medial branch** forms the **second dorsal metatarsal or common digital artery** while the **lateral branch** forms the **third and fourth dorsal metatarsal or common digital arteries**. Each of the common digital artery runs down the interdigital space and divides into two **proper digital arteries** supplying the adjacent digits. The **caudal branch of saphenous** descends on the medial face of the gastrocnemius and the long head of the deep digital flexor muscles, gives out the lateral tarsal artery and continues as the **medial tarsal artery** to the plantar surface of the tarsus. Here it gives off the **medial and lateral plantar arteries** which descend on either sides of the tendon of deep digital flexor muscle and anastomose with the perforating metatarsal artery to form the **plantar arch**. From this arch extend down three **deep caudal metatarsal arteries** which descend into the corresponding interdigital space. The **medial tarsal artery** continues its descending course and after reaching the metatarso-phalangeal joint divides into **second, third and fourth superficial caudal digital arteries.** These arteries anastomose with similar arteries given out by the plantar arch and those of the dorsal metatarsal arteries. From this anastomosis, extend three **caudal digital arteries** which descend the interdigital spaces and join the **proper digital arteries** of the corresponding digits and supply the structures of the adjoining digits. The **cranial tibial artery** runs down the lateral aspect of the dorsal (cranial) surface of tibia obliquely under cover of the extensor muscles, detaches three **deep metatarsal arteries** and continues between the second and third metatarsal bones as **perforating metatarsal artery**. The deep metatarsal arteries pass down between the metatarsal bones and unite with the three cranial metatarsal arteries and the caudal metatarsal arteries.

The **veins** of hind limb in dog are mostly the satellites of the arteries like that in ox. The **digital veins** are cranial (dorsal) and caudal (plantar). The **cranial (dorsal) proper digital** veins unite to form the cranial (dorsal) common digital veins which ascend and unite to form a single **dorsal metatarsal vein**. It ascends to the distal extremity of leg and divides into two branches, the medial and lateral. The medial branch passes upward to the medial face of the proximal part of the leg and joins the caudomedial metatarsal vein to form the **medial saphenous vein** while the lateral branch forms the **lateral saphenous vein**. The **caudal (plantar) proper digital veins** unite to form three **caudal (plantar) common digital veins** which cause the formation of **superficial venous arch** at the metatarso-phalangeal articulation. From this arch, arise the caudomedial and caudolateral metatarsal veins. The **caudomedial metatarsal vein** in its upward course joins the medial branch of the dorsal metatarsal vein at the proximal third of the leg to form the caudal root of the medial saphenous vein. In the same way, the **caudolateral metatarsal vein** forms the caudal root of the medial saphenous vein. The cranial root of the medial saphenous vein is formed by the medial branch of the cranial tibial vein while that of the lateral saphenous vein is formed by the lateral branch of the cranial tibial vein. **The medial and the lateral saphenous veins** are thus formed by union of the cranial and caudal roots which extend from the medial and lateral metatarsal veins respectively. The **cranial and caudal tibial veins** unite in the proximal part of the leg to form the **popliteal vein** which in its upward course forms the **femoral** vein that joins the **external iliac vein.**

The **lymphatics** of the hind limb of dog are comprised of **deep inguinal and popliteal lymph nodes**. The gross features including the afferents and efferents of these lymph nodes are similar to those of ox. The popliteal lymph node is, however, more superficial in position in dog than that in ox. The coxal and epigastric lymph nodes are absent.

Sheep and Goat

The arteries of the hind limb of sheep and goat are in general similar to those of ox with the following variations.

The **external iliac artery** originates from the abdominal aorta ventral to and between the fifth and sixth lumbar vertebrae in sheep and ventral to sixth lumbar vertebra in goat as against its position at the level of sixth lumbar vertebra in general or at the fourth or fifth vertebra occasionally in ox. The **cranial branch of circumflex iliac artery** extends to the dorsal border of rectus abdominis muscle in goat. The **cremasteric artery** originates invariably from the pudendoepigastric trunk (a common trunk of caudal epigastric and external pudic arteries) in ox and sheep while in the goat it's origin is variable either from the caudal epigastric, the external pudic or from the deep femoral arteries. The **medial plantar artery** in sheep and goat receives the proximal perforating branch from the dorsal metatarsal artery on the tarsometatarsal joint. The **lateral plantar artery** in sheep and goat contributes to only deep plantar arch as against its contribution to both, the superficial plantar arch and deep plantar arch in ox. The **caudal femoral artery** arises from popliteal artery in sheep and goat as against its origin from femoral artery in ox.

The **veins** of the hind limb in sheep and goat are satellites of the arteries and have no remarkable differences from those of ox.

The **lymphatics** are comprised of only popliteal lymph node in sheep and the popliteal and deep inguinal lymph nodes in goat. The general morphological features including the afferents and efferents are similar to those of ox. The popliteal lymph node is prominent and deeply situated.

Pig

The arteries of hind limb of pig more or less resemble those of ox. The external iliac artery originates from the abdominal aorta ventral to the last lumbar vertebra and somewhat cranial to the sacral promontory. It leaves the abdominal cavity through the femoral ring (triangle) and continues as femoral artery passing through the femoral canal under the deep surface of the sartorius. Its major branches are the deep circumflex iliac and the deep femoral arteries. The caudal epigastric and the external pudic arteries arise in a common trunk as pudendoepigastric trunk from the deep femoral artery. The femoral artery after descending the femoral canal continues in the popliteal region as popliteal artery. The saphenous artery is the most extensive branch of the femoral. It gives out medial malleolar branches which ramify on the dorsomedial aspect of the tarsus. At the level of sustentaculum tali it divides into the medial and lateral plantar arteries. From the distal plantar arch arise four digital arteries which descend and supply the two accessory digits and two main digits.

The **veins** are the satellites of the arteries and need no separate description about their course, branching and distribution.

The **lymphatics** are comprised of three lymph nodes. These are the iliofemoral, superficial popliteal and deep popliteal lymph nodes. The deep inguinal and coxal lymph nodes are absent. The **iliofemoral lymph node** is situated near the origin of pudendoepigastric trunk from the deep femoral artery. The **superficial popliteal lymph node** is situated on the dorsocaudal surface of the gastrocnemius muscle. The **deep popliteal lymph node** is smaller than the superficial popliteal lymph node and is located craniocaudal to it on the gastrocnemius muscle. The afferents to these nodes are from the structures in the surrounding area while the efferents join the medial iliac or the ischiatic lymph node.

Fowl

The arteries of the hind limb of fowl mainly include the **iliac (external iliac)** and **sciatic (ischiatic) arteries**. Each **external iliac artery** originates directly from the aorta, passes laterally in the middle of the renal tissue between the cranial and middle lobes of the kidney and after reaching the lateral wall of the pelvis gives out **pubic artery**. It leaves the pelvis through the inguinal hiatus. After getting exit from the pelvis the external iliac artery continues as **femoral artery**. It distributes branches to the musculature and skin over the preacetabular ilium and thigh and gives out cranially the **cranial coxal artery** and caudally the **medial femoral artery**. The **femoral artery** descends femorotibialis (tibialis anticus) muscle and terminates cranial to the knee. The paired **ischiatic arteries** extend laterad from the descending aorta in the region of kidneys and leave the pelvis through the ilio-ischiatic foramen. On entering the thigh, the artery runs under the cover of the iliotibialis and iliofibularis muscles and at the distal end of the femur it continues as popliteal artery. The **popliteal artery** gives off muscular branches on the caudal aspect of the leg, descends the groove between the tibia and fibula, detaches medial tibial artery and is continued as **cranial tibial artery**. The **cranial tibial artery** courses distally over the cranial surface of tibia gives out the **peroneal artery** and then the **lateral tibial artery** and after reaching the proximal end of tarso-metatarsus continues as **dorsal common**

metatarsal artery which in its proximal course gives out **plantar tarsal arteries** and then the **plantar metatarsal arteries**. These arteries form the **plantar arch** at the metatarso-phalangeal articulation. From this arch extend the **proper digital arteries.**

The **veins** are the satellites of the arteries and need no separate description about their course, branching and distribution.

The **lymphatics** in fowl comprise only lymphatic ducts (vessels). There are no lymph nodes in fowl. The main lymphatic vessels of the hind limb of fowl follow the digital, metatarsal and tibial veins into the coelom.

SECTION-C
NERVES

102

Nerves of Hind Limb

Pelvic (Lumbosacral) plexus

The hind limb is supplied by the nerve branches extending from the Pelvic (lumbosacral) plexus (Fig. 6-4 A and B) which is formed by the convergence of the ventral divisions of the last three lumbar and first two sacral nerves. It is formed in two parts, the cranial and caudal. The two parts are connected by anastomotic branches. The cranial (lumbar) part is formed by the fourth and fifth lumbar nerves and lies between the psoas major and psoas minor muscles while the caudal (sacral) part is formed by the sixth lumbar and first and second sacral nerves. Some times a root from third sacral also joins this part. It lies on the pelvic surface of the sacrosciatic (ischial) ligament. The nerves extending from the cranial part of the plexus are the lateral cutaneous femoral, the femoral and the obturator. The nerves extending from the caudal part are the cranial gluteal, caudal gluteal and the sciatic (ischiatic).

Lateral cutaneous femoral nerve

The lateral cutaneous femoral nerve while leaving the cranial part of the plexus, receives fibres from the fourth lumbar nerve, passes caudally between the psoas major and psoas minor muscles and reaches the tuber coxae. Here it perforates the obliquus abdominis externus muscle in company with the circumflex iliac artery and reaches the skin of the lateral aspect of the thigh. In this course, the nerve supplies the psoas major, psoas minor, iliacus and external oblique muscles of the abdomen and the skin and cutaneous muscle on the lateral face of the thigh.

Femoral nerve

The femoral nerve is formed by the roots of the fifth and sixth lumbar nerves, receives fibres from fourth lumbar nerve and then emerges through the cranial part of the plexus. It passes ventrally and caudally between the psoas muscles, crosses the lateral face of the psoas minor, gets under the cover of the sartorius, crosses the tendon of iliopsoas, supplies a branch to that muscle, gives out the medial saphenous nerve and deeps between the rectus femoris and vastus internus divisions of the quadriceps femoris and terminates in this muscle supplying branches to it and the articularis genu.

The medial saphenous nerve arises from the femoral nerve a little above the pelvic brim, crosses the tendon of the psoas minor, passes along the caudal border of the sartorius between that muscle and the vastus internus in the femoral canal, and gives off a long branch that passes caudally and terminates into the head of the pectineus. The medial saphenous nerve gains exit through the femoral canal with the medial saphenous artery and vein by emerging through the sartorius and gracilis at about the level of stifle joint. Here it supplies branches to the sartorius and gracilis and divides into two groups of branches that descend the medial aspect of the leg and terminate by penetrating the fascia and skin of this region at the level of the distal third of the leg.

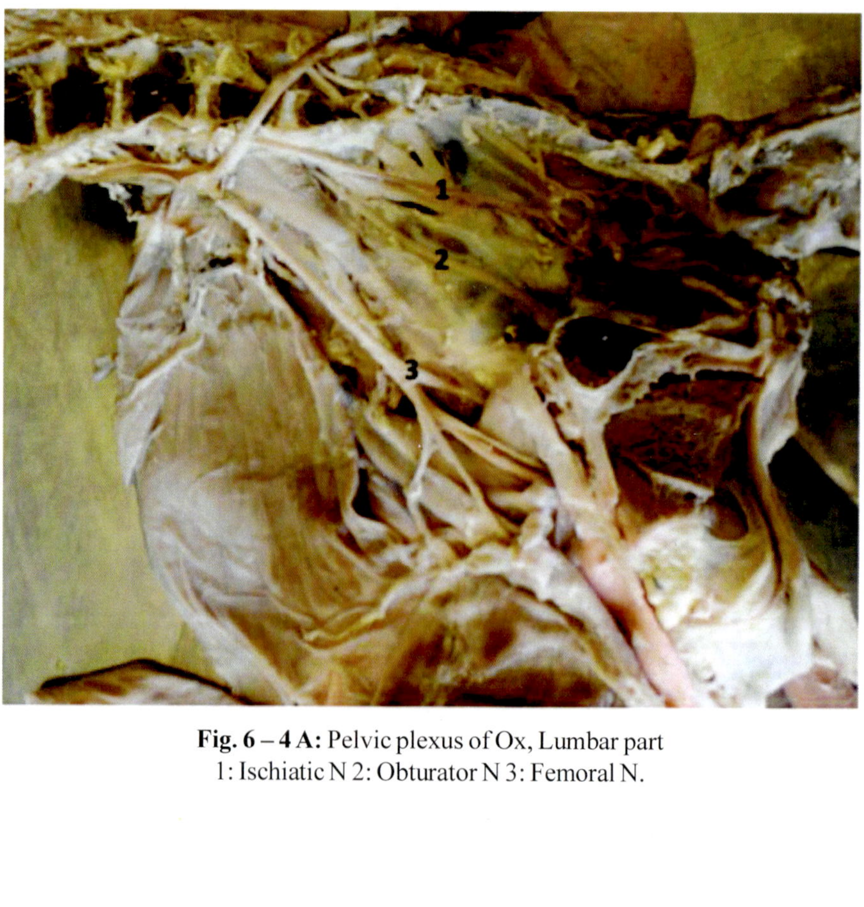

Fig. 6 – 4 A: Pelvic plexus of Ox, Lumbar part
1: Ischiatic N 2: Obturator N 3: Femoral N.

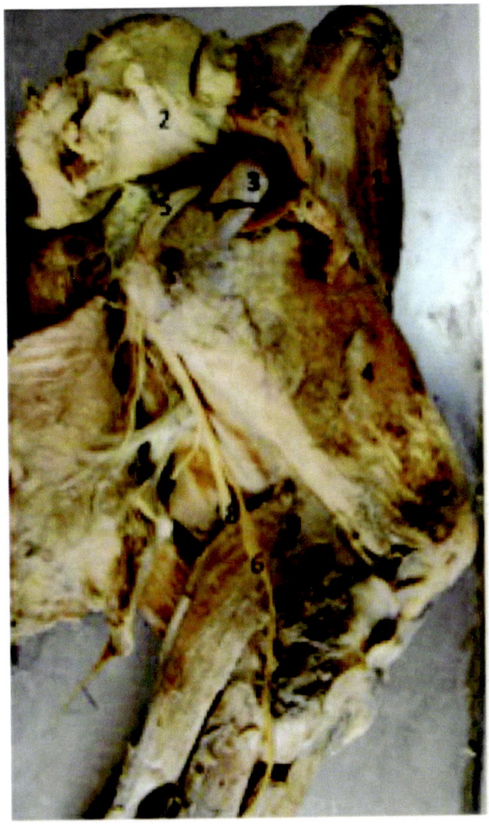

Fig. 6 – 4 B: Pelvic plexus of Ox, Sacral part and nerves of hindlimb
1. Tensor fasciae lata m. 2. Middle gluteus m 3. Gluteus accessorius 4. Quadriceps femoris m. 5. Sciatic nerve 6. External popliteal nerve (Peroneal nerve) 7. External Saphenous nerve (Posterior cutaneous nerve) 8. Internal Popliteal nerve 9. Gastrocnemius m

Obturator nerve

The obturator nerve derives fibres from the fourth, fifth and sixth lumbar nerves. It passes caudally under the wing of the sacrum, crosses the iliacus, then on the medial surface of the ilium that is covered by peritoneum. Here it turns down on the shaft of the ilium towards the obturator foramen, gives out a branch to obturator internus, passes out through the obturator foramen and terminates into the obturator externus muscle by supplying branches to the pectineus, adductor and gracilis muscles.

Cranial gluteal nerve

The cranial gluteal nerve is the first and the cranial most nerves extending from the second (sacral) part of the lumbosacral plexus. Its fibres are derived from the sixth lumbar and first sacral nerves. Following a short course it divides into several branches which leave the cavity through the greater sciatic (ischiatic) foramen in company with the cranial gluteal vessels along the cranial side of the sciatic (ischiatic) nerve and supply the middle and deep gluteus and tensor fasciae latae muscles.

Caudal gluteal nerve

The caudal gluteal nerve derives its fibres from the first and second sacral nerves and additionally in some subjects from the third sacral nerve. It leaves the pelvic cavity along the caudal border of the sciatic nerve through the greater sciatic foramen, turns caudally leaving the company of the sciatic nerve and divides into dorsal and ventral branch. The dorsal branch supplies the middle gluteus muscle and the ventral branch passes towards the tuber ischii and supplies the biceps femoris muscle.

Sciatic (ischiatic) nerve

The sciatic nerve is often called as greater sciatic or ischiatic nerve. It is the largest and longest nerve of the body. It is formed by the fibres derived from the ventral branches of the last lumbar and first two sacral nerves. It passes caudoventrally on the pelvic surface of the sacrosciatic (ischiatic) ligament and gets exit from the pelvic cavity through the greater sciatic (ischiatic) foramen. After emerging through this foramen it lies on the lateral surface of the broad sacrosciatic (sacrotuberal) ligament. In this initial course it is a wide, flat band and gives out several muscular branches to the gluteus, biceps femoris, the semimembranosus and the semitendinosus muscles. From here, it turns downward between the middle and deep gluteus muscles, gains the hollow between the trochanter and the tuber ischii behind the hip joint, runs over the gamellus and quadratus femoris under cover of the biceps femoris muscles. On reaching the thigh the nerve descends the muscular canal bounded by the biceps femoris and semitendinosus laterally and adductor and semimembranosus medially, deeps between the two heads of the gastrocnemius, runs for a short distance through popliteal region as popliteus nerve and then is continued down as the tibial nerve. The following are the major branches of this nerve.

1. A **small slender muscular branch** arises from the caudal border of the sciatic nerve in its pelvic course. It passes through the lesser sciatic foramen and supplies to the obturator internus, quadratus femoris and gemellus muscles.

2. A **large muscular branch** arises from the caudal border of the sciatic nerve after emerging through the greater sciatic foramen at the level of hip joint and divides into three branches. These supply the biceps femoris, semitendinosus and semimembranosus muscles.

3. **The caudal cutaneous nerve** of the leg arises from the caudal border of the sciatic nerve near the middle of the thigh. It descends on the deep surface of the biceps femoris and between this muscle and the semitendinosus. On reaching the lateral surface of leg in the hollow just cranial to the Achille's tendon it crosses the lateral surface of the tarsus and terminates in the metatarsal region. It supplies the skin on the lateral surface of leg, tarsus and metatarsus.

4. The **peroneal (fibular) nerve** is a large trunk arising from the sciatic nerve in the middle two third of the thigh. It descends with the sciatic to the origin of gastrocnemius at the distal end of thigh, separates from it, crosses the lateral face of the gastrocnemius under cover of the biceps femoris and divides into the superficial and deep branches. Before this division, it gives out the **lateral cutaneous nerve of the leg** which supplies the skin on the dorsolateral aspect of the leg. The **superficial peroneal nerve** supplies a branch to lateral digital extensor and descends in the groove between the lateral digital extensor and peroneus longus muscle and terminates by ramifications in the skin on the dorsal and lateral face of the tarsus, metatarsus and around the whole fetlock joint. The **deep peroneal nerve** passes between the lateral digital extensor and peroneus longus muscles, gives branches to these and the tibialis anticus (cranialis) and peroneus tertius muscles, descends along the tendons of lateral and long digital extensors and divides on the dorsal aspect of the hock into the lateral and medial branches. The **lateral branch** passes down subcutaneously on the dorsal face of metatarsus and supplies a cutaneous branch to the skin of this region. The **lateral branch** supplies muscular branch to extensor bravis and articular branch to the tarsus and descends the dorsal groove of the metatarsus in company with the dorsal metatarsal vein, reaches the interdigital space and divides into cranial (dorsal) and caudal (plantar) branches. The **cranial branch** joins the superficial peroneal nerve and forms the **cranial (dorsal) common digital nerve**, while the **caudal branch** joins the medial plantar nerve and forms the **caudal (plantar) common digital nerve.**

5. The **popliteus nerve** passes along the caudal border of the popliteal muscle on the caudal surface of the proximal third of the leg and furnishes muscular branches to the medial and lateral heads of the gastrocnemius, popliteus, superficial digital flexor, deep digital flexor and the soleus muscles.

Tibial nerve

The tibial nerve is the continuation of the sciatic nerve next to the popliteal nerve. It emerges from beneath the medial head of the gastrocnemius, becomes subcutaneous, descends the medial face of the leg in front of the Achille's tendon and on reaching the hock it divides into medial and lateral plantar nerves.

The **medial plantar nerve** descends under cover of the deep fascia of metatarsus between the tendon of superficial digital flexor muscle and suspensory ligament, passes along the medial border of the tendon of deep digital flexor and in the distal third of metatarsus divides into two branches, the medial and lateral. The **medial branch** supplies twigs to the rudimentary digit and is continued down as **plantar medial digital nerve**. The lateral branch turns round the tendon of deep digital flexor, enters the interdigital space and joins the branch of the deep peroneal nerve and forms the **plantar common digital nerve.**

The **lateral plantar nerve** runs laterad and descends on the lateral border of the tendon of superficial digital flexor, gives out a branch to suspensory ligament and the lateral rudimentary digit and continues down on the lateral side of the flexor tendon of lateral digit as the **plantar lateral digital nerve.**

103

Comparative Anatomy of Nerves of Hind Limb

Horse

The **lumbosacral plexus** in horse is formed by last three lumbar and first two sacral nerves, similar to that in ox. The **caudal gluteal nerve** divides into two branches. The **medial branch** supplies the superficial gluteal muscle in addition to the middle and deep gluteal and biceps femoris muscles. The **lateral branch** reaches the level of tuber ischii and terminates into the semitendinosus muscle at the perineal region. The **sciatic nerve** is almost similar to that of ox in the disposition and distribution of its branches. The **superficial and deep peroneal nerves** are also similar to those of ox. The **tibial nerve** divides at the distal third of the leg into **medial and lateral plantar** nerves. Each plantar nerve divides at the fetlock into **cranial, middle and caudal digital nerves.**

Dog

The **lumbosacral plexus** in dog is formed by the last four or five lumbar and first two or three sacral nerves. The **cranial gluteal nerve** receives fibres from sixth and seventh lumbar and first and second sacral nerves. The **caudal gluteal nerve** arises from sixth and seventh lumbar and first sacral nerves. The **sciatic nerve** derives fibres from sixth and seventh lumbar and first and second sacral nerves. The **lateral cutaneous nerve** arises either from sciatic or from the peroneal nerve. The **peroneal nerve** divides into superficial and deep branches, similar to those of ox. The **tibial nerve** divides into medial and lateral plantar nerves at the level of distal third of the leg. The **medial plantar** nerve divides at the metatarsus into medial and lateral branches. The **medial branch** becomes the first plantar common digital nerve. It divides to form the plantar proper digital nerves of the first and second digits. The **lateral branch** divides into three **plantar metatarsal nerves** which unite, in the intermetatarsal space with the three **plantar common digital nerves** of the lateral plantar nerve. Each of these **united plantar common digital nerves** descends and after reaching at the metatarso-phalangeal articulation into three **plantar proper digital nerves**. The **lateral plantar nerve,** divides into three plantar common digital nerves which join the three plantar metatarsal nerves and form the **plantar (caudal) proper digital nerves**. The **united proper digital nerves** supply the second to fifth digit and terminate into the corresponding intermetatarsal space.

Sheep and Goat

The sciatic nerve in sheep receives major contribution of fibres from the first and second sacral nerves and a little from the sixth lumbar nerve while in goat it is mainly from the sixth lumbar and first sacral nerves with a small contribution from second sacral nerve. The caudal cutaneous femoral nerve arises as a slender branch of sciatic nerve in sheep and goat. The sciatic nerve and its pattern of branching and distribution in the hind limb of sheep and goat is almost similar to that in ox.

Pig

The **lumbosacral plexus** in pig is formed on the medial surface of the sciatic ligament. The femoral nerve extends from the cranial (lumbar) part of the plexus. The origin of this nerve is variable. The main contribution is from the fifth lumbar nerve while the fibres from third to sixth lumbar nerves may contribute for its formation. Its first branch, the **saphenous** nerve supplies the fascia and skin over the stifle, medial aspect of the thigh and leg and the dorsomedial aspect of the tarsus. The **femoral nerve**, after reaching the fetlock, divides into medial and lateral branch. The medial branch descends along the dorsomedial aspect of the leg metatarsus as medial (abaxial) dorsal digital nerve while the lateral branch joins the medial branch of superficial peroneal nerve and forms the dorsal common digital nerve. The **obturator nerve** receives contribution from the same lumbar nerves as those of the femoral nerve. It supplies the obturator externus, gracilis, pectineus and adductor muscles. The **sciatic nerve** is formed by the fibres received from fifth and sixth lumbar and second sacral nerves. The branching, distribution and further continuation of this nerve in pig is same as that in ox. The distribution of digital nerves, however, differs because of four instead of two digits of the limb in pig.

Fowl

The **lumbosacral plexus** in fowl is formed by the last two lumbar and first four sacral nerves. The plexus is formed in two, the cranial (lumbar) and caudal (pelvic) parts, similar to that in mammals. The **cranial part** is formed by the last two lumbar and first sacral nerves. It furnishes the **femoral, saphenous**

and obturator nerves and a nerve to tensor fasciae latae. The **caudal part** is formed by a major contribution from first sacral nerve and a variable contribution from sacral nerves second to fourth. This part releases the **gluteal and sciatic nerves** for distribution to the muscles and other structures in the hind limb (leg) in birds.

SECTION-D

APPLIED ANATOMY

104

Applied Anatomy of Hind Limb

Sites for surgical interventions

Luxation of patella in cattle and horses

The luxation of patella is a condition wherein the patella of the stifle joint (femoropatellar articulation) is locked above the medial ridge of the trochlea of the femur.

Anatomy of femoropatellar articulation of the stifle joint

The **stifle joint** is a composite joint formed in two parts. One of these is an articulation between the condyles of distal extremity of femur and the condyles of the proximal extremity of tibia (**femoro-tibial articulation**) and the other is the articulation between the trochlea of the distal extremity of the femur and the articular surface of the patella (**femoro-patellar articulation**).

The **trochlea of the femur** consists of two asymmetrical ridges separated by a groove. The medial ridge is more prominent, wider and a little more extended dorsally than the lateral ridge. The two ridges converge ventrally. The **articular surface of the patella** is more or less quadrilateral or triangular with the base above and apex below. It has a vertical ridge in the middle and it separates the two concave areas of which the medial one is larger than the lateral. The patella is fastened against the trochlea with the help of three types of ligaments. One of these is the capsular ligament which is attached to the periphery of the articular areas of the two segments of the joint. The other one is the medial and lateral collateral ligaments. The third set of ligaments is the patellar (straight) ligaments.

The **patellar ligaments** are three in number, the medial, middle and the lateral. These are strong and wide bands of ligaments. The medial patellar ligament extends from the medial border of the patellar fibrocartilage and terminates on the medial side of the cranial tuberosity of the tibia. The middle patellar ligament extends from the apex of the patella and terminates on the tibial crest and the cranial tuberosity of tibia. The lateral patellar ligament extends from the lateral part of the cranial surface of the patella and terminates on the lateral part of the cranial tuberosity of the tibia. A bursa is interposed between the medial patellar ligament and the upper part of the trochlea and another bursa is interposed between the lateral patellar ligament and the cranial tuberosity of the tibia. The tendon of insertion of the gluteobiceps muscle inserts on the base and the cranial surface of the patella.

Anatomical reasons of luxation of patella

While walking, the patella glides over the trochlea of femur. In contraction of the biceps femoris (gluteobiceps) muscle the patella is pulled up and in relaxation of the muscle it glides down. Some times, in the extreme extension, the patella is locked on the upper end of the medial ridge of the trochlea because of its greater size and higher level than the lateral ridge. As a result, the medial patellar ligament becomes tense.

Symptoms

The intermittent fixation of patella on the upper part of the trochlea results in a characteristic jumping action of the hind limb. Many times the limb remains in caudal extension for a longer period than normal. Some times the limb is dragged for a few steps before clicking forward to a normal posture.

Remedy and surgical procedure

The best and simple remedy to relieve the animal of this condition is desmotomy of patella (patellar desmotomy). The surgery is preferred to perform under hygienic conditions and local anaesthetic infiltration at the stifle joint, either in standing or recumbent position. The site is identified by palpating the tibial crest by the tip of thumb and gradually sliding the thumb and gently pressing the soft space between the median and middle patellar ligaments. The incision is made at about 4 to 5 cm proximal to the most cranial bulging of cranial tuberosity at the groove between medial and middle patellar ligaments. The space in this groove is normally occupied by fat and is covered by fascia. The blade of the scalpel is inserted in the skin in dorsoventral direction with the blade facing downward and ones it reaches the space, the scalpel is turned to horizontal position. The medial ligament is about 2.5 cm in width and it is cut horizontally. The two cut ends of the medial patellar ligaments are completely separated. With proper post operative care, the animal starts walking normally within 15 to 21 days after the operation.

Stringhalt in horses

Stringhalt is a sudden flexion of one or both hind limbs in the horse. It is most easily seen while the horse is walking or trotting. This condition is because of spasmodic contraction of the lateral digital extensor muscle of the hind limb. It occurs when the digital extensor muscle of hind limb contracts extensively or digital flexor muscle lacks sufficient opposition.

The clinical signs are usually more extensive when the horse is turning or backing up. In severe condition, some horses kick themselves in the abdomen when they are trying to walk.

Resection of the tendon of lateral digital extensor as it is running over the hock is one of the remedial measures for this condition.

Anatomical site and procedure for resection

The tendon of the lateral digital extensor muscle runs over the lateral surface of the hock. It joins the tendon of long digital extensor muscle at about the middle third of the dorsal surface of the metatarsal bone. As they pass over the hock under the annular ligament, the tendons of both of these muscles are enclosed in a common sheath. These tendons can be palpated subcutaneously after they emerge through the common sheath. The tendon of lateral digital extensor is identified by tracing it back up to its muscular belly and ones it is confirmed, the same tendon is traced down by palpation sufficiently below the point of their emergence through the common sheath. The site for resection of the tendon is about 3 cm proximal to the junction of the two tendons. Under hygienic conditions a skin incision of about 3 cm is made at this point and then The tendon (of lateral digital extensor) is cut horizontally.

Nerve blocks

In most of the affections of hind limb, the epidural anaesthesia is commonly used. In rare cases the peroneal and the tibial nerve blocks are performed for specific purposes in the hind limb of large animals.

Peroneal nerve block

Anatomy of peroneal nerve

The peroneal nerve block is performed for surgical procedures below the hock in the hind limb. The peroneal nerve is one of the two terminal branches of the sciatic nerve. It arises from sciatic at the middle of the thigh, passes distally under the gluteobiceps and later between this muscle and the lateral head of the gastrocnemius muscle. Further down it descends between the peroneus longus and lateral digital extensor muscles over the caudal border of the lateral condyle of tibia and divides into the superficial and deep branches at the proximal part of the metatarsus. The superficial peroneal nerve passes subcutaneously over the dorsal surface of the metatarsal bone and reaches the digits to become the dorsal common digital nerve that supplies the dorsal aspect of the digits. The deep peroneal nerve passes down through the vascular groove and is covered by the tendons of the extensor muscles and the fascia on the dorsal surface of the metacarpus. After reaching the digits it supplies the dorsal aspect of the digits of the hind limb.

Site for nerve block

The peroneal nerve block is performed on this nerve before its division into superficial and deep branches. The best site is on the caudal border of the lateral condyle of tibia where the nerve is subcutaneous and is separated away from the vessels. A bony prominence on the caudal edge of the lateral condyle of tibia is palpated and the needle is inserted through the skin and the aponeurotic sheet of the biceps femoris muscle until the point of needle touches the caudal edge of the lateral condyle of tibia.

The effect of this nerve block is to desensitize the dorsal (extensor) aspect of the digits of the hind limb.

Tibial nerve block

Anatomy of tibial nerve

The tibial nerve, following its separation from the peroneal nerve as a branch of sciatic nerve at the middle of the thigh, continues between the two heads of the gastrocnemius. It further descends between the lateral head of gastrocnemius and superficial digital flexor and at a distal third of the leg lies cranial to the tuber calcis. Passing down from the tuber calcis, it divides into two branches which become the medial and lateral plantar nerves. These nerves, after passing down the plantar surface of the metatarsus reach the digits and supply the plantar surface of the digits.

Site for nerve block

The radial nerve block is performed on this nerve before it division into medial and lateral plantar nerves. The nerve is superficial in position along the tendons of gastrocnemius muscle on the cranial aspect of the tuber calcis. The tendons of the gastrocnemius muscles are grasped between the thumb and the index finger of one hand about 10 to 12 cm above the summit of the tuber calcis. The needle is inserted just below the thumb until the point of needle can be felt by index finger just below the skin on the other side of the tendon.

The effect of this nerve block is to desensitize the plantar aspect of the digits of the hind limb.

Bibliography

Akers, R. M. and D. M. Denbow. 2013. Anatomy and Physiology of Domestic Animals. 2nd ed., Wiley- Blackwell.

Bhamburkar, V. R. 1987. Anatomical Studies on the Sympathetic Nervous System in Goat. Ph.D. Thesis Submitted to G. B. Pant University, Pantnagar (Nainital) U.P. India.

Bhamburkar, V. R. and R. V. Pandit. 1989. Localization of the central neurons of cranial cervical ganglion in buffalo. Indian J. Vet. Anat. 1: 14-16.

Bhamburkar, V. R. and Prem Prakash. 1990. Anatomical disposition of the thoracic sympathetic nervous system in goat. Indian J. Vet. Anat. 2: 50-51.

Bhamburkar, V. R. and Prem Prakash. 1990. Distribution of sympathetic nerves to the stomach in goat. Indian J. Vet. Anat. 2: 51

Bhamburkar, V. R. and Prem Prakash. 1991. Autonomic innervation of pelvic organs in goat. Indian J. Vet. Anat. 3: 51

Bhamburkar, V. R. and R. S. Dalvi. 1994. Comparative gross and histomorphological study of the external ear of domestic animals. Indian J. Vet. Anat. 6: 45- 46.

Bhardwaj, R. L., R. Rajput and K. S. Roy. 2002. Applied Anatomy of Domestic Animals. Kalyani Publishers, Ludhiana, New Delhi, India.

Colville, T. and J. M. Bassert. 2009. Clinical Anatomy and Physiology: A Laboratory Manual. Mosby. Elsevier. St. Louis, Missouri.

de Lahunta, A. and R. E. Habel. 1986. Applied Veterinary Anatomy. W. B. Saunders Company, Philadelphia.

Dyce, K. M., W. O. Sack and T. G. Wensing. 2010. Text Book of Veterinary Anatomy. 4th ed. Elsevier.

Evans, H. E. and de Lahunta. 2013. Miller's Anatomy of the Dog. Elsevier. Saunders, St. Louis. Missouri.

Getty, R. 2002. The Anatomy of the Domestic Animals. 5th ed. (First East-West Press Edition) Affiliated East-West Press Pvt. Ltd. New Delhi, India.

Ghoshal, N. G., T. Koch and P. Popesko. 1981. The Venous Drainage of the Domestic Animals. W. B. Saunders Company. Philadelphia.

Habel, R. E. 1963. Applied Anatomy: A Laboratory Guide for Veterinary Students. Published by Author Ithaca, New York.

Habel, R. E. 1970. Guide to the dissection of Domestic Ruminants. Published by the Author. Ithaca, New York.

Kaupp, B. F. 1918. The Anatomy of the Domestic Fowl. W. B. Saunders Co. , Philadelphia.

Lumb, W. V. and E. W. Jones. 1984. Veterinary Anaesthesia. 2nd ed. Lea and Febiger, Philadelphia.

May, N. D. S. 1970. The Anatomy of the Sheep. 3rd ed. University of Queensland Press, Brisbane, Australia.

McFadyean, J. 1922. The Anatomy of the Horse. A Dissection Guide. 3rd ed. W. & A. K. Johnston Ltd. Edinburgh.

McFadyean, J. 1953. Osteology and Arthrology of the Domesticated Animals. 4th ed. Edited by H. V. Hughes and J. W. Dransfield. Bailliere Tindal & Cox. London.

McKibben, J. and R. Getty. 1968. A comparative morphologic study of the cardiac innervation in domestic animals: I Canine. Am. J. Anat. 122(2): 533-544.

McKibben, J. and R. Getty. 1968. A comparative morphologic study of the cardiac innervation in domestic animals: II Feline. Am. J. Anat. 122(2): 545-554.

McKibben, J. and R. Getty. 1969. A study of the cardiac innervation in domestic animals: Cattle. Anat. Rec. 165 (2): 141-152.

McKibben, J. and R. Getty. 1969. Innervation of heart of domestic animals: Horse. Am. J. Vet. Res. 30 (2): 193-202.

McKibben, J. and R. Getty. 1969. Innervation of heart of domestic animals: Pig. Am. J. Vet. Res. 30 (5): 793-789.

McLeod, W. M. 1958. Bovine Anatomy. Burgess Publishing Co. Minneapolis- Minnesota.

Miller, M. E. , G. L. Cristenson and H. E. Evans. 1964. Anatomy of the dog. W. B. Saunders Co. Philadelphia.

Mysore Veterinary College. 1959. Anatomy Lecture Notes. Personal collection.

Nickel, R., A. Schummer and E. Seiferle. 1986. The Anatomy of the Domestic Animals. Verlag Paul Parey, Berlin. Hamburg. Springer-Verlag, New York. Berlin.

Nomina Anatomica Veterinaria. 1973. 2nd ed. International Committee on Veterinary Anatomical Nomenclature. World Association of Veterinary Anatomists. Vienna.

Pasquini, C., T. Spurgeon and S. Pasquini. 2011. Anatomy of Domestic Animals: Systemic and Regional. Studz Publishing, Australia.

Raghavan, D. 1964. Ed. The Anatomy of the Ox. Indian Council of Agricultural Research. New Delhi. India.

Sack W. O. and Hamilton, W. P. 1982. Essentials of Pig Anatomy. Veterinary Textbooks Cop. Springer, Ithaca, New York.

Sisson, S. and J. D. Grossman. 1940. The Anatomy of the Domestic Animals. 3rd ed. W. B. Saunders Co. Philadelphia.

Wingerd, B. D. 2006. Pig Anatomy and Dissection Guide. Bluedoor Publishing, Minneapolis, Minnesota.